Current Research in Immunology

Current Research in Immunology

Edited by Ashley Crawford

STATES
ACADEMIC PRESS
www.statesacademicpress.com

States Academic Press,
109 South 5th Street,
Brooklyn, NY 11249, USA

Visit us on the World Wide Web at:
www.statesacademicpress.com

ISBN: 978-1-63989-138-2

Cataloging-in-Publication Data

Current research in immunology / edited by Ashley Crawford.
p. cm.
Includes bibliographical references and index.
ISBN 978-1-63989-138-2
1. Immunology--Research. 2. Serology--Research. I. Crawford, Ashley.
QR182.5 .C87 2022
616.079 072--dc23

Table of Contents

Preface

This book has been a concerted effort by a group of academicians, researchers and scientists, who have contributed their research works for the realization of the book. This book has materialized in the wake of emerging advancements and innovations in this field. Therefore, the need of the hour was to compile all the required researches and disseminate the knowledge to a broad spectrum of people comprising of students, researchers and specialists of the field.

The complex system of processes and structures which protect an organism from disease is known as the immune system. The area of study within biology which focuses on the immune systems in organisms is known as immunology. It analyzes the relationship between pathogens, body systems and immunity. Some of the major areas of study within immunology are clinical immunology, ecoimmunology and developmental immunology. The disorders of the immune system are studied within clinical immunology. These disorders are categorized into immunodeficiency and autoimmunity. Ecoimmunology studies the relationship between an organism's immune system, and the biotic and abiotic environment. This book unfolds the innovative aspects of immunology which will be crucial for the progress of this field in the future. While understanding the long-term perspectives of the topics, it makes an effort in highlighting their impact as a modern tool for the growth of the discipline. This book includes contributions of experts and scientists which will provide innovative insights into this field.

At the end of the preface, I would like to thank the authors for their brilliant chapters and the publisher for guiding us all-through the making of the book till its final stage. Also, I would like to thank my family for providing the support and encouragement throughout my academic career and research projects.

Editor

1

Theories and quantification of thymic selection

Andrew J. Yates*

Departments of Systems and Computational Biology, Microbiology and Immunology, Albert Einstein College of Medicine, New York, NY, USA

Edited by:
Rob J. De Boer, Utrecht University, Netherlands

Reviewed by:
Anton van der Merwe, University of Oxford, UK
Viktor Müller, Hungarian Academy of Sciences and Eötvös Loránd University, Hungary
Johannes Textor, Utrecht University, Netherlands

****Correspondence:***
Andrew J. Yates, Departments of Systems and Computational Biology, Microbiology and Immunology, Albert Einstein College of Medicine, 1300 Morris Park Avenue, New York, NY 10461, USA
e-mail: andrew.yates@einstein.yu.edu

The peripheral T cell repertoire is sculpted from prototypic T cells in the thymus bearing randomly generated T cell receptors (TCR) and by a series of developmental and selection steps that remove cells that are unresponsive or overly reactive to self-peptide–MHC complexes. The challenge of understanding how the kinetics of T cell development and the statistics of the selection processes combine to provide a diverse but self-tolerant T cell repertoire has invited quantitative modeling approaches, which are reviewed here.

Keywords: thymic selection, T cells, mathematical modeling, repertoire selection, theoretical biology

INTRODUCTION

Conventional ($CD4^+$ and $CD8^+$) T cells are an integral part of adaptive immune systems in vertebrates. A key stage in their development is the creation of the T cell receptor (TCR) through a stochastic process of gene rearrangement. The resulting pre-selection TCR repertoire has the potential to recognize a very large array of peptides derived both from self and from foreign organisms, presented on Major Histocompatibility Complex (MHC) molecules on the surfaces of other cells. Much of T cell development occurs in a specialized organ in the chest called the thymus, within which this diverse potential repertoire of TCR is vetted. A process referred to as positive selection removes cells with TCR conformations that are generally non-responsive to self-peptide–MHC ligands (self-pMHC), and negative selection removes cells that are overly reactive to self-pMHC and pose a threat of autoimmune responses. The post-selection repertoire exported from the thymus comprises T cells that are largely non-responsive to self, yet capable of responding with remarkable specificity to foreign peptides.

There is a very extensive literature relating to thymic development and selection [for reviews, see for example Ref. (1–3)], but here we summarize the key ideas briefly (**Figure 1**). Conventional T cells begin life as lymphoid progenitors, which migrate from the bone marrow to the inner, cortical region of the thymus and begin a process of proliferation and maturation. Early in development in the cortex thymocytes are referred to as double negative (DN), lacking expression of the CD4 and CD8 co-receptors that are involved in TCR signaling. The TCR comprises two chains and is formed by a multi-step gene rearrangement process that first generates the TCRβ, γ, and δ chains (a small proportion of cells diverge at this stage to seed the $\gamma\delta$ T cell lineage) and then the TCRα chain at around the transition from the DN to $CD4^+CD8^+$ (double positive, DP) stage. TCR$\alpha\beta$ cells then migrate among cortical thymic epithelial cells and dendritic cells, auditioning for the ability to recognize self-pMHC. There is evidence that DP cells with non-functional TCR can undergo repeated TCRα rearrangements (4) to re-audition. Positively-selected cortical thymocytes begin negative selection and eventually move to the outer capsule of the thymus, the medulla. There they complete negative selection through interactions with medullary thymic epithelial cells and dendritic cells. TCR$\alpha\beta$ thymocytes, which recognize self-peptides presented on MHC class I or class II below an acceptable threshold of reactivity develop into the CD8 SP (single-positive, $CD4^-CD8^+$) or CD4 SP ($CD4^+CD8^-$) lineages, respectively, and are eventually exported into the peripheral circulation as naive T cells.

The topic of thymic selection has received substantial attention from the immunological modeling community, perhaps for two main reasons. First, selection has widely been viewed as a well-delineated optimization problem – how to craft a TCR repertoire that covers the space of possible pMHC ligands as widely as possible, while preserving sufficient specificity to discriminate between self and foreign (and between different foreign) peptides? This question naturally invites quantitative arguments. Second, the biology is well-characterized – a relatively small number of cell types and modes of interaction appear to be involved, and large amounts of experimental data are available. These simplify and constrain the construction of models.

Modeling studies have focused on many aspects of thymic selection but many questions and uncertainties remain. What are the rates and efficiencies of passage through the different phases of development and selection, and in what thymic microenvironments do each take place? How do thymocytes integrate signals received from interactions with pMHC to make fate decisions?

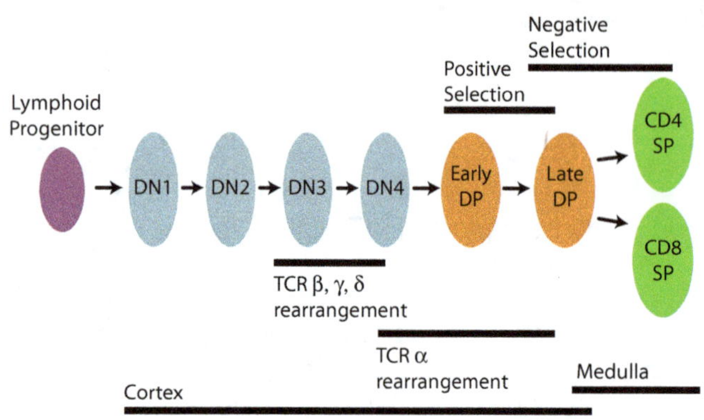

FIGURE 1 | Stages in the development of CD4 and CD8 T cells in the thymus.

What are the relative contributions of the MHC itself and its associated peptide to TCR signaling and fate determination? What influence do each of these have on the post-selection repertoire's diversity and coverage of the pMHC universe, and its ability to discriminate between self and foreign? How complete is the removal of potentially self-reactive clones? How many TCR interactions contribute to a thymocyte's fate decisions? What evolutionary pressures have determined the typical number of MHC alleles we possess? There have been many different theoretical approaches to these questions – from mean-field population dynamic models of progression through developmental stages, to probabilistic models of selection, to explicitly spatial models of migration within the thymus.

This review groups studies of these topics into broadly labeled categories, but in some cases the grouping is arbitrary – many of these questions are related and have been addressed either alone or in combination. The review has a bottom-up structure, beginning with an overview of experimental quantification of selection and modeling of thymocyte population dynamics. It then moves to studies of higher-level properties of the T cell repertoire, such as TCR cross-reactivity, and concludes with the problem of optimal within-individual MHC diversity.

THE POPULATION DYNAMICS OF THYMOCYTES

Basic elements of a quantitative understanding of thymic development are the steady-state population sizes of different developmental stages, the mean times to transit between them and the proportion surviving at each stage, which we refer to as the efficiencies of selection. While some quantities can be experimentally determined, mathematical models have helped us develop a more complete description of the kinetics of selection, both for the thymocyte population as a whole and for the CD4 and CD8 lineages in isolation.

To estimate the parameters of a dynamical system usually involves observing its response to perturbations. One method is to follow cohorts of cells as they progress through development using intra-thymic injection of a dye or radioisotope label (5–8). Arguably this method is less disruptive than cell transfers, but the uptake of marker can be heterogeneous (5, 7) and measurements of death rates using injected dyes rather than congenic markers may be confounded by loss of label (9). More recently, methods have included using GFP (green fluorescent protein) expressed during TCR rearrangement, its decaying intensity then a marker for time spent in development (10); inducible TCR signaling can be used to arrest, release, and follow cohorts of cells from the early DP stage (11); and small numbers of labeled thymocytes isolated at different developmental states can be followed after intra-thymic injection (11, 12). The population dynamics have also been exposed by transiently depleting thymocytes and observing the system's return to equilibrium (13). Various experimental systems, with or without associated dynamical models, are in general agreement over several quantitative aspects of thymic development but inconsistencies and uncertainties remain.

SELECTION EFFICIENCIES AND CELL FLUXES

Thymocytes begin to select against self-pMHC ligands at the DP stage following TCR rearrangement and so we focus on survival, proliferation, and differentiation from this stage onward. The proportion of DP cells that reach maturity (that is, survive both positive and negative selection) is widely agreed to be 5% or less (6, 11, 13–16). Within this pruning process, the general view is that positive selection is the most stringent, with 75–80% of cells failing to progress from the earliest DP stage, suggesting the majority of TCR generated are unable to recognize peptides in conjunction with MHC class I or II to any useful degree (11, 13, 15, 17, 18). Many studies have estimated that between 20 and 50% of positively-selected thymocytes then survive negative selection (11, 17, 19–22), although Itano and Robey (8) estimated a selection efficiency as high as 90% for DP cells into the CD4 SP lineage.

The rate of production of mature CD4 and CD8 cells in the thymi of young adult mice is roughly 1% of total thymocytes or $1-3\times10^6$ cells/day, a figure arrived at by a variety of labeling methods (5–7). Egerton et al. (6) estimated this to be just over 3% of the rate of entry into the DP population, meaning that fueling this trickle of output requires that roughly 30% of all thymocytes enter the DP stage each day. This again illustrates the extent of the filtering of the pre-selection repertoire that appears to be required to produce a functional and self-tolerant population of naive T cells. The thymus gradually involutes and its rate of output declines with age in both mice (23) and in humans (24), indicating that the bulk of the peripheral T cell repertoire is probably generated early in life.

THE MAJORITY OF THYMOCYTE DIVISION LIKELY OCCURS PRE-SELECTION

Labeled nucleotide uptake assays have revealed that substantial proliferation of thymocytes occurs before selection on self-pMHC ligands begins, stopping at or around the time of TCR rearrangement at the late DN/early DP stage (6, 25, 26). However, it is proliferation following TCR rearrangement that is most relevant for understanding how repertoire diversity is generated. Division during selection means a smaller proportion of TCR clonotypes may pass selection than measures of percentage survival suggest (27). The extent of division early in selection is unclear – estimates of the proportion of newly generated DP cells that are dividing have ranged from 11 to 68% (6, 25, 28), and CFSE labeling in *in vitro* thymic organ cultures showed up to 5 divisions from DP onward (29). However, the DP population comprises cells pre- and post-TCR rearrangement, and there appears to be very little proliferation within the more mature DP population (6, 11, 15). There is a low level of proliferation during or just before the SP stage (11, 13, 25, 30), with CD8 SP more prone to division than CD4 SP (10).

Perhaps the most reliable experimental measure of average levels of proliferation during selection uses T cell receptor excision circles (TRECs). TRECs are circular DNA fragments that are stable remnants of the recombination events that generate the TCR and are shared randomly between daughter cells on division. The mean TREC content per cell is a rough measure of the mean number of divisions that have taken place since the TCR was generated. One caveat is that TREC studies are used most commonly in humans and much of what we discuss here derive from studies in mice. Another is that standard TREC measurements contain no information about the variance of the division number, and may gloss over even quite extreme heterogeneity in division patterns. Nevertheless a study of human infants observed 1–2 divisions on average between TCR rearrangement at the $CD3^{low}$ $CD4^+CD8^+$ stage and mature CD4 or CD8 SP; once shortly after TCR rearrangement, and another at the CD8 (but not CD4) SP stage (31). The high TREC content they observed at the early DP stage may reflect multiple rearrangements taking place in order to generate a functional TCRα-chain. In line with these results, the TREC content of naive $CD31^+CD4^+$ recent thymic emigrants in human infants is ~0.1–0.9/cell (32), suggesting that up to three divisions take place on average between TCR rearrangement and export to the periphery, although this may include some post-thymic proliferation and so is an upper limit on the extent of intra-thymic division.

TURNOVER RATES AND TRANSIT TIMES

Experimental estimates of the times taken to transit different developmental stages (immature DP $\rightarrow$ mature DP $\rightarrow$ SP $\rightarrow$ Export) are variable, particularly within the SP population (6, 10, 12, 25). Possible reasons for these discrepancies include different labeling protocols, different gating strategies defining thymic subpopulations, heterogeneity of cell populations, and differences in the kinetics of MHC class I-restricted and class II-restricted lineages. It has also been unclear whether selection is a "conveyor belt," first-in first-out, or has a more stochastic "lucky dip" nature (25). From a modeling perspective these are two points on a continuum. If an experimentally identifiable developmental stage comprises several shorter, sequential differentiation steps, the variance in the transit time through that stage is lowered with respect to a single-step model of transit. The more obligate steps, the more conveyor-belt-like the system appears.

There is general agreement that the transition from non-dividing mature DP to SP takes on average 3–4 days (6, 12, 15, 28), although it has been argued that it takes significantly longer to reach CD8 SP than CD4 SP (33). This transition is dependent on TCR signaling (15, 34). Observing a well-defined delay in the appearance of labeled SP cells, Egerton et al. (6) argued for a first-in-first-out kinetic in the DP population. This suggests DP cells must transit through a number of obligate steps. Subsequent experimental and modeling studies have addressed this, and are discussed below. The same study estimated a mean SP residence time of ~12 days, comparable to other estimates of the medullary residence time (6, 28). McCaughtry et al. (10) argued that this is an overestimate of the time mature conventional SP T cells take to develop, because the SP population is heterogeneous, also containing Treg, NKT, and $\gamma\delta$ T cells, which turn over more slowly. They estimated SP CD4/CD8 residence times to be 4.4/4.6 days. Saini et al. (33) arrived at similar estimates. As for DP cells, there are may be several developmental stages within the SP population and so it seems unlikely that SP residence times are exponentially distributed.

Stritesky et al. (12) estimated the total rate (cells per unit time) at which cells are negatively selected to be almost six times greater than the rate of positive selection, and found that both processes occur predominantly at the DP stage. Converting these figures into the relative efficiencies of positive and negative selection requires knowledge of how long cells spend in each selecting phase. If indeed positive selection is the more stringent, their result indicates that negative selection must take place over a relatively short timescale within the DP compartment. This is supported by a recent study observing negative selection of DP thymocytes taking place over ~12 h (35).

Interpreting data on transit or residence times can be problematic when both death and differentiation are taking place, as they clearly are at the DP stage(s) of development. If death and differentiation are modeled as independent processes, then at equilibrium transit rates through a compartment are not necessarily the same as turnover rates. If cells are maturing at rate μ and dying at rate δ, the population turns over at rate $\mu + \delta$ and the expected time a cell spends in that compartment is $1/(\mu + \delta)$. However, the mean time that successfully differentiating cells spend in each compartment is shorter because it is conditioned on survival, and is $\mu/(\mu + \delta)^2$ (if cells are capable of maturing but are simultaneously at risk of dying, those that successfully mature tend to do so early). This difference can be quite substantial, as we see below.

KINETIC MODELS OF THYMIC DEVELOPMENT

Data from these experimental studies and others have invited the use of population dynamic models to infer the kinetics of development. In the first studies to model thymic development, Mehr and collaborators utilized ordinary differential equation (ODE) models of the flow from DN $\rightarrow$ early DP $\rightarrow$ late DP $\rightarrow$ CD4/CD8 SP (36, 37). They utilized measures of steady-state population sizes and parameters either inferred from data or explored systematically to ask questions about the underlying dynamics. Mehr et al. (36) argued that positive selection likely involves triggering of proliferation as well as rescue from death, and while they were unable to use the steady-state data to make strong statements about the timing of positive versus negative selection, they inferred that most death at the DP stage is due to failure to positively select, consistent with many experimental and subsequent modeling studies.

There is evidence from fetal thymic organ cultures that populations of mature $CD4^+$ T cells resident in the thymus may enrich for the CD4 lineage while reducing thymic output. Mehr et al. (37) used a similar model with these data to propose that the mature resident cells increase survival of developing single-positive CD4 T cells while reducing proliferation or increasing the rate of differentiation of DP cells. They suggest that mature CD4 T cells exert their influence by restricting the number of available pMHC ligands in the thymus, which could simultaneously reduce proliferation of DP cells (lowering thymic output) and decrease the stringency of negative selection (increasing the efficiency of maturation into the mature SP state). Again, these conclusions were reached using data from the thymus at steady-state.

Mehr and collaborators also studied the seeding of the cortical stroma with bone marrow-derived progenitor cells using a combination of modeling and experiment. They showed how migration between niche sites explained the competitive advantage of younger progenitors over older (38, 39), and that reconstitution of the progenitor population following irradiation is limited by damage to stromal niches and incumbent, surviving cells (40).

Thomas-Vaslin et al. (13) studied naive T cell homeostasis from the thymus through to the periphery. They induced systemic depletion of T cells for 7 days through expression of a suicide gene in dividing cells, and followed the kinetics of reconstitution. To interpret these data they developed a multi-compartment ODE model of T cell development, with a finer-grained treatment of transit through the DN, DP, and SP stages. In their model extensive proliferation occurs through the DN to early DP, with the latter population dividing 5 times. Their best-fitting model assumes all cell death (positive and negative selection) takes place at the late DP stage. They estimated 5% of total thymocytes (DN, DP, and SP) or ~3×10^6 are exported as naive SP cells per day, and that 93% of DP thymocytes are lost, in line with existing estimates, and again suggesting that the bulk of negative selection occurs at DP. The mean times spent overall in the early DP (dividing), late DP (selecting), and SP compartments were estimated to be 1.2, 2.7, and 5.8 days respectively.

Sinclair et al. (11) used a different experimental system, with controllable TCR signaling that allowed arrest and release of cells at the early DP stage, and used a multi-compartment ODE model to quantify transit dynamics and selection efficiencies. Rather than simply early or late, they broke the DP stage into a branched developmental progression defined by the expression levels of CD5 and the TCR (33). In their schema, DP1 thymocytes are pre-selection; progression to DP2 requires a positively-selecting TCR signal; DP2 thymocytes consist of class I- and class II-restricted thymocytes in the first 12–48 h of development; and DP3 thymocytes are predominantly MHC class I-restricted cells that can select into CD8SP only. Thus cells destined for CD4SP transit DP1-DP2 only, and CD8SP transit through DP1, DP2, and DP3.

Sinclair et al. (11) estimated that ~75% in DP1 fail to progress to DP2, reflecting failure to positively select and dying of neglect. Overall, 5% of DP cells become CD4SP and ~2% become CD8SP, and so ~94% of DP cells are lost. They also saw relatively low levels of cell death in the SP compartment. These results suggest again that the bulk of negative selection occurs before cells transition to SP. They saw very little proliferation in their system, using a variety of methods, and so did not model cell division. Mean residence times in DP1 and DP2 were 3.5 and 1.4 days, respectively, with the smaller CD8 lineage spending an additional 7 days in DP3. They estimated 23% of all thymocytes at DP and SP enter the DP compartment per day. These selection efficiencies and the net flux agree with other estimates. Accounting for the selection bias on maturing cells, the model predicts that successful thymocytes spend on average 1.3 days in DP1 + DP2, 4.5 days in DP3. SP4 and SP8 residence times were 5 and 3.7 days, respectively, with very little cell death occurring. Their analysis therefore suggests that CD4SP/CD8SP cells take ~6.3/9.5 days from entry into DP1 to export.

MIGRATION WITHIN THE THYMUS AND THE TIMING OF POSITIVE AND NEGATIVE SELECTION

From the perspective of modelers attempting to connect models of thymocyte dynamics to data, it is important to understand when and where the different phases of development and selection occur. Selection begins in the thymic cortex, where the majority of thymocytes perform undirected random walks (41) encountering pMHC on cortical thymic epithelial cells. Sensitivity to medullary chemokine receptor signals begins to increase immediately following receipt of a positive selection signal and positively-selected cortical thymocytes eventually display rapid, directed motion toward the medulla (41), where they encounter pMHC on medullary thymic epithelial cells and dendritic cells. Negative selection takes place in the medulla (35, 42–44) but also late in migration through the cortex (45) and possibly even throughout development (46). The mapping between these migratory and selecting processes to developmental stages is not clearly defined. Cells undergoing negative selection in the medulla include DP populations (35), indicating that maturation from DP to SP does not coincide precisely with the cortical–medullary transition but further supporting the conclusion that the extensive cell loss at the DP stage comes from failure of both positive and negative selection. Further, antigen-presenting cells in the cortex and medulla appear to differ in their ability to provide positive or negative selection signals, either through differences in pMHC expression or diversity, or levels of co-stimulation (47–51). It seems therefore that negative selection at the DP stage takes place in at least two distinct spatial and TCR-stimulatory environments.

MODELS OF SELECTION WITHIN THE CORTEX AND MEDULLA

Motivated by this, Faro et al. (52) took a different perspective; rather than partitioning selecting thymocytes into developmental stages, they used a probabilistic model to describe selection within the cortex and the medulla. They aimed to quantify the number of selecting events, the number of selecting APC encounters and pMHC engagements, and the efficiencies of positive and negative selection in each region. Using the experimental estimates of overall selection efficiencies, and one experimental estimate of the efficiency of negative selection in the medulla, they inferred that most thymocyte death occurs by failure to positive select in the cortex, and cells are ~10 times more likely to be deleted (negatively selected) in the medulla than in the cortex. With these efficiencies, through a parameter search, they were able to infer the number of ligands each thymocyte selects on in each spatial compartment. They came to the striking conclusion that for each cortical thymocyte selection takes places on <60 pMHC ligand interactions, likely in order to achieve in their model the required high level of failure to positively select. However, this needs to be reconciled with the ~3-day mean lifetime of cells at DP1, which suggests cells have far more opportunities to positively select, either through repeated encounters with APC or through repeated rearrangements of the TCRα chain [see Ref. (53) and refs therein], before dying of neglect.

IDENTIFYING THE SOURCE OF THE CD4:CD8 LINEAGE BIAS IN THYMUS

CD4 SP outnumber CD8 SP by roughly 4:1 in the thymi of many species. Using time courses of development in control mice and those lacking MHC class I or class II, Sinclair et al. (11) estimated the CD4 and CD8 lineage-specific selection efficiencies. In control animals, the highest death rate was at the positively-selected DP2 stage, and was substantially greater for MHC class I-restricted cells. MHC class I- and class II-restricted cells are indistinguishable at DP1 and DP2, but they were able to back-calculate the rates of production of precursors of the two lineages after TCR rearrangement, and found they were comparable. This suggests that the CD4:CD8 asymmetry in the thymus derives in large part from more stringent selection acting on MHC class I-restricted cells and not from any significant asymmetry in the predisposition of randomly generated TCR to recognize MHC class I or class II. Theirs is a model of CD4/CD8 lineage commitment in which the ability of a DP thymocyte to recognize MHC class I or class II dictates whether it will progress to the CD8 or CD4 lineages, respectively (8, 54). This is contrast to a less efficient, selective process in which a thymocyte's decision to downregulate either CD4 or CD8 expression is stochastic and decoupled from MHC preference, such that potentially viable TCR may fail positive selection [see, for example Ref. (55, 56); and Ref. (57) for a discussion of a hybrid mechanism]. Mehr et al. (36) proposed a purely instructive model of selection, in which pre-selection thymocytes are in principle able to recognize both MHC class I or II, and concluded that the most likely explanation of the CD4 bias is a difference in the *per capita* rates of maturation from DP into the two lineages, rather than differences in death rates.

The majority of models discussed here assume that thymocytes undergo screening independently. Mehr et al. (36, 37) implicitly allowed for competition with density-dependent proliferation rates at each developmental stage. However, there is some evidence that the probabilities of maturation can be impacted by competition between thymocytes, both globally and in lineage-specific ways. The efficiency of selection of transgenic TCRs varies with their abundance and with the availability of cognate pMHC (15, 58–60), and the selection of polyclonal MHC class I-restricted thymocytes is more efficient in the absence of MHC class II and vice versa (11). These observations suggest that selection efficiencies may be limited by competition both within and between lineages for access to pMHC or other resources needed for selection, and so may impact on the CD4:CD8 ratio emerging from the thymus. Two studies have used explicitly spatial, agent-based models of thymocyte migration and development to investigate this issue. Souza-e Silva et al. (61) modeled the movement of DN, DP, and CD4 SP and CD8 SP populations and their interactions with thymic epithelial cells (TEC) and chemokine gradients, using a 2D model. The structure of the epithelial networks was derived from histological samples from both mice and infant humans. Parameters were chosen to give agreement with published data regarding the repopulation of the thymus after sublethal irradiation, although a sensitivity analysis was not performed. In their model the CD4:CD8 ratio emerges as a result of competition for access to TEC and stochastic variation in the duration of signaling, which has been associated with CD4/CD8 lineage commitment (62). Their simulations also reproduce an observed variation in the CD4:CD8 ratio as irradiated thymi reconstitute and, in their model, the degree of competition increases. Efroni et al. (63) also took an agent-based approach and concluded that MHC class I and class II ligands on TECs are limiting. If continued access to pMHC stimulation is required for survival, and class I restricted cells stay conjugated to MHC for longer than MHC class II-restricted cells, exclusion of competitors leads to a higher death rate of cells developing into the CD8 lineage and a skewing of the CD4:CD8 ratio. Such a competitive model is an experimentally testable explanation of the differential death rates observed by Sinclair et al. (11).

CHARACTERISTICS OF THE TCR REPERTOIRE

Various summary statistics can be used to describe T cell populations pre- or post-selection. The *diversity* (or the *repertoire*) usually denotes the total number of distinct TCR sequences or clonotypes. The *cross-reactivity* measures a TCR's capacity for discrimination, and is quoted as either the average number or the proportion of different pMHC that one TCR responds to above some defined functional threshold. *Specificity* is inversely related to cross-reactivity. A mirror quantity is the *precursor frequency*, also referred to as the response frequency – the average proportion of all TCR capable of recognizing one pMHC. Further, selection operates in the context of an individual's own MHC alleles. *MHC restriction* measures the degree to which a given TCR is limited to recognizing peptides presented by one or more self-MHC; and *alloreactivity* is the proportion of TCR that respond to a foreign MHC, which is relevant for transplantation of tissues from one individual to another. In the sections that follow we describe how theoretical models have been used to understand how these quantities are linked and constrained by thymic selection.

TCR CROSS-REACTIVITY

A diverse TCR repertoire seems to be a requirement for coverage of pMHC shape space. However, the number of theoretically possible pMHC complexes appears to be far greater than any individual's capacity for unique TCR clonotypes (64–66); a simple calculation for just one MHC class I variant, assuming it presents 2% of all possible 9-residue peptides, yields $20^9 \times 0.02 \simeq 10^{10}$ possible pMHC, compared with the roughly 5×10^7 naive CD8 T cells in a mouse. To minimize the probability that any given foreign pMHC will escape detection by the immune system, some degree of TCR cross-reactivity therefore seems beneficial. Mason (64) used a variety of methods and data sources to estimate that one MHC class I-restricted T cell responds to between 10^6 and 10^7 nonamer peptides, or one in 10^3 to 10^4 pMHC using the theoretical estimate of the potential pMHC diversity; and Ishizuka et al. (65) used peptide libraries to estimate more directly that one CD8 T cell clone responds to roughly 1 in 3×10^4 peptide–MHC class I ligands. On the other hand, the average degree of cross-reactivity seems necessarily constrained from above, to avoid excessive deletion of the repertoire and to preserve specificity for self/non-self discrimination. It therefore seems plausible that evolutionary pressures might have optimized this trade-off and determined the degree to which TCR can respond to multiple pMHC.

OPTIMAL LEVELS OF TCR CROSS-REACTIVITY – PROBABILISTIC ARGUMENTS

Several variants of essentially the same argument predict that the diversity of self-peptides involved in selection is the strongest influence on the optimum level of TCR cross-reactivity (64, 67–70). One version of the argument is as follows. The proportion of the positively-selected T cell repertoire R_0 that avoids deletion, f, decreases with both the number of self antigens N_s and the cross-reactivity r, $f = (1-r)^{N_s}$ which is approximately $\exp(-rN_s)$ for $r \lesssim 1/N_s$. A pathogen escapes immune recognition if all fR_0 surviving unique clonotypes fail to recognize (cross-react with) all x epitopes it generates, with probability

$$P_E = (1-r)^{fR_0x} \simeq \exp(-rfR_0x) \tag{1}$$

where again the approximation holds if $r \lesssim 1/(fR_0x)$. This ignores MHC restriction, but including this refinement yields similar conclusions (67). Using the expression for f,

$$R_0 \simeq -\log(P_E)\frac{\exp(rN_s)}{rx}. \tag{2}$$

This equation connects the repertoire before negative selection R_0, the probability of immune escape P_E and the pre-selection cross-reactivity r. R_0 is relatively insensitive to P_E but very sensitive to the diversity of self, N_s. In this model, then, the strongest determinant of the size of the pre-selection repertoire is the diversity of self antigens, N_s, and not the requirement for minimizing the probability that a pathogen escapes detection (67).

The three-way relation expressed by equation (2) can then be used to estimate the optimal cross-reactivity under different evolutionary constraints. Suppose the potential repertoire size R_0 is relatively conserved and evolution has selected for the smallest P_E by tuning TCR cross-reactivity; in this case, the optimal cross-reactivity is simply the inverse of the number of distinct self-pMHC involved in selection, $r = 1/N_s$. The same value of r arises if evolution is assumed to minimize the required repertoire size R_0, whatever the value of P_E (67). Thus the more diverse the self-peptides involved in thymic selection, the more specific (less cross-reactive) the TCR needs to be. The same result can be derived in a very general way using extreme-value theory (70), requiring only the assumption that the negative selection threshold in the thymus is equal to the activation threshold in the periphery.

The induction of tolerance in the thymus is likely incomplete and there may be mature lymphocytes that are able to recognize self-peptides not involved in thymic selection. Borghans and De Boer (71) argued that to minimize the probability of these cells mounting a cross-reactive autoimmune response to this "ignored self" while responding to a pathogen demands higher levels of specificity than predicted by the simplest models. In this model, optimal cross-reactivity is then modulated by the potential diversity of the repertoire; the greater the number of possible T cell clonotypes, the lower cross-reactivity is required.

Percus et al. (72) took a different approach to studying optimal cross-reactivity, prompted by the observation that the sizes of the binding sites of the TCR and the B cell receptor (antibodies) are similar, at roughly 15 amino acids. They concluded that this size is large enough to provide discriminatory power but small enough that there is sufficient cross-reactivity for coverage of foreign antigen shape space. Interestingly this result does not arise from the demand for self–non-self discrimination, but rather from the constraint of the observation that the B and T cell repertoires comprise $\sim 10^7$ different receptors. However, this diversity itself may be derived from the self-tolerance arguments described above (64, 67–69). It has since been established that substantially fewer peptide residues are involved in TCR recognition. Burroughs et al. (73) analyzed the proteomes of humans and several microorganisms and showed that even the seven exposed (non-anchor) residues of the nine-mer peptides bound to one MHC class I allele may promote self/non-self discrimination, with <0.5% overlap in these sequences between humans and different microorganisms.

CONVERGENT ESTIMATES OF LEVELS OF NEGATIVE SELECTION

Several of these studies concluded that at the optimal level of cross-reactivity the probability of negative selection is roughly 63%, making various assumptions regarding the magnitude of parameters and maximizing the probability that the post-selection repertoire mounts a response to a foreign pMHC. However, the probability of negative selection can be derived without any assumptions regarding parameter values. From above, the fraction of the positively-selected repertoire with cross-reactivity r that survives deletion on N_s self-peptides is $f = (1-r)^{N_s}$. The probability that the post-selection repertoire $R = fR_0$ fails to recognize one given foreign pMHC is given by equation (1) with $x = 1$,

$$P_E = (1-r)^{fR_0} = (1-r)^{R_0(1-r)^{N_s}}. \tag{3}$$

This is minimized with respect to r at $r = 1 - \exp(-1/N_s)$, exactly (the optimal cross-reactivity $r \simeq 1/N_s$ then obtains if $N_s \gg 1$). So if evolution acts on cross-reactivity to minimize the probability of foreign pMHC escaping detection, the fraction of the positively-selected repertoire that survives negative selection is then simply $f = (1-r)^{N_s} = \exp(-1) \simeq 0.37$, or $\simeq 63\%$ of positively-selected thymocytes are deleted.

Mason (64) arrived at the same result assuming heuristically that the quantity to be maximized is the "reactivity" of the repertoire, proportional to the number of peptides each T cell can recognize multiplied by the proportion surviving negative selection;

$$\begin{aligned}&\text{Reactivity} \sim \text{Cross-reactivity}\\&\quad\times \text{P(survive negative selection)} \sim r \times (1-r)^{N_s}.\end{aligned}$$

Maximizing this reactivity is equivalent to minimizing the probability of escape in equation (3) when r is assumed to be small. There, using the Taylor expansion gives $P_E \simeq 1 - rR_0(1-r)^{N_s}$, and so the probability of responding $(1-P_E)$ is $\sim rR_0(1-r)^{N_s}$, or Mason's reactivity. Since r is small, the probability of negative selection is $(1-r)^{N_s} \simeq \exp(-rN_s)$ and so the reactivity is proportional to $r\exp(-rN_s)$, which is maximal with respect to r when argument of the exponential is -1. Thus again $f \simeq 0.37$ and the optimal cross-reactivity $r \simeq 1/N_s$.

An essentially identical argument applies to negative selection of B cells (67, 69). This estimate of f is remarkably consistent with estimates of levels of negative selection in the thymus from several experimental and population dynamic modeling studies (11, 17, 19–22).

ALTERNATIVE TREATMENTS OF CROSS-REACTIVITY

These models assume a universal cross-reactivity parameter r, but T cells may have the capacity to modulate their activation thresholds in response to their signaling environment (74, 75). Motivated by this, Scherer et al. (76) developed a model in which T cells tune their activation thresholds (and thus their cross-reactivity) to the level of their strongest interaction with self-pMHC during selection. If combined with a deletion mechanism that removes cells with activation thresholds so high as to be judged functionally inert, this model appears to be a more efficient mechanism of thymic selection than the standard clonal deletion model. Scherer et al. showed that the tuning model increases the probability of mounting an immune response to a given pathogen epitope, given a pre-selection repertoire size R_0, and the number of self-pMHC ligands involved in selection, N_s. The improvement offered by the tuning model is most striking for small pre-selection repertoires, $R_0 \ll N_s$, but disappears for $R_0 \gg N_s$. The latter inequality likely holds for mice and humans; the potential number of unique TCR sequences exceeds the estimated 10^3–10^5 self-peptides able to be presented by a given MHC allele (73, 77, 78). Further, equation (1) predicts that at the optimal cross-reactivity $r = 1/N_s$, the probability of one epitope ($x = 1$) escaping recognition is $P_E = \exp(-R_0/eN_s)$ where e is the base of the natural logarithm. For $P_E < 0.05$, expected in humans and mice, requires $R_0 \gtrsim 10N_s$. Despite this, Scherer et al. (76) argue that the tuning model is a more parsimonious mechanism of self-tolerance in the thymus than the standard model of deletion based on evolutionarily optimized cross-reactivity.

Finally, many of these arguments assumed thymic selection alone optimizes cross-reactivity, but the requirement for memory T cells to discriminate between different pathogens may impose a further constraint of its own (79, 80).

EXPLORING CROSS-REACTIVITY WITH SEQUENCE-BASED MODELS OF THYMIC SELECTION

A series of related papers by Detours, Perelson, and Mehr (27, 81–83) used a model of TCR–pMHC interactions to understand at a more mechanistic level how cross-reactivity, alloreactivity, and MHC restriction emerge in the post-selection repertoire. Here we focus on their treatment of TCR cross-reactivity, and return to alloreactivity and MHC restriction in the next section. Their starting point was an established model of protein binding (81, 84). They described the interaction between the variable region of the TCR and its pMHC ligand with strings of digits, and binding strengths between each digit pair were determined by the degree of complementarity between their binary representations (81). MHC and peptide contributed additively to the affinity of the interaction, the quantity assumed to drive selection. Given the number of digits ascribed to the polymorphic MHC residues in contact with the TCR, and the number of digits representing the peptide, selection could be performed on a randomly generated TCR repertoire using randomly generated peptide–MHC complexes. Affinity thresholds were then adjusted to give stringencies of positive and negative selection similar to those observed experimentally.

To circumvent the computational costs of selection using realistic numbers of peptides and unique pre-selection TCRs, they derived expressions for the mean-field predictions of the model for given parameter sets. This has the advantage of yielding population-level statements, which average over all possible TCR, MHC, and peptide sequences.

Detours and Perelson (82) estimated the precursor frequency, the proportion of naive T cells able to respond to a particular foreign pMHC. Experimental estimates of this quantity lie in the range 10^{-6}–10^{-4} (85–89). They term this the response frequency, R, and found it to be strongly and inversely related to the number of selecting self-pMHC ligands. Since precursor frequency is positively correlated with cross-reactivity (64), this result is in keeping with the theoretical studies discussed above (64, 67–70). It is also consistent with observations that repertoires selected on a restricted range of peptides exhibit higher cross-reactivity than normal (90–92). For R to lie in the observed range constrains the number of distinct peptides each MHC can present to be of the order 10^3–10^5, in line with estimates for murine MHC class I (77), MHC class II (78), and human MHC class I (73).

To explore the effect of thymic selection on specificity in more detail, Chao et al. (93) revisited the complementary digit-string model. Again peptide and MHC were assumed to contribute additively to an antigenic distance from the TCR, which was inversely related to affinity or the strength of a selecting signal. They confirmed that negative selection reduced the coverage of peptide space, defined as the proportion of peptides that are recognized on the selecting MHC. This was equivalent to a reduction in the cross-reactivity of the repertoire; it reduced the mean antigenic distance to foreign pMHC complexes.

Chao et al. (93) then used the model to address the question of why the number of pMHC that one T cell is able to respond to varies widely across TCR (94). Their simulations suggested that the degree of cross-reactivity to a foreign peptide was inversely related to the peptide's similarity to self, which can be understood with the following argument. In their model, in the pre-selection repertoire a TCR's affinity for the MHC and peptide portions of its ligand are uncorrelated. Selection introduces an inverse correlation between a TCR's affinity for its selecting MHC and its strongest affinity for self-peptide; to select, a TCR's strongest interaction with self must lie between the positive and negative selecting thresholds. (The narrower the range of affinities defining the selecting region, the stronger this correlation will be.) Selected T cells with high affinity for MHC then have a relatively low affinity for the self-peptide component and require only weak binding to foreign peptide to be activated (activation in their model is defined to be an interaction above the negative selection threshold). These cells are therefore cross-reactive to foreign peptides. Conversely, selected TCR that bind relatively weakly to MHC have higher affinity to self and require strong binding to foreign peptide for activation, and therefore have more specificity for foreign antigen. Thus it emerges from their model that a TCR's specificity to foreign peptide is positively correlated to its affinity for self-peptide; or equivalently, a TCR's cross-reactivity is positively correlated with its affinity for MHC.

The effect of negative selection on cross-reactivity can be understood with a similar argument. A TCR with high affinity for MHC will survive negative selection only if it has low affinity to all self-peptides, which is unlikely. Negative selection therefore enriches for cells with lower affinity for MHC, which from the argument above tend to be less cross-reactive. This reduction in coverage means specificity to foreign peptide must be increased.

Kosmrlj et al. (95) used a more physical, mechanistic approach to understanding how negative selection increases specificity, with the aim of characterizing the properties of the amino acid sequences of specific and cross-reactive TCR. Using the Miyazawa–Jernigan matrix (96) to quantify the interaction energies of pairs of amino acids, they extended the digit-string model to calculate the binding affinities between the peptide and the CDR3 region of the TCR, with a constant contribution from the MHC. (The variable peptide element of the pMHC ligand can be assumed to include the polymorphic MHC residues; thus their model may allow for MHC restriction, although this was not discussed.) Košmrlj et al. (97) presents an analytical treatment of the model.

They observed that TCRs selected against multiple peptides on the same MHC had peptide contact residues enriched in weakly interacting amino acids. In their model this arises by a sort of buffering mechanism – such sequences are able to withstand multiple substitutions in the peptide sequence to which they bind most strongly, and so are more resistant to negative selection than those TCR with strongly binding residues. For these TCR to survive selection requires that the invariant MHC contribution to the binding energy is of moderate strength – contributing sufficiently to favor positive selection but well below the negative selection threshold.

Kosmrlj et al. (95) argue that it is this enrichment for weakly binding TCR driven by negative selection that underlies antigen specificity. Antigen recognition is assumed to occur when a TCR signal exceeds the negative selection threshold made up by several interactions. This requires the peptide to contain several amino acids capable of binding the most strongly to the generally weakly binding TCR contact residues. Each contributes significantly to the total binding energy, and so any mutation to the peptide sequence has a high probability of abrogating recognition. Thus there is a restricted peptide signature or "barcode" required to trigger the TCR. In their model, TCR selected against a single pMHC were enriched slightly for strongly interacting amino acids. For these TCR, they argue, fewer amino acids contribute on average to the binding energy, triggering is more robust to mutations in the peptide sequence, and so the TCR is more cross-reactive. Thus again the argument emerges that the cross-reactivity is inversely related to the diversity of self driving selection. Kosmrlj et al. (98) employed this idea to put forward an explanation of why the population of elite-controllers of HIV infection is enriched for the HLA-B57 allele. Using a predictive peptide binding algorithm they argued that HLA-B*5701 binds a lower diversity of self-peptides than average. Cytotoxic T cells restricted to this allele are then expected to be more cross-reactive than average and so are more resistant to virus mutations that might otherwise escape CTL control.

Chao et al. (93) and Kosmrlj et al. (95) took different approaches to the problem of how negative selection increases specificity. They came to the common conclusion that the most specific TCR are those with low to intermediate affinity to MHC – high enough to have a reasonable probability of passing positive selection, but low enough to avoid negative selection by allowing headroom for the additional contribution from the peptide component. The greater this headroom, the smaller the proportion of peptides that can trigger activation and so the greater the specificity.

THE EMERGENCE OF SPECIFICITY IN AVIDITY-BASED MODELS OF SELECTION

Van den Berg et al. (99) developed a statistical framework to study the question of how specificity and self-tolerance can derive from a pre-selection repertoire of relatively promiscuous TCR. In their formalism, T cell activation is avidity-based and related to the rate of TCR triggering. Their starting point is that TCRs are degenerate and low affinity, binding weakly to many pMHC. TCR perceive an average signal derived from endogenous self-pMHC, and are triggered only by pMHC with sufficiently high prevalence and affinity to be visible above this background. The authors introduce the concept of an antigen presentation profile (APP), characterizing the abundances of different pMHC on antigen-presenting cells (APC). Positively-selected cells are selected against a given number of APC each with distinct APPs. In their framework, negative selection acts only on ubiquitous peptides presented on all APCs, and decisions are made on the basis of the entire APP of one APC. TCR that are triggered by this constitutive self-background are deleted. This filtering acts to sharpen the boundary between triggering rates, which give low and high activation probabilities, and so specificity can emerge even from a highly degenerate TCR. Interestingly they predict that negative selection does not have to be particularly stringent to generate an acceptably self-tolerant repertoire. Nevertheless in this model the selected repertoire may still be reactive to self-peptides expressed heterogeneously in the thymus, and in particular to peptides expressed at high levels only on certain cell types. Van den Berg and Rand (100) review avidity-based models of ligand discrimination.

ALLOREACTIVITY AND MHC RESTRICTION

A high proportion (1–24%) of peripheral T cells are reactive to peptides presented on a foreign MHC allele (101–103), reflected clinically by acute T cell mediated rejection of grafts from MHC-mismatched donors. These promiscuous "allogenic" responses contrast with the low precursor frequency (10^{-6}–10^{-4}) in normal immune responses to peptides presented by an individual's own MHC. Allogenic responses are also apparently counter to the notion of MHC restriction. Reconciling these results may tell us great deal about the relative contributions of peptide and MHC binding motifs to the TCR signals driving selection, and how this breakdown influences the coverage and cross-reactivity of the T cell repertoire.

Detours and Perelson (82) used their digit-string model of TCR–pMHC interactions, described above, to show how the probabilities of responsiveness to self and foreign MHC emerge.

Mean alloreactivities of 1–2% arose naturally, at the lower end of the range of experimental estimates, and they showed that the alloreactivities of the pre- and post-selection repertoires are similar, as observed experimentally (17, 22). In essence, the modeling supports the hypothesis that the greater degree of alloreactivity than response frequency arises simply because many more pMHC ligands can be generated from one MHC than can be generated from one peptide (104). In other words, each TCR is triggered by ligands in a subset of pMHC shape space; one particular MHC along with its associated diversity of peptides will cover a far greater region of shape space than covered by one peptide and all the self-MHC alleles capable of presenting it; a given MHC will then stimulate far more of the T cell repertoire than will a given peptide.

They found that alloreactivity correlates with the extent of negative selection and inversely to the degree of MHC restriction. It can be seen intuitively how this emerges from their model. If negative selection is weak, positive selection must be correspondingly stringent in order to yield the selection efficiencies observed experimentally (3–5%). Stringent positive selection imposes an imprint of self-MHC on the repertoire – only those TCRs that bind strongly to self-MHC residues survive. The strength of binding to a randomly generated MHC not involved in selection (i.e., a foreign MHC) is then on average lower to that of self-MHC in the post-selection repertoire. This difference increases, and thus alloreactivity decreases, as the required strength of binding to self-MHC increases.

This trade-off between alloreactivity and restriction might be expected as they appear to be in conflict. However, experimental estimates of these two quantities are variable. The conclusions described above were derived analytically from a model capturing the mean-field behavior of the digit-string selection process, but did not deal with the variance in these measures of the repertoire outputs across specific simulations or experimental systems. The final study of the series (83) took a simulation-based approach, explicitly performing repertoire selection on random TCR and pMHC populations. This confirmed the inverse correlation between alloreactivity and MHC restriction and yielded sufficient variability to account for restriction ranging from absolute to partial in different settings.

Overall the digit-string model explored by Detours and colleagues yields remarkable agreement with many observations. Their model of TCR–pMHC binding is highly abstracted, but appears to be a powerful one. In part this might be because the relevant quantities for selection in their model are the minimum and maximum binding affinities that each TCR experiences during exposure to large samples of randomly generated pMHC strings. These two quantities will be drawn from extreme-value distributions, which should be insensitive to the distribution of binding strengths of randomly chosen TCR–pMHC pairs (70, 105). The additivity of the MHC and peptide contributions to the fate-determining signal is likely the most questionable assumption, as the authors point out. Fate decisions may be based on the sum of several TCR interactions (which means for example that positive selection may occur though proximal binding of multiple low-affinity ligands) and so an avidity-based model may be more appropriate. Another caveat is that the population-average model assumes that positive selection takes place on at most one MHC allele, which we will also return to.

INSIGHTS INTO FATE DETERMINATION MECHANISMS FROM STOCHASTICITY IN SELECTION

Regulatory T cells (Treg) are a distinct lineage of CD4SP cells thought to lie at the higher end of the spectrum of acceptable self-reactivity and play a crucial role in the control of autoimmunity and tolerance to innocuous antigens. Many experimental studies of Treg development have shown that cells with the same TCR can develop into conventional and regulatory T cells within the same selecting environment [see, for example, Ref. (58, 106)], illustrating again, as represented in so many models, the stochastic nature of selection. There are at least two possible sources of this stochasticity. In a purely selective model precursors with identical TCR might be predisposed to the conventional or Treg fates through natural variation in expression of factors involved in lineage commitment. In a purely instructive model, cells within a clone are uncommitted, and intra-clonal heterogeneity in fate may derive from variation in the experience of each thymocyte during selection – most likely because each encounters a different random sample of self-peptides.

Bains et al. (107) used a probabilistic, instructive model that reflects this view of fate determination driven entirely by antigenic experience during selection, in conjunction with data from Ref. (58) to infer the number of pMHC binding events involved in fate determination. In that study, the numbers of conventional and Treg cells with a transgenically expressed TCR were measured for varying abundances of that TCR's agonist peptide on thymic epithelial cells. Conventional cell numbers declined monotonically with agonist abundance, while Treg increased and then decreased. Thus as agonist abundance increased, it appeared that T cells were initially diverted into the Treg lineage, before the risk of deletion through exposure to agonist dominated. Using this information and a simple graphical argument they were able to infer that fate decisions could not be affinity-driven (that is, made on the basis of a single pMHC interaction) unless TCR sensitivity varies during development, for which there is evidence [see Ref. (107) and references therein]. This model also explains apparently paradoxical observations regarding the effect of partial and full TCR agonists on the efficiency of Treg production (108).

THE LIMITS OF NEGATIVE SELECTION

The potentially very large number of unique self-pMHC prompts the question of whether it is possible to tolerize thymocytes to all self-peptides within the timescale of thymic development. Müller and Bonhoeffer (109) studied this problem. Using constraints from the mouse proteome and the efficiencies of peptide production and binding to MHC, they estimated an upper limit of approximately 5×10^6 possible self-pMHC class I complexes. Notably, this diversity of self is several orders of magnitude lower than figures derived from the simple combinatoric arguments (64, 66) and is more closely aligned with an estimate that $\sim 10^5$ different nine-mers derived from the human proteome are expected to bind to one human MHC class I allele (73). The key quantity in Müller and Bonhoeffer's calculation is the probability P that a given self-pMHC is presented by any given APC in sufficient numbers for negative selection to occur. The probability that a thymocyte specific for this (and only this) self-pMHC escapes negative selection is P_E in their notation – distinct from the probability of immune escape discussed above – and $P_E = (1-P)^n$, where n is the number of unique APC encountered during selection. In this model, P_E is extremely sensitive to the number of copies h of a given self-pMHC that an APC needs to present in order to cause deletion – varying h between 15 and 1500 gives values of P_E between 10^{-11} and 0.8. Favoring the higher estimates of h, Müller and Bonhoeffer (109) concluded that negative selection on the potential diversity of self is likely to be very leaky. Instead, they suggest thymic selection operates on a restricted subset of self-pMHC, a constraint imposed by the number of APCs encountered during selection. This requires that further tolerogenic mechanisms operate in the periphery to prevent autoimmune response to self antigens not encountered in the thymus (53, 70).

To support their argument, Müller and Bonhoeffer (109) reverted to the older model of cross-reactivity and selection to generate another estimate of the number of selecting ligands using the observed efficiency of negative selection. Recall that the probability of thymocyte with cross-reactivity r escaping negative selection on N_s unique selecting ligands is $P = (1-r)^{N_s} \simeq e^{-rN_s}$. Using the estimate of $r = 2 \times 10^{-5}$ (88), and $P \simeq 0.33$, they obtain $N_s \simeq 10^5$ unique selecting self-pMHC, or ~4% of the putative total number of self-pMHC. This estimate is consistent with those of Detours et al. (27). Both studies assume that this cross-reactivity r of thymocytes with self-pMHC is equal to the cross-reactivity of mature naive T cells to foreign pMHC. Since negative selection likely acts as a filter to reduce cross-reactivity in the post-selection repertoire (see above), this assumption is moot. But the need to meet the empirical constraint $e^{-rN_s} \simeq 0.33$ implies that higher values of r would reduce the number of unique selecting ligands N_s even further.

A subsequent exchange (110, 111) discussed the assumption that each TCR negatively selects only on a single self-pMHC ligand. Müller and Bonhoeffer (111) argued that in the Bernoulli trial model of cross-reactivity and selection, a 33% probability of survival implies that another third of all thymocytes were reactive to one self-pMHC only, giving some quantitative support to their original model. The discussion also addressed whether N_s is constrained by the residence time in the thymus or is a result of restricted presentation of self antigens. Müller and Bonhoeffer (111) favored the latter, presuming that evolution has optimized the thymic residence time for the purposes of efficient selection on a subset of self-peptides. More recently it has been argued that incomplete depletion of self-reactive cells in the thymus may be sufficient for robust self/non-self discrimination in the periphery, if interactions facilitating consensus between T cells are required for the initiation or suppression of immune responses (70).

OPTIMALITY OF INDIVIDUAL MHC DIVERSITY – CONSTRAINTS ARISING FROM THYMIC SELECTION

The polymorphism of the MHC is huge, with hundreds of alleles identified at the HLA-A, HLA-B, and HLA-DR loci in humans (MHC is referred to as HLA in humans but hereon the term MHC is generally used, for simplicity). This diversification is thought not to have occurred by genetic drift but by two non-exclusive mechanisms. Heterozygote advantage (112, 113) suggests that individuals expressing more unique MHC alleles gain fitness by being able to present a larger array of pathogen peptides. Overall the evidence for heterozygote advantage in experimental models of infection is equivocal, though, and it has been argued with a quantitative model that this mechanism alone is insufficient to explain the extent of allelic diversity (114). Another theory is that MHC polymorphism is maintained by frequency-dependent selection under pathogen pressure, in which rare alleles confer protection against pathogen subversion of peptide presentation by commonly expressed alleles (115).

Intriguingly, individuals possess only a small proportion of all MHC alleles. Heterozygous humans possess six at the major HLA-A, HLA-B, and HLA-C loci, which code for MHC class I molecules that present peptides to $CD8^+$ T cells, and six to eight at the HLA-DP, HLA-DQ, and HLA-DR MHC class II loci, which present to $CD4^+$ T cells. A common explanation for this restricted within-individual diversity is that it derives from the need to generate a broad, functional, and self-tolerant TCR repertoire in the thymus without excessive negative selection (116, 117). The qualitative argument is as follows. If n is the number of MHC alleles per person, then increasing n both increases the diversity of pathogen-derived peptides that can be presented and increases the probability that a thymocyte will be able to obtain positively-selecting signals. On the other hand, higher n will also increase the range of self-peptides that can be presented. This will increase the stringency of negative selection, leading to inefficient generation of T cells in the thymus and potential gaps in the repertoire's coverage of peptide space. The observed number of different MHC molecules per individual may result from a trade-off between these demands.

The nature of MHC restriction needs to be considered carefully in these arguments. If restriction is absolute and each TCR recognizes only one MHC allele, increasing the number of alleles per person simply increases the size and diversity of the T cell repertoire with no cost because selection operates on each MHC-restricted subset of the pre-selection repertoire independently. In this case an upper limit to within-host MHC diversity might derive only from the need for APC to display sufficient numbers of peptides in conjunction with each MHC molecule to reliably mediate selection or immune activation. The trade-off evident in the qualitative argument above arises when MHC restriction is not absolute and thymocytes are capable of being positively and/or negatively selected on more than one allele.

Woelfing et al. (118) provide an excellent review of theoretical approaches to understanding intra-individual MHC diversity, but we outline the key results here. Nowak et al. (119) were the first to assess the qualitative trade-off argument using a mathematical model. In their analysis they defined h and f to be the proportions of T cells capable of being positively and negatively selected, respectively, by a given MHC allele. If an individual expresses n distinct MHC alleles, they argue that the proportion of the T cell repertoire surviving selection is

$$(1-(1-h)^n)(1-f)^n.$$

The first term represents positive selection; $(1-h)^n$ is the probability that a TCR fails to be selected by any MHC. The second term represents negative selection; $(1-f)^n$ is the probability that a TCR is not negatively selected by any MHC. The proportion of the repertoire surviving is maximized at $n=(1/h)\log(1+h/f)$. They argue that $h \leq f$, supported by the experimental and modeling consensus is that positive selection is more stringent than negative selection. This gives $n \sim 1/f$. However, using only the assumptions that $hn \ll 1$, or that it is rare for a TCR to be positively selected on more than one MHC allele, and that the proportion of all peptides that can bind to a given MHC is $\ll 1$, they calculate that $n=2/f$ maximizes the probability of a response to a randomly chosen foreign pMHC.

Borghans et al. (120) pointed out that this model contains an inconsistency, which allows for cells that fail to be positively selected on one MHC to be negatively selected by the same MHC. They denoted p and n to be the unconditional probabilities that one TCR is positively and negatively selected by a given MHC molecule. Then $n < p$, because the number of cells that fail negative selection on one MHC is necessarily smaller than the number that audition for it following positive selection on that same MHC. The proportion of the original repertoire that survives is then

$$(1-n)^M - (1-p)^M. \quad (4)$$

This model effectively lowers the stringency of negative selection expressed in Nowak et al. (119) and so reduces the cost of increasing the number of MHC alleles. They estimated the probabilities p and n were 0.01 and 0.005 respectively, using the known efficiencies of positive and negative selection in mice with known numbers of MHC alleles. The optimal value of M for these parameter values is far larger than observed allele numbers; conversely, asking what values of p and n correspond to the observed ranges of M being optimal leads to unrealistic levels of positive and negative selection. Their analysis therefore questions the trade-off hypothesis as an explanation of limited MHC diversity.

They suggest alternatives. They estimate that existing typical numbers of MHC alleles together with TCR cross-reactivity may be "good enough" for maximizing the probability of responding to a foreign peptide on self-MHC – in this case the selective pressure for increasing MHC alleles is weak or absent. Alternatively, increased numbers of MHC alleles may increase the risk of autoimmunity through cross-reactivity of T cells responding to antigen that have not been fully tolerized to self. Finally, limited numbers of MHC alleles may allow for sufficient densities of pMHC on the surface of antigen-presenting cells to be able to efficiently select and activate MHC-restricted T cells.

MHC restriction is not absolute in the models described above, although it holds approximately for positive selection when the per-allele positive selection probability p is small. However, there is evidence to suggest that MHC restriction is not manifest strongly at the positive selection stage. Zerrahn et al. (22) observed that a relatively large proportion of TCR still positively select when a single type of pMHC was expressed in the thymus. In that study, pre-selection TCRs had approximately a 5% chance of responding to a given class II MHC, independently for different alleles, validating one of the assumptions of these simple probabilistic selection models. On similar lines, Huseby et al. (92) found that the positively-selected repertoire contains TCR with a high degree of cross-reactivity across MHC alleles, and suggested that MHC restriction emerges as a result of negative selection. Finally, the high degree of alloreactivity suggests that positive selection is only weakly MHC-restricted, and that failure to positive select reflects a generic inability to bind to MHC.

Motivated by this possibility, Woelfing et al. (118) revisited these probabilistic models. They assumed positive selection is highly degenerate with respect to MHC and that even very weak cross-reactivity with any allele is sufficient. Under this assumption, one of the presumed advantages of high MHC diversity is removed. Maximizing the probability of mounting an immune response, they estimated the optimal MHC diversity to be in a physiological range of 3–25.

Van den Berg and Rand (121) used a very different and sophisticated approach to the same optimality problem using a mechanistic, stochastic model of TCR triggering rather than the probabilistic repertoire-based models described above. Considering negative selection only, they concluded that limited individual MHC diversity is beneficial for self–non-self discrimination. The essence of their mathematical argument is that restricting the "diversity of foreign" is the key to increasing the signal-to-noise ratio for aTCR attempting to discriminate a foreign peptide from the background of self. This is achieved with a combination of limiting the number of MHC alleles each TCR can recognize (MHC restriction) and limiting the number of peptides that can be presented from one protein on one MHC allele ("peptide selectivity") to be roughly one. However, the need to ensure that every foreign protein is represented requires multiple MHC alleles, placing a theoretical lower bound on their number. An upper bound comes from the requirement that the density of relevant pMHC ligands must not fall too low on the surface of an APC, similar to the suggestion in Borghans et al. (120) – if a given pMHC is diluted by too many MHC, the relevant TCR will experience fluctuations in signaling that may reduce its discriminatory power. They conclude that of the order 10 MHC alleles is optimal. Notably, as in Ref. (118), this estimate arises without any constraints from positive selection.

SUMMARY

This review has outlined how several relatively simple descriptions of single TCR–pMHC interactions have been used to understand aspects of TCR repertoire development. However, the discussion is necessarily incomplete. In particular, there is an extensive literature exploring the molecular mechanisms by which individual or collections of TCR discriminate between ligands of different affinities [see, for example, Ref. (100, 122–126)], which has direct relevance to thymic selection. It remains unclear how proximal TCR signals derived from multiple and diverse pMHC ligands can drive the emergence of specificity and MHC restriction in the post-selection repertoire, although the models of selection on ensembles of ligands have made steps in this direction (99, 121). Are repeated super-threshold contacts required for negative selection, or is a single encounter with a high affinity ligand sufficient to cause deletion?

Many of the models discussed here assume that a single interaction above a minimum signaling threshold is sufficient for positive selection. However, there is evidence that repeated or sustained TCR signaling is required during the DP stage for positive selection to occur [see, for example, Ref. (17, 127)]. This may explain findings that positive and negative selection take place concurrently (46).

Overall it is remarkable how much insight into the quantitative aspects of thymic selection has emerged from highly abstracted models. However, there remain a lot of open areas for research, and many of the questions raised in the introduction are still unresolved. Regulatory T cell development in particular has received very little attention from modelers, and already it appears that the simplest extension to the simple probabilistic fixed-threshold model to include a fixed range of affinity or avidity for Treg selection is not sufficient to explain many experimental observations (107). The task of synthesizing and reconciling the huge diversity of experimental data related to thymic development is a daunting one, but the information available is perhaps currently underexploited by theorists.

ACKNOWLEDGMENTS

The author thanks Charles Sinclair and the reviewers for helpful comments. This work was supported by the NIH (R01AI093870).

REFERENCES

1. Paul WE, editor. *Fundamental Immunology.* 6 ed. Philadelphia: Lippincott Williams & Wilkins (2008).
2. Starr TK, Jameson SC, Hogquist KA. Positive and negative selection of T cells. *Annu Rev Immunol* (2003) **21**:139–76. doi:10.1146/annurev.immunol.21.120601.141107
3. Moran AE, Hogquist KA. T-cell receptor affinity in thymic development. *Immunology* (2012) **135**(4):261–7. doi:10.1111/j.1365-2567.2011.03547.x
4. Petrie HT, Livak F, Schatz DG, Strasser A, Crispe IN, Shortman K. Multiple rearrangements in T cell receptor alpha chain genes maximize the production of useful thymocytes. *J Exp Med* (1993) **178**(2):615–22. doi:10.1084/jem.178.2.615
5. Scollay RG, Butcher EC, Weissman IL. Thymus cell migration. Quantitative aspects of cellular traffic from the thymus to the periphery in mice. *Eur J Immunol* (1980) **10**(3):210–8. doi:10.1002/eji.1830100310
6. Egerton M, Scollay R, Shortman K. Kinetics of mature T-cell development in the thymus. *Proc Natl Acad Sci U S A* (1990) **87**(7):2579–82. doi:10.1073/pnas.87.7.2579
7. Graziano M, St-Pierre Y, Beauchemin C, Desrosiers M, Potworowski EF. The fate of thymocytes labeled in vivo with CFSE. *Exp Cell Res* (1998) **240**(1):75–85. doi:10.1006/excr.1997.3900
8. Itano A, Robey E. Highly efficient selection of CD4 and CD8 lineage thymocytes supports an instructive model of lineage commitment. *Immunity* (2000) **12**(4):383–9. doi:10.1016/S1074-7613(00)80190-9
9. Quackenbush RC, Shields AF. Local re-utilization of thymidine in normal mouse tissues as measured with iododeoxyuridine. *Cell Tissue Kinet* (1988) **21**(6):381–7.
10. McCaughtry TM, Wilken MS, Hogquist KA. Thymic emigration revisited. *J Exp Med* (2007) **204**(11):2513–20. doi:10.1084/jem.20070601
11. Sinclair C, Bains I, Yates AJ, Seddon B. Asymmetric thymocyte death underlies the CD4:CD8 T-cell ratio in the adaptive immune system. *Proc Natl Acad Sci U S A* (2013) **110**(31):E2905–14. doi:10.1073/pnas.1304859110
12. Stritesky GL, Xing Y, Erickson JR, Kalekar LA, Wang X, Mueller DL, et al. Murine thymic selection quantified using a unique method to capture deleted T cells. *Proc Natl Acad Sci U S A* (2013) **110**(12):4679–84. doi:10.1073/pnas.1217532110
13. Thomas-Vaslin V, Altes HK, de Boer RJ, Klatzmann D. Comprehensive assessment and mathematical modeling of T cell population dynamics and homeostasis. *J Immunol* (2008) **180**(4):2240–50.
14. Shortman K, Vremec D, Egerton M. The kinetics of T cell antigen receptor expression by subgroups of CD4+8+ thymocytes: delineation of CD4+8+3(2+) thymocytes as post-selection intermediates leading to mature T cells. *J Exp Med* (1991) **173**(2):323–32. doi:10.1084/jem.173.2.323
15. Huesmann M, Scott B, Kisielow P, von Boehmer H. Kinetics and efficacy of positive selection in the thymus of normal and T cell receptor transgenic mice. *Cell* (1991) **66**(3):533–40. doi:10.1016/0092-8674(81)90016-7
16. von Boehmer H. Positive selection of lymphocytes. *Cell* (1994) **76**(2):219–28. doi:10.1016/0092-8674(94)90330-1
17. Merkenschlager M, Graf D, Lovatt M, Bommhardt U, Zamoyska R, Fisher AG. How many thymocytes audition for selection? *J Exp Med* (1997) **186**(7):1149–58. doi:10.1084/jem.186.7.1149
18. Monteiro MC, Couceiro S, Penha-Gonçalves C. The multigenic structure of the MHC locus contributes to positive selection efficiency: a role for MHC class II gene-specific restriction. *Eur J Immunol* (2005) **35**(12):3622–30. doi:10.1002/eji.200535190
19. Ignatowicz L, Rees W, Pacholczyk R, Ignatowicz H, Kushnir E, Kappler J, et al. T cells can be activated by peptides that are unrelated in sequence to their selecting peptide. *Immunity* (1997) **7**(2):179–86. doi:10.1016/S1074-7613(00)80521-X
20. van Meerwijk JP, Marguerat S, Lees RK, Germain RN, Fowlkes BJ, MacDonald HR. Quantitative impact of thymic clonal deletion on the T cell repertoire. *J Exp Med* (1997) **185**(3):377–83. doi:10.1084/jem.185.3.377
21. Tourne S, Miyazaki T, Oxenius A, Klein L, Fehr T, Kyewski B, et al. Selection of a broad repertoire of CD4+ T cells in H-2Ma0/0 mice. *Immunity* (1997) **7**(2):187–95. doi:10.1016/S1074-7613(00)80522-1
22. Zerrahn J, Held W, Raulet DH. The MHC reactivity of the T cell repertoire prior to positive and negative selection. *Cell* (1997) **88**(5):627–36. doi:10.1016/S0092-8674(00)81905-4
23. Hale JS, Boursalian TE, Turk GL, Fink PJ. Thymic output in aged mice. *Proc Natl Acad Sci U S A* (2006) **103**(22):8447–52. doi:10.1073/pnas.0601040103
24. Steinmann GG, Klaus B, Muller-Hermelink HK. The involution of the ageing human thymic epithelium is independent of puberty. A morphometric study. *Scand J Immunol* (1985) **22**(5):563–75. doi:10.1111/j.1365-3083.1985.tb01916.x
25. Scollay R, Godfrey DI. Thymic emigration: conveyor belts or lucky dips? *Immunol Today* (1995) **16**(6):268–73. doi:10.1016/0167-5699(95)80179-0
26. Porritt HE, Gordon K, Petrie HT. Kinetics of steady-state differentiation and mapping of intrathymic-signaling environments by stem cell transplantation in nonirradiated mice. *J Exp Med* (2003) **198**(6):957–62. doi:10.1084/jem.20030837
27. Detours V, Mehr R, Perelson AS. Deriving quantitative constraints on T cell selection from data on the mature T cell repertoire. *J Immunol* (2000) **164**(1):121–8.
28. Lucas B, Vasseur F, Penit C. Production, selection, and maturation of thymocytes with high surface density of TCR. *J Immunol* (1994) **153**(1):53–62.
29. Hare KJ, Wilkinson RW, Jenkinson EJ, Anderson G. Identification of a developmentally regulated phase of postselection expansion driven by thymic epithelium. *J Immunol* (1998) **160**(8):3666–72.
30. Pénit C, Vasseur F. Expansion of mature thymocyte subsets before emigration to the periphery. *J Immunol* (1997) **159**(10):4848–56.
31. Okamoto Y, Douek DC, McFarland RD, Koup RA. Effects of exogenous interleukin-7 on human thymus function. *Blood* (2002) **99**(8):2851–8. doi:10.1182/blood.V99.8.2851
32. Junge S, Kloeckener-Gruissem B, Zufferey R, Keisker A, Salgo B, Fauchere J-C, et al. Correlation between recent thymic emigrants and CD31+ (PECAM-1) CD4+ T cells in normal individuals during aging and in lymphopenic children. *Eur J Immunol* (2007) **37**(11):3270–80. doi:10.1002/eji.200636976
33. Saini M, Sinclair C, Marshall D, Tolaini M, Sakaguchi S, Seddon B. Regulation of Zap70 expression during thymocyte development enables temporal separation of CD4 and CD8 repertoire selection at different signaling thresholds. *Sci Signal* (2010) **3**(114):ra23. doi:10.1126/scisignal.2000702
34. Liu X, Adams A, Wildt KF, Aronow B, Feigenbaum L, Bosselut R. Restricting Zap70 expression to CD4+CD8+ thymocytes reveals a T cell receptor-dependent proofreading mechanism controlling the completion of positive selection. *J Exp Med* (2003) **197**(3):363–73. doi:10.1084/jem.20021698
35. Dzhagalov IL, Chen KG, Herzmark P, Robey EA. Elimination of self-reactive T cells in the thymus: a timeline for negative selection. *PLoS Biol* (2013) **11**(5):e1001566. doi:10.1371/journal.pbio.1001566
36. Mehr R, Globerson A, Perelson AS. Modeling positive and negative selection and differentiation processes in the thymus. *J Theor Biol* (1995) **175**(1):103–26. doi:10.1006/jtbi.1995.0124

37. Mehr R, Perelson AS, Fridkis-Hareli M, Globerson A. Feedback regulation of T cell development in the thymus. *J Theor Biol* (1996) **181**(2):157–67. doi:10.1006/jtbi.1996.0122
38. Mehr R, Abel L, Ubezio P, Globerson A, Agur Z. A mathematical model of the effect of aging on bone marrow cells colonizing the thymus. *Mech Ageing Dev* (1993) **67**(1–2):159–72. doi:10.1016/0047-6374(93)90120-G
39. Mehr R, Segel L, Sharp A, Globerson A. Colonization of the thymus by T cell progenitors: models for cell-cell interactions. *J Theor Biol* (1994) **170**(3):247–57. doi:10.1006/jtbi.1994.1185
40. Mehr R, Fridkis-Hareli M, Abel L, Segel L, Globerson A. Lymphocyte development in irradiated thymuses: dynamics of colonization by progenitor cells and regeneration of resident cells. *J Theor Biol* (1995) **177**(2):181–92. doi:10.1006/jtbi.1995.0237
41. Witt CM, Raychaudhuri S, Schaefer B, Chakraborty AK, Robey EA. Directed migration of positively selected thymocytes visualized in real time. *PLoS Biol* (2005) **3**(6):e373. doi:10.1371/journal.pbio.0030373
42. Surh CD, Sprent J. T-cell apoptosis detected in situ during positive and negative selection in the thymus. *Nature* (1994) **372**(6501):100–3. doi:10.1038/372100a0
43. Sprent J, Kishimoto H. The thymus and negative selection. *Immunol Rev* (2002) **185**:126–35. doi:10.1034/j.1600-065X.2002.18512.x
44. Le Borgne M, Ladi E, Dzhagalov I, Herzmark P, Liao YF, Chakraborty AK, et al. The impact of negative selection on thymocyte migration in the medulla. *Nat Immunol* (2009) **10**(8):823–30. doi:10.1038/ni.1761
45. McCaughtry TM, Baldwin TA, Wilken MS, Hogquist KA. Clonal deletion of thymocytes can occur in the cortex with no involvement of the medulla. *J Exp Med* (2008) **205**(11):2575–84. doi:10.1084/jem.20080866
46. Baldwin KK, Trenchak BP, Altman JD, Davis MM. Negative selection of T cells occurs throughout thymic development. *J Immunol* (1999) **163**(2):689–98.
47. Lorenz RG, Allen PM. Thymic cortical epithelial cells lack full capacity for antigen presentation. *Nature* (1989) **340**(6234):557–9. doi:10.1038/340557a0
48. Mizuochi T, Kasai M, Kokuho T, Kakiuchi T, Hirokawa K. Medullary but not cortical thymic epithelial cells present soluble antigens to helper T cells. *J Exp Med* (1992) **175**(6):1601–5. doi:10.1084/jem.175.6.1601
49. Gray DHD, Seach N, Ueno T, Milton MK, Liston A, Lew AM, et al. Developmental kinetics, turnover, and stimulatory capacity of thymic epithelial cells. *Blood* (2006) **108**(12):3777–85. doi:10.1182/blood-2006-02-004531
50. Hogquist KA, Xing Y. Why CD8+ T cells need diversity when growing up. *Immunity* (2010) **32**(1):5–6. doi:10.1016/j.immuni.2010.01.005
51. Nitta T, Murata S, Sasaki K, Fujii H, Ripen AM, Ishimaru N, et al. Thymoproteasome shapes immunocompetent repertoire of CD8+ T cells. *Immunity* (2010) **32**(1):29–40. doi:10.1016/j.immuni.2009.10.009
52. Faro J, Velasco S, González-Fernández A, Bandeira A. The impact of thymic antigen diversity on the size of the selected T cell repertoire. *J Immunol* (2004) **172**(4):2247–55.
53. Mason D. Some quantitative aspects of T-cell repertoire selection: the requirement for regulatory T cells. *Immunol Rev* (2001) **182**:80–8. doi:10.1034/j.1600-065X.2001.1820106.x
54. Borgulya P, Kishi H, Müller U, Kirberg J, von Boehmer H. Development of the CD4 and CD8 lineage of T cells: instruction versus selection. *EMBO J* (1991) **10**(4):913–8.
55. Corbella P, Moskophidis D, Spanopoulou E, Mamalaki C, Tolaini M, Itano A, et al. Functional commitment to helper T cell lineage precedes positive selection and is independent of T cell receptor MHC specificity. *Immunity* (1994) **1**(4):269–76. doi:10.1016/1074-7613(94)90078-7
56. Itano A, Kioussis D, Robey E. Stochastic component to development of class I major histocompatibility complex-specific T cells. *Proc Natl Acad Sci U S A* (1994) **91**(1):220–4. doi:10.1073/pnas.91.1.220
57. Germain RN. T-cell development and the CD4-CD8 lineage decision. *Nat Rev Immunol* (2002) **2**(5):309–22. doi:10.1038/nri798
58. van Santen H-M, Benoist C, Mathis D. Number of T reg cells that differentiate does not increase upon encounter of agonist ligand on thymic epithelial cells. *J Exp Med* (2004) **200**(10):1221–30. doi:10.1084/jem.20041022
59. Bautista JL, Lio C-WJ, Lathrop SK, Forbush K, Liang Y, Luo J, et al. Intraclonal competition limits the fate determination of regulatory T cells in the thymus. *Nat Immunol* (2009) **10**(6):610–7. doi:10.1038/ni.1739
60. Lee H-M, Bautista JL, Scott-Browne J, Mohan JF, Hsieh C-S. A broad range of self-reactivity drives thymic regulatory T cell selection to limit responses to self. *Immunity* (2012) **37**(3):475–86. doi:10.1016/j.immuni.2012.07.009
61. Souza-e Silva H, Savino W, Feijóo RA, Vasconcelos ATR. A cellular automata-based mathematical model for thymocyte development. *PLoS One* (2009) **4**(12):e8233. doi:10.1371/journal.pone.0008233
62. Liu X, Bosselut R. Duration of TCR signaling controls CD4-CD8 lineage differentiation in vivo. *Nat Immunol* (2004) **5**(3):280–8. doi:10.1038/ni1040
63. Efroni S, Harel D, Cohen IR. Emergent dynamics of thymocyte development and lineage determination. *PLoS Comput Biol* (2007) **3**(1):e13. doi:10.1371/journal.pcbi.0030013
64. Mason D. A very high level of crossreactivity is an essential feature of the T-cell receptor. *Immunol Today* (1998) **19**(9):395–404. doi:10.1016/S0167-5699(98)01299-7
65. Ishizuka J, Grebe K, Shenderov E, Peters B, Chen Q, Peng Y, et al. Quantitating T cell cross-reactivity for unrelated peptide antigens. *J Immunol* (2009) **183**(7):4337–45. doi:10.4049/jimmunol.0901607
66. Sewell AK. Why must T cells be cross-reactive? *Nat Rev Immunol* (2012) **12**(9):669–77. doi:10.1038/nri3279
67. De Boer RJ, Perelson AS. How diverse should the immune system be? *Proc Biol Sci* (1993) **252**(1335):171–5. doi:10.1098/rspb.1993.0062
68. Whitaker L, Renton AM. On the plausibility of the clonal expansion theory of the immune system in terms of the combinatorial possibilities of amino-acids in antigen and self-tolerance. *J Theor Biol* (1993) **164**(4):531–6. doi:10.1006/jtbi.1993.1171
69. Nemazee D. Antigen receptor 'capacity' and the sensitivity of self-tolerance. *Immunol Today* (1996) **17**(1):25–9. doi:10.1016/0167-5699(96)80565-2
70. Butler TC, Kardar M, Chakraborty AK. Quorum sensing allows T cells to discriminate between self and nonself. *Proc Natl Acad Sci U S A* (2013) **110**(29):11833–8. doi:10.1073/pnas.1222467110
71. Borghans JA, De Boer RJ. Crossreactivity of the T-cell receptor. *Immunol Today* (1998) **19**(9):428–9. doi:10.1016/S0167-5699(98)01317-6
72. Percus JK, Percus OE, Perelson AS. Predicting the size of the T-cell receptor and antibody combining region from consideration of efficient self-nonself discrimination. *Proc Natl Acad Sci U S A* (1993) **90**(5):1691–5. doi:10.1073/pnas.90.5.1691
73. Burroughs NJ, de Boer RJ, Kesmir C. Discriminating self from nonself with short peptides from large proteomes. *Immunogenetics* (2004) **56**(5):311–20. doi:10.1007/s00251-004-0691-0
74. Grossman Z, Singer A. Tuning of activation thresholds explains flexibility in the selection and development of T cells in the thymus. *Proc Natl Acad Sci U S A* (1996) **93**(25):14747–52. doi:10.1073/pnas.93.25.14747
75. Anderton SM, Wraith DC. Selection and fine-tuning of the autoimmune T-cell repertoire. *Nat Rev Immunol* (2002) **2**(7):487–98. doi:10.1038/nri842
76. Scherer A, Noest A, de Boer RJ. Activation-threshold tuning in an affinity model for the T-cell repertoire. *Proc Biol Sci* (2004) **271**(1539):609–16. doi:10.1098/rspb.2003.2653
77. Cox AL, Skipper J, Chen Y, Henderson RA, Darrow TL, Shabanowitz J, et al. Identification of a peptide recognized by five melanoma-specific human cytotoxic T cell lines. *Science* (1994) **264**(5159):716–9. doi:10.1126/science.7513441
78. Hunt DF, Michel H, Dickinson TA, Shabanowitz J, Cox AL, Sakaguchi K, et al. Peptides presented to the immune system by the murine class II major histocompatibility complex molecule I-Ad. *Science* (1992) **256**(5065):1817–20. doi:10.1126/science.1319610
79. Borghans JA, Noest AJ, De Boer RJ. How specific should immunological memory be? *J Immunol* (1999) **163**(2):569–75.
80. Borghans JAM, De Boer RJ. Memorizing innate instructions requires a sufficiently specific adaptive immune system. *Int Immunol* (2002) **14**(5):525–32. doi:10.1093/intimm/14.5.525
81. Detours V, Sulzer B, Perelson AS. Size and connectivity of the idiotypic network are independent of the discreteness of the affinity distribution. *J Theor Biol* (1996) **183**(4):409–16. doi:10.1006/jtbi.1996.0231
82. Detours V, Perelson AS. Explaining high alloreactivity as a quantitative consequence of affinity-driven thymocyte selection. *Proc Natl Acad Sci U S A* (1999) **96**(9):5153–8. doi:10.1073/pnas.96.9.5153
83. Detours V, Perelson AS. The paradox of alloreactivity and self MHC restriction: quantitative analysis and statistics. *Proc Natl Acad Sci U S A* (2000) **97**(15):8479–83. doi:10.1073/pnas.97.15.8479
84. Perelson AS, Weisbuch G. Immunology for physicists. *Rev Mod Phys* (1997) **69**:1219–68. doi:10.1103/RevModPhys.69.1219
85. Stockinger H, Pfizenmaier K, Hardt C, Rodt H, Röllinghoff M, Wagner H. H-2 restriction as a consequence of intentional priming: T cells of fully allogeneic

chimeric mice as well as of normal mice respond to foreign antigens in the context of H-2 determinants not encountered on thymic epithelial cells. *Proc Natl Acad Sci U S A* (1980) **77**(12):7390–4. doi:10.1073/pnas.77.12.7390
86. Merkenschlager M, Terry L, Edwards R, Beverley PC. Limiting dilution analysis of proliferative responses in human lymphocyte populations defined by the monoclonal antibody UCHL1: implications for differential CD45 expression in T cell memory formation. *Eur J Immunol* (1988) **18**(11):1653–61. doi:10.1002/eji.1830181102
87. Zinkernagel RM. Immunology taught by viruses. *Science* (1996) **271**(5246): 173–8. doi:10.1126/science.271.5246.173
88. Blattman JN, Antia R, Sourdive DJD, Wang X, Kaech SM, Murali-Krishna K, et al. Estimating the precursor frequency of naive antigen-specific CD8 T cells. *J Exp Med* (2002) **195**(5):657–64. doi:10.1084/jem.20001021
89. Moon JJ, Chu HH, Pepper M, McSorley SJ, Jameson SC, Kedl RM, et al. Naive CD4(+) T cell frequency varies for different epitopes and predicts repertoire diversity and response magnitude. *Immunity* (2007) **27**(2):203–13. doi:10.1016/j.immuni.2007.07.007
90. Huseby ES, Crawford F, White J, Kappler J, Marrack P. Negative selection imparts peptide specificity to the mature T cell repertoire. *Proc Natl Acad Sci U S A* (2003) **100**(20):11565–70. doi:10.1073/pnas.1934636100
91. Slifka MK, Blattman JN, Sourdive DJD, Liu F, Huffman DL, Wolfe T, et al. Preferential escape of subdominant CD8+ T cells during negative selection results in an altered antiviral T cell hierarchy. *J Immunol* (2003) **170**(3):1231–9.
92. Huseby ES, White J, Crawford F, Vass T, Becker D, Pinilla C, et al. How the T cell repertoire becomes peptide and MHC specific. *Cell* (2005) **122**(2):247–60. doi:10.1016/j.cell.2005.05.013
93. Chao DL, Davenport MP, Forrest S, Perelson AS. The effects of thymic selection on the range of T cell cross-reactivity. *Eur J Immunol* (2005) **35**(12):3452–9. doi:10.1002/eji.200535098
94. Kraj P, Pacholczyk R, Ignatowicz L. Alpha beta TCRs differ in the degree of their specificity for the positively selecting MHC/peptide ligand. *J Immunol* (2001) **166**(4):2251–9.
95. Kosmrlj A, Jha AK, Huseby ES, Kardar M, Chakraborty AK. How the thymus designs antigen-specific and self-tolerant T cell receptor sequences. *Proc Natl Acad Sci U S A* (2008) **105**(43):16671–6. doi:10.1073/pnas.0808081105
96. Miyazawa S, Jernigan RL. Residue-residue potentials with a favorable contact pair term and an unfavorable high packing density term, for simulation and threading. *J Mol Biol* (1996) **256**(3):623–44. doi:10.1006/jmbi.1996.0114
97. Košmrlj A, Chakraborty AK, Kardar M, Shakhnovich EI. Thymic selection of T-cell receptors as an extreme value problem. *Phys Rev Lett* (2009) **103**:068103. doi:10.1103/PhysRevLett.103.068103
98. Kosmrlj A, Read EL, Qi Y, Allen TM, Altfeld M, Deeks SG, et al. Effects of thymic selection of the T-cell repertoire on HLA class I-associated control of HIV infection. *Nature* (2010) **465**(7296):350–4. doi:10.1038/nature08997
99. van den Berg HA, Rand DA, Burroughs NJ. A reliable and safe T cell repertoire based on low-affinity T cell receptors. *J Theor Biol* (2001) **209**(4):465–86. doi:10.1006/jtbi.2001.2281
100. van den Berg HA, Rand DA. Quantitative theories of T-cell responsiveness. *Immunol Rev* (2007) **216**:81–92. doi:10.1111/j.1600-065X.2006.00491.x
101. Bevan MJ, Langman RE, Cohn M. H-2 antigen-specific cytotoxic T cells induced by concanavalin A: estimation of their relative frequency. *Eur J Immunol* (1976) **6**(3):150–6. doi:10.1002/eji.1830060303
102. Ashwell JD, Chen C, Schwartz RH. High frequency and nonrandom distribution of alloreactivity in T cell clones selected for recognition of foreign antigen in association with self class II molecules. *J Immunol* (1986) **136**(2): 389–95.
103. Suchin EJ, Langmuir PB, Palmer E, Sayegh MH, Wells AD, Turka LA. Quantifying the frequency of alloreactive T cells in vivo: new answers to an old question. *J Immunol* (2001) **166**(2):973–81.
104. Matzinger P, Bevan MJ. Hypothesis: why do so many lymphocytes respond to major histocompatibility antigens? *Cell Immunol* (1977) **29**(1):1–5. doi:10.1016/0008-8749(77)90269-6
105. Fisher RA, Tippet LHC. Limiting forms of the frequency distribution of the largest or smallest member of a sample. *Proc Camb Philos Soc* (1928) **24**:180–90. doi:10.1017/S0305004100015681
106. Picca CC, Oh S, Panarey L, Aitken M, Basehoar A, Caton AJ. Thymocyte deletion can bias Treg formation toward low-abundance self-peptide. *Eur J Immunol* (2009) **39**(12):3301–6. doi:10.1002/eji.200939709
107. Bains I, van Santen HM, Seddon B, Yates AJ. Models of self-peptide sampling by developing T cells identify candidate mechanisms of thymic selection. *PLoS Comput Biol* (2013) **9**(7):e1003102. doi:10.1371/journal.pcbi.1003102
108. Picca CC, Simons DM, Oh S, Aitken M, Perng OA, Mergenthaler C, et al. CD4+ CD25+ Foxp3+ regulatory T cell formation requires more specific recognition of a self-peptide than thymocyte deletion. *Proc Natl Acad Sci U S A* (2011) **108**(36):14890–5. doi:10.1073/pnas.1103810108
109. Müller V, Bonhoeffer S. Quantitative constraints on the scope of negative selection. *Trends Immunol* (2003) **24**(3):132–5. doi:10.1016/S1471-4906(03)00028-0
110. Bandeira A, Faro J. Quantitative constraints on the scope of negative selection: robustness and weaknesses. *Trends Immunol* (2003) **24**(4):172–3. doi:10.1016/S1471-4906(03)00055-3
111. Müller V, Bonhoeffer S. Response to Bandeira and Faro: closing the circle of constraints. *Trends Immunol* (2003) **24**(4):173–5. doi:10.1016/S1471-4906(03)00056-5
112. Doherty PC, Zinkernagel RM. Enhanced immunological surveillance in mice heterozygous at the H-2 gene complex. *Nature* (1975) **256**(5512):50–2. doi:10.1038/256050a0
113. McClelland EE, Penn DJ, Potts WK. Major histocompatibility complex heterozygote superiority during coinfection. *Infect Immun* (2003) **71**(4):2079–86. doi:10.1128/IAI.71.4.2079-2086.2003
114. De Boer RJ, Borghans JAM, van Boven M, Kesmir C, Weissing FJ. Heterozygote advantage fails to explain the high degree of polymorphism of the MHC. *Immunogenetics* (2004) **55**(11):725–31. doi:10.1007/s00251-003-0629-y
115. Borghans JAM, Beltman JB, De Boer RJ. MHC polymorphism under host-pathogen coevolution. *Immunogenetics* (2004) **55**(11):732–9. doi:10.1007/s00251-003-0630-5
116. Vidovic D, Matzinger P. Unresponsiveness to a foreign antigen can be caused by self-tolerance. *Nature* (1988) **336**(6196):222–5. doi:10.1038/336222a0
117. Lawlor DA, Zemmour J, Ennis PD, Parham P. Evolution of class-I MHC genes and proteins: from natural selection to thymic selection. *Annu Rev Immunol* (1990) **8**:23–63. doi:10.1146/annurev.iy.08.040190.000323
118. Woelfing B, Traulsen A, Milinski M, Boehm T. Does intra-individual major histocompatibility complex diversity keep a golden mean? *Philos Trans R Soc Lond B Biol Sci* (2009) **364**(1513):117–28. doi:10.1098/rstb.2008.0174
119. Nowak MA, Tarczy-Hornoch K, Austyn JM. The optimal number of major histocompatibility complex molecules in an individual. *Proc Natl Acad Sci U S A* (1992) **89**(22):10896–9. doi:10.1073/pnas.89.22.10896
120. Borghans JAM, Noest AJ, De Boer RJ. Thymic selection does not limit the individual MHC diversity. *Eur J Immunol* (2003) **33**(12):3353–8. doi:10.1002/eji.200324365
121. van den Berg HA, Rand DA. Antigen presentation on MHC molecules as a diversity filter that enhances immune efficacy. *J Theor Biol* (2003) **224**(2):249–67. doi:10.1016/S0022-5193(03)00162-0
122. Altan-Bonnet G, Germain RN. Modeling T cell antigen discrimination based on feedback control of digital ERK responses. *PLoS Biol* (2005) **3**(11):e356. doi:10.1371/journal.pbio.0030356
123. Prasad A, Zikherman J, Das J, Roose JP, Weiss A, Chakraborty AK. Origin of the sharp boundary that discriminates positive and negative selection of thymocytes. *Proc Natl Acad Sci U S A* (2009) **106**(2):528–33. doi:10.1073/pnas.0805981105
124. Palmer E, Naeher D. Affinity threshold for thymic selection through a T-cell receptor-co-receptor zipper. *Nat Rev Immunol* (2009) **9**(3):207–13. doi:10.1038/nri2469
125. Govern CC, Paczosa MK, Chakraborty AK, Huseby ES. Fast on-rates allow short dwell time ligands to activate T cells. *Proc Natl Acad Sci U S A* (2010) **107**(19):8724–9. doi:10.1073/pnas.1000966107
126. Currie J, Castro M, Lythe G, Palmer E, Molina-París C. A stochastic T cell response criterion. *J R Soc Interface* (2012) **9**(76):2856–70. doi:10.1098/rsif.2012.0205
127. Wilkinson RW, Anderson G, Owen JJ, Jenkinson EJ. Positive selection of thymocytes involves sustained interactions with the thymic microenvironment. *J Immunol* (1995) **155**(11):5234–40.

2

Combinatorial cytokine code generates anti-viral state in dendritic cells

Boris M. Hartmann[1], Nada Marjanovic[1], German Nudelman[1], Thomas M. Moran[2] and Stuart C. Sealfon[1]*

[1] Department of Neurology, Mount Sinai School of Medicine, Center for Translational Systems Biology, New York, NY, USA
[2] Department of Microbiology, Mount Sinai School of Medicine, Center for Translational Systems Biology, New York, NY, USA

Edited by:
Penelope Anne Morel, University of Pittsburgh, USA

Reviewed by:
Robert Adam Harris, Karolinska Institutet, Sweden
Hans Acha-Orbea, Center for Immunity and Infection Lausanne, Switzerland
Giovanna Schiavoni, Istituto Superiore di Sanità, Italy

****Correspondence:***
Stuart C. Sealfon, Department of Neurology, Mount Sinai School of Medicine, Center for Translational Systems Biology, One Gustave L Levy Place, MSH Box 1137, New York, NY 10029, USA
e-mail: stuart.sealfon@mssm.edu

The physiological function of the immune system and the response to therapeutic immunomodulators may be sensitive to combinatorial cytokine micro-environments that shape the responses of specific immune cells. Previous work shows that paracrine cytokines released by virus-infected human dendritic cells (DC) can dictate the maturation state of naïve DCs. To understand the effects of paracrine signaling, we systematically studied the effects of combinations cytokines in this complex mixture in generating an anti-viral state. After naïve DCs were exposed to either IFNβ or to paracrine signaling released by DCs infected by Newcastle disease virus (NDV), microarray analysis revealed a large number of genes that were differently regulated by the DC-secreted paracrine signaling. In order to identify the cytokine mechanisms involved, we identified 20 cytokines secreted by NDV infected DCs for which the corresponding receptor gene is expressed in naïve DCs. By exposing cells to all combinations of 19 cytokines (leave-one-out studies), we identified five cytokines (IFNβ, TNFα, IL-1β, TNFSF15, and IL28) as candidates for regulating DC maturation markers. Subsequent experiments identified IFNβ, TNFα, and IL1β as the major contributors to this anti-viral state. This finding was supported by infection studies *in vitro*, by T-cell activation studies and by *in vivo* infection studies in mouse. Combination of cytokines can cause response states in DCs that differ from those achieved by the individual cytokines alone. These results suggest that the cytokine microenvironment may act via a combinatorial code to direct the response state of specific immune cells. Further elucidation of this code may provide insight into responses to infection and neoplasia as well as guide the development of combinatorial cytokine immunomodulation for infectious, autoimmune, and immunosurveillance-related diseases.

Keywords: TNFa, IL1b, IFNb, anti-viral signaling, DC maturation, combinatorial effect

INTRODUCTION

The limitations of single cytokine therapy have motivated interest in evaluating the effects of combinatorial treatment. Individual therapeutic cytokines often fail to achieve full or sustained clinical benefits for many patients. For example, IFNα, which is the current therapy for chronic hepatitis C infection, fails to clear HCV titers in half of treated patients (1). The cytokine interferon beta (IFNβ) has limited activity against multiple sclerosis in a large segment of patients (2). Cytokine combination therapy, where two or more cytokine-based medications are simultaneous administered to treat a single disease, has shown promise in multiple medical conditions, such as cancer (3), myocardial infarction (4), and osteoporosis (5). Recent studies have also begun to reveal how combined extracellular stimuli can synergistically direct the responses of immune cells. Retinoic acid combined with IL-15 causes dendritic cells (DCs) to skew the T-cell polarization toward TH17 cells (6). SCF and IL-2 have a synergistic effect on the proliferation NK cells (7). TNFα and IFNγ act together on smooth airway cells to enhance CXCL-10 expression (8). IL17 together with TNFα or IL1β induces MCP-1 and MIP-2 in murine mesangial cells (9). Despite its potential, studying combinations of cytokines is experimentally difficult and relatively little systematic exploration in this important area has been reported.

We previously reported that paracrine signaling mediated by the complex mixture of cytokines secreted by virus-infected DCs in culture causes naïve uninfected DCs to develop an anti-viral state characterized by upregulation of DC maturation markers, increased phagocytic activity, and greater resistance to viral infection (10). Since the discovery of type I interferon, paracrine cytokine signaling has been recognized as a crucial component in orchestrating the immune responses to virus infection. However, IFNβ pretreatment alone is not sufficient to induce this paracrine induction of anti-viral activated DCs (10). In the present study, we investigate the combinatorial cytokine code underlying this effect, by studying combinations of the single components of the secretome of virus-infected DCs. Understanding how this combinatorial cytokine code modulates immune responses may guide the development of better combination therapy approaches and help elucidate how the microenvironment directs appropriate responses in specific cell types during infection.

MATERIALS AND METHODS

DIFFERENTIATION OF DCs

All human research protocols for this work have been reviewed and approved by the IRB of the Mount Sinai School of Medicine. Monocyte-derived DCs were obtained from healthy human blood donors following a standard protocol described elsewhere (11). Briefly, human peripheral blood mononuclear cells were isolated from buffy coats by Ficoll density gradient centrifugation (Histopaque, Sigma Aldrich) at 1450 rpm and CD14^{+} monocytes were immunomagnetically purified by using a MACS CD14 isolation kit (Miltenyi Biotech). Monocytes were then differentiated into naïve DCs by 5–6 days incubation at 37°C and 5% CO_2 in DC growth media, which contains RPMI Medium 1640 (Invitrogen/Gibco) supplemented with 10% fetal calf serum (Hyclone), 2 mM of L-glutamine, 100 U/mL penicillin and 100 g/mL streptomycin (Pen/Strep) (Invitrogen), 500 U/mL hGM-CSF (Preprotech), and 1000 U/mL hIL-4 (Preprotech). All experiments were replicated using cells obtained from different donors. Overall, we used DCs from 21 different donors for this study.

VIRUS PREPARATION AND VIRAL INFECTION

The Newcastle disease virus (NDV) (rNDV/B1) was generated in Prof. Peter Palese's laboratory (12). NDV-RFP, Influenza A/California/04/09 (H1N1), and A/Puerto Rico/8/1934 (H1N1) were obtained from Prof. Adolfo Garcia-Sastre's laboratory (13). For infection, virus stocks were diluted in serum free medium and added directly onto pelleted DCs at a multiplicity of infection of 1.

GENERATION OF AVDCs

Anti-viral activated dendritic cells (AVDCs) were generated by employing a trans-well system. The trans-well system consists of an upper and a lower chamber separated by a 0.4 μm PET membrane (Millipore) that allows diffusion of cytokines and chemokines through the membrane but avoids the interaction of the cells in both chambers. To generate the AVDCs, naïve DCs were infected as described above. After the 40 min incubation, the cells were washed with PBS, and cultured in the trans-well system. Infected and non-infected DCs were allocated in the upper and lower chamber, respectively. Two independent wells were set-up with infected or naïve non-infected DCs as positive and negative controls. The cultures were incubated at 37°C in 5% CO_2 for 18 h. All cells were then washed in PBS and harvested for flow cytometry analysis and RNA isolation. The supernatant was kept at −80°C for ELISA analysis of cytokines/chemokines.

MICROARRAY ANALYSIS

Samples from AVDCs, DCs infected with NDV, and DCs treated with IFNβ for 8 h were used for microarray analysis. Naive DCs served as negative control. Three samples were taken per treatment. RNA was extracted with the RNeasy plus kit (Qiagen) following the manufacturer's protocol. Gene expression was assayed using broad human genome specific HG-U133_Plus_2 GeneChip expression probe arrays (Affymetrix). Raw data was processed with the Partek Pro software using the RMA background correction, with an adjustment of GC content as pre-background adjustment. Data was normalized to its quantile, data was log transformed to a base of two, and probe sets were summarized to its mean. Principal component analysis (PCA) of samples plotted in genespace was performed for all probe sets. Robustness of the PCA was tested by randomization (Figure S1 in Supplementary Material). One-way ANOVA was calculated by using Method of Moments (14). Fisher's least significant difference with FDR as multiple testing correction was used to calculate the following contrasts AVDC vs. IFNβ, AVDC vs. CTRL, IFNβ vs. CTRL, NDV vs. CTRL. List were generated by a fold change and *p*-value (FDR adjusted) criteria. Bioinformatic analysis was performed using Ingenuity software. The data used are deposited in NCBI's gene expression omnibus (15) and are accessible through GEO series accession number GSE52081 (http://www.ncbi.nlm.nih.gov/geo/query/acc.cgi?acc=GSE52081).

ELISA

In order to minimize the supernatant volume to assay, a Beadlyte Human Multiplex ELISA analysis (Millipore) was used following manufacturer instructions. Briefly, 100 μl from each compartment/well was incubated in a 96-well filter PVDF 1.2 μm plate specially designed to retain cytokines/chemokines, with a mixture of anti-cytokine IgG conjugated beads for the different cytokines/chemokines assayed. After 2 h incubation, the plate was filtered and washed three times with Assay solution (PBS pH 7.4 containing 1% BSA, 0.05% Tween-20, and 0.05% sodium azide). The washes were followed by 1.5 h incubation with biotin-conjugated anti-cytokine IgG. After Assay solution washing, Streptavidin–Phycoerythrin, was added followed by addition after 30 min Stop solution [0.2% (v/v) formaldehyde in PBS pH 7.4]. The plate was then filtered and each well resuspended in 125 μl of Assay buffer, and read in a Luminex 100 machine. Single cytokine ELISA (IFNβ) was also performed according to manufacturers protocol (PBL).

CYTOKINE TREATMENTS

Dendritic cells were exposed to 1.3 μg/mL TNFα (Symansis), 9 μg/mL CCL3 (Symansis), 3.8 μg/mL IL8 (Symansis), 20 μg/mL CXCL10 (Peprotech), 0.5 μg/mL CCL5 (Peprotech), 9 μg/mL IL6 (Peprotech), 2.8 μg/mL IFNα2 (PBL InterferonSource), 0.03 μg/mL CXCL12 (Peprotech), 2 μg/mL IFNALPHA16 (PBL InterferonSource), 0.03 μg/mL IL12a (Symansis), 4.4 μg/mL IL18 (R&D SYSTEMS), 0.2 μg/mL IL1a (R&D SYSTEMS), 1 μg/mL IL1RA (R&D SYSTEMS), 4 μg/mL IL28a (AbD Serotec), 4 μg/mL IL29 (R&D SYSTEMS), 0.1 μg/mL TNFSF15 (AbD Serotec), 0.1 μg/mL TNFSF4 (R&D Systems), 0.1 μg/mL TNFSF10 (R&D Systems), 0.2 μg/mL IL1β (eBiosciences), and 8.89 μg/mL IFNβ (PBL InterferonSource) in various combinations for 8 h. For the first screening with 20 cytokines, we used cells from three different donors. To adjust for overall differences between individuals, we normalized data of each individual to the median of all treatments. All other cytokine screening experiments were carried out with replicated from the same donor and then repeated with at least two additional donors.

FLOW CYTOMETRY ANALYSIS

Cells were washed with FACS staining buffer (Beckman Coulter) and stained with monoclonal antibodies for HLA-DR and CD86 (BD Biosciences). NDV-GFP cells were analyzed without any additional staining. Cells were assayed on an LSRII flow cytometer (BD Biosciences) and analyzed with Cytobank software (16). Raw data as well as analyses can be downloaded at: https://www.cytobank.org/cytobank/experiments?project=565

IMAGING FLOW CYTOMETRY ANALYSIS OF BEAD UPTAKE AND APOPTOSIS

For analysis for apotosis and infectivity cells were fixed after treatment with 1% paraformaldehyde (Electron Microscopy Science), permeabilized with Methanol (Sigma), and washed in PBS and stained with influenza NP specific antibodies (Abcam) and Hoechst 33342 (Invitrogen) as nuclear dye. Single cell images were acquired using the IS 100 Imaging flow cytometer (Amnis). Apoptotic cells were identified by fragmentation of nucleus (intensity of nuclear image at a 30% threshold) and shape of the bright-field image (contrast) using IDEAS software (Amnis). To detect phagocytosis, 1 μm 488 nm fluorescence labeled latex microspheres (Polysciences Corp.) at a concentration of 50 beads per cell were co-cultured for 2 h at 37°C with cytokine pretreated cells. Single cell images were acquired using extended depth field imaging distortion in order to identify beads in different focal planes within a cell. The numbers of beads incorporated by cells were quantified in the images captured using image analysis software (IDEAS Software, Amnis Corp).

REAL-TIME PCR

mRNA expression levels were quantified by real-time reverse transcriptase polymerase chain reaction (PCR). RNA was isolated from cells using Qiagen Micro RNeasy kit following the manufactures protocol (QIAGEN). cDNA was synthesized from total RNA with AffinityScript™ Multi-Temp RT (Stratagene) with oligo dT_{18} as primer. For real-time PCR PlatinumTaq DNA polymerase (Invitrogen) and a SYBR green (Molecular Probes) containing buffer were used. The real-time PCRs were performed using a thermocycler (ABI7900HT; Applied Biosystems) as previously described (21). The RNA levels for the house keeping genes ribosomal protein S11, tubulin, and β-actin were also assayed in all samples to be used as an internal controls. mRNA measurements were normalized using a robust global normalization algorithm. All control crossing threshold (Ct) values were corrected by the median difference in all samples from Actb. All samples were then normalized by the difference from the median Ct of the three corrected control gene Ct levels in each sample, with the value converted to a nominal copy number per cell by assuming 2500 Actb mRNA molecules per cell and an amplification efficiency of 93% for all reactions. PCR results from DCs exposed to combinations of cytokines were normalized to values from untreated cells and log 2 transformed prior further statistical analysis. To get a picture of overall induction of those genes assayed, we summarized the log transformed expression levels on the most right column of **Figure 7**. Primers for genes can be found in the Table S3 in Supplementary Material.

T-CELL ACTIVATION ASSAY

PBMCs were exposed to inactivated native measles virus for 4 days. From these samples, CD3 cells were isolated by negative selection using the Pan T-Cell Isolation Kit II (Miltenyi) and stained with CFSE (Invitrogen). Those cells were then co-cultured with cytokine pretreated DCs which were also pulsed with inactivated native measles virus. T-cell proliferation was measured by the reduction of CFSE intensity of cells.

IN VIVO EXPERIMENTATION

Animal studies were performed in compliance with the U.S. Department of Health and Human Services Guide for the Care and Use of Laboratory Animals and protocols were approved by the Institutional Animal Care and Use Committee (IACUC) of the Mount Sinai School of Medicine. Animals were pretreated with murine 3.5 mg/kg BW IFNβ (PBL InterferonSource), murine 1.3 mg/kg BW TNFα (Peprotech), and 0.5 mg/kg IL1β (Peprotech) 6 and 3 h prior infection with the influenza A strain PR8 in an inhalation chamber.

STATISTICAL ANALYSIS

Micro array analysis was performed with the Partek Pro software 1-way ANOVA was calculated by using Method of Moments (14). Genes were compared by asymptotic unpaired *t*-test comparisons followed by a Benjamini–Hochberg multiple testing correction. All other data was analyzed with R. Maturation marker expression, apoptosis induction, and infectivity levels were first analyzed with ANOVA, followed with pairwise comparisons using the Tukey's "Honest Significant Difference" method. PCR of the gene expression after combinatorial treatment was also analyzed with ANOVA followed Tukey's "Honest Significant Difference" method and an additional Bonferroni multiple testing correction for the summarized data. Bead uptake data were analyzed with a pairwise Wilcoxon Rank Sum Test with the Bonferroni method for multiple testing correction. Survival of mice was analyzed with a Mantel–Haenszel test for survival analysis. Data as well as the R analysis can de downloaded from the supplementary data.

RESULTS

EXPOSURE TO PARACRINE SIGNALING FROM INFECTED DCs INDUCES GENE EXPRESSION PROFILE DISTINCT FROM THAT CAUSED BY IFNβ ALONE

The effects of paracrine signaling from infected DCs on naive DCs, transforming them to what we have previously referred to as anti-viral activated DCs [AVDC, Ref. (6)], were studied using microarrays (**Figure 1**). To compare the effects of paracrine signaling to the effects of a single cytokine treatment, we exposed naive DCs either to paracrine signaling from NDV infected cells (which generates AVDCs) or to IFNβ at a concentration found in the supernatants of NDV infected DCs. RNA samples from naive cells (CTRL) and NDV infected cells (NDV) were also assayed.

A PCA on the samples was performed in order to test how much individual samples are similar to the biological replicates within a group and how the different groups relate to each other. The PCA showed that cells exposed to paracrine signaling from infected DCs had a different overall expression profile than cells exposed to IFNβ alone (**Figure 1A**). Top genes for vectors were CXCL11, ISG20, ISG20, IDO1, IFI27, IFITM1, IFIT2, OASL, and CXCL9 for principal component (PC) 1; IFIT2, CXCL11, CCDC88A, NEXN, MALAT1, TNFSF10, P2RY12, SAMD9L, SMCHD1, and NEXN for PC2 PPBP, MMP1, ADAM12, IRG1, AKAP12, SLC28A3, DNAJC6, FABP4, ITGA9, and FABP4 for PC3. ANOVA (FDR $p < 0.05$) and

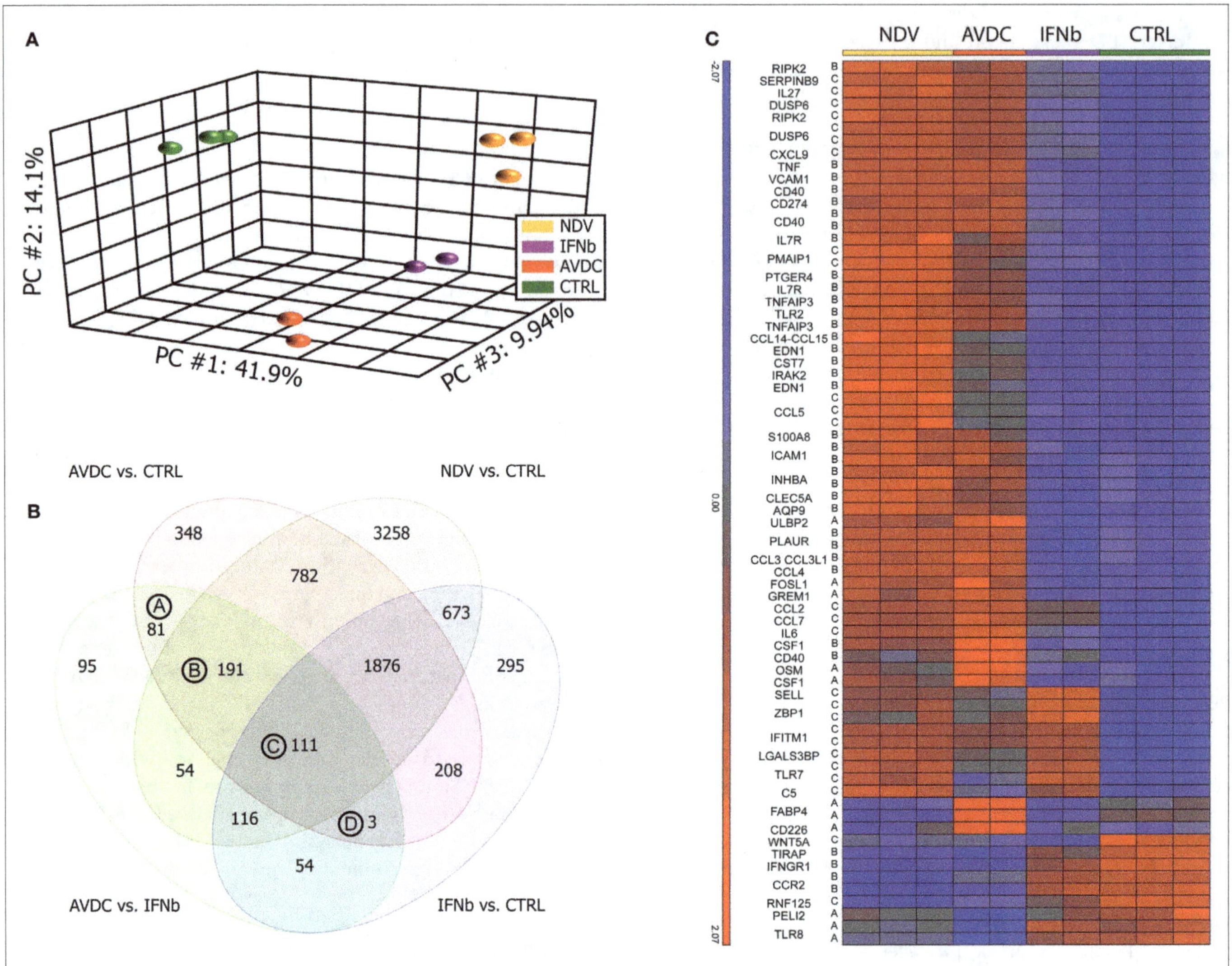

FIGURE 1 | Paracrine signaling from virus-infected DCs cells induce a different gene expression pattern compared to cells exposed to IFNβ alone. Microarray profiles were obtained from human monocyte-derived DCs exposed to paracrine signaling from NDV infected DCs or to IFNβ alone. Sample groups: NDV: DCs infected with NDV; IFNβ: DCs exposed to IFNβ alone; AVDCs: DCs exposed to paracrine signaling from NDV infected cells in a trans-well system; CTRL: naive unexposed and uninfected DCs. **(A)** Principal component analysis of samples on all genes represented on the microarray. First three principal components showing 41.9% (PC1), 14.1% (PC2), and 9.94% (PC3) of the overall change in gene expression in the data set. **(B)** Venn diagram comparing genes which differed (twofold, FDR $p < 0.05$) between each pair of conditions. **(C)** Genes which are differed between AVDC vs. CTRL and AVDC vs. IFNβ and have a gene ontology association with anti-viral immune processes.

twofold change threshold relative to control cells identified 7088 genes altered by NDV infection, 3600 genes altered by paracrine signaling (AVDC), and 3336 genes changed by IFNβ alone.

The number of genes differentially expressed between each pair of the four groups studied is indicated in **Figure 1B**. A comparison between cells exposed to paracrine signaling and IFNβ alone showed 705 differentially expressed genes. From those 705 transcripts, which showed a significant change between exposure to paracrine signaling and single cytokine IFNβ treatment, 81 were significantly altered by the paracrine signaling but did not show significant induction by NDV infection or IFNβ treatment when compared to control [Group (A) in **Figure 1B**], 191 genes were significantly induced by paracrine signaling and NDV infection but not IFNβ treatment when compared to control [Group (B) in **Figure 1B**] and 111 genes were significantly induced by paracrine signaling, NDV infection, and IFNβ treatment when compared to control [Group (C) in **Figure 1B**]. Three genes were changed by paracrine signaling and IFNβ treatment when compared to control but still differed significantly when compared between exposure to paracrine signaling and IFNβ treatment. Heat maps of all genes in groups A, B, C, and D can be seen in the supplementary material (Figure S2 in Supplementary Material). Fifty genes from the list of 389 transcripts being significantly different when exposed to paracrine signaling vs. IFNβ alone, as well as when exposed to paracrine signaling and naive cells could be linked to anti-viral immunity (**Figure 1C**). Among those, 50 genes were regulators of inflammation and immune response including *VCAM-1* (17), *AQP9* (18), *RIPK2* (19), *IRAK2* (20), *CCL3L1* (21); cytokines like *IL6*, *OSM* (22); genes linked to anti-viral immunity *CCL3L3* (23), *CSF1* (24), *CD274* (25), *CD40* (26), *IL7R* (27); immune cell activation *CLEC5A* (28), *EDN* (29), *CST7* (30), and also a suppressor of apoptosis *PTGER4* (31).

BYSTANDER DCs ARE EXPOSED TO A COMPLEX CYTOKINE ENVIRONMENT

To identify cytokines and chemokines induced during NDV infection, to which uninfected bystander DC cells are exposed, we analyzed the 7088 transcripts induced by NDV. Seventy-eighty transcripts could be associated to the gene ontology terms cytokine activity or chemokine activity (**Figure 2A**). We further narrowed this list by setting an expression threshold of 6.5 based on the intersection of the two populations of expressed and non-expressed genes (**Figure 2B**) and identifying which cytokines/chemokines could be associated with receptor genes also expressed in DCs. This analysis linked CCL4 to CCR5 (32, 33), CCL3 to CCR5 (34), CCL3 to CCR1 (35), CCL2 to CCR2 (36, 37), CCL7 to CCR5 (33), CCL7 to CCR3 (38), CCL8 to CCR2 (39), CXCL10 to CCR3 (40), CXCL9 to CCR3 (40), CXCL11 to CCR3 (40), CCL15 to CCR3 (41), CCL15 to CCR1 (41), CCL5 to CCR3 (36), CCL5 to CCR5 (42, 43), CXCL12 to CXCR4 (44), CXCL3 to CXCR2 (36), CXCL5 to CXCR2 (45), CXCL1 to CXCR2 (46), IL6 to IL6R (47), IL1a to IL1R1 (48), IL1β to IL1R2 (49), IL1β to IL1R1 (50), TNF to TNFRSF1B (51), TNF to FAS (52), TNF to TNFRSF1A (53), IL15 to IL15RA (54), IL7 to IL7R (55), IL7 to IL2RG (56), IFNβ to IFNAR1 (57), IFNβ to IFNAR2 (58), IFNW1 to IFNAR1 (59), IFNA2 to IFNAR (60), IFNE to IFNAR1 (61), TNFSF10 to TNFRS10B (62), CCL19 to CCR7 (63), TNFSF15 to TNFRSF6B (64), IL28A to IL10RB (65), IL29 to IL10RB (65), IL12A to IL12RB1 (66), IL12A to IL12RB1 (67), and CSF1 to CSF1R (68) (**Figure 2C**).

The level of expression of cytokines and chemokines identified by this bioinformatics analysis was measured in an 18-h time course experiment (1) in supernatant from DCs infected by NDV, (2) in the supernatant associated with AVDCs in trans-well experiments, and (3) in supernatant of cells exposed to IFNβ alone by ELISA (**Figure 3A**) or in cellular mRNA by real-time PCR (**Figure 3B**). Cytokines which did not exhibit detectable expression by ELISA or PCR (not shown) were excluded for further screening. This led to the selection of the following 20 cytokines and chemokines for further study that were induced in NDV infected DCs: TNFα, CCL3, IL8, CXCL10, CCL5, IL6, IFNα CXCL12, IFNALPHA16, IL12a, IL18, IL1RA, IL28, IL29, TNFSF15, TNFSF4, TNFSF10, IL1α, IL1β, and IFNβ.

IDENTIFICATION OF INDIVIDUAL CYTOKINES CONTRIBUTING TO COMBINATORIAL EFFECTS

We next studied the combinatorial effects of the 20 cytokines identified above on the induction of maturation marker expression in naïve DCs. Because studying all combinations of 20 cytokines was impractical, we identified combinatorial cytokine candidates by comparing the effect of all 20 cytokines on naïve DCs to the effects of all possible 19-cytokine combinations lacking one of the cytokines. These experiments used the maximum concentration measured by ELISA or, for cytokines measured by PCR, the concentration was estimated from transcript levels by comparing the PCR and ELISA levels of IFNβ. Many cytokines peaked at about 10 h during the 18 h time course. Therefore, we expose DCs to the cytokine mixtures for 8 h to best approximate the conditions of the paracrine signaling during viral infection. In this experiment, we used cells from three different donors for biological replicates, which resulted in a high variance of marker expression between donors. To adjust for differences between individuals, we normalized data to the overall median values.

The absence of TNFα, IL18, IL28, and IFNalpha16 reduced the expression of CD86, when compared to the exposure to all 20 cytokines (**Figure 4**). The absence of IFNa2, IL18, IL1α, TNFSF15, IL1β, and IFNβ reduced the expression of HLA-DR (**Figure 4**). We studied nine cytokines (IFNα, IFNALPHA16, IFNβ, IL1α, IL1β, IL18, IL28, TNFα, TNFSF15) in similar leave one cytokine out experiments as well as single cytokine exposure studies. These nine cytokines gave the same responses as the original 20, indicating that the 11 cytokines excluded from further study are not major contributors to maturation marker induction during paracrine signaling (**Figure 5**). The cytokine minus one studies with the remaining nine cytokines suggested the importance of IFNβ, for CD86 upregulation and IFNβ, IL28, and TNFSF15 for HLA-DR upregulation. When DCs were exposed to individual cytokines, IFNβ and IL1β induced CD86 and IFNβ and TNFα induced HLA-DR. Therefore five cytokines (IFNβ, IL28, TNFSF15, TNFα, IL1β) were selected for further study.

TNFα, IFNβ, AND IL1β INDUCE A PARACRINE ACTIVATED ANTI-VIRAL STATE

We studied the effects of combinations of the five cytokines on maturation marker expression, viral resistance, and phagocytic activity. For the maturation marker expression studies, human DCs were exposed to combinations of the five cytokines for 8 h and the levels of CD86 and HLA-DR were measured by flow cytometry. IFNb alone increases the expression of both markers. The additional increases observed with all combinations of cytokines did not achieve statistical significance in comparison to IFNb alone with tight control for family wise error. IL28 did not cause any trend toward an increase in maturation marker expression (**Figure 6A**). To improve statistical power, we performed maturation marker induction experiments using four cytokines IFNβ, TNFSF15, TNFα, and IL1b. Here, the combinations of IFNβ with either TNFα or IL1b showed a significantly higher induction of CD86 when compared to the effects of IFNβ alone (**Figure 6B**). The combination of IFNβ with IL1b showed a significantly higher HLA-DR induction when compared to IFNb alone (**Figure 6C**).

As one of the most important features observed in paracrine activated AVDCs is resistance to viral infection (6), we pretreated DCs with combinations of the five cytokines for 8 h and subsequently infected them with an RFP expressing NDV for 8 h. Infectivity was measured by using flow cytometry to quantify RFP expression. Because infectivity by RFP-NDV is so sensitive to IFNβ, its concentration was reduced for this study. Still, due to the effect of the RFP insertion which makes the virus less viable and more susceptible to the effects of IFNβ, changes observed with cytokine

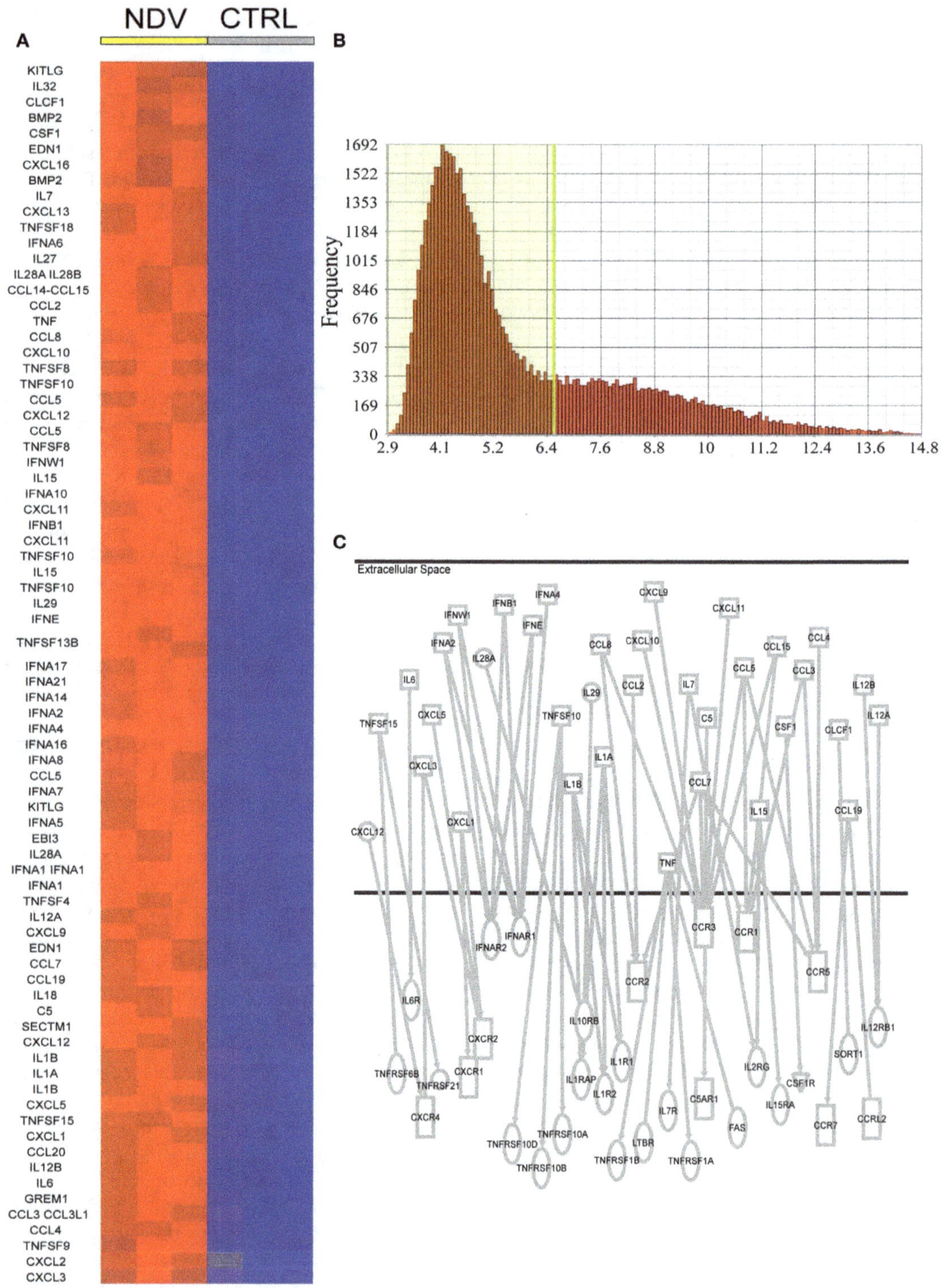

FIGURE 2 | Candidate NDV induced cytokines in DCs for a paracrine effect on DCs. **(A)** Cytokines and chemokines induced by NDV (twofold FDR $p < 0.05$) compared to naive DCs. **(B)** Expression level of all genes expressed in naive DCs. A cutoff of expression above 6.5 was used to identify potentially expressed cytokine and chemokine receptors. **(C)** Ingenuity analysis linking induced cytokines/chemokines to receptor genes also expressed in DCs.

combinations were statistically not significant when compared to single cytokine IFNβ exposure. The combination of IFNβ and IL1β showed the largest reduction of infection (**Figure 6D**).

Another feature of AVDCs is the heightened phagocytic activity (10). Therefore, we tested fluorescent bead phagocytosis following exposure to combinations of IFNβ, TNFSF15, TNFα, and IL1β.

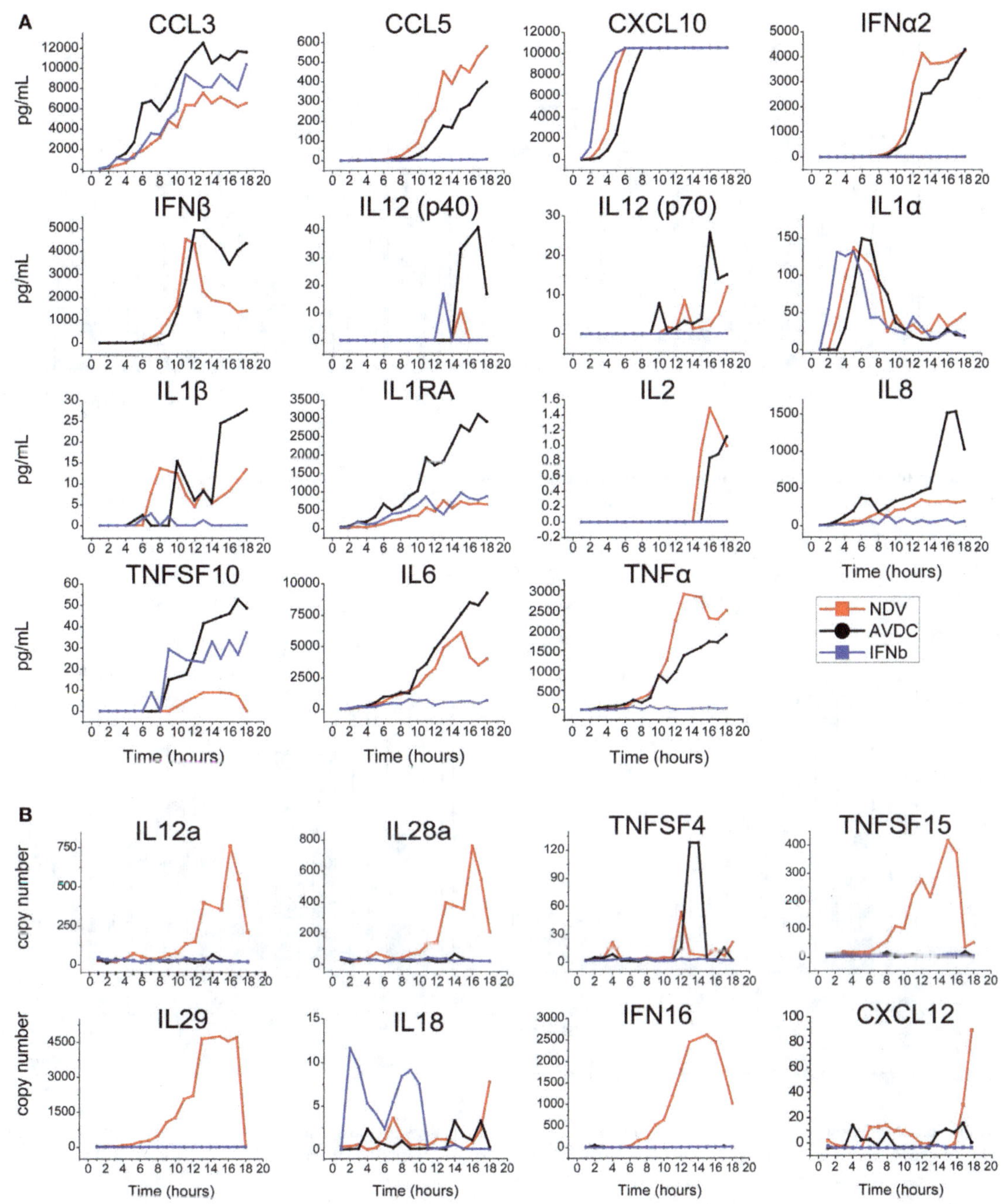

FIGURE 3 | Time course of expression of cytokines/chemokines in NDV infected DCs, AVDC, and IFNβ exposed DCs determined by (A) multiplex ELISA or IFNβ ELISA or (B) real-time PCR over an 18 h period. NDV (red line) indicates measurements from supernatants (ELISA) or cells (PCR) which were infected with NDV at an MOI of 1. AVDC (black line) indicates measurements from supernatants from infected and co-cultured naïve DCs at a 1:1 ratio (ELISA) or naïve DCs which were co-cultured with infected cells (PCR). IFNβ (blue line) indicates measurements from supernatants (ELISA) or cells (PCR) from naïve DCs exposed to IFNβ alone.

To improve statistical power and in view of the lack of effect on maturation markers, IL28 was excluded from this study. Cells were pretreated with cytokine combinations for 8 h, and then co-cultured with fluorescent beads for 4 h. The number of beads in each cell was then counted using imaging flow cytometry. The highest rates of phagocytosis were seen with all four cytokines exposed together and with exposure to IFNβ with either IL1β or TNFSF15 (**Figure 6E**).

We also looked at the capacity of combinations of the five cytokines to regulate 16 immune related genes that had been identified as preferentially induced by paracrine signaling in comparison with IFNβ exposure alone (see **Figure 1C**). Here, we exposed

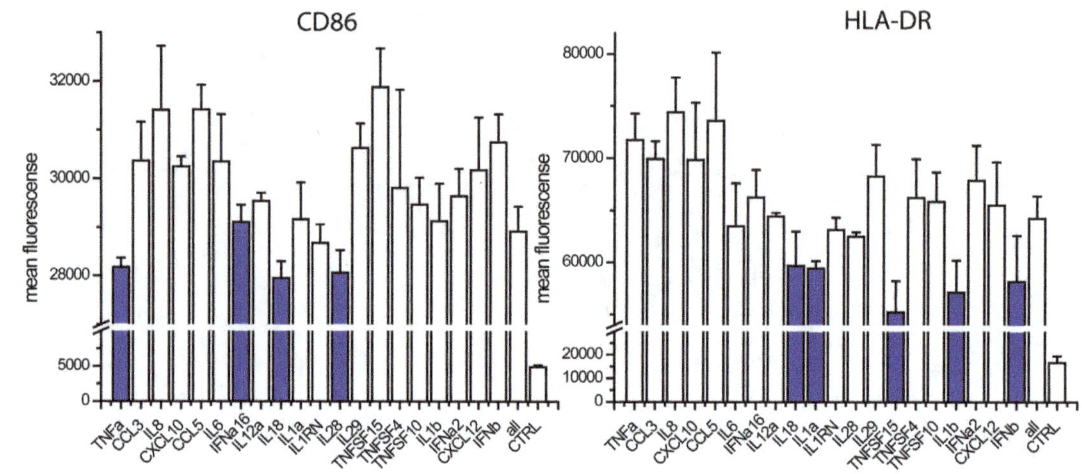

FIGURE 4 | Contribution of individual cytokines in 20 cytokine paracrine signal. Maturation marker expression of DCs after 8 h to exposure to all 20 cytokines (all) or the leave-one-out combinations of 19 cytokines. Note that a reduction in expression with a cytokine absent indicates that the cytokine may contribute to induction.

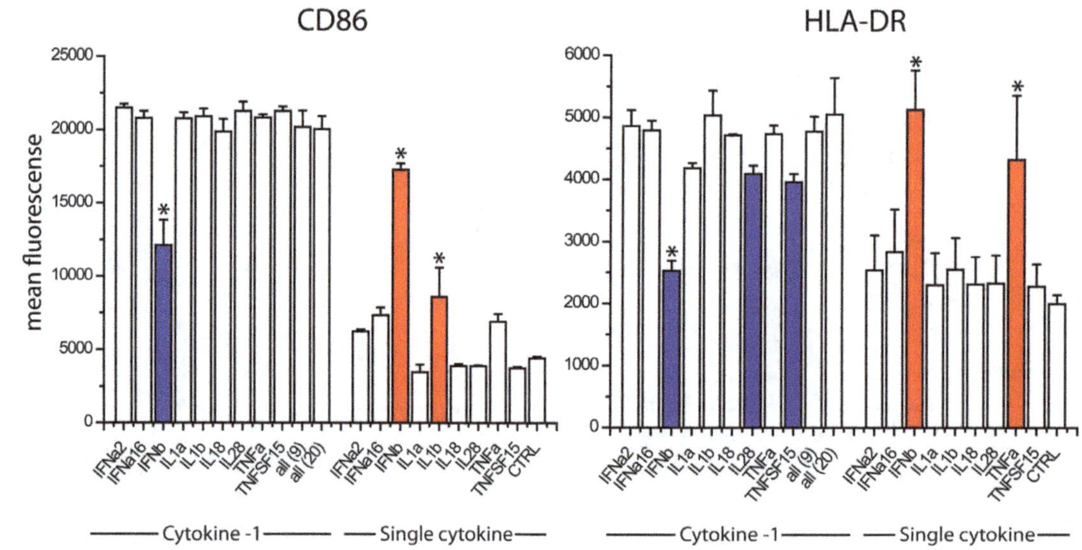

FIGURE 5 | Contribution of individual cytokines in nine cytokine paracrine signal. Maturation marker expression of DCs after 8 h to exposure to all nine cytokines, all leave-one-out combination of eight cytokines and each individual cytokine treatment (Single cytokine) (*$p \leq 0.002$ to cells exposed to all nine cytokines in Cytokine-1 treatment and to untreated cells in the single cytokine treatments).

DCs for 8 h to all possible combinations of IFNβ, IL28, TNFSF15, TNFα, IL1β, mRNA, and performed qPCR. Gene expression is plotted on a heatmap (**Figure 7**). The genes assayed were *VCAM-1, AQP9, RIPK2, IRAK2, CCL3L1, IL6, OSM, CCL3L3, CSF1, CD274, CD40, IL7R, CLEC5A, EDN, CST7*, and *PTGER4*). Nine of these genes showed the highest induction when treated with the triple combination of IFNβ, TNFα, and IL1β (**Figure 7**). The genes showing combinatorial cytokine preferences are associated with anti-viral immunity (*CCL3L3, CSF1, IL7R*), regulation of inflammation (*AQP9, IRAK2, RIPK2*), and immune cell activation (*CST7, EDN*, cytokine *OSM*). The induction of IL6 was also high with the triple cytokine treatment. Overall, these experiments demonstrate that IFNβ, TNFα, and IL1β acting together are the principal drivers of the paracrine induced anti-viral state in DCs.

We next performed concentration response studies to determine if the combinatorial effects of the cytokines were synergistic. At lower concentrations, all three cytokines together produced the highest levels of both CD86 expression although at higher concentrations, equivalent levels could be achieved with the combination of TNFα and IFNβ alone (**Figure 8**). For HLA-DR expression, the combination of all three cytokines at lower concentrations produced the highest levels, although at higher concentrations TNFα and IL1β induced similar levels. For both maturation markers, the effects of combinatorial

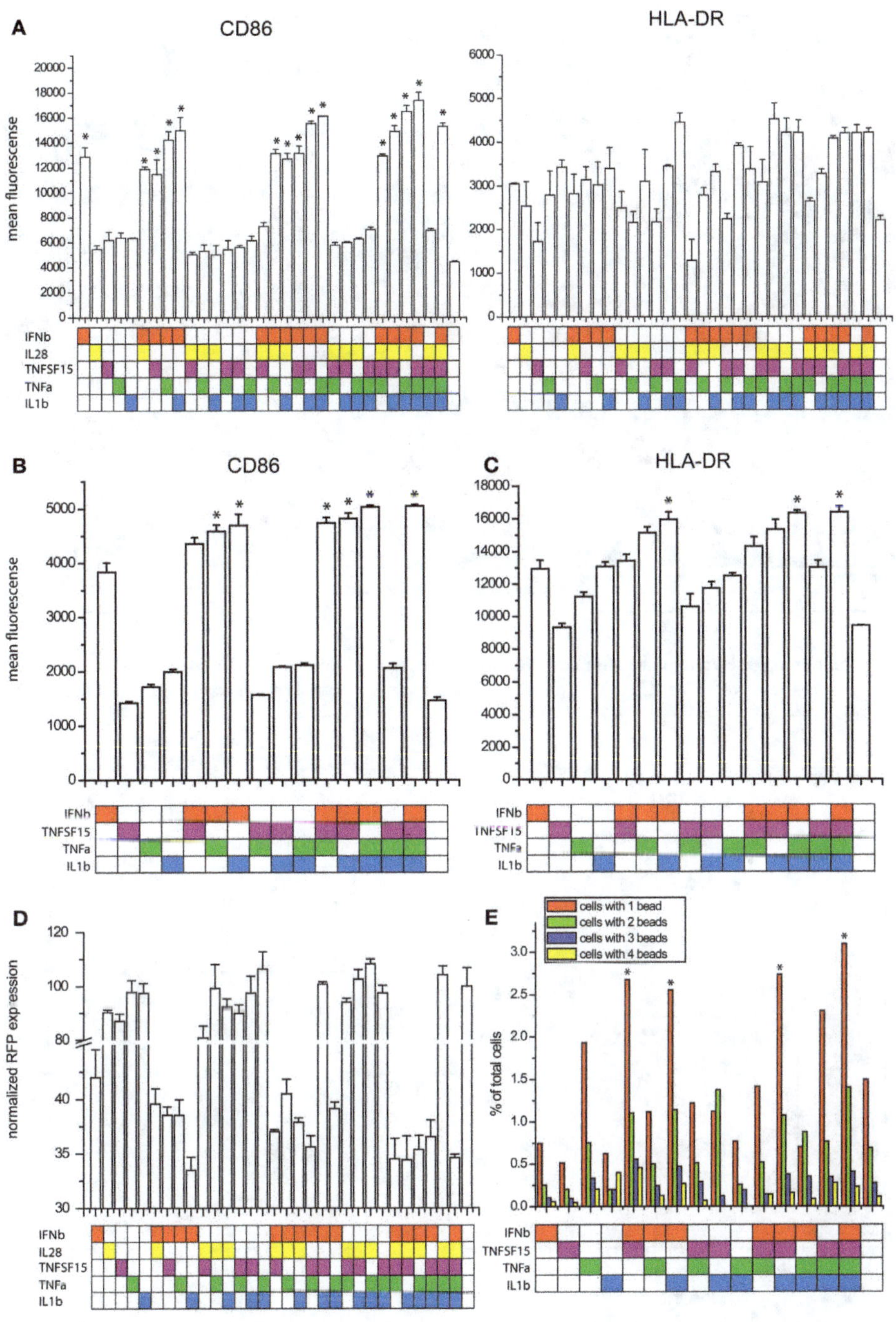

FIGURE 6 | Effects of combinatorial cytokine treatment. (A) Maturation marker expression after exposure to combinations of IFNβ, IL28, TNFSF15, TNFα and IL1β, measured by flow cytometry (*$p \leq 0.05$ compared to untreated cells). **(B)** CD86 expression after exposure to combinations of IFNβ, TNFSF15, TNFα and IL1β, measured by flow cytometry (*$p \leq 0.05$ compared to cells treated with IFNβ alone). **(C)** HLA-DR expression after exposure to combinations of IFNβ, TNFSF15, TNFα and IL1β, measured by flow cytometry (*$p \leq 0.05$ compared to cells treated with IFNβ alone). **(D)** Infectivity of NDV after cytokine combination pretreatment for 8 h in DCs measured by RFP expression. **(E)** Phagocytosis assay measured by bead uptake by imaging flow cytometry (*$p \leq 0.05$ compared to untreated cells).

exposure dramatically exceeded the effects of any individual cytokine. Statistical values for pairwise comparisons within each dilution step are shown in Tables S1 and S2 in Supplementary Material. We also investigated the effect of combinations of various combinations of the two cytokines IFNβ and TNFα, which showed a synergistic induction with CD86 (Figure S3 in Supplementary Material). These results support the view that the effects of combinatorial exposure produce a qualitatively different cellular effect than do the individual cytokines.

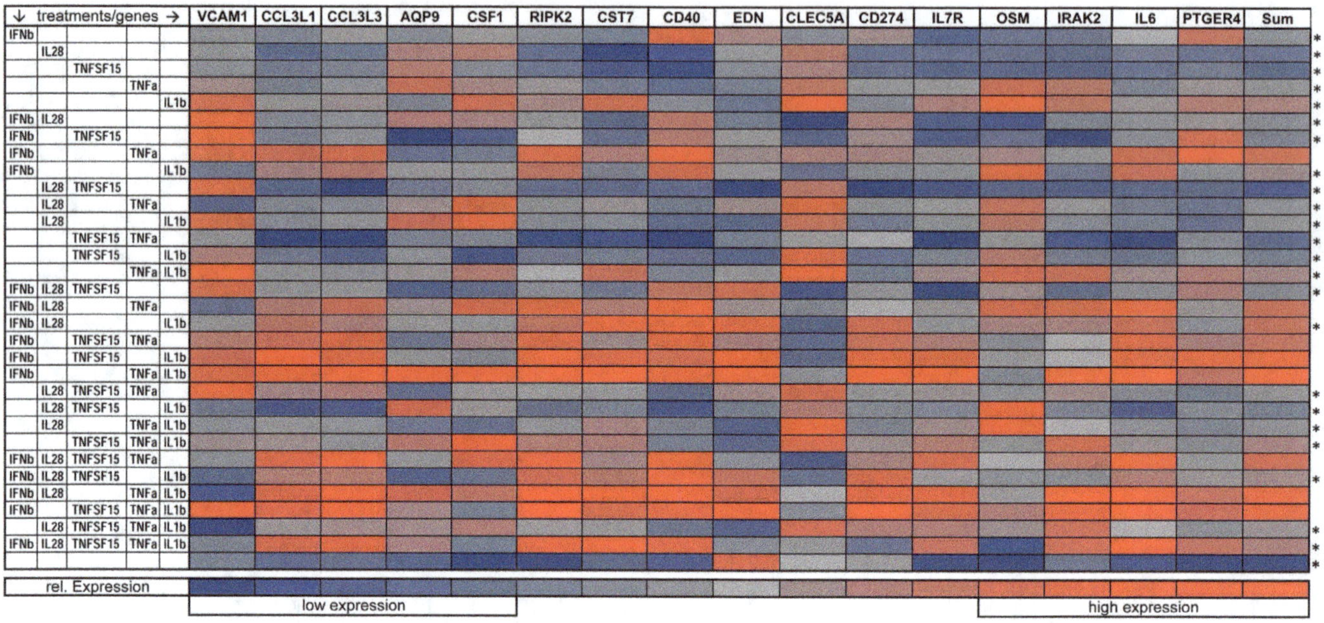

FIGURE 7 | Gene expression of immune relevant genes after combinatorial IFNβ, IL28, TNFSF15, TNFα, and IL1β treatment. Heat map is normalized to the lowest (blue) and highest (red) expression level for each individual gene (*$p \leq 0.05$ compared to cells exposed to the triple combination of TNFα, IFNβ, and IL1b).

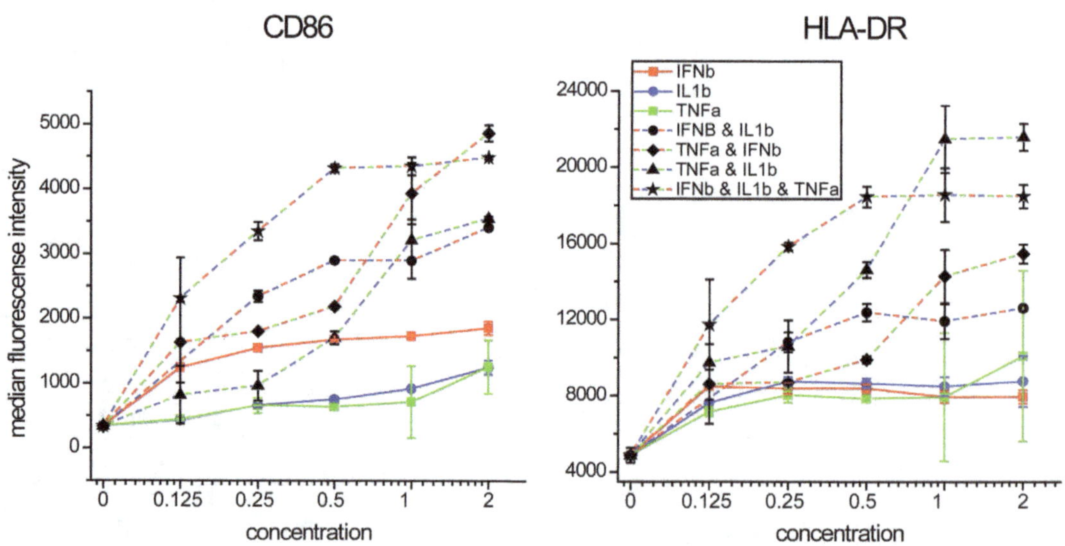

FIGURE 8 | Maturation marker expression by combinations of IFNβ, TNFα, and IL1β. DCs were exposed to combinations of three cytokines at a range of concentrations relative to that found in supernatants of NDV infected DCs.

COMBINATORIAL EFFECTS OF TNFα, IL1β, AND IFNβ ON PATHOGENIC VIRUSES

The studies described above rely on NDV, which is not pathogenic in humans and does not express immune antagonists having activity in human cells. We were interested in studying the effects of combination cytokine exposure on a human pathogen and studied the recent pandemic Influenza A virus Cal/09. We pretreated DCs with all combinations of IFNβ, TNFα, and IL1β for 8 h and subsequently infected them with influenza A/California/7/2009 and measured infectivity, maturation marker induction as well as induction of apoptosis. The triple combination of all three cytokines as well as the dual cytokine mixture of IL1β and IFNβ significantly increased the suppression of infectivity when compared to IFNβ pretreatment alone (**Figure 9A**). The triple combination also caused the highest induction of CD86, HLA-ABC, and HLA-DR in virus NP-expressing cells (**Figures 9B–D**).

Apoptosis was assayed in the same samples using imaging flow cytometry to measure nuclear fragmentation (**Figures 9F,G**). Interestingly, pretreatment with single cytokines did not reduce influenza-induced apoptosis, whereas the triple combination as well as the dual cytokine combinations with IFNβ could reduce cell death (**Figure 9E**). These data suggests that the triple combination of cytokines improves DC survival, resistance to infectivity, and increases costimulatory marker expression for T-cell activation.

COMBINATORIAL EFFECT OF TNFα, IL1β, AND IFNβ ON INDUCTION OF VIRUS SPECIFIC T-CELL RESPONSE

In order to see if the induction of the costimulatory markers by the triple combination of IFNβ, TNFα, and IL1β has an effect on T-cell activation, we studied the induction of measles specific T-cell proliferation after co-culture with cytokine pretreated and measles primed T-cells. We exposed the CD14 depleted PBMCs from the same donors which were used for DC generation to measles vaccine and harvested T-cell 5 days later. Those T-cells were co-cultured for 3 days with measles primed DCs exposed to combinations of IFNβ, TNFα and IL1β. Proliferation was measured by the dilution of the membrane bound dye CFSE by flow cytometry. The triple combination of IFNβ, TNFα, and IL1β significantly increased cell proliferation compared to non-pretreated DCs (**Figure 10**). These results indicate that the costimulatory marker upregulation also affects activation of the adaptive immune system.

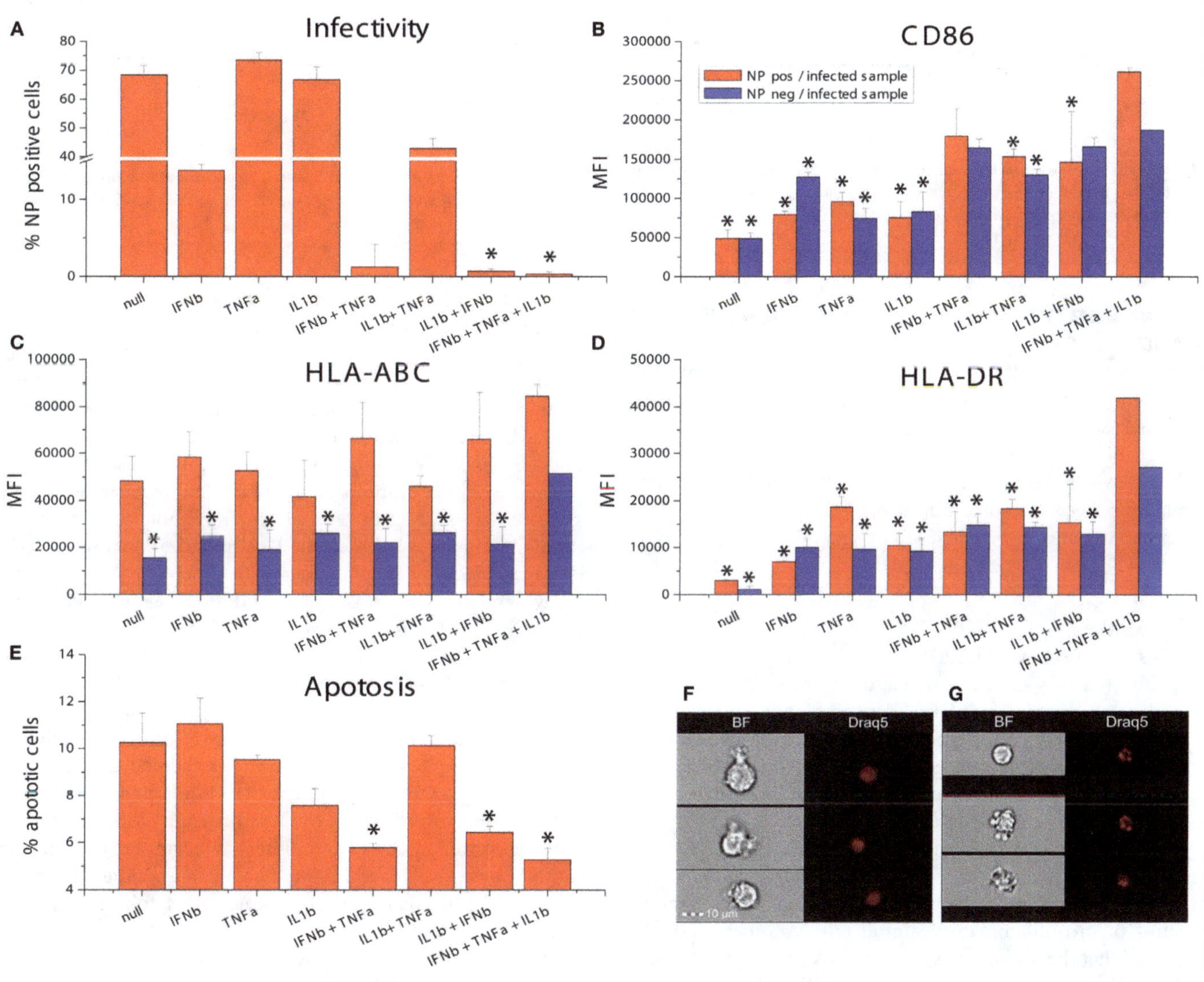

FIGURE 9 | Effects of combinatorial of IFNβ, TNFα, and IL1β treatment on DCs infected with the pandemic influenza A Cal/09 strain. **(A)** Infectivity assayed by NP expression (*$p \leq 0.05$ compared to cells exposed to IFNβ). **(B)** Expression of the maturation marker CD86. **(C)** Expression of the maturation marker HLA-ABC. **(D)** Expression of the maturation marker HLA-DR (*$p \leq 0.05$ compared to cells exposed to the triple combination of TNFα, IFNβ, and IL1b). **(E)** Apoptosis assayed by assessing nuclear fragmentation and cell granularity by imaging flow cytometry (*$p \leq 0.05$ compared to untreated cells). **(F)** Sample images of non-apoptotic cells. **(G)** Sample images of apoptotic cells.

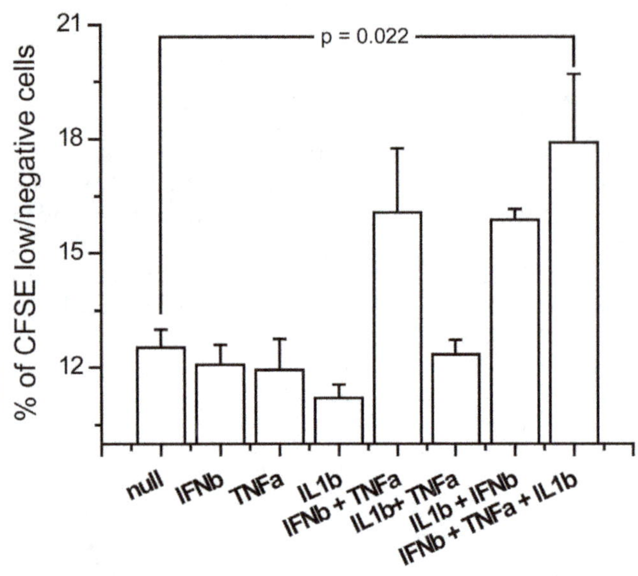

FIGURE 10 | Antigen specific proliferation of T-cells exposed to cytokine pretreated DCs. Measles antilogous specific T-cells were co-cultured with cytokine pretreated DCs which were also pulsed with measles vaccine. Proliferation was measured by the dilution of CFSE.

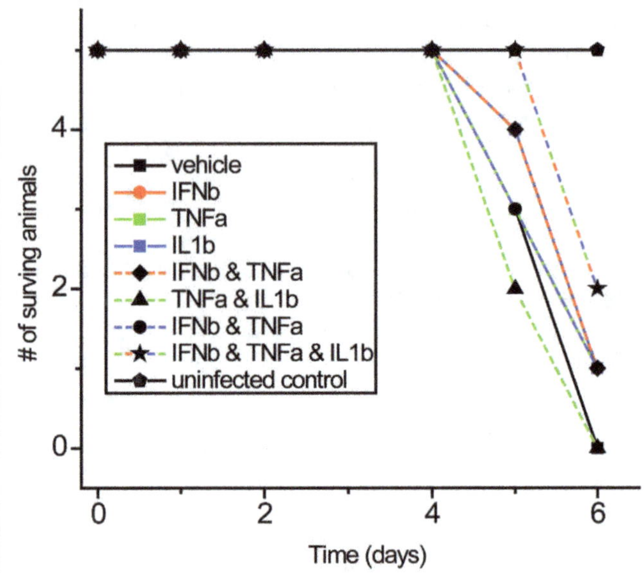

FIGURE 11 | Effects of IFNβ, TNFα, and IL1β combinations on mortality with PR8 virus *in vivo*. Mice received cytokine injection i.p. 6 h before and 6 h after infection with PR8 virus.

COMBINATORIAL EFFECT OF TNFα, IL1β, AND IFNβ ON INFLUENZA MORBIDITY *IN VIVO*

We next studied the effects of IFNβ, TNFα, and IL1β on influenza virus pathogenicity *in vivo* using a well-characterized aerosolized-virus mouse infection model (69). Cytokines were injected intraperitoneally both 3 h before and after inhalation infection with PR8 virus. While the differences were modest, the triple combination was found to improve survival times significantly compared to control (p: 0.0456) following PR8 infection in mice (**Figure 11**).

DISCUSSION

In this study, we show that IFNβ, TNFα, and IL1β are secreted by virus-infected DCs and act combinatorially to alter the anti-viral response state of uninfected DCs. This combination is responsible for maturation marker upregulation in naive as well as in infected cells, reduction of virus induced apoptosis, heightened phagocytic activity, specific autologous T-cell activation, and resistance to viral infection *in vitro* as well as in *in vivo*.

The importance of cellular micro-environments in dictating immune cell responses is supported by the report that the inflammatory state of macrophages can be reprogramed by exposure to an anti- or pro-inflammatory stimuli (70). Another report has suggested that the initial exposure to a cytokine signal determines and fixes the final state of the macrophage (71). These reports, as well as the finding that the combination of IL-4, IL-10, and TGFb skew the development of myeloid cells into M2 macrophages, support the importance of combinatorial cytokine signals in immune regulation (72). DCs themselves are differentiated into different lineages by exposure to different cytokines including GMCSF and Flt3 (73).

Since the discovery of type I interferon, paracrine cytokine signaling has been recognized as a crucial component in orchestrating the immune responses to virus infection. Recent studies have begun to reveal the importance of combinatorial extracellular stimuli in directing the responses of immune cells. For example, when DCs are exposed to lipopolysaccharide in the context of apoptotic cells, they induce TH17 cells, a response that is not achieved by either stimulus alone (74). Retinoic acid acts alone on T-cells to induce Treg cells. However, retinoic acid combined with IL-15 causes DCs to skew the T-cell polarization toward TH17 cells (6). TLR7/8 ligand combined with either TLR3 or TLR4 ligands synergistically increases IFNβ and IFNλ1 expression in DCs (75). SCF and IL-2 have a synergistic effect on the proliferation NK cells (7). TNFα and IFNγ act together on smooth airway cells to enhance CXCL-10 expression (8). IL17 together with TNFα or IL1β induces MCP-1 and MIP-2 in murine mesangial cells (9). These combinatorial effects are likely to prove clinically relevant, for example, by contributing to individual differences in the response to cytokine treatment (76). While beyond the scope of the present investigation, the role of relative timing of combinatorial cytokine signals is another important area for further study. We have also not addressed the potential combinatorial role of alarmins, which can work in concert with cytokines to induce different cell states (77).

To our knowledge, this is the first report of IFNβ, TNFα, and IL1β working in concert to alter the response state of any immune cell. Previous studies have implicated pairs of this triad in influencing immune responses. The combination of IL-1β and IFNβ has been reported to promote immune control of West Nile virus infection in the CNS (78). TNFα and IFNβ have also been found to affect macrophages and fibroblasts in reducing the infectivity of poxviruses (79, 80).

Several of the transcripts that are preferentially induced in DCs by the exposure to all three cytokines have been found to serve important roles in inflammation and immunity: CCL3L3 suppresses HIV proliferation (23); AQP9 is a marker for inflammation (81); CSF1 is a biomarker for respiratory syncytial virus infection (24); RIPK2 knockout in mice causes hyper-susceptibility to infection with influenza A virus (82); EDN possesses anti-viral activity against single stranded RNA viruses like respiratory syncytial virus, Hepatitis and HIV (83); IL7R expression inversely correlates with FoxP3 and suppressive function of human $CD4^+$ T reg cells (84); OSM is a pro-inflammatory cytokine (22); and IRAK2 is needed to sustain cytokine production during prolonged activation of the TLR signaling pathway (85). When maturation marker induction was studied by cytokine induction alone, we found that CD86 is most strongly driven by IFNβ with synergistic effects of TNFα or IL1β. HLA-DR was little changed by individual cytokines but was strongly induced by TNFα and IL1β together. The gene VCAM-1 was most induced by the TNFα and IL1β together and PTGER4 was most induced by IFNβ and TNFα. While the overall DC cell state observed requires all three cytokines, the differences in the cytokines most important for various components of these DC responses provides the basis for future studies to dissect the underlying signaling and transcriptional mechanisms involved in these combinatorial effects.

Surprisingly, the triple combination of IFNβ, TNFα, and IL1β reduced influenza-induced cell death in infected DCs. This is interesting as IFNβ is known to be an inducer of apoptosis in DCs (86), and indicates how the effects of one cytokine may be very different depending on which other cytokines are stimulating a cell. Maturation marker induction as well as cell survival are important for the activation of the adaptive immune system. The observation of a heightened proliferation of virus specific T-cells when exposed to DCs pretreated with the triple combination supports this view. The modestly increased survival of mice to PR8 infection when treated with the three cytokines suggests the combinatorial coding of cell responses has significance *in vivo*.

The large number of cytokines secreted by infected DCs is remarkable. We identify combinatorial effects involving only three of these secreted factors on DCs. It is probable that combinatorial signaling of different cytokine mixtures influences the activation state of other immune cells and that other immune cells also serve as the source of complex cytokine signals. The specific activation state of any immune cell can depend on both the cytokine mixture present and their concentration (see **Figure 8**). Thus the immune system can potentially generate many distinct micro-environments that shape the local activation state of various immune cells. This provides the potential for a dynamic and spatially distributed complexity of the set point of the immune system that could be crucial in organizing the local and system responses to infection, neoplasia, and injury. Unraveling this combinatorial code may have benefits in guiding combination immunotherapy for autoimmune diseases, for chronic infections and for other immune system influenced diseases as well as for personalizing interventions in relationship to individual variation in background cytokine expression.

ACKNOWLEDGMENT

This work was supported by NIAID contract HHSN27220100-0054C.

REFERENCES

1. Chang DY, Shin EC. Immune-based therapy for chronic hepatitis C. *J Leukoc Biol* (2009) **86**:33–9. doi:10.1189/jlb.1208772
2. Stübgen JP. Recombinant interferon-beta therapy and neuromuscular disorders. *J Neuroimmunol* (2009) **212**:132–41. doi:10.1016/j.jneuroim.2009.04.015
3. Kalaaji AN, Lu J, Markovic SN, Celis E, Pittelkow MR. Combination cytokine therapy inhibits tumor growth by generation of tumor-specific T-cell responses in a murine melanoma model. *Cytokine* (2010) **49**:287–93. doi:10.1016/j.cyto.2009.11.016
4. Sanganalmath SK, Stein AB, Guo Y, Tiwari S, Hunt G, Vincent RJ, et al. The beneficial effects of postinfarct cytokine combination therapy are sustained during long-term follow-up. *J Mol Cell Cardiol* (2009) **47**:528–35. doi:10.1016/j.yjmcc.2009.07.009
5. Sun X, Su J, Bao J, Peng T, Zhang L, Zhang Y, et al. Cytokine combination therapy prediction for bone remodeling in tissue engineering based on the intracellular signaling pathway. *Biomaterials* (2012) **33**:8265–76. doi:10.1016/j.biomaterials.2012.07.041
6. DePaolo RW, Abadie V, Tang F, Fehlner-Peach H, Hall JA, Wang W, et al. Co-adjuvant effects of retinoic acid and IL-15 induce inflammatory immunity to dietary antigens. *Nature* (2011) **471**:220–4. doi:10.1038/nature09849
7. Benson DM, Yu J, Becknell B, Wei M, Freud AG, Ferketich AK, et al. Stem cell factor and interleukin-2/15 combine to enhance MAPK-mediated proliferation of human natural killer cells. *Blood* (2009) **113**:2706–14. doi:10.1182/blood-2008-05-159285
8. Clarke DL, Clifford RL, Jindarat S, Proud D, Pang L, Belvisi M, et al. TNFα and IFNγ synergistically enhance transcriptional activation of CXCL10 in human airway smooth muscle cells via STAT-1, NF-κB, and the transcriptional coactivator CREB-binding protein. *J Biol Chem* (2010) **285**:29101–10. doi:10.1074/jbc.M109.0999952
9. Iyoda M, Shibata T, Kawaguchi M, Hizawa N, Yamaoka T, Kokubu F, et al. IL-17A and IL-17F stimulate chemokines via MAPK pathways (ERK1/2 and p38 but not JNK) in mouse cultured mesangial cells: synergy with TNF-alpha and IL-1beta. *Am J Physiol Renal Physiol* (2010) **298**:F779–87. doi:10.1152/ajprenal.00198.2009
10. Bordería AV, Hartmann BM, Fernandez-Sesma A, Moran TM, Sealfon SC. Antiviral-activated dendritic cells: a paracrine-induced response state. *J Immunol* (2008) **181**:6872–81.
11. Fernandez-Sesma A, Marukian S, Ebersole BJ, Kaminski D, Park MS, Yuen T, et al. Influenza virus evades innate and adaptive immunity via the NS1 protein. *J Virol* (2006) **80**:6295–304. doi:10.1128/JVI.02381-05
12. Park MS, Garcia-Sastre A, Cros JF, Basler CF, Palese P. Newcastle disease virus V protein is a determinant of host range restriction. *J Virol* (2003) **77**:9522–32. doi:10.1128/JVI.77.17.9522-9532.2003
13. Chou YY, Albrecht RA, Pica N, Lowen AC, Richt JA, García-Sastre A, et al. The M segment of the 2009 new pandemic H1N1 influenza virus is critical for its high transmission efficiency in the guinea pig model. *J Virol* (2011) **85**:11235–41. doi:10.1128/JVI.05794-11
14. Eisenhart C. The assumptions underlying the analysis of variance. *Biometrics* (1947) **3**:1–21. doi:10.2307/3001534
15. Edgar R, Domrachev M, Lash AE. Gene Expression Omnibus: NCBI gene expression and hybridization array data repository. *Nucleic Acids Res* (2002) **30**:207–10. doi:10.1093/nar/30.1.207
16. Kotecha N, Krutzik PO, Irish JM. Web-based analysis and publication of flow cytometry experiments. *Curr Protoc Cytom* (2010) **Chapter 10**:Unit10.17. doi:10.1002/0471142956.cy1017s53
17. Ou R, Zhang M, Huang L, Flavell RA, Koni PA, Moskophidis D. Regulation of immune response and inflammatory reactions against viral infection by VCAM-1. *J Virol* (2008) **82**:2952–65. doi:10.1128/JVI.02191-07

18. Suárez-Fariñas M, Fuentes-Duculan J, Lowes MA, Krueger JG. Resolved psoriasis lesions retain expression of a subset of disease-related genes. *J Invest Dermatol* (2011) **131**:391–400. doi:10.1038/jid.2010.280
19. Moreira LO, Zamboni DS. NOD1 and NOD2 signaling in infection and inflammation. *Front Immunol* (2012) **3**:328. doi:10.3389/fimmu.2012.00328
20. Yin W, Wan Y, Kim TW, Yao P, Xiao H, Zhou H, et al. The kinase activity of interleukin-1 receptor-associated kinase 2 is essential for lipopolysaccharide-mediated cytokine and chemokine mRNA stability and translation. *J Interferon Cytokine Res* (2011) **31**:415–22. doi:10.1089/jir.2010.0094
21. McKinney C, Merriman ME, Chapman PT, Gow PJ, Harrison AA, Highton J, et al. Evidence for an influence of chemokine ligand 3-like 1 (CCL3L1) gene copy number on susceptibility to rheumatoid arthritis. *Ann Rheum Dis* (2008) **67**:409–13. doi:10.1136/ard.2007.075028
22. Malik N, Kallestad JC, Gunderson NL, Austin SD, Neubauer MG, Ochs V, et al. Molecular cloning, sequence analysis, and functional expression of a novel growth regulator, oncostatin M. *Mol Cell Biol* (1989) **9**:2847–53.
23. Miyakawa T, Obaru K, Maeda K, Harada S, Mitsuya H. Identification of amino acid residues critical for LD78beta, a variant of human macrophage inflammatory protein-1alpha, binding to CCR5 and inhibition of R5 human immunodeficiency virus type 1 replication. *J Biol Chem* (2002) **277**:4649–55. doi:10.1074/jbc.M109198200
24. Huang YC, Li Z, Hyseni X, Schmitt M, Devlin RB, Karoly ED, et al. Identification of gene biomarkers for respiratory syncytial virus infection in a bronchial epithelial cell line. *Genomic Med* (2008) **2**:113–25. doi:10.1007/s11568-009-9080-y
25. Tsuda M, Matsumoto K, Inoue H, Matsumura M, Nakano T, Mori A, et al. Expression of B7-H1 and B7-DC on the airway epithelium is enhanced by double-stranded RNA. *Biochem Biophys Res Commun* (2005) **330**:263–70. doi:10.1016/j.bbrc.2005.02.161
26. Ballesteros-Tato A, León B, Lund FE, Randall TD. CD4+ T helper cells use CD154-CD40 interactions to counteract T reg cell-mediated suppression of CD8+ T cell responses to influenza. *J Exp Med* (2013) **210**:1591–601. doi:10.1084/jem.20130097
27. Bengsch B, Spangenberg HC, Kersting N, Neumann-Haefelin C, Panther E, von Weizsäcker F, et al. Analysis of CD127 and KLRG1 expression on hepatitis C virus-specific CD8+ T cells reveals the existence of different memory T-cell subsets in the peripheral blood and liver. *J Virol* (2007) **81**:945–53. doi:10.1128/JVI.01354-06
28. Batliner J, Mancarelli MM, Jenal M, Reddy VA, Fey MF, Torbett BE, et al. CLEC5A (MDL-1) is a novel PU.1 transcriptional target during myeloid differentiation. *Mol Immunol* (2011) **48**:714–9. doi:10.1016/j.molimm.2010.10.016
29. Yang D, Rosenberg HF, Chen Q, Dyer KD, Kurosaka K, Oppenheim JJ. Eosinophil-derived neurotoxin (EDN), an antimicrobial protein with chemotactic activities for dendritic cells. *Blood* (2003) **102**:3396–403. doi:10.1182/blood-2003-01-0151
30. Magister S, Obermajer N, Mirkovic B, Svajger U, Renko M, Softic A, et al. Regulation of cathepsins S and L by cystatin F during maturation of dendritic cells. *Eur J Cell Biol* (2012) **91**:391–401. doi:10.1016/j.ejcb.2012.01.001
31. Nishihara H, Kizaka-Kondoh S, Insel PA, Eckmann L. Inhibition of apoptosis in normal and transformed intestinal epithelial cells by cAMP through induction of inhibitor of apoptosis protein (IAP)-2. *Proc Natl Acad Sci U S A* (2003) **100**:8921–6. doi:10.1073/pnas.1533221100
32. Combadiere C, Ahuja SK, Tiffany HL, Murphy PM. Cloning and functional expression of CC CKR5, a human monocyte CC chemokine receptor selective for MIP-1(alpha), MIP-1(beta), and RANTES. *J Leukoc Biol* (1996) **60**:147–52.
33. Blanpain C, Migeotte I, Lee B, Vakili J, Doranz BJ, Govaerts C, et al. CCR5 binds multiple CC-chemokines: MCP-3 acts as a natural antagonist. *Blood* (1999) **94**:1899–905.
34. Rossi Paccani S, Tonello F, Patrussi L, Capitani N, Simonato M, Montecucco C, et al. Anthrax toxins inhibit immune cell chemotaxis by perturbing chemokine receptor signalling. *Cell Microbiol* (2007) **9**:924–9. doi:10.1111/j.1462-5822.2006.00840.x
35. Jensen PC, Thiele S, Ulven T, Schwartz TW, Rosenkilde MM. Positive versus negative modulation of different endogenous chemokines for CC-chemokine receptor 1 by small molecule agonists through allosteric versus orthosteric binding. *J Biol Chem* (2008) **283**:23121–8. doi:10.1074/jbc.M803458200
36. Yamagata T, Ichinose M. Agents against cytokine synthesis or receptors. *Eur J Pharmacol* (2006) **533**:289–301. doi:10.1016/j.ejphar.2005.12.046
37. Pamer EG. Tipping the balance in favor of protective immunity during influenza virus infection. *Proc Natl Acad Sci U S A* (2009) **106**:4961–2. doi:10.1073/pnas.0901574106
38. Ponath PD, Qin S, Post TW, Wang J, Wu L, Gerard NP, et al. Molecular cloning and characterization of a human eotaxin receptor expressed selectively on eosinophils. *J Exp Med* (1996) **183**:2437–48. doi:10.1084/jem.183.6.2437
39. Proudfoot AE. Chemokine receptors: multifaceted therapeutic targets. *Nat Rev Immunol* (2002) **2**:106–15. doi:10.1038/nri722
40. Loetscher P, Pellegrino A, Gong JH, Mattioli I, Loetscher M, Bardi G, et al. The ligands of CXC chemokine receptor 3, I-TAC, Mig, and IP10, are natural antagonists for CCR3. *J Biol Chem* (2001) **276**:2986–91. doi:10.1074/jbc.M005652200
41. Lee JS, Kim IS. Leukotactin-1/CCL15 induces cell migration and differentiation of human eosinophilic leukemia EoL-1 cells through PKCdelta activation. *Mol Biol Rep* (2010) **37**:2149–56. doi:10.1007/s11033-009-9687-z
42. Tyner JW, Uchida O, Kajiwara N, Kim EY, Patel AC, O'Sullivan MP, et al. CCL5-CCR5 interaction provides antiapoptotic signals for macrophage survival during viral infection. *Nat Med* (2005) **11**:1180–7. doi:10.1038/nm1303
43. Wong M, Uddin S, Majchrzak B, Huynh T, Proudfoot AE, Platanias LC, et al. Rantes activates Jak2 and Jak3 to regulate engagement of multiple signaling pathways in T cells. *J Biol Chem* (2001) **276**:11427–31. doi:10.1074/jbc.M010750200
44. Doranz BJ, Orsini MJ, Turner JD, Hoffman TL, Berson JF, Hoxie JA, et al. Identification of CXCR4 domains that support coreceptor and chemokine receptor functions. *J Virol* (1999) **73**:2752–61.
45. White JR, Lee JM, Young PR, Hertzberg RP, Jurewicz AJ, Chaikin MA, et al. Identification of a potent, selective non-peptide CXCR2 antagonist that inhibits interleukin-8-induced neutrophil migration. *J Biol Chem* (1998) **273**:10095–8. doi:10.1074/jbc.273.17.10095
46. Schraufstatter IU, Chung J, Burger M. IL-8 activates endothelial cell CXCR1 and CXCR2 through Rho and Rac signaling pathways. *Am J Physiol Lung Cell Mol Physiol* (2001) **280**:L1094–103.
47. Nagafuchi H, Suzuki N, Mizushima Y, Sakane T. Constitutive expression of IL-6 receptors and their role in the excessive B cell function in patients with systemic lupus erythematosus. *J Immunol* (1993) **151**:6525–34.
48. Dinarello CA. Biologic basis for interleukin-1 in disease. *Blood* (1996) **87**:2095–147.
49. Neumann D, Kollewe C, Martin MU, Boraschi D. The membrane form of the type II IL-1 receptor accounts for inhibitory function. *J Immunol* (2000) **165**:3350–7.
50. Barksby HE, Lea SR, Preshaw PM, Taylor JJ. The expanding family of interleukin-1 cytokines and their role in destructive inflammatory disorders. *Clin Exp Immunol* (2007) **149**:217–25. doi:10.1111/j.1365-2249.2007.03441.x
51. Nagata S. Apoptosis by death factor. *Cell* (1997) **88**:355–65. doi:10.1016/S0092-8674(00)81874-7
52. Gisslinger H, Kurzrock R, Gisslinger B, Jiang S, Li S, Virgolini I, et al. Autocrine cell suicide in a Burkitt lymphoma cell line (Daudi) induced by interferon alpha: involvement of tumor necrosis factor as ligand for the CD95 receptor. *Blood* (2001) **97**:2791–7. doi:10.1182/blood.V97.9.2791
53. Pincheira R, Castro AF, Ozes ON, Idumalla PS, Donner DB. Type 1 TNF receptor forms a complex with and uses Jak2 and c-Src to selectively engage signaling pathways that regulate transcription factor activity. *J Immunol* (2008) **181**:1288–98.
54. Mortier E, Bernard J, Plet A, Jacques Y. Natural, proteolytic release of a soluble form of human IL-15 receptor alpha-chain that behaves as a specific, high affinity IL-15 antagonist. *J Immunol* (2004) **173**:1681–8.
55. Olosz F, Malek TR. Three loops of the common gamma chain ectodomain required for the binding of interleukin-2 and interleukin-7. *J Biol Chem* (2000) **275**:30100–5. doi:10.1074/jbc.M004976200
56. Noguchi M, Nakamura Y, Russell SM, Ziegler SF, Tsang M, Cao X, et al. Interleukin-2 receptor gamma chain: a functional component of the interleukin-7 receptor. *Science* (1993) **262**:1877–80. doi:10.1126/science.8266077
57. Russell-Harde D, Wagner TC, Perez HD, Croze E. Formation of a uniquely stable type I interferon receptor complex by interferon beta is dependent upon particular interactions between interferon beta and its receptor and independent of tyrosine phosphorylation. *Biochem Biophys Res Commun* (1999) **255**:539–44. doi:10.1006/bbrc.1998.0105
58. Chuntharapai A, Gibbs V, Lu J, Ow A, Marsters S, Ashkenazi A, et al. Determination of residues involved in ligand binding and signal transmission in the human IFN-alpha receptor 2. *J Immunol* (1999) **163**:766–73.

59. Thomas C, Moraga I, Levin D, Krutzik PO, Podoplelova Y, Trejo A, et al. Structural linkage between ligand discrimination and receptor activation by type I interferons. *Cell* (2011) **146**:621–32. doi:10.1016/j.cell.2011.06.048
60. Coccia EM. IFN regulation and functions in myeloid dendritic cells. *Cytokine Growth Factor Rev* (2008) **19**:21–32. doi:10.1016/j.cytogfr.2007.10.005
61. O'Sullivan LA, Liongue C, Lewis RS, Stephenson SE, Ward AC. Cytokine receptor signaling through the Jak-Stat-Socs pathway in disease. *Mol Immunol* (2007) **44**:2497–506. doi:10.1016/j.molimm.2006.11.025
62. Lemke J, Noack A, Adam D, Tchikov V, Bertsch U, Röder C, et al. TRAIL signaling is mediated by DR4 in pancreatic tumor cells despite the expression of functional DR5. *J Mol Med (Berl)* (2010) **88**:729–40. doi:10.1007/s00109-010-0619-0
63. Rossi D, Zlotnik A. The biology of chemokines and their receptors. *Annu Rev Immunol* (2000) **18**:217–42. doi:10.1146/annurev.immunol.18.1.217
64. Migone TS, Zhang J, Luo X, Zhuang L, Chen C, Hu B, et al. TL1A is a TNF-like ligand for DR3 and TR6/DcR3 and functions as a T cell costimulator. *Immunity* (2002) **16**:479–92. doi:10.1016/S1074-7613(02)00283-2
65. Uzé G, Monneron D. IL-28 and IL-29: newcomers to the interferon family. *Biochimie* (2007) **89**:729–34. doi:10.1016/j.biochi.2007.01.008
66. Trinchieri G. Interleukin-12 and the regulation of innate resistance and adaptive immunity. *Nat Rev Immunol* (2003) **3**:133–46. doi:10.1038/nri1001
67. Watford WT, Moriguchi M, Morinobu A, O'Shea JJ. The biology of IL-12: coordinating innate and adaptive immune responses. *Cytokine Growth Factor Rev* (2003) **14**:361–8. doi:10.1016/S1359-6101(03)00043-1
68. Fantl WJ, Johnson DE, Williams LT. Signalling by receptor tyrosine kinases. *Annu Rev Biochem* (1993) **62**:453–81. doi:10.1146/annurev.biochem.62.1.453
69. Moltedo B, López C, Pazos M, Becker M, Hermesh T, Moran T. Cutting edge: stealth influenza virus replication precedes the initiation of adaptive immunity. *J Immunol* (2009) **183**:3569–73. doi:10.4049/jimmunol.0900091
70. Gratchev A, Kzhyshkowska J, Köthe K, Muller-Molinet I, Kannookadan S, Utikal J, et al. Mphi1 and Mphi2 can be re-polarized by Th2 or Th1 cytokines, respectively, and respond to exogenous danger signals. *Immunobiology* (2006) **211**:473–86. doi:10.1016/j.imbio.2006.05.017
71. Erwig LP, Kluth DC, Walsh GM, Rees AJ. Initial cytokine exposure determines function of macrophages and renders them unresponsive to other cytokines. *J Immunol* (1998) **161**:1983–8.
72. Parsa R, Andresen P, Gillett A, Mia S, Zhang XM, Mayans S, et al. Adoptive transfer of immunomodulatory M2 macrophages prevents type 1 diabetes in NOD mice. *Diabetes* (2012) **61**:2881–92. doi:10.2337/db11-1635
73. Watowich SS, Liu YJ. Mechanisms regulating dendritic cell specification and development. *Immunol Rev* (2010) **238**:76–92. doi:10.1111/j.1600-065X.2010.00949.x
74. Jorens PG, Delvigne CR, Hermans CR, Haber I, Holvoet J, De Deyn PP. Cerebral arterial thrombosis preceding ulcerative colitis. *Stroke* (1991) **22**:1212. doi:10.1161/01.STR.22.9.1212
75. Mäkelä SM, Osterlund P, Julkunen I. TLR ligands induce synergistic interferon-β and interferon-λ 1 gene expression in human monocyte-derived dendritic cells. *Mol Immunol* (2011) **48**:505–15. doi:10.1016/j.molimm.2010.10.005
76. Axtell RC, de Jong BA, Boniface K, van der Voort LF, Bhat R, De Sarno P, et al. T helper type 1 and 17 cells determine efficacy of interferon-beta in multiple sclerosis and experimental encephalomyelitis. *Nat Med* (2010) **16**:406–12. doi:10.1038/nm.2110
77. Yang D, de la Rosa G, Tewary P, Oppenheim JJ. Alarmins link neutrophils and dendritic cells. *Trends Immunol* (2009) **30**:531–7. doi:10.1016/j.it.2009.07.004
78. Ramos HJ, Lanteri MC, Blahnik G, Negash A, Suthar MS, Brassil MM, et al. IL-1β signaling promotes CNS-intrinsic immune control of West Nile virus infection. *PLoS Pathog* (2012) **8**:e1003039. doi:10.1371/journal.ppat.1003039
79. Wang F, Gao X, Barrett J, Shao Q, Bartee E, Mohamed M, et al. RIG-I mediates the co-induction of tumor necrosis factor and type I interferon elicited by myxoma virus in primary human macrophages. *PLoS Pathog* (2008) **4**:e1000099. doi:10.1371/journal.ppat.1000099
80. Bartee E, Mohamed MR, Lopez MC, Baker HV, McFadden G. The addition of tumor necrosis factor plus beta interferon induces a novel synergistic antiviral state against poxviruses in primary human fibroblasts. *J Virol* (2009) **83**:498–511. doi:10.1128/JVI.01376-08
81. Mesko B, Poliska S, Szegedi A, Szekanecz Z, Palatka K, Papp M, et al. Peripheral blood gene expression patterns discriminate among chronic inflammatory diseases and healthy controls and identify novel targets. *BMC Med Genomics* (2010) **3**:15. doi:10.1186/1755-8794-3-15
82. Lupfer C, Thomas PG, Anand PK, Vogel P, Milasta S, Martinez J, et al. Receptor interacting protein kinase 2-mediated mitophagy regulates inflammasome activation during virus infection. *Nat Immunol* (2013) **14**:480–8. doi:10.1038/ni.2563
83. Malik A, Batra JK. Antimicrobial activity of human eosinophil granule proteins: involvement in host defence against pathogens. *Crit Rev Microbiol* (2012) **38**:168–81. doi:10.3109/1040841X.2011.645519
84. Liu W, Putnam AL, Xu-Yu Z, Szot GL, Lee MR, Zhu S, et al. CD127 expression inversely correlates with FoxP3 and suppressive function of human CD4+ T reg cells. *J Exp Med* (2006) **203**:1701–11. doi:10.1084/jem.20060772
85. Pauls E, Nanda SK, Smith H, Toth R, Arthur JS, Cohen P. Two phases of inflammatory mediator production defined by the study of IRAK2 and IRAK1 knock-in mice. *J Immunol* (2013) **191**:2717–30. doi:10.4049/jimmunol.1203268
86. Yen JH, Ganea D. Interferon beta induces mature dendritic cell apoptosis through caspase-11/caspase-3 activation. *Blood* (2009) **114**:1344–54. doi:10.1182/blood-2008-12-196592

3

Embryonic stem cells promoting macrophage survival and function are crucial for teratoma development

Tianxiang Chen[1,2†], Xi Wang[1,3†], Lei Guo[4,5†], Mingmei Wu[1], Zhaoxia Duan[1], Jing Lv[4], Wenjiao Tai[4], Hemamalini Renganathan[1], Ruth Didier[4], Jinhua Li[6], Dongming Sun[1], Xiaoming Chen[7], Xijing He[5], Jianqing Fan[8], Wise Young[1] and Yi Ren[4]*

[1] W. M. Keck Center for Collaborative Neuroscience, Rutgers, The State University of New Jersey, New Jersey, NJ, USA
[2] Department of Thoracic Surgery, First Affiliated Hospital, School of Medicine, Zhejiang University, Hangzhou, China
[3] Institute of Neurosciences, The Fourth Military Medical University, Xian, China
[4] Department of Biomedical Sciences, Florida State University College of Medicine, Tallahassee, FL, USA
[5] Department of Orthopedic Surgery, The Second Hospital of Xian Jiaotong University, Xian, China
[6] Department of Anatomy and Developmental Biology, Monash University, Clayton, VIC, Australia
[7] Institute of Translational Medicine, First Affiliated Hospital, Wenzhou Medical University, Wenzhou, China
[8] Statistics Laboratory, Princeton University, Princeton, NJ, USA

Edited by:
Fang-Ping Huang, Imperial College London, UK

Reviewed by:
Ralf Dressel, University Medical Center Göttingen, Germany
Laura Eugenia Velazquez, Université Paris 13, France
Armel Hervé Nwabo Kamdje, University of Ngaoundéré, Cameroon

***Correspondence:**
Yi Ren, Department of Biomedical Sciences, College of Medicine, Florida State University, 1115 West Call Street, Tallahassee, FL 32306, USA
e-mail: yi.ren@med.fsu.edu

†Tianxiang Chen, Xi Wang and Lei Guo have contributed equally to this work.

Stem cell therapies have had tremendous potential application for many diseases in recent years. However, the tumorigenic properties of stem cells restrict their potential clinical application; therefore, strategies for reducing the tumorigenic potential of stem cells must be established prior to transplantation. We have demonstrated that syngeneic transplantation of embryonic stem cells (ESCs) provokes an inflammatory response that involves the rapid recruitment of bone marrow-derived macrophages (BMDMs). ESCs are able to prevent mature macrophages from macrophage colony-stimulating factor (M-CSF) withdrawal-induced apoptosis, and thus prolong macrophage lifespan significantly by blocking various apoptotic pathways in an M-CSF-independent manner. ESCs express and secrete IL-34, which may be responsible for ESC-promoted macrophage survival. This anti-apoptotic effect of ESCs involves activation of extracellular signal-regulated kinase (ERK)1/2 and PI3K/Akt pathways and thus, inhibition of ERK1/2 and PI3K/AKT activation decreases ESC-induced macrophage survival. Functionally, ESC-treated macrophages also showed a higher level of phagocytic activity. ESCs further serve to polarize BMDMs into M2-like macrophages that exhibit most tumor-associated macrophage phenotypic and functional features. ESC-educated macrophages produce high levels of arginase-1, Tie-2, and TNF-α, which participate in angiogenesis and contribute to teratoma progression. Our study suggests that induction of M2-like macrophage activation is an important mechanism for teratoma development. Strategies targeting macrophages to inhibit teratoma development would increase the safety of ESC-based therapies, inasmuch as the depletion of macrophages completely inhibits ESC-induced angiogenesis and teratoma development.

Keywords: angiogenesis, apoptosis, embryonic stem cells, macrophages, teratoma

INTRODUCTION

Stem cell-based therapies possess promising outcomes for many conditions, including spinal cord injury and other neurological degenerative disorders. However, this powerful therapeutic strategy is problematic because the pluripotency of stem cells is accompanied by a large risk of tumor formation after transplantation. Theoretically, three classes of tumors can be envisaged to arise from pluripotent stem cells (PSCs) including embryonic stem cells (ESCs) and induced pluripotent stem cells (iPSCs); viz. teratomas, teratocarcinomas, and secondary tumors (1). Teratoma is constituted by cells from endodermal, mesodermal, and ectodermal lineages (2–4). Not only ESCs but also ESC-derived neuronal progenitors can induce teratomas in animal models (5). The tumorigenicity of stem cells is the major obstacle to the successful application of stem cell-based therapies (6). The safety issue of stem cells must be evaluated properly and the adverse consequences of teratoma formation from these stem cells must be overcome before stem cell therapy can be used for clinical application.

Various strategies developed to reduce this risk of teratoma formation include prolonged pre-differentiation of ESCs *in vitro*, blocking signaling pathways that promote proliferation, induction of apoptosis of proliferative ESCs, sorting cells expressing precursor markers, and deleting undifferentiated ESCs immunologically, genetically, and chemically (7–18). However, it is difficult to obtain a yield of 100% pure differentiated stem cells for transplantation: the contamination of grafts with undifferentiated cells can give rise to teratoma formation (19–21). Furthermore, teratoma could potentially develop into highly malignant teratocarcinoma, which constitutes of persistent and undifferentiated stem cells (22). Therefore, efforts must be made to ensure safe transplantation of a PSC-based cell treatment. We used undifferentiated ESCs as a worst-case model for teratoma formation by stem cells and studied the role of macrophages and niche microenvironment of stem cell growth in the progression of teratomas.

The interplay of immune cells, especially macrophages and ESCs, causes alterations in the microenvironment and potential for tumorigenicity, which regulate the initiation, progression, angiogenesis, and metastasis of tumor. Thus, targeting this immune response can significantly inhibit the evolution of tumors (23, 24). Our previous data also demonstrated that interaction between transplanted ESCs and macrophages creates a microenvironment that facilitates the initiation and progression of teratomas (24). Infiltrated macrophages deliver macrophage migration inhibitory factor (MIF) and other angiogenic factors to stimulate endothelial cell proliferation and pericyte differentiation (24). There is growing evidence to suggest that macrophages promote tumorigenesis and that the tumor microenvironment polarizes macrophages toward an M2 (pro-tumor) phenotype, with properties that differ from the M1 phenotype (25–28). However, the role of macrophages in ESC growth and teratoma development is not clear. In this study, we demonstrate that ESCs promote macrophage survival and M2-like activation are critically important for teratoma angiogenesis and development. Significantly, we show that depletion of macrophages inhibits teratoma growth tremendously. Therefore, ESC-educated macrophages are considered attractive targets for an anti-teratoma strategy after ESC transplantation.

MATERIALS AND METHODS

REAGENTS AND ANTIBODIES

All the chemicals were purchased from Sigma (St. Louis, MO, USA) and cell culture media were purchased from Invitrogen (Carlsbad, CA, USA) unless specifically noted. The F4/80 hybridoma cell line was from American Tissue Culture Collection (ATCC, Manassas, VA, USA). Recombinant mouse IL-34 was from R&D Systems (Minneapolis, MN, USA). The primary antibodies used in the study are listed in **Table 1**. All Alexa Fluor- or HRP-conjugated secondary antibodies were from Invitrogen.

Table 1 | Antibodies included in the study.

Protein name	Antibody ID	Manufacturer
AKT	4685	Cell Signaling
Arginase-1	sc-18354	Santa Cruz
Caspase-9	9504	Cell Signaling
CD31	553708	BD Biosciences
CD45	103108	BioLegend
Cytochrome *c*	4272	Cell Signaling
ERK1/2	4695	Cell Signaling
GAPDH	2118	Cell Signaling
IBA-1	019-19741	Wako
IL-34	PAB13397	Abnova
M-CSF	3155	Cell Signaling
PI3K p85	4257	Cell Signaling
Iκbα (Ser32)	2859	Cell Signaling
Phospho-Akt	9271	Cell Signaling
Phospho-ERK1/2	4370	Cell Signaling
Phospho-PI3K p85	4228	Cell Signaling
Tie-2	sc-9026	Santa Cruz
YM1	01404	Stem Cell Technologies

MICE

C57BL/6 mice and transgenic CX3CR1^{GFP} mice from Jackson Laboratory (Bar Harbor, ME, USA) were maintained in the pathogen-free animal facility in Rutgers, the State University of New Jersey. All animal experimental protocols were authorized by the Animal Care and Facilities Committee of Rutgers, the State University of New Jersey and Florida State University.

PREPARATION OF MOUSE BONE MARROW-DERIVED MACROPHAGES

Mouse bone marrow-derived macrophages (BMDMs) from C57BL/6 mice were prepared as described (24). Briefly, BM cells from mice 6–8 weeks of age were collected from femoral shafts by flushing the marrow cavity of femurs with Dulbecco's modified eagle medium (DMEM) supplemented with 1% fetal bovine serum (FBS). The cell suspensions were passed through an 18-gage needle to disperse cell clumps. Cells were cultured for 7 days at a cell density of 1×10^6/ml in 100 mm polystyrene tissue culture dishes (BD Biosciences) containing DMEM supplemented with 15% conditioned medium from L929 cells [a source of macrophage colony-stimulating factor (M-CSF)] and 10% FBS. Cell morphology was analyzed by image capture (Carl Zeiss, Germany) and using LSM 510 software (Nikon, Japan). The long axis, defined as the longest length of the cells, was manually traced and measured.

ESC CULTURE AND PREPARATION OF ESC-CONDITIONED MEDIUM

The mouse green fluorescent protein (GFP)-expressing -ESC line (F12) derived from C57BL/6 mouse was a kind gift from Professor Melitta Schachner (Rutgers University). Freshly thawed ESCs (P0) were seeded into a 10-cm tissue culture dish in the presence of mitomycin-treated murine embryo fibroblast (MEF) feeder layer, in ESC media [10^3 U/ml LIF (Millipore, CA, USA), 15% FBS, 1% non-essential amino acids solution (MEM), 200 mM L-glutamine, 1% nucleoside solution, 1% 100 nM Na-Pyruvate, and 0.2% 2-Mercaptoethanol in DMEM]. LIF was added every day into the culture medium. After 3–4 passages, ESCs were maintained only on a 0.1% gelatin-coated tissue culture dish without a feeder layer. ESC colonies were sub-cultured for every 2–3 days and their supernatant was collected as conditioned medium. ESC-conditioned medium (ESC-CM) was prepared by spinning the ESCs at 1,000 rpm for 5 min to pellet the cells, while the supernatant was again spun at 2,500 rpm for 10 min to remove any debris. Supernatant was then filtered through a 0.4-μ filter (Corning, USA). Supernatant collected from multiple passages was pooled together and stored at −80°C. Regular culture medium without ESCs was incubated in the same way and used as control medium (Con-M).

HISTOLOGY AND IMMUNOFLUORESCENCE

Mice were transcardially perfused with 0.9% saline followed by 4% paraformaldehyde. A segment of tissue encompassing the transplantation site was removed and fixed in 4% paraformaldehyde for 3 h and then cryoprotected in 20% sucrose overnight at 4°C. For histologic examination, the sections were stained with hematoxylin and eosin (H&E). For immunofluorescence staining, the sections were incubated with primary antibodies overnight at room temperature (RT) followed by secondary antibodies at RT for 2 h. Non-specific binding was excluded by using secondary antibody only. Samples were examined and microphotographs were taken using a Zeiss AxioCam microscope and an AxioPhot image collection system (Carl Zeiss, Germany), and Confocal Laser Scanning Microscopy (Nikon, Japan). Tumor volume was determined as follows: short diameter^2 × long diameter × 1/2.

TRANSPLANTATION AND ESCs IN SPINAL CORD AND LIVER

Laminectomy was performed on WT and chimerical mice at the T9–T10 level to expose the spinal cord. GFP–ESCs (50,000 in 1 μl DMEM) were injected slowly at this segment of each mouse's spinal cord using a microliter syringe (Hamilton Company, NV, USA) fixed in a stereotaxic frame. ESCs (100,000 in 5.0 μl DMEM) were also injected slowly via microliter syringe into the left lobe of mouse liver. Mice were sacrificed and perfused at different time points after cell transplantation.

MTT ASSAY

To determine cell viability the colorimetric MTT metabolic activity assay was used. BMDMs were seeded in a 96-well plate at a density of 8,000 cell per well and cells were treated with Con-M and ESC-M for 48 h. MTT [3-(4,5-dimethylthiazolyl-2)-2,5-diphenyltetrazolium bromide] was added to each well and plate was incubated for 4 h. Finally, the absorbance was measured at 540 nm by using a microplate reader. The relative MTT uptake (% cell viability) was expressed as a percentage relative to the control cells.

PHAGOCYTIC FUNCTION TEST

Mature BMDMs were seeded in a 96-well culture plate at a density of 1×10^4 cells/well and incubated with Con-M and ESC-M for 24 h. BMDMs were incubated with carboxylate-modified fluorescent red Latex beads and apoptotic cells for 1 h, respectively. Non-ingested particles were washed away and phagocytosis was imaged by a Zeiss Axiovert 200 M Microscope (Carl Zeiss) and software AxioVision 4.6 (Carl Zeiss).

ARGINASE ACTIVITY ASSAY

To prepare the cell lysate for assay of arginase activity, BMDMs were rinsed with PBS after each specific treatment and 1×10^5 BMDMs from each group were lysed in 100 μl of lysis buffer containing 10 mM Tris-HCl (pH 7.4), proteinase inhibitor cocktail, and 0.4% Triton-X 100 for 10 min. Arginase activity of various cell lysate was measured by quantitative colorimetric assay of arginase activity (Bioassay Systems, CA, USA) according to the manufacturer's instructions. One unit of arginase activity is defined as 1 μmol of L-arginine converted to ornithine and urea per minute at pH 9.5 and 37°C. Urea concentration, as the degree of arginase activity, was measured at 520 nm at RT by spectrometer.

ANNEXIN V AND PROPIDIUM IODIDE STAINING

Bone marrow-derived macrophages were rinsed with PBS after each specific treatment and the apoptosis of BMDMs was measured by PE Annexin V Apoptosis Detection Kit I (BD Biosciences, CA, USA) according to the manufacturer's instructions. Binding of Annexin V and PI was measured by a flow cytometer (BD Biosciences, CA, USA) and analyzed using FlowJo software (FlowJo, NJ, USA).

RNA ISOLATION AND QUANTITATIVE REAL-TIME-PCR

Bone marrow-derived macrophages were incubated with Con-M and ESC-M for 6 and 12 h, respectively. Total RNA was isolated by TRIZOL and reverse-transcribed into cDNA by using oligo-dT primers and SuperScript II Reverse Transcriptase. The TNF-α primer pair (5′-ATGCTGGGACAGTGACCTGG-3′ and 5′-CCTTGATGGTGGTGCATGAG-3′) was specifically designed for mRNA. The ABI7900HT detection system (Applied Biosystems, UK) was used for quantitative real-time (qRT)-PCR. SYBR Green dye (Applied Biosystems) was used to monitor the replication of PCR products. Quantification of products were obtained by standard curve and then normalized to GAPDH amount. The gene expression level was represented by the ratio of gene TNF-α/GAPDH.

WESTERN BLOT

Western blot assay was performed following the standard procedure. Briefly, after washing with ice-cold PBS, cells were lysed with RIPA buffer containing phosphatase inhibitor and proteinase inhibitor cocktail. Total cellular proteins were loaded onto SDS-polyacrylamide gel electrophoresis (SDS-PAGE) and then transferred to PVDF membranes (GE Healthcare, UK). After blocking in 5% milk or BSA (according to antibody manufacturer's instructions) in Tris-buffered saline containing 0.1% Tween 20 (TBST) for 1 h at RT, membranes were incubated with appropriate primary antibody solution overnight at 4°C. Membranes were placed in appropriate secondary antibody for 1 h after rinsing in TBST. Subsequently, proteins were visualized by ECL plus western blot detection system (GE Healthcare, UK).

EX VIVO MOUSE AORTIC RING ASSAY

Mouse aortic ring assay was carried out as described (29) using C57BL/6 mice (8–12 weeks). Briefly, thoracic aortic segments were cut into 1-mm rings and carefully placed with the lumen of the rings opened up on Matrigel (BD Biosciences) with Con-M or ESC-M and then overlaid with an additional Matrigel. Aortic rings were examined daily and digital images were taken at day 6 for quantitative analysis of the area of vessel outgrowth by the SPOT Advanced program (Media Cybernetics, Sterling Heights, MI, USA). Microvessel outgrowth was calculated by circling the extent of microvessel outgrowth at 6 days and subtracting the area of the aortic ring (29).

DEPLETION OF MACROPHAGES *IN VIVO*

Liposomes containing either dichloromethylene diphosphonate (clodronate, a gift from Roche Diagnostics, Germany) or PBS were prepared as described (30). Mice were injected with clodronate liposomes (CL-Lip) or PBS liposomes (PBS-Lip) at 100 mg/kg body weight by intraperitoneal (i.p.) injection twice a week for up to 4 weeks.

STATISTICAL ANALYSIS

Results showed in figures were presented as mean ± SEM with *n* representing the frequency of experiments. Student's unpaired

t-test was used to evaluate statistical significance with a p value <0.05 considered significant.

RESULTS

TERATOMA DEVELOPMENT AFTER ESC INJECTION INTO SPINAL CORD

Undifferentiated enhanced gene fluorescent protein (EGFP)–ESCs were stereotaxically injected into the spinal cord of mice exposed by a T9–T10 laminectomy. During the first week after ESC injection, hindlimb function, as reflected by the Basso Mouse Scale (BMS), was normal. However, the BMS score decreased rapidly at 10 days after ESC injection and all mice were paralyzed at day 17 after cell transplantation (**Figure 1A**) because of rapid tumor growth (**Figure 1B**). The mice survived for only 3 weeks after ESC transplantation (data not shown). Histological examination revealed that these tumors were teratomas since they consisted of structures derived from all three embryonic germ lineages (**Figure 1C**). While most teratomas are benign, malignant teratomas do occur. Prognosis is inversely related to stage and histological grade, which is based on the amount of neurepithelium and immature neural tubes present according to the World Health Organization (WHO) classification (31). Teratomas of grade 0–1 are classified as benign or low grade, while grade 3 is malignant. We found that the median teratoma grade in mice was 3.0 (**Figure 1D**), indicating that these teratomas in mice were teratocarcinomas.

ESCs STIMULATE MACROPHAGE INFILTRATION

We observed the early infiltration of a large population of Mac-2^+/IBA-1^+ macrophages within the teratomas (**Figure 1E**). Macrophages can be detected as early as 1 day after ESC injection, with peak macrophage infiltration occurring after 1 week (**Figures 1E,F**). **Figure 1F** shows the mean density of macrophages (IBA-1^+) recruited at the ESC implantation site at different time points after ESC injection. Interestingly, there was a significant reduction in macrophage distribution after 2 weeks. The numbers of macrophages at 2 and 3 weeks were significantly less than those at any earlier time points and the difference between 2 and 3 weeks was no longer significant (**Figure 1F**). This suggests that macrophages may play an important role in teratoma initiation. By contrast, injection of PBS alone in the spinal cord did not induce macrophage infiltration (data not shown).

TERATOMA DEVELOPMENT IN THE TISSUE OUTSIDE OF SPINAL CORD

To better exclude the effect of neural and glial cells in spinal cord on teratoma growth and differentiation, an examination of teratomas induced by ESC transplantation in non-neural sites could support the role of signals produced by macrophages vs. other tissue types. ESCs were injected into liver and representative teratoma at week 4 is shown in **Figure 1G**. A large teratoma had formed in the liver and an enormous number of macrophages was detected (**Figure 1G**).

ESC-SECRETED FACTORS ACT AS MACROPHAGE SURVIVAL FACTORS

The ESC-induced macrophage distribution could result from either increased recruitment of these cells into the teratoma or cell survival. We first examined the function of ESCs in macrophage growth. It has been well-documented that M-CSF is a hematopoietic growth factor necessary for monocyte survival, proliferation, and differentiation (32, 33). L929 conditioned medium is the source for M-CSF. Mouse ESC-CM (without direct cell–cell contact) and control medium (Con-M, medium to culture ESCs) were used in the study. Day 7 BMDMs were cultured with DMEM alone, Con-M and ESC-M and DMEM with M-CSF for 48 h and cell viability was measured by monitoring metabolic activity of the cells using MTT assay. Incubation of BMDMs in the presence of M-CSF and ESC-M caused a significant increase in cell viability compared to medium without M-CSF (DMEM alone) and Con-M treatment (**Figure 2A**). These data suggest that ESC-M can partially prevent the loss of macrophage viability after M-CSF withdrawal, although to a lesser extent than did M-CSF. Furthermore, heat-inactivated ESC-M by boiling for 10 min failed to increase macrophage viability (data not shown).

ESCs PROTECT MACROPHAGES FROM M-CSF WITHDRAWAL-INDUCED APOPTOSIS *IN VITRO*

To further evaluate whether the survival effect of ESCs was due to the inhibition of apoptosis, apoptosis of macrophages was assessed by surface Annexin V staining using FACS and caspase-9 activation. When mature BMDMs were cultured with M-CSF, <10% of cells were Annexin V-positive (**Figures 2B,C**). However, when cells were subjected to medium without M-CSF or Con-M, more than 25% of the cells underwent apoptosis (**Figures 2B,C**). Propidium iodide (PI) staining revealed that M-CSF withdrawal or Con-M treatment for 24 h did not increase PI-positive macrophages significantly compared to M-CSF or ESC-M treatment (**Figure 2C**). Furthermore, Con-M treatment induced activation of caspase-9, assessed by the appearance of the cleaved caspase-9 (**Figure 2D**). Treatment of cells with ESC-M significantly protected M-CSF withdrawal-induced caspase-9 activation and apoptosis (**Figures 2B–D**). These results suggest that the anti-apoptotic effect of ESCs on macrophages resulted in enhanced cell survival. In order to identify whether ESC-mediated cell survival is induced directly by mediators in ESC-M or indirectly by stimulating the release of secondary mediators acting in an autocrine manner, we detected M-CSF and IL-34, the two most well-documented cytokines that regulate macrophage survival and differentiation (34). ESCs did not produce M-CSF (data not shown) but expressed a high level of IL-34 (**Figure 2E**) and secreted into the ESC-M (16.034 ± 4.56 ng/ml, $n = 3$). BMDM treated with ESCs did not further increase M-CSF and IL-34 expression (data not shown), suggesting that ESC-induced BMDM survival is M-CSF-independent and that IL-34 from ESCs may promote macrophage survival.

ACTIVATION OF PI3K/Akt AND ERK IS NECESSARY FOR ESC-INDUCED MACROPHAGE SURVIVAL

The PI3K pathway is one of the most potent intracellular mechanisms for promoting cell survival, and PI3K/Akt and extracellular regulated kinase1/2 (ERK1/2) regulate macrophage survival in response to M-CSF and IL-34 (35–37). We therefore examined whether activation of PI3K and ERK1/2 was required for ESC-mediated macrophage survival. As shown in **Figures 3A,B**, ESC-M stimulated phosphorylation of p85 regulatory subunit of PI3K and ERK1/2 as early as 3 min, and a persistent phosphorylation level was maintained up to 30 min. ESCs also induced activation of

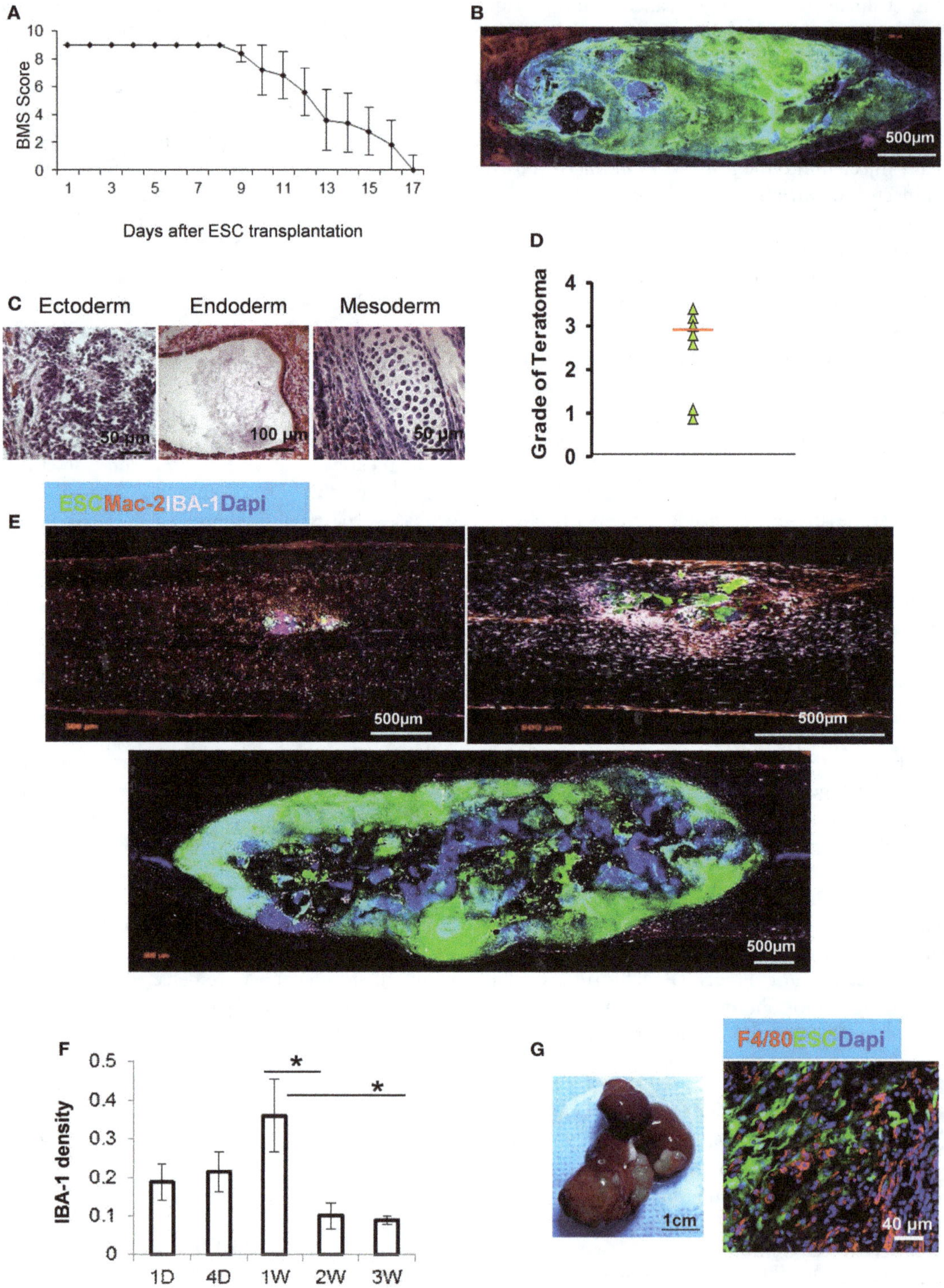

FIGURE 1 | Teratoma formation and macrophage infiltration after ESC injection into spinal cord. **(A)** ESCs were stereotaxically injected into the spinal cord in C57BL/6 mice and the function of the hindlimbs was evaluated by BMS score ($n = 7$, data are represented as mean ± SEM). A score of 0 indicates complete paralysis of the hind limbs and 9 denotes full mobility. **(B)** Tumor formation in spinal cord at 3 weeks after GFP–ESC injection. **(C)** Histological staining of spinal cord sections at 2 weeks after ESC injection showing structures derived from three embryonic germ lineages. **(D)** Median of teratoma grade in mice ($n = 6$). **(E)** Representative micrographs showing macrophage recruitment during teratoma progression. Macrophages in the sections of spinal cord at 1 day (upper left), 1 week (upper right), and 3 weeks after ESC transplantation (lower) were detected by antibodies to IBA-1 (purple) and Mac-2 (red). **(F)** Quantification of IBA-1⁺ macrophages at indicated time points after ESC transplantation ($n = 10$, $*p < 0.05$, two-sided Wilcoxon test. Data are represented as mean ± SEM). **(G)** Representative gross morphology of teratoma in liver (left) and F4/80⁺ macrophages in teratoma at 4 weeks after ESC transplantation in liver.

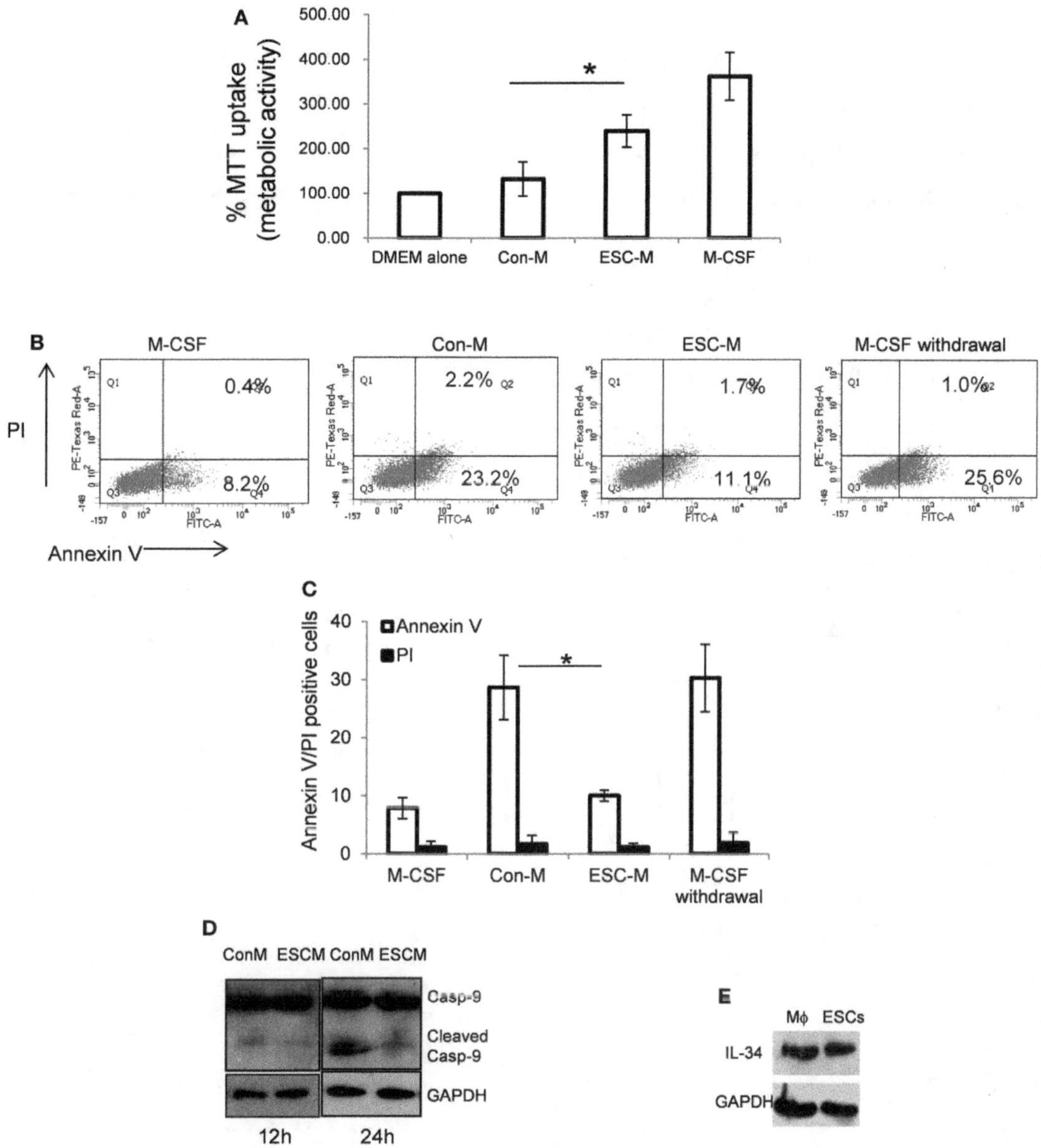

FIGURE 2 | Embryonic stem cells enhance BMDM survival. **(A)** Day 7 BMDMs were incubated with DMEM alone in absence of M-CSF, Con-M, ESC-M, and DMEM in the presence of M-CSF for 48 h. The metabolic activity of the cells was analyzed by the MTT assay and is presented relative to the activity of cells treated with DMEM alone ($n = 3$). **(B,C)** Flow cytometric analysis of annexin V/propidium iodide (PI) staining of BMDMs treated with ESC-M, Con-M, DMEM with M-CSF, and DMEM alone for 24 h, respectively ($n = 3$). **(D)** Effect of ESCs on caspase-9 activation. BMDMs were treated with Con-M and ESC-M for 12 and 24 h, respectively and whole cell lysates were analyzed by Western blotting for caspase-9 activation. **(E)** IL-34 in BMDMs and ESCs was detected by Western blot analysis. $*p < 0.05$, two-sided Wilcoxon test. Data are represented as mean ± SEM.

the major downstream kinase Akt of PI3K by phosphorylating residue Ser473 (**Figure 3C**). It is interesting to note that ESC-M also induced NF-κB activation by enhancing IκBα phosphorylation (**Figure 3C**). We further determined whether LY-294002 and PD98059, specific inhibitors of PI3K and ERK1/2, can reverse the protective role of ESC-M on macrophage survival. Both LY-294002 and PD98059 significantly reduced ESC-mediated macrophage survival (**Figure 3D**), suggesting that PI3K and ERK1/2 activation are required for ESC-mediated macrophage survival. Moreover, the activation of PI3K and ERK1/2 was inhibited by LY-294002 and PD98059, respectively, which parallels their effect on macrophage survival (**Figure 3E**).

We showed that ESCs produce IL-34 (**Figure 2E**) and the concentration of IL-34 in ESC-M was 16.034 ± 4.56 ng/ml. We therefore examined the ability of mouse recombinant IL-34 to promote macrophage survival on BMDMs. IL-34 simulated macrophage survival in a dose-dependent manner (**Figure 3F**). IL-34 at low as 10 ng/ml increased macrophage survival. Furthermore, IL-34

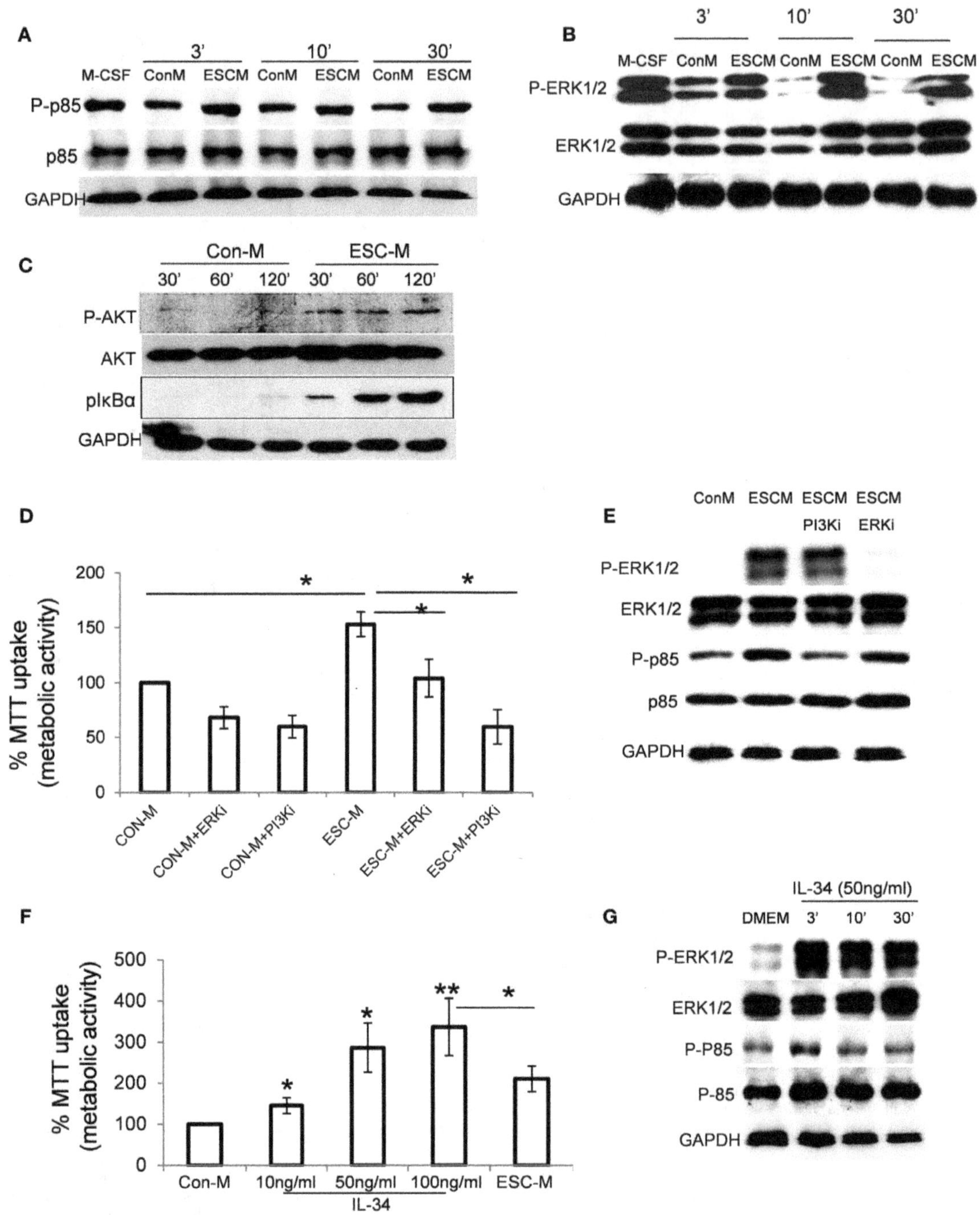

FIGURE 3 | Effect of ESCs on activation of PI3K/Akt, ERK1/2, and NF-κB pathways. Phosphorylation of p85 **(A)**, p-ERK1/2 **(B)**, and pAkt and NF-κB **(C)** in BMDMs treated with Con-M and ESC-M for the indicated time. **(D)** Effect of inactivation of PI3K and ERK1/2 in ESC-induced cell survival. BMDMs were pretreated with PI3K inhibitor LY-294002 (20 μM) and ERK inhibitor PD98059 (10 μM) for 30 min and then treated with Con-M and ESC-M for 48 h. The metabolic activity of the cells was analyzed by the MTT assay and is presented relative to the activity of cells treated with Con-M ($n = 3$, $*p < 0.05$, two-sided Wilcoxon test. Data are represented as mean ± SEM). **(E)** BMDMs were pretreated with PI3K inhibitor LY-294002 (20 μM) and ERK inhibitor PD98059 (10 μM) for 30 min and then treated with Con-M and ESC-M for 30 min. Phosphorylation of p85 and p-ERK1/2 was detected by Western Blot assay. **(F)** Effect of IL-34 on macrophage survival. BMDMs were incubated with mouse recombinant IL-34 at the indicated concentration for 48 h. The metabolic activity of the cells was analyzed by the MTT assay and is presented relative to the activity of cells treated with Con-M ($n = 3$, $*p < 0.05$; $**p < 0.001$, ANOVA, data are represented as mean ± SEM). **(G)** Phosphorylation of p85 and p-ERK1/2 in BMDMs treated with IL-34 (50 ng/ml) for the indicated time.

stimulated phosphorylation of ERK1/2 and PI3K in macrophages to a similar degree, with similar kinetics, compared to ESC-M treatment (**Figure 3G**).

ESCs INDUCES TYPICAL SHAPE CHANGE

We next examined how ESCs modulate macrophage function. We exposed mature BMDMs to interferon γ (IFN-γ), IL-4, ESC-M, Con-M, and IL-34 for 72 h, respectively. BMDMs present a unique morphology, depending on the stimulation used. Cells treated with IL-4, which stimulates M2 activation, adopted a spindle-shape morphology (**Figure 4A**). M1 macrophages induced by IFN-γ had a relatively round shape with large filopodia. Con-M treatment exhibited the typical bipolar, spindle-shaped morphology of BMDMs. In contrast, ESC-M led to a majority of elongated fibroblast-like-shaped cells and some of the macrophages showed a long, single process or bipolar processes (**Figure 4A**). IL-34 treated cells demonstrated a wider range of cell length whereas the ESC-M treated cells displayed a relatively shorter range because the cells were all approximately the same length (**Figure 4A**). Quantitative analysis showed that ESC-M-treated macrophages exhibited a

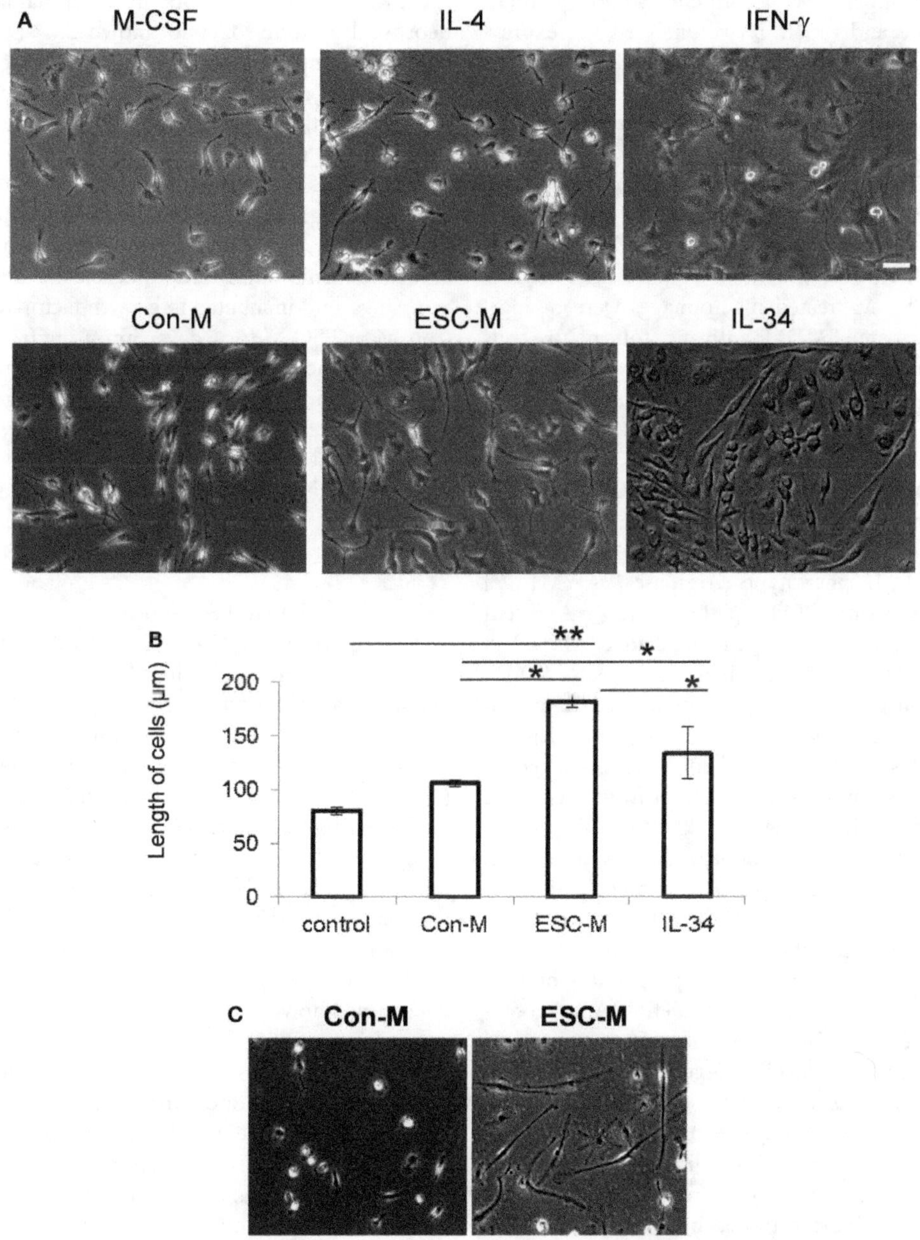

FIGURE 4 | Effect of ESCs on macrophage activation. (A) Representative phase-contrast photomicrographs of BMDMs (original magnification, ×400). BMDMs were cultured with M-CSF, IL-4, IFN-γ, IL-34, Con-M, and ESC-M for 72 h. **(B)** Length of BMDMs incubated with IL-34, Con-M, and ESC-M for 72 h was measured by ImageJ ($n = 6$, $^*p < 0.05$, $^{**}p < 0.001$, two-sided Wilcoxon test. Data are represented as mean ± SEM). **(C)** Representative phase-contrast photomicrographs of primary microglial cells incubated with Con-M and ESC-M for 72 h. Original magnification, ×400.

significantly higher degree of elongation compared either to Con-M treated or untreated macrophages (**Figure 4B**). The average length of cells treated with IL-34 was longer than that of Con-M treated cells but shorter than that of ESC-M, suggesting that other factors produced by ESC-M may have contributed to cell elongation. To further demonstrate that the ESC-induced phenotypic characteristic was not restricted to BMDMs, we isolated primary microglial cells from brain. ESC-M also resulted in remarkable elongation in microglial cells (**Figure 4C**).

ESCs MAINTAIN MACROPHAGE PHENOTYPE AND FUNCTION

In order to know whether ESC treatment would maintain macrophage phenotype and function, we analyzed the expression of macrophage markers such as F4/80 and Mac-2 on cells treated with ESC-M. BMDMs were treated with Con-M and ESC-M for 3 days and expression of macrophage markers was confirmed by flow cytometry and Western Blot analysis, respectively. Both Con-M and ESC-M treatment maintained macrophages expressing a high level of F4/80 (**Figure 5A**). Mac-2 expression was enhanced by ESC-M treatment and the expression level was higher compared with Con-M treatment (**Figure 5B**). To further study, whether ESC-M-treated macrophages were biologically functional, we incubated BMDMs with apoptotic neutrophils (PMNs) and latex beads for 30 min. The results showed that ESC-M-treated BMDMs displayed active functional phagocytosis of apoptotic cells and latex beads (**Figures 5C,D**).

ESCs POLARIZE MACROPHAGES INTO UNIQUE M2-LIKE CELLS

In addition to the role of ESCs promoting macrophage infiltration and survival, ESCs are able to activate BMDMs and stew them toward the M2 phenotype (Arginase-1^{high}YM1^{high}) via activation of STAT3 and STAT6 pathways (24). A recent study showed that macrophage elongation enhanced the effect of M2-inducing cytokines and inhibited the effect of M1-inducing cytokines, suggesting that cell shape has an important role in modulating macrophage activation (38). We demonstrated in the present study that the phenotypic characterizations of ESC-treated macrophages were distinct from classic M2 macrophages induced by IL-4 (**Figure 4A**). We thus further evaluated whether ESC-treated macrophages are different from "alternatively activated" M2 macrophages. Treatment with ESC-M significantly enhanced arginase-1 (Arg-1) activity in BMDMs in a time-dependent manner, compared to treatment with Con-M using a colorimetric assay that detects production of urea (**Figure 5E**). The distributions of angiopoietin (Ang) receptor (Tie)-2^{+} (Tie-2) cells and F4/80^{+}/arginase-1^{+} macrophages were detected in the teratoma *in vivo* (**Figure 5F**). It has been shown that M2 express a very low level of TNF-α (39, 40). However, we showed that macrophages expressed only minimal TNF-α mRNA in the absence of ESC-M (**Figure 5G**). Upon co-culture with ESC-M, TNF-α expression increased significantly in macrophages (**Figure 5G**). Furthermore, the amount of TNF-α secreted into the culture medium was significantly increased in BMDMs treated with ESC-M compared to the amount present in supernatants of Con-M-treated macrophages (**Figure 5H**). In summary, ESC-macrophages exhibited an Arg-1^{high}Tie-2^{high}TNF-α^{high} phenotype, which differs from conventional M2 phenotypes.

ESCs EXERTS ANGIOGENIC ACTIVITY *EX VIVO* AND *IN VIVO*

It is widely accepted that tumor growth requires angiogenesis. Therefore, fast teratoma growth is supposedly induced by increased angiogenesis. ESCs were injected into the spinal cord and images were taken at 3 weeks after cell transplantation. Spinal cords with teratoma appeared reddish or brownish, suggesting an increased permeability (**Figure 6A**). Immunohistochemical analysis of teratoma tissue with anti-CD31 antibody showed a massively branched intratumoral vascular network at 3 weeks after cell injection (**Figure 6A**). This high density of "plexus-like" vascularity in teratoma may be important for teratoma growth. By contrast, injection of PBS alone in the spinal cord did not produce neovascularization (data not shown).

To better understand the contribution of macrophages to vascular development during teratoma progression, we performed a ring sprouting *ex vivo* assay. A 3D-culture of aortic rings in Matrigel was used to evaluate the outgrowth of linear endothelial structures from the preexisting vessel (41). The aorta ring assay is thought to more closely mimic multiple stages of *in vivo* angiogenesis, including endothelial cell proliferation, migration, and tube formation. Mouse thoracic aorta was sectioned into 1-mm rings, and incubated in growth factor-reduced matrigel with Con-M or ESC-M for 6 days. Sprouting from the rings was photographed and outgrowth area was quantitated. ESC-M treatment significantly increased the areas of sprouting (1.81 ± 0.03 mm^2) at 6 days, whereas Con-M-treated ring segments showed little sprouting (**Figures 6B,C**). Qualitatively, the arborization of endothelial networks emanating from aortic rings was also more complex in the rings treated with ESC-M. Together, these data demonstrated an important role for ESC-mediated angiogenesis in aortic rings *ex vivo*.

We showed that ESC-educated macrophages (SEM) exhibited an Arg-1^{high}Tie-2^{high}TNF-α^{high} phenotype (**Figures 5E–H**). In order to know whether TNF-α is responsible for ESC-enhanced angiogenesis, aortic rings were cultured with TNF-α at 10 ng/ml for 6 days. A significant increase in angiogenic spouting was observed in aortic rings in response to TNF-α treatment (**Figures 6B,C**). Therefore, we consider that TNF-α contributed, at least partially, to ESC-induced angiogenesis.

It has been shown that macrophages are found around sprouting neovessels and are particularly abundant at the root of the vascular outgrowth (42). Pharmacologic ablation of macrophages from aortic explants blocked formation of neovessels *in vitro* and reduced aortic ring-induced angiogenesis *in vivo* (42). We further determined how crucial macrophages are to the enhanced angiogenic ability of ESCs. We applied a well-documented approach to deleted macrophages by treating mice with liposome-encapsulated clodronate (Cl-Lip) or control liposomes (PBS-Lip) (43). We used CX3CR1 $^{GFP/-}$ mice, in which one (CX3CR1$^{GFP/+}$) copy of the CX3CR1 gene was interrupted by EGFP (44). CX3CR1 is highly expressed by human and mouse macrophages (45). Intraperitoneal injection of mice with Cl-Lip but not control liposomes (PBS-Lip) resulted in complete depletion of macrophages in the aortic ring tissue (**Figure 6D**). Depletion of macrophages by Cl-Lip led to a markedly reduced angiogenic response to ESC-M (**Figure 6E**). However, we cannot rule out the direct effect of ESC-M on aortic ring sprouting, because Cl-Lip treatment did not completely inhibit the vascularization (**Figure 6E**).

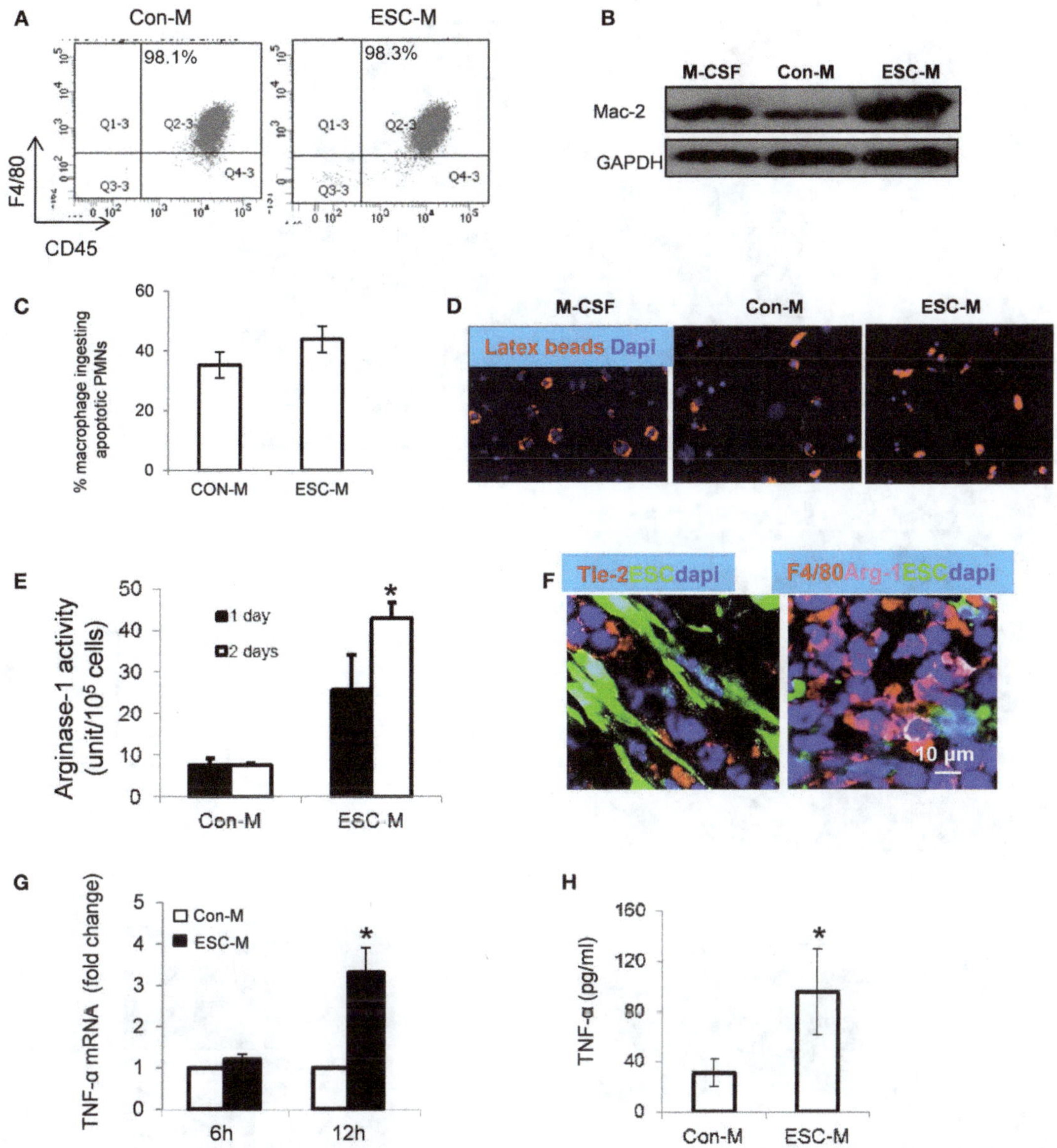

FIGURE 5 | Effect of ESCs on macrophage activation. BMDMs were incubated with Con-M or ESC-M for 72 h and F4/80 (macrophage marker), CD45 (hematopoietic marker), and Mac-2 (macrophage marker) were assessed by flow cytometry **(A)** and Western Blot **(B)**, respectively. **(C)** BMDMs were pretreated with Con-M and ESC-M for 48 h and then incubated with apoptotic neutrophils for 30 min. The number of macrophages ingesting apoptotic cells was counted ($n = 4$, data are represented as mean ± SEM). **(D)** BMDMs pretreated with Con-M and ESC-M ingestion of latex beads (red, original magnification, ×400). **(E)** BMDMs were treated with Con-M and ESC-M for 1 and 2 days and arginase-1 activity was detected by colorimetric assay ($n = 3$, $*p < 0.05$, two-sided Wilcoxon test. Data are represented as mean ± SEM). **(F)** Representative confocal images of immunostaining of sections from mice at 2 weeks after ESC injection showing positive staining for Tie-2 (red, left) and F4/80 (red, right) Arginase-1 (purple), respectively. **(G)** TNF-α mRNA in BMDMs treated with Con-M and ESC-M for 6 and 12 h was detected by real time RT-PCR ($n = 4$, $*p < 0.05$, two-sided Wilcoxon test. Data are represented as mean ± SEM). **(H)** TNF-α in the supernatants of BMDMs treated with Con-M and ESC-M for 48 h was detected by ELISA ($n = 3$, $*p < 0.05$, two-sided Wilcoxon test. Data are represented as mean ± SEM).

TARGETING MACROPHAGES INHIBITS ESC-INDUCED ANGIOGENESIS AND TERATOMA DEVELOPMENT

A large amount of macrophage infiltration and phenotype of M2-like macrophages in the teratoma suggested that macrophages may create a microenvironment for teratoma development. We depleted macrophage populations from mice to verify the contribution of macrophages to teratoma growth. We demonstrated that i.p. injection of Cl-Lip twice a week after ESC transplantation into liver resulted in near-complete depletion of macrophages in liver and teratoma when assayed at 4 weeks (**Figures 7A,B**). We also quantified the blood vessel density by counting the percentage of the area occupied by cross-section of all blood vessels in an image. We observed that blood vessel density in teratoma from mice treated with

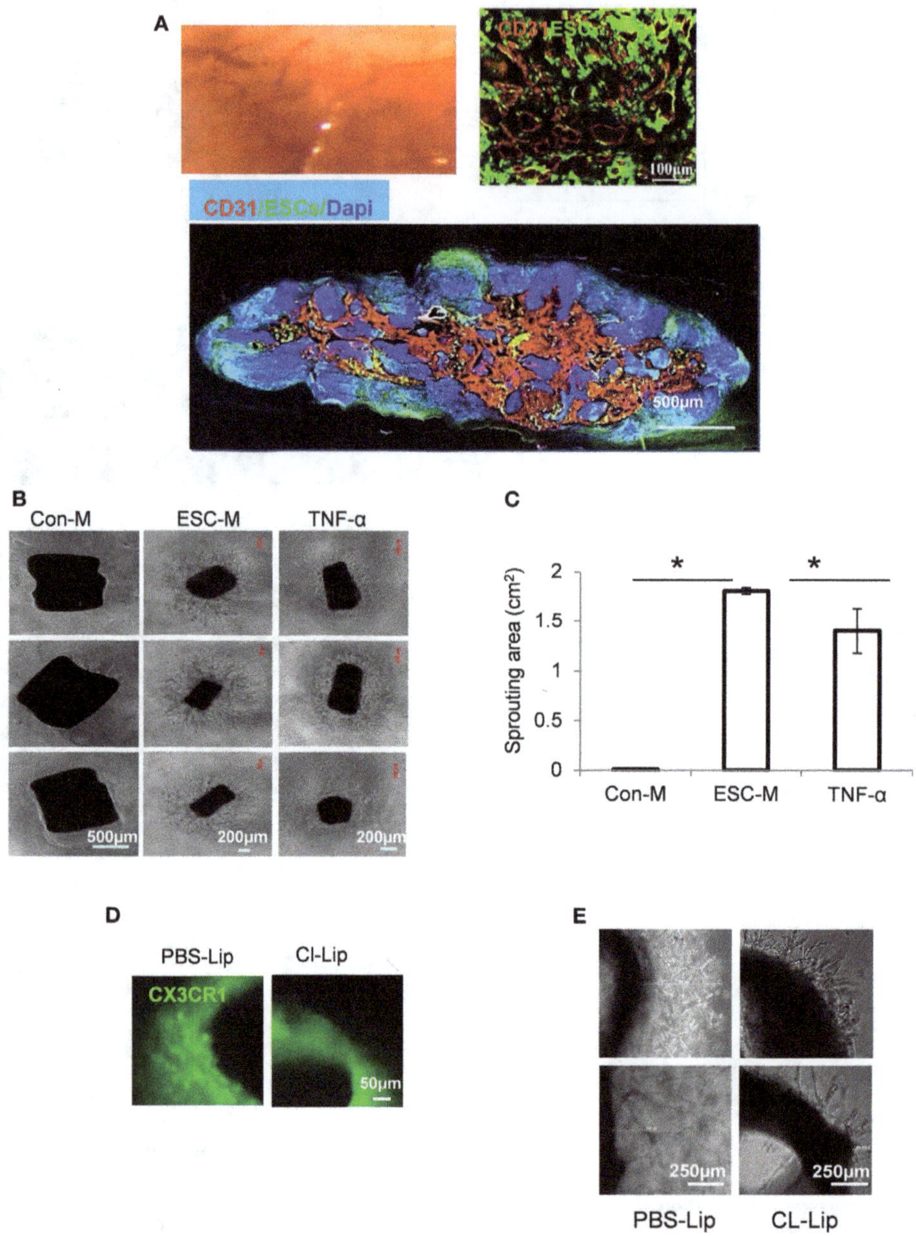

FIGURE 6 | Embryonic stem cells induced an angiogenic switch in macrophages. (A) Representative gross morphology micrograph showing blood vessel development during teratoma progression (top left) and immunostaining by endothelial marker CD31 (red) in sections from mice at 3 weeks after ESC injection (top right and bottom). **(B)** Representative gross morphology of aortic rings in Matrigel containing Con-M (left panel), ESC-M (middle panel), or TNF-α at 10 ng/ml (right panel) at day 6. **(C)** Area of vascular sprouting at day 6 in Con-M, ESC-M, and TNF-α was measured by ImageJ ($n = 6$, $^*p < 0.05$, two-sided Wilcoxon test. Data are represented as mean ± SEM). **(D)** Representative gross morphology of aortic ring from CX3CR1$^{GFP/+}$ mice treated with PBS-Lip (left) and CL-Lip for 4 weeks (right). **(E)** Mice were treated with PBS-Lip (left) and CL-Lip (right) for 4 weeks and aortic rings were cultured in Matrigel containing ESC-M for 6 days. Representative gross morphology of aortic ring sprouting was taken.

Cl-Lip was significantly lower than that of control treatment (**Figure 7C**). Blood vessels were significantly smaller in Cl-Lip-treated teratoma compared to control treatment (**Figure 7C**). Depletion of macrophages did not affect the pluripotency of ESCs, as all three germ layers can be observed in macrophage-deleted teratoma (**Figure 7D**). Teratomas from mice treated with PBS-Lip appeared much darker and were filled with blood, indicating that functional vasculature had formed via angiogenesis (**Figure 7E**). In contrast, tumor tissue from mice treated with Cl-Lip was transparent (**Figure 7E**). Subsequently, ablation of macrophages significantly inhibited teratoma growth, with a mean tumor size of 83.13 ± 60.81 mm^3 in Cl-Lip group vs. 2502.75 ± 1410.02 mm^3 in mice treated with PBS-Lip ($n = 5$, $p < 0.05$, **Figure 7F**).

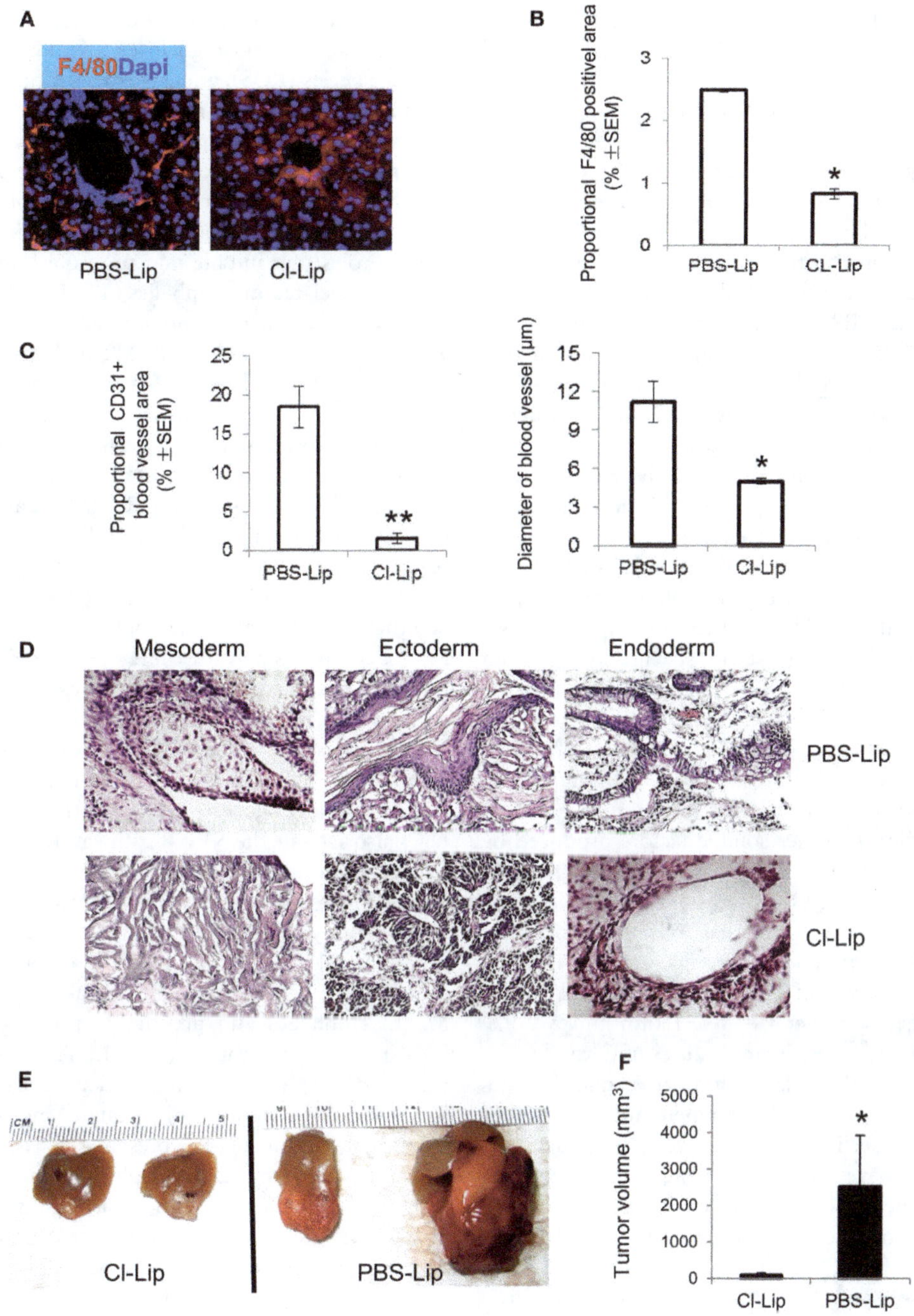

FIGURE 7 | Depletion of macrophages inhibiting angiogenesis and teratoma growth. (A) Cl-Lip was administrated i.p. at the day for ESC injection and twice a week for 4 weeks. PBS-Lip was used as control. Liver tissues were stained with F4/80. Note that Cl-Lip treatment completely depleted F4/80$^+$ macrophages in liver harvested from the Cl-Lip-treated group (left) and control group (treated with PBS-Lip) at 4 weeks after ESC transplantation. Quantification of F4/80$^+$ macrophages **(B)**, density of blood vessels stained for CD31 [**(C)**, left], size of blood vessels [**(C)**, right], HE staining **(D)**, and representative images of teratomas **(E)** in teratomas from Cl-Lip- or PBS-Lip-treated mice at 4 weeks after ESC transplantation. **(F)** Average teratoma size at 4 weeks after ESC transplantation in the Cl-Lip and PBS-Lip treated groups. $^*p < 0.05$, $^{**}p < 0.001$, $n = 5$, two-sided Wilcoxon test. Data are represented as mean ± SEM.

DISCUSSION

In this study, we demonstrated for the first time that BMDMs can be guided by ESCs to migrate to the site of ESC implantation while soluble factor(s) produced by ESCs polarize macrophages into a novel Arg-1^{high}Tie-2^{high}TNF-α^{high} phenotype. Furthermore, ESCs can prevent BMDM apoptosis induced by M-CSF-withdrawal through PI3K/Akt and ERK1/2 activation. We demonstrated that these ESC-educated macrophages (SEM) exhibit an elongated morphology and produce high level of TNF-α, which participates in angiogenesis and contributes to teratoma progression. Depletion of macrophages completely inhibits ESC-induced angiogenesis and teratoma development. These studies provide a novel rationale for the control of teratoma development by targeting macrophage growth or activation.

Macrophage colony-stimulating factor is known to regulate monocyte/macrophage survival (32, 33). PI3K/Akt and ERK or MARK are the major signaling pathways triggered by M-CSF stimulation (35, 46, 47). We showed that ESCs promote the survival of cultured BMDMs after M-CSF withdrawal, and that activation of both PI3K/Akt and ERK1/2 MAP kinase are required for the survival effect of ESCs, which is similar to that activated by M-CSF. ESC-maintained macrophage survival and function was independent of M-CSF, because M-CSF was detectable neither in ESC-M nor in ESC-M-treated macrophages (24). In the present study, we studied whether other factors are involved as autocrine or paracrine effectors to induce macrophage survival. For example, GM-CSF and IL-4 are known to regulate monocyte/macrophage survival (48). Our results ruled out the requirement for GM-CSF and IL-4, as these cytokines were undetectable in ESC-M (24). Recent studies reported that IL-34 is an alternative ligand for M-CSF receptor (CSF-1R) (34, 49). IL-34 binds specifically to human and mouse myeloid cells, induces ERK1/2 activation, and supports macrophage proliferation and differentiation (34). We showed that IL-34 is highly expressed by ESCs. IL-34 promotes macrophage survival and activates ERK and PI3K pathways. Although IL-34 also results in cell elongation, its effect is not as strong as that of ESC-M. It is possible that other soluble factors produced by ESCs play a role in cell shape change. It has been reported recently that IL-34-activated macrophages exhibit an IL-10^{high} IL-12^{low} M2 profile in response to LPS stimulation (50). Therefore, it is likely that IL-34 produced by ESCs play a pivotal role in ESC-induced macrophage survival and M2 polarization. More studies are needed to investigate whether IL-34 secretion and M2-like polarization of macrophages are general features of ESCs.

It is interesting to note that a large number of macrophages exist in the early stage of teratoma development and the number of macrophages rapidly declines at 2 weeks after ESC injection. We reasoned that ESCs have ability to regulate macrophage survival and activation. The inhibition of macrophage apoptosis by ESCs at an early stage may favor teratoma initiation and development. However, the effect of ESCs on macrophage may be reduced once ESCs are differentiated into its three germ layer structures. It will be important to determine whether fully differentiated tissues lose the ability to maintain macrophage function or have the capacity to inhibit macrophage survival. Beside IL-34, the factors produced by ESCs that promote macrophage growth and program M2-like phenotype remain unknown. It is possible that the function/phenotypes of macrophages are regulated by coordinated action of different classes of molecules secreted by ESCs. However, more detailed studies will be necessary to determine whether additional molecules either alone or in combination contribute to macrophage survival. The identification of these factors appears crucial in the development of strategies to prevent and/or reverse macrophage phenotype and thereby increase the safety of stem cell applications in clinical settings.

Beside mediation of macrophage survival, ESCs are able to regulate macrophage activation. It is well-documented that M1 macrophages express high levels of nitric oxide (NO), reactive oxygen species (ROS), and TNF-α, contributing to tissue inflammation and damage. In contrast, M2 macrophages produce anti-inflammatory factors and have a reduced capacity to produce pro-inflammatory molecules, thereby contributing to wound healing and tissue remodeling, as well as tumor progression (51–53). Tumor microenvironment educates macrophages to perform supportive roles that initiate and promote tumor progression (28). Tumor-associated macrophages (TAMs) have many properties of M2 phenotype such as impaired expression of IL-12 and TNF-α, and up-regulated levels of M2 markers including Arg-1 and YM1 (54–58). However, TAMs from several tumor models also exhibit typical M1 cytokines such as TNF-α and IL-1β (59). We previously showed that ESC-treated macrophages express higher levels of M2 markers such as PPAR-γ, Arg-1, YM1, as well as M2 cytokines including VEGF, MMP9, and MCP-1 (24), suggesting that ESCs induced the M2-like phenotype. In the present study, we demonstrated that ESCs not only increased Arg-1 and Tie-2^{+} expression but also triggered TNF-α expression, implying that ESC-educated macrophages are different from classic M2 macrophages and resemble more TAMs. ESCs–macrophages not only exhibited M2 characteristics (expression of M2 markers and STAT3/6 activation) but also acquired properties of M1 macrophages (activation of NF-κB) and TAMs (high levels of Tie-2 and TNF-α), exhibiting enhanced neovasculation in an *in vitro* and *ex vivo* angiogenesis assay. Another point of interest is that ESCs also activate the NF-κB pathway. Defective NF-κB activation within macrophages leads to the development of an M2 activation. Although ESCs are not oncogenically transformed, they have potent ability to regulate macrophage function and induce the unique Arg-1^{high}Tie-2^{high}TNF-α^{high} phenotype. Tie-2-expressing monocytes/macrophages (TEM) share some characteristics with M2 macrophages and are highly pro-angiogenic cells critical for tumor vascularization (59, 60). Tie-2 expression can be up-regulated by TNF-α (61). Specific depletion of TEM or conditional *Tie2* knockdown inhibits tumor angiogenesis. (62–64). Within the ESC implantation site, the presence of Tie-2^{+} macrophages and TNF-α secreted by ESC-macrophages stimulates angiogenesis and supports teratoma growth. Several angiogenic molecules may be linked to ESC-induced angiogenesis. We previously showed that ESCs increased macrophage MIF, MMP9, VEGF, and MCP-1. MIF secretion is tightly regulated by TNF-α (65, 66) and MIF can also increase TNF-α expression (67, 68). Therefore, TNF-α may be the key factor in ESC-induced angiogenesis. Anti-TNF-α agents such as infliximab (IFX), etanercept (ETA), adalimumab (ADA), golimumab (GLM), and certolizumab pegol (CZP) have been widely used for the treatment of a variety of chronic inflammatory diseases. Thus targeting TNF-α by administration of TNF-α antagonists may be a promising option to suppress teratoma angiogenesis. However, side effects such as increasing frequency of infection and promoting tumor growth by induction of T cell apoptosis make anti-TNF-α treatment a difficult balance. Administration of CZP can minimize this side effect since it does not induce T cell apoptosis but remains an efficacious treatment for inflammatory diseases because of the lack of an Fc region (69).

Embryonic stem cells can attract macrophages, induce M2 activation, and promote macrophage survival, and consequently, inhibition of any of these three functions could potentially offer a therapeutic solution to prevent teratoma development. A few strategies are developed to target macrophages: inhibiting macrophage migration, suppressing macrophage survival, promoting M1 activation, and blocking M2 polarization (70). Our data suggested that IL-34 maybe important to maintain macrophage survival via activation of PI3K and ERK1/2. Therefore, targeting IL-34 and the PI3K/ERK pathways could decrease macrophage number effectively and alter the microenvironment involved in teratoma angiogenesis and development. Because IL-34 was recently discovered (34), no antagonists are currently available to inhibit IL-34 activity. Thus, in turn, the antagonists of IL-34 receptor (CSF-1R) can be applied to block IL-34 binding to its receptor. Anti-CSF-1R treatment to inhibit tumor growth *in vitro* and *in vivo* has been well-documented (71, 72). Similar strategies can be applied to target macrophages in teratoma models. In addition, combined targeting of the ERK1/2 and PI3K pathways in teratoma may be a potential therapeutic strategy. Numerous small molecule inhibitors of specific PI3K and ERK1/2 pathways have been developed to exhibit promising anti-tumor activity *in vitro* and *in vivo* (73). For example, therapy with a dual PI3K (ZSTK474) and MEK inhibitor (CI-1040) combination is more effective than either inhibitor alone in cancer treatment (74). Combination of the PI3K inhibitor GDC-094 and the MEK inhibitor PD 0325901 induced marked tumor growth inhibition *in vivo* (75). Further study is required to demonstrate whether the dual PI3K and ERK inhibition have anti-teratoma activity *in vivo*, either through direct inhibition of macrophage survival, or ESC growth because PI3K is implicated in regulation of ESC proliferation (76).

Specifically, targeting M2 or TAM-like cells remains challenging. It has been shown that pharmacological skewing of TAM polarization from an M2 macrophage phenotype to a full M1 macrophage phenotype sustains anti-tumor immunity (57). It is possible to re-polarize TAMs. The recent report showed that M2pep, a peptide, can preferentially binds to M2 macrophages with low affinity for other leukocytes. Systemical administration of an M2pep fusion peptide with a proapoptotic peptide specifically reduced M2-like macrophages (77). A combination of CpG oligodeoxynucleotides and an IL-10 receptor-specific antibody switched TAMs from an M2 to an M1 type and triggered an innate response that was able to cure the majority of mice bearing large tumors (78).

One therapeutic option is to target STAT3. Numerous studies demonstrated that constitutive activation of STAT3 promotes initiation and development of tumors by inducing cell proliferation, angiogenesis, and metastasis in a wide variety of tumors (79). Furthermore, STAT3 is a critical mediator of LIF-induced signaling pathways that regulate ES cell self-renewal and proliferation (80). STAT3 also contributes to M2 macrophage activation. Therefore, STAT3 could be an attractive target to control teratoma development by direct effects on ESC growth and macrophage M2-like activation. Numerous strategies to suppress STAT3 activation have been developed such as anti-sense oligonucleotide targeting STAT3, synthetic drugs, small molecules, and gene therapy techniques (79).

In conclusion, our present findings show an important link between ESC-induced macrophage infiltration, growth and activation, initiation of angiogenesis, and teratoma development. ESCs induce BMDM accumulation and stew novel pro-angiogenic phenotype and thus accelerate teratoma development. A better understanding of the regulation and function of macrophages in the tumorigenicity of ESCs may yield useful therapies for the safe transplantation of ESCs. Targeting of the host microenvironment of the transplantation site such as modulating macrophage phenotype and function rather than ESCs directly could be a more efficient approach for suppressing angiogenesis and teratoma progression without affecting the pluripotency of ESCs.

AUTHOR CONTRIBUTIONS

The author(s) have made the following declarations about their contributions: conceived and designed the experiments: Yi Ren. Performed the experiments: Tianxiang Chen, Xi Wang, Lei Guo, Mingmei Wu, Zhaoxia Duan, Jing Lv, Wenjiao Tai, Hemamalini Renganathan, and Ruth Didier. Analyzed the data: Tianxiang Chen, Xi Wang, Jianqing Fan, and Yi Ren. Contributed reagents/materials/analysis tools: Jinhua Li, Xiaoming Chen, Dongming Sun, Xijing He, Jianqing Fan, and Wise Young. Wrote the first draft of the paper: Yi Ren. Contributed to the writing of the paper: Yi Ren.

ACKNOWLEDGMENTS

The authors acknowledge Dr. M. Schachner for providing mouse EGFP–ESCs and help from Dr. N. Goldsmith. The authors also thank Dr. B. Watson for proofreading the manuscript. Financial disclosure: this work was supported by the National Science Foundation (DMS-0714589 to Yi Ren), National Institutes of Health (R01GM100474-01 to Jianqing Fan and Yi Ren), a Joyce and Les Goodman scholarship (to Yi Ren), National Natural Science Foundation of China (81301996 to Tianxiang Chen; 81171156 to Xi Wang), and Zhejiang Provincial Natural Science Foundation of China (LQ13H160012 to Tianxiang Chen). The funders had no role in study design, data collection and analysis, decision to publish, or preparation of the manuscript.

REFERENCES

1. Sharpe ME, Morton D, Rossi A. Nonclinical safety strategies for stem cell therapies. *Toxicol Appl Pharmacol* (2012) **262**(3):223–31. doi:10.1016/j.taap.2012.05.007
2. Nussbaum J, Minami E, Laflamme MA, Virag JA, Ware CB, Masino A, et al. Transplantation of undifferentiated murine embryonic stem cells in the heart: teratoma formation and immune response. *FASEB J* (2007) **21**(7):1345–57. doi:10.1096/fj.06-6769com
3. Swijnenburg RJ, Tanaka M, Vogel H, Baker J, Kofidis T, Gunawan F, et al. Embryonic stem cell immunogenicity increases upon differentiation after transplantation into ischemic myocardium. *Circulation* (2005) **112**(9 Suppl):166–72. doi:10.1161/circulationaha.104.525824
4. Reubinoff BE, Pera MF, Fong CY, Trounson A, Bongso A. Embryonic stem cell lines from human blastocysts: somatic differentiation in vitro. *Nat Biotechnol* (2000) **18**(4):399–404. doi:10.1038/74447
5. Chaudhry GR, Fecek C, Lai MM, Wu WC, Chang M, Vasquez A, et al. Fate of embryonic stem cell derivatives implanted into the vitreous of a slow retinal degenerative mouse model. *Stem Cells Dev* (2009) **18**(2):247–58. doi:10.1089/scd.2008.0057
6. Lee AS, Tang C, Rao MS, Weissman IL, Wu JC. Tumorigenicity as a clinical hurdle for pluripotent stem cell therapies. *Nat Med* (2013) **19**(8):998–1004. doi:10.1038/nm.3267

7. Kim JH, Auerbach JM, Rodriguez-Gomez JA, Velasco I, Gavin D, Lumelsky N, et al. Dopamine neurons derived from embryonic stem cells function in an animal model of Parkinson's disease. *Nature* (2002) **418**(6893):50–6. doi:10.1038/nature00900
8. Chung S, Shin BS, Hedlund E, Pruszak J, Ferree A, Kang UJ, et al. Genetic selection of sox1GFP-expressing neural precursors removes residual tumorigenic pluripotent stem cells and attenuates tumor formation after transplantation. *J Neurochem* (2006) **97**(5):1467–80. doi:10.1111/j.1471-4159.2006.03841.x
9. Fukuda H, Takahashi J, Watanabe K, Hayashi H, Morizane A, Koyanagi M, et al. Fluorescence-activated cell sorting-based purification of embryonic stem cell-derived neural precursors averts tumor formation after transplantation. *Stem Cells* (2006) **24**(3):763–71. doi:10.1634/stemcells.2005-0137
10. Ben-David U, Benvenisty N. Chemical ablation of tumor-initiating human pluripotent stem cells. *Nat Protoc* (2014) **9**(3):729–40. doi:10.1038/nprot.2014.050
11. Bieberich E, Silva J, Wang G, Krishnamurthy K, Condie BG. Selective apoptosis of pluripotent mouse and human stem cells by novel ceramide analogues prevents teratoma formation and enriches for neural precursors in ES cell-derived neural transplants. *J Cell Biol* (2004) **167**(4):723–34. doi:10.1083/jcb.200405144
12. Choo AB, Tan HL, Ang SN, Fong WJ, Chin A, Lo J, et al. Selection against undifferentiated human embryonic stem cells by a cytotoxic antibody recognizing podocalyxin-like protein-1. *Stem Cells* (2008) **26**(6):1454–63. doi:10.1634/stemcells.2007-0576
13. Schuldiner M, Itskovitz-Eldor J, Benvenisty N. Selective ablation of human embryonic stem cells expressing a "suicide" gene. *Stem Cells* (2003) **21**(3):257–65. doi:10.1634/stemcells.21-3-257
14. Tang C, Lee AS, Volkmer JP, Sahoo D, Nag D, Mosley AR, et al. An antibody against SSEA-5 glycan on human pluripotent stem cells enables removal of teratoma-forming cells. *Nat Biotechnol* (2011) **29**(9):829–34. doi:10.1038/nbt.1947
15. Ben-David U, Gan QF, Golan-Lev T, Arora P, Yanuka O, Oren YS, et al. Selective elimination of human pluripotent stem cells by an oleate synthesis inhibitor discovered in a high-throughput screen. *Cell Stem Cell* (2013) **12**(2):167–79. doi:10.1016/j.stem.2012.11.015
16. Ben-David U, Nudel N, Benvenisty N. Immunologic and chemical targeting of the tight-junction protein claudin-6 eliminates tumorigenic human pluripotent stem cells. *Nat Commun* (2013) **4**:1992. doi:10.1038/ncomms2992
17. Lee MO, Moon SH, Jeong HC, Yi JY, Lee TH, Shim SH, et al. Inhibition of pluripotent stem cell-derived teratoma formation by small molecules. *Proc Natl Acad Sci U S A* (2013) **110**(35):E3281–90. doi:10.1073/pnas.1303669110
18. Suzuki DE, Nakahata AM, Okamoto OK. Knockdown of E2F2 inhibits tumorigenicity, but preserves stemness of human embryonic stem cells. *Stem Cells Dev* (2014) **23**(11):1266–74. doi:10.1089/scd.2013.0592
19. Lee AS, Tang C, Cao F, Xie X, van der Bogt K, Hwang A, et al. Effects of cell number on teratoma formation by human embryonic stem cells. *Cell Cycle* (2009) **8**(16):2608–12. doi:10.4161/cc.8.16.9353
20. Hentze H, Soong PL, Wang ST, Phillips BW, Putti TC, Dunn NR. Teratoma formation by human embryonic stem cells: evaluation of essential parameters for future safety studies. *Stem Cell Res* (2009) **2**(3):198–210. doi:10.1016/j.scr.2009.02.002
21. Rong Z, Fu X, Wang M, Xu Y. A scalable approach to prevent teratoma formation of human embryonic stem cells. *J Biol Chem* (2012) **287**(39):32338–45. doi:10.1074/jbc.M112.383810
22. Goldring CE, Duffy PA, Benvenisty N, Andrews PW, Ben-David U, Eakins R, et al. Assessing the safety of stem cell therapeutics. *Cell Stem Cell* (2011) **8**(6):618–28. doi:10.1016/j.stem.2011.05.012
23. Dressel R, Schindehutte J, Kuhlmann T, Elsner L, Novota P, Baier PC, et al. The tumorigenicity of mouse embryonic stem cells and in vitro differentiated neuronal cells is controlled by the recipients' immune response. *PLoS One* (2008) **3**(7):e2622. doi:10.1371/journal.pone.0002622
24. Wang X, Chen T, Leng L, Fan J, Cao K, Duan Z, et al. MIF produced by bone marrow-derived macrophages contributes to teratoma progression after embryonic stem cell transplantation. *Cancer Res* (2012) **72**(11):2867–78. doi:10.1158/0008-5472.can-11-3247
25. Biswas SK, Sica A, Lewis CE. Plasticity of macrophage function during tumor progression: regulation by distinct molecular mechanisms. *J Immunol* (2008) **180**(4):2011–7. doi:10.4049/jimmunol.180.4.2011
26. Allavena P, Sica A, Garlanda C, Mantovani A. The Yin-Yang of tumor-associated macrophages in neoplastic progression and immune surveillance. *Immunol Rev* (2008) **222**:155–61. doi:10.1111/j.1600-065X.2008.00607.x
27. Lewis CE, Pollard JW. Distinct role of macrophages in different tumor microenvironments. *Cancer Res* (2006) **66**(2):605–12. doi:10.1158/0008-5472.can-05-4005
28. Pollard JW. Tumour-educated macrophages promote tumour progression and metastasis. *Nat Rev Cancer* (2004) **4**(1):71–8. doi:10.1038/nrc1256
29. Tian Y, Jain S, Kelemen SE, Autieri MV. AIF-1 expression regulates endothelial cell activation, signal transduction, and vasculogenesis. *Am J Physiol Cell Physiol* (2009) **296**(2):C256–66. doi:10.1152/ajpcell.00325.2008
30. Van Rooijen N, Sanders A. Liposome mediated depletion of macrophages: mechanism of action, preparation of liposomes and applications. *J Immunol Methods* (1994) **174**(1–2):83–93. doi:10.1016/0022-1759(94)90012-4
31. Mostofi FK, Sesterhenn I. Histological classification of testis tumours. *Histological Typing of Testis Tumours.* Berlin Heidelberg: Springer-Verlag (1998). p. 3–5.
32. Jaworowski A, Wilson NJ, Christy E, Byrne R, Hamilton JA. Roles of the mitogen-activated protein kinase family in macrophage responses to colony stimulating factor-1 addition and withdrawal. *J Biol Chem* (1999) **274**(21):15127–33. doi:10.1074/jbc.274.21.15127
33. Hundal RS, Gomez-Munoz A, Kong JY, Salh BS, Marotta A, Duronio V, et al. Oxidized low density lipoprotein inhibits macrophage apoptosis by blocking ceramide generation, thereby maintaining protein kinase B activation and Bcl-XL levels. *J Biol Chem* (2003) **278**(27):24399–408. doi:10.1074/jbc.M209179200
34. Lin H, Lee E, Hestir K, Leo C, Huang M, Bosch E, et al. Discovery of a cytokine and its receptor by functional screening of the extracellular proteome. *Science* (2008) **320**(5877):807–11. doi:10.1126/science.1154370
35. Kelley TW, Graham MM, Doseff AI, Pomerantz RW, Lau SM, Ostrowski MC, et al. Macrophage colony-stimulating factor promotes cell survival through Akt/protein kinase B. *J Biol Chem* (1999) **274**(37):26393–8. doi:10.1074/jbc.274.37.26393
36. Bhatt NY, Kelley TW, Khramtsov VV, Wang Y, Lam GK, Clanton TL, et al. Macrophage-colony-stimulating factor-induced activation of extracellular-regulated kinase involves phosphatidylinositol 3-kinase and reactive oxygen species in human monocytes. *J Immunol* (2002) **169**(11):6427–34. doi:10.4049/jimmunol.169.11.6427
37. Wang Y, Zeigler MM, Lam GK, Hunter MG, Eubank TD, Khramtsov VV, et al. The role of the NADPH oxidase complex, p38 MAPK, and Akt in regulating human monocyte/macrophage survival. *Am J Respir Cell Mol Biol* (2007) **36**(1):68–77. doi:10.1165/rcmb.2006-0165OC
38. McWhorter FY, Wang T, Nguyen P, Chung T, Liu WF. Modulation of macrophage phenotype by cell shape. *Proc Natl Acad Sci U S A* (2013) **110**(43):17253–8. doi:10.1073/pnas.1308887110
39. Sica A, Schioppa T, Mantovani A, Allavena P. Tumour-associated macrophages are a distinct M2 polarised population promoting tumour progression: potential targets of anti-cancer therapy. *Eur J Cancer* (2006) **42**(6):717–27. doi:10.1016/j.ejca.2006.01.003
40. Mantovani A, Schioppa T, Porta C, Allavena P, Sica A. Role of tumor-associated macrophages in tumor progression and invasion. *Cancer Metastasis Rev* (2006) **25**(3):315–22. doi:10.1007/s10555-006-9001-7
41. Masson VV, Devy L, Grignet-Debrus C, Bernt S, Bajou K, Blacher S, et al. Mouse aortic ring assay: a new approach of the molecular genetics of angiogenesis. *Biol Proced Online* (2002) **4**:24–31. doi:10.1251/bpo30
42. Gelati M, Aplin AC, Fogel E, Smith KD, Nicosia RF. The angiogenic response of the aorta to injury and inflammatory cytokines requires macrophages. *J Immunol* (2008) **181**(8):5711–9. doi:10.4049/jimmunol.181.8.5711
43. Qian B, Deng Y, Im JH, Muschel RJ, Zou Y, Li J, et al. A distinct macrophage population mediates metastatic breast cancer cell extravasation, establishment and growth. *PLoS One* (2009) **4**(8):e6562. doi:10.1371/journal.pone.0006562
44. Jung S, Aliberti J, Graemmel P, Sunshine MJ, Kreutzberg GW, Sher A, et al. Analysis of fractalkine receptor CX(3)CR1 function by targeted deletion and green fluorescent protein reporter gene insertion. *Mol Cell Biol* (2000) **20**(11):4106–14. doi:10.1128/MCB.20.11.4106-4114.2000
45. Geissmann F, Manz MG, Jung S, Sieweke MH, Merad M, Ley K. Development of monocytes, macrophages, and dendritic cells. *Science* (2010) **327**(5966):656–61. doi:10.1126/science.1178331

46. Sengupta A, Liu WK, Yeung YG, Yeung DC, Frackelton AR Jr, Stanley ER. Identification and subcellular localization of proteins that are rapidly phosphorylated in tyrosine in response to colony-stimulating factor 1. *Proc Natl Acad Sci U S A* (1988) **85**(21):8062–6. doi:10.1073/pnas.85.21.8062
47. Hamilton JA. CSF-1 signal transduction. *J Leukoc Biol* (1997) **62**(2):145–55.
48. Sieweke MH, Allen JE. Beyond stem cells: self-renewal of differentiated macrophages. *Science* (2013) **342**(6161):1242974. doi:10.1126/science.1242974
49. Wei S, Nandi S, Chitu V, Yeung YG, Yu W, Huang M, et al. Functional overlap but differential expression of CSF-1 and IL-34 in their CSF-1 receptor-mediated regulation of myeloid cells. *J Leukoc Biol* (2010) **88**(3):495–505. doi:10.1189/jlb.1209822
50. Foucher ED, Blanchard S, Preisser L, Garo E, Ifrah N, Guardiola P, et al. IL-34 induces the differentiation of human monocytes into immunosuppressive macrophages. Antagonistic effects of GM-CSF and IFNgamma. *PLoS One* (2013) **8**(2):e56045. doi:10.1371/journal.pone.0056045
51. Mantovani A, Sica A, Sozzani S, Allavena P, Vecchi A, Locati M. The chemokine system in diverse forms of macrophage activation and polarization. *Trends Immunol* (2004) **25**(12):677–86. doi:10.1016/j.it.2004.09.015
52. Martinez FO, Sica A, Mantovani A, Locati M. Macrophage activation and polarization. *Front Biosci* (2008) **13**:453–61. doi:10.2741/2692
53. Gordon S. Alternative activation of macrophages. *Nat Rev Immunol* (2003) **3**(1):23–35. doi:10.1038/nri978
54. Gordon S, Martinez FO. Alternative activation of macrophages: mechanism and functions. *Immunity* (2010) **32**(5):593–604. doi:10.1016/j.immuni.2010.05.007
55. Biswas SK, Gangi L, Paul S, Schioppa T, Saccani A, Sironi M, et al. A distinct and unique transcriptional program expressed by tumor-associated macrophages (defective NF-kappaB and enhanced IRF-3/STAT1 activation). *Blood* (2006) **107**(5):2112–22. doi:10.1182/blood-2005-01-0428
56. Sica A, Mantovani A. Macrophage plasticity and polarization: in vivo veritas. *J Clin Invest* (2012) **122**(3):787–95. doi:10.1172/jci59643
57. Sica A, Bronte V. Altered macrophage differentiation and immune dysfunction in tumor development. *J Clin Invest* (2007) **117**(5):1155–66. doi:10.1172/jci31422
58. Martinez FO, Helming L, Gordon S. Alternative activation of macrophages: an immunologic functional perspective. *Annu Rev Immunol* (2009) **27**:451–83. doi:10.1146/annurev.immunol.021908.132532
59. Biswas SK, Mantovani A. Macrophage plasticity and interaction with lymphocyte subsets: cancer as a paradigm. *Nat Immunol* (2010) **11**(10):889–96. doi:10.1038/ni.1937
60. Lewis CE, De Palma M, Naldini L. Tie2-expressing monocytes and tumor angiogenesis: regulation by hypoxia and angiopoietin-2. *Cancer Res* (2007) **67**(18):8429–32. doi:10.1158/0008-5472.can-07-1684
61. Chen JX, Chen Y, DeBusk L, Lin W, Lin PC. Dual functional roles of Tie-2/angiopoietin in TNF-alpha-mediated angiogenesis. *Am J Physiol Heart Circ Physiol* (2004) **287**(1):H187–95. doi:10.1152/ajpheart.01058.2003
62. Capobianco A, Monno A, Cottone L, Venneri MA, Biziato D, Di Puppo F, et al. Proangiogenic Tie2(+) macrophages infiltrate human and murine endometriotic lesions and dictate their growth in a mouse model of the disease. *Am J Pathol* (2011) **179**(5):2651–9. doi:10.1016/j.ajpath.2011.07.029
63. De Palma M, Venneri MA, Galli R, Sergi Sergi L, Politi LS, Sampaolesi M, et al. Tie2 identifies a hematopoietic lineage of proangiogenic monocytes required for tumor vessel formation and a mesenchymal population of pericyte progenitors. *Cancer Cell* (2005) **8**(3):211–26. doi:10.1016/j.ccr.2005.08.002
64. Mazzieri R, Pucci F, Moi D, Zonari E, Ranghetti A, Berti A, et al. Targeting the ANG2/TIE2 axis inhibits tumor growth and metastasis by impairing angiogenesis and disabling rebounds of proangiogenic myeloid cells. *Cancer Cell* (2011) **19**(4):512–26. doi:10.1016/j.ccr.2011.02.005
65. Bernhagen J, Calandra T, Bucala R. Regulation of the immune response by macrophage migration inhibitory factor: biological and structural features. *J Mol Med (Berl)* (1998) **76**(3–4):151–61. doi:10.1007/s001090050204
66. Calandra T, Bernhagen J, Metz CN, Spiegel LA, Bacher M, Donnelly T, et al. MIF as a glucocorticoid-induced modulator of cytokine production. *Nature* (1995) **377**(6544):68–71. doi:10.1038/377068a0
67. Donnelly SC, Haslett C, Reid PT, Grant IS, Wallace WA, Metz CN, et al. Regulatory role for macrophage migration inhibitory factor in acute respiratory distress syndrome. *Nat Med* (1997) **3**(3):320–3. doi:10.1038/nm0397-320
68. Mitchell RA, Liao H, Chesney J, Fingerle-Rowson G, Baugh J, David J, et al. Macrophage migration inhibitory factor (MIF) sustains macrophage proinflammatory function by inhibiting p53: regulatory role in the innate immune response. *Proc Natl Acad Sci U S A* (2002) **99**(1):345–50. doi:10.1073/pnas.012511599
69. Nesbitt A, Fossati G, Bergin M, Stephens P, Stephens S, Foulkes R, et al. Mechanism of action of certolizumab pegol (CDP870): in vitro comparison with other anti-tumor necrosis factor alpha agents. *Inflamm Bowel Dis* (2007) **13**(11):1323–32. doi:10.1002/ibd.20225
70. Tang X, Mo C, Wang Y, Wei D, Xiao H. Anti-tumour strategies aiming to target tumour-associated macrophages. *Immunology* (2013) **138**(2):93–104. doi:10.1111/imm.12023
71. Hume DA, MacDonald KP. Therapeutic applications of macrophage colony-stimulating factor-1 (CSF-1) and antagonists of CSF-1 receptor (CSF-1R) signaling. *Blood* (2012) **119**(8):1810–20. doi:10.1182/blood-2011-09-379214
72. Pyonteck SM, Akkari L, Schuhmacher AJ, Bowman RL, Sevenich L, Quail DF, et al. CSF-1R inhibition alters macrophage polarization and blocks glioma progression. *Nat Med* (2013) **19**(10):1264–72. doi:10.1038/nm.3337
73. Britten CD. PI3K and MEK inhibitor combinations: examining the evidence in selected tumor types. *Cancer Chemother Pharmacol* (2013) **71**(6):1395–409. doi:10.1007/s00280-013-2121-1
74. Jokinen E, Laurila N, Koivunen JP. Alternative dosing of dual PI3K and MEK inhibition in cancer therapy. *BMC Cancer* (2012) **12**:612. doi:10.1186/1471-2407-12-612
75. Haagensen EJ, Thomas HD, Wilson I, Harnor SJ, Payne SL, Rennison T, et al. The enhanced in vivo activity of the combination of a MEK and a PI3K inhibitor correlates with [18F]-FLT PET in human colorectal cancer xenograft tumour-bearing mice. *PLoS One* (2013) **8**(12):e81763. doi:10.1371/journal.pone.0081763
76. Welham MJ, Kingham E, Sanchez-Ripoll Y, Kumpfmueller B, Storm M, Bone H. Controlling embryonic stem cell proliferation and pluripotency: the role of PI3K- and GSK-3-dependent signalling. *Biochem Soc Trans* (2011) **39**(2):674–8. doi:10.1042/bst0390674
77. Cieslewicz M, Tang J, Yu JL, Cao H, Zavaljevski M, Motoyama K, et al. Targeted delivery of proapoptotic peptides to tumor-associated macrophages improves survival. *Proc Natl Acad Sci U S A* (2013) **110**(40):15919–24. doi:10.1073/pnas.1312197110
78. Guiducci C, Vicari AP, Sangaletti S, Trinchieri G, Colombo MP. Redirecting in vivo elicited tumor infiltrating macrophages and dendritic cells towards tumor rejection. *Cancer Res* (2005) **65**(8):3437–46. doi:10.1158/0008-5472.can-04-4262
79. Siveen KS, Sikka S, Surana R, Dai X, Zhang J, Kumar AP, et al. Targeting the STAT3 signaling pathway in cancer: role of synthetic and natural inhibitors. *Biochim Biophys Acta* (2014) **1845**(2):136–54. doi:10.1016/j.bbcan.2013.12.005
80. Yang J, van Oosten AL, Theunissen TW, Guo G, Silva JC, Smith A. Stat3 activation is limiting for reprogramming to ground state pluripotency. *Cell Stem Cell* (2010) **7**(3):319–28. doi:10.1016/j.stem.2010.06.022

Conflict of Interest Statement: The authors declare that the research was conducted in the absence of any commercial or financial relationships that could be construed as a potential conflict of interest.

4

From pre-DP, post-DP, SP4, and SP8 thymocyte cell counts to a dynamical model of cortical and medullary selection

Maria Sawicka[1†], Gretta L. Stritesky[2†], Joseph Reynolds[1], Niloufar Abourashchi[1], Grant Lythe[1], Carmen Molina-París[1]* and Kristin A. Hogquist[2]*

[1] Department of Applied Mathematics, School of Mathematics, University of Leeds, Leeds, UK
[2] Department of Laboratory Medicine and Pathology, Center for Immunology, University of Minnesota, Minneapolis, MN, USA

Edited by:
Ramit Mehr, Bar-Ilan University, Israel

Reviewed by:
Ramit Mehr, Bar-Ilan University, Israel
Ruy Ribeiro, Los Alamos National Laboratory, USA
Christian Schönbach, Nazarbayev University, Kazakhstan

***Correspondence:**
Carmen Molina-París, Department of Applied Mathematics, School of Mathematics, University of Leeds, Leeds LS2 9JT, UK
e-mail: carmen@maths.leeds.ac.uk;
Kristin A. Hogquist, Department of Laboratory Medicine and Pathology, Center for Immunology, University of Minnesota, 2101 6th Street SE, Minneapolis, MN 55414, USA
e-mail: hogqu001@umn.edu

†Maria Sawicka and Gretta L. Stritesky have contributed equally to this work.

Cells of the mature $\alpha\beta$ T cell repertoire arise from the development in the thymus of bone marrow precursors (thymocytes). $\alpha\beta$ T cell maturation is characterized by the expression of thousands of copies of identical $\alpha\beta$ T cell receptors and the CD4 and/or CD8 co-receptors on the surface of thymocytes. The maturation stages of a thymocyte are: (1) double negative (DN) (TCR^-, $CD4^-$ and $CD8^-$), (2) double positive (DP) (TCR^+, $CD4^+$ and $CD8^+$), and (3) single positive (SP) (TCR^+, $CD4^+$ or $CD8^+$). Thymic antigen presenting cells provide the appropriate micro-architecture for the maturation of thymocytes, which "sense" the signaling environment via their randomly generated TCRs. Thymic development is characterized by (i) an extremely low success rate, and (ii) the selection of a functional and self-tolerant T cell repertoire. In this paper, we combine recent experimental data and mathematical modeling to study the selection events that take place in the thymus after the DN stage. The stable steady state of the model for the pre-DP, post-DP, and SP populations is identified with the experimentally measured cell counts from 5.5- to 17-week-old mice. We make use of residence times in the cortex and the medulla for the different populations, as well as recently reported asymmetric death rates for CD4 and CD8 SP thymocytes. We estimate that 65.8% of pre-DP thymocytes undergo death by neglect. In the post-DP compartment, 91.7% undergo death by negative selection, 4.7% become CD4 SP, and 3.6% become CD8 SP. Death by negative selection in the medulla removes 8.6% of CD4 SP and 32.1% of CD8 SP thymocytes. Approximately 46.3% of CD4 SP and 27% of CD8 SP thymocytes divide before dying or exiting the thymus.

Keywords: thymocytes, negative selection, positive selection, death by neglect, mathematical model, steady state

1. INTRODUCTION

T cells are a major component of the adaptive immune system that play a crucial role in protection against a wide variety of pathogens. The T cell receptor (TCR) is generated by somatic recombination and has a vast potential to recognize foreign organisms. T cells do not recognize pathogens directly, but rather through binding pathogen fragments displayed by major histocompatibility complex (MHC) proteins on the surface of antigen presenting cells (APCs). Since MHC molecules are highly polymorphic, useful T cells must be selected for in each individual of the species. These T cells must have lineage specific effector functions that may include direct lysis, production of cytokines, and ability to regulate immune responses. Furthermore, some T cells have the potential to drive dangerous autoimmune responses (1). For all of these reasons, the development of a T cell repertoire is a highly specialized and tightly regulated process (2, 3). It takes place in a dedicated organ, the thymus, where unique properties of the microenvironment ensure the production of functional, yet self-tolerant T cells (4–6).

Multi-potent precursors travel from the bone marrow to the thymus through the blood. When they enter the thymus, the precursors that commit to the T cell lineage [or canonical early T cell progenitors (7)], after a 2 week period on average, transition from the double negative (DN) stage, where they do not express the co-receptors CD4 and CD8, to the double positive (DP) stage, where they express both co-receptors (6). At this stage, the majority of the cells have made productive TCR gene rearrangements and express a fully formed $\alpha\beta$ TCR on the cell surface. DP cells are located in the cortex region of the thymus, where they use their TCR to survey self-peptides presented by MHCs on cortical thymic epithelial cells (cTECs) (8). DPs that recognize self-peptide-MHC complexes with low affinity undergo positive selection, whereas those with high affinity are deleted by negative selection (3). Those DP that fail to recognize self-peptide-MHC will undergo apoptosis in a process referred to as death by neglect. The DP cells that are positively selected will then transition to the single positive (SP) stage, where they express either the CD4 or CD8 co-receptor, depending upon their MHC class specificity (9). MHC class specificity also dictates gene expression changes that will ultimately determine the effector functions of that T cell: generally, cytotoxicity for CD8 T cells and cytokine production for CD4 T cells. All positively selected cells, whether MHC class I or class II specific, up-regulate the chemokine receptor CCR7, which facilitates their migration to the medulla, where they undergo further selection events. The medulla contains medullary epithelial cells (mTECs) that express tissue-restricted antigens regulated by the nuclear factor Aire (10).

Exposure to tissue-restricted antigens allows for further deletion of T cells specific for self-antigens they may encounter in the periphery. Finally, those cells that have been positively selected, yet have avoided negative selection, will mature and migrate to the periphery (11).

Previous efforts to develop mathematical models of thymic selection have been based on deterministic approaches or cellular automata simulations. These studies have shown the importance of (i) thymic antigen diversity on the size of the selected T cell repertoire (12), (ii) death rates for the more differentiated thymocyte subsets (13), (iii) thymocyte proliferation and residence times (14), (iv) epithelial networks for thymocyte development and migration (15), (v) thymocyte competition for antigen (16), (vi) self-pMHC complexes expressed on dendritic cells (DCs) (17), (vii) receptor–ligand binding affinity (18), and (viii) a sharp threshold in TCR-ligand binding affinity that defines the boundary between negative and positive selection (19). Recent work by Ribeiro and Perelson (20) supports the need to develop appropriate mathematical models to interpret T cell receptor excision circles (or TREC) data, which are used to quantify thymic export (20). Sinclair et al. in Ref. (21) bring together experimental immunology with mathematical modeling to conclude that CD8 precursor thymocytes are more susceptible to death than CD4 precursors. This asymmetry in the death rates underlies the experimentally observed CD4:CD8 T cell ratio in the periphery.

Previous experimental studies have tried to determine the number of cells going through positive and negative selection in the thymus. However, reports estimating the relative number of cells undergoing negative selection compared to positive selection have been widely variable. Some find that very few cells undergo negative selection; others find that two times more cells undergo negative selection than positive selection (22–25). In this report, we develop a deterministic mathematical model of T cell development in the thymus. Some of us recently published a report where we used a novel approach (Bim$^{-/-}$Nur77^{GFP} mice) that allowed us to calculate the number of cells undergoing positive and negative selection (26). Using previously published data on the relative life-span of DP and SP cells, we estimated the hourly rate of both positive and negative selection (26). In this manuscript, we make use of (i) a subset of this experimental data, and (ii) the asymmetric death rates observed for CD4 and CD8 precursor thymocytes (21), to develop two mathematical models that will enable us to estimate selection rates in the cortex and the medulla, and provide a quantitative measure for the stringency of thymic selection. The first model (see Section 2.1) allows the identification of the following parameters: DN thymocyte influx into the cortex, pre-DP and post-DP death rates, and pre-DP and post-DP differentiation rates. Under the assumption of asymmetric death rates for the CD4 and CD8 SP thymocytes (21), we extend the first model to provide estimates for the following medullary rates (see Section 2.2): CD4 and CD8 SP death, proliferation, and maturation rates.

2. MATERIALS AND METHODS

2.1. A FIRST MODEL OF THYMIC DEVELOPMENT AFTER THE DN STAGE

In this section, we introduce a deterministic model of thymocyte development after the DN stage. This first model will be required to calibrate the parameter values of the second model introduced in Section 2.2. In particular, and as described in Section 3.2, the first model allows the identification of parameter values for the following rates: ϕ, μ_1, μ_2, φ_1, and φ_2.

This mathematical model makes use of a data set obtained from the analysis of eight C57BL/6 wild type and Bim deficient mice (average age 9 weeks), that express a Nur77^{GFP} transgene to indicate TCR signal strength experience (26). Flow cytometric analysis, as described in that study, used standard markers to define various stages of T cell development in the thymus. The Nur77^{GFP} reporter and Bim deficiency were novel modifications that allowed us to quantify cells that normally would be deleted by strong TCR signaling. In the mathematical model, we consider the following thymocyte populations: n_1, the population of pre-selection DP thymocytes (double positive), that are TCRβ^{low} and CD69^{low} (26), n_2, the population of post-selection DP thymocytes, that are TCRβ^{+} and CD69^{high} (26), and n_3, the population of mature SP (single positive) thymocytes.

We assume that DN thymocytes differentiate to become pre-selection DP thymocytes with rate (cells/day) ϕ. We further assume that after the DN stage, thymocyte cell fate is determined by the TCR signal, which a given thymocyte has received. Sinclair et al. used CFSE labeling to show that there is no proliferation at the post-DP stage (see Figure A1 of their manuscript) (21). Stritesky et al. looked at proliferation in the post-DP pool with BrdU labeling, and found no evidence (26). We have, thus, only included proliferation in the SP thymocyte population (21, 26). The three populations, n_1, n_2, and n_3, are involved in the following selection events in the cortex and the medulla (see **Figure 1**):

- $\emptyset \xrightarrow{\phi} n_1$ – flux of DN thymocytes into compartment n_1,
- $n_1 \xrightarrow{\varphi_1} n_2$ – differentiation from pre-DP (n_1) to post-DP (n_2) thymocytes induced by TCR signal,
- $n_1 \xrightarrow{\mu_1} \emptyset$ – death by neglect of pre-DP thymocytes due to lack of (or weak) TCR signal,
- $n_2 \xrightarrow{\varphi_2} n_3$ – differentiation from post-DP (n_2) to SP (n_3) thymocytes sustained by intermediate TCR signal,
- $n_2 \xrightarrow{\mu_2} \emptyset$ – apoptosis of post-DP (n_2) thymocytes due to strong TCR signal,
- $n_3 \xrightarrow{\varphi_3}$ periphery – exit of SP thymocytes (n_3) to the periphery (thymic maturation),
- $n_3 \xrightarrow{\lambda_3} 2\, n_3$ – proliferation of SP thymocytes (n_3) in the medulla, and
- $n_3 \xrightarrow{\mu_3} \emptyset$ – apoptosis of SP (n_3) thymocytes due to strong TCR signal.

The time evolution of the three populations can be described by the following set of ordinary differential equations (ODEs), which are based on the selection events described above:

$$\begin{cases} \dfrac{dn_1}{dt} = \phi - \varphi_1 n_1 - \mu_1 n_1\,, \\ \dfrac{dn_2}{dt} = \varphi_1 n_1 - \varphi_2 n_2 - \mu_2 n_2\,, \\ \dfrac{dn_3}{dt} = \varphi_2 n_2 - \varphi_3 n_3 - \mu_3 n_3 + \lambda_3 n_3\,. \end{cases} \tag{1}$$

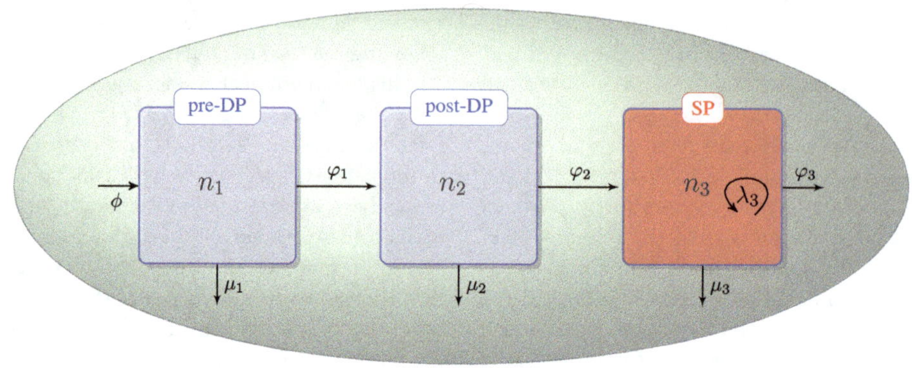

FIGURE 1 | Thymic development as hypothesized in the first model. The flux, ϕ, represents the differentiation of DNs into pre-DPs. Pre-DP thymocytes have two fates: further differentiation into the post-DP pool (φ_1) or death by neglect (μ_1). Post-DP thymocytes have two fates: further differentiation into the SP pool (φ_2) or death by apoptosis (μ_2). Finally, SP thymocytes have three fates: maturation and exit into the periphery (φ_3), death by apoptosis (μ_3), or proliferation (λ_3).

We are interested in studying the steady state of these populations, as the experimental data correspond to population cell numbers in the three stages (pre-DP, post-DP, and SP) for a steady state thymus (26). The steady state of the system of equations [equation (1)] is given by:

$$n_1^* = \frac{\phi}{\varphi_1 + \mu_1}, \quad n_2^* = \frac{n_1^*\varphi_1}{\varphi_2 + \mu_2}, \quad n_3^* = \frac{n_2^*\varphi_2}{\varphi_3 + \mu_3 - \lambda_3}. \quad (2)$$

This unique steady state exists if and only if $\varphi_3 + \mu_3 - \lambda_3 > 0$, so that we have $n_3^* > 0$. In order to study the linear stability of the steady state, we calculate A, the Jacobian matrix of equation (1), as follows:

$$A = \begin{pmatrix} -(\varphi_1 + \mu_1) & 0 & 0 \\ \varphi_1 & -(\varphi_2 + \mu_2) & 0 \\ 0 & \varphi_2 & -(\varphi_3 + \mu_3 - \lambda_3) \end{pmatrix}. \quad (3)$$

A is also the Jacobian matrix at the steady state $n^* = (n_1^*, n_2^*, n_3^*)$, as the system of ODEs [equation (1)] is linear. The three eigenvalues of A are given by (as the matrix is lower triangular):

$$\beta_1 = -(\varphi_1 + \mu_1), \quad \beta_2 = -(\varphi_2 + \mu_2), \quad \beta_3 = -(\varphi_3 + \mu_3 - \lambda_3).$$

Therefore, the steady state [equation (2)] is stable, if and only if, $\varphi_3 + \mu_3 - \lambda_3 > 0$, which is also the condition for its existence. We conclude this section with the analytical solution of the system of ODEs [equation (1)], given initial conditions, which provides the time evolution of the three thymocyte populations:

$$n_1(t) = n_1^* + n_1(0)\, e^{-(\varphi_1+\mu_1)t},$$

$$n_2(t) = n_2^* + \frac{n_1(0)\,\varphi_1}{[(\varphi_2 + \mu_2) - (\varphi_1 + \mu_1)]} e^{-(\varphi_1+\mu_1)t} + n_2(0)\, e^{-(\varphi_2+\mu_2)t},$$

$$n_3(t) = n_3^* + \frac{n_1(0)\,\varphi_1}{[(\varphi_2 + \mu_2) - (\varphi_1 + \mu_1)]} \times \frac{\varphi_2}{[(\varphi_3 + \mu_3 - \lambda_3) - (\varphi_1 + \mu_1)]} e^{-(\varphi_1+\mu_1)t} + \frac{n_2(0)\,\varphi_3}{[(\varphi_3 + \mu_3 - \lambda_3) - (\varphi_2 + \mu_2)]} e^{-(\varphi_2+\mu_2)t} + n_3(0)\, e^{-(\varphi_3+\mu_3-\lambda_3)t}, \quad (4)$$

where $n_1(0)$, $n_2(0)$, $n_3(0)$ represent the initial conditions for the thymocyte populations. Note that in the late time limit, that is, if $t \to +\infty$ and $\varphi_3 + \mu_3 - \lambda_3 > 0$, then $n_1(t) \to n_1^*$, $n_2(t) \to n_2^*$ and $n_3(t) \to n_3^*$, as it is the unique stable steady state.

2.2. A SECOND MODEL OF THYMIC DEVELOPMENT AFTER THE DN STAGE: CD4 AND CD8 SP THYMOCYTES

As described in Section 2.1, the first deterministic model will allow us to calibrate some of the parameters of a more comprehensive model, which we now introduce. We subdivide the SP thymocyte population in two classes: CD4 SP and CD8 SP thymocytes. This is an extension of the model introduced in the previous section, and is motivated by the fact that experimentally, SP thymocytes express either the CD4 or the CD8 co-receptor. We now have four different thymocyte populations to consider: n_1, the population of pre-selection DP (double positive) thymocytes, n_2, the population of post-selection DP thymocytes, n_4, the population of mature $CD4^+$ SP (single positive) thymocytes, and n_8, the population of mature $CD8^+$ SP (single positive) thymocytes.

As described in the previous section, we assume that DN thymocytes differentiate to become pre-selection DP thymocytes with rate (cells/day) ϕ, and that after the DN stage, thymocyte cell fate is determined by the TCR signal, which a given thymocyte has received. Thus, the four populations, n_1, n_2, n_4, and n_8, with $n_3 = n_4 + n_8$, are involved in the following selection events in the cortex and the medulla (see **Figure 2**):

- $\emptyset \xrightarrow{\phi} n_1$ – flux of DN thymocytes into compartment n_1,
- $n_1 \xrightarrow{\varphi_1} n_2$ – differentiation from pre-DP (n_1) to post-DP (n_2) thymocytes induced by TCR signal,

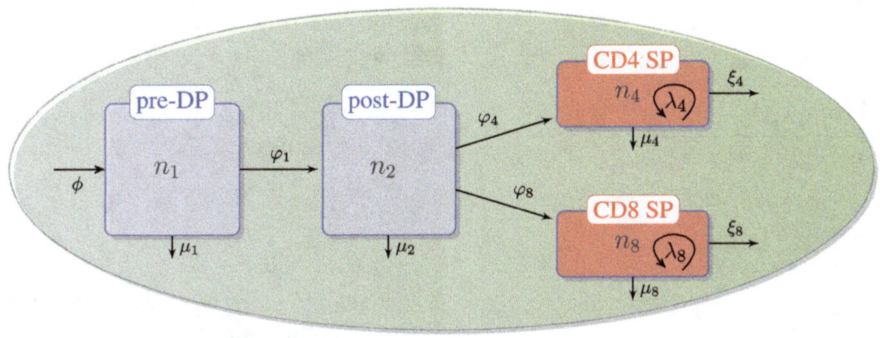

FIGURE 2 | Thymic development as hypothesized in the second model. We assume there is a flux, ϕ, that represents the differentiation of DNs into pre-DPs. Pre-DP thymocytes have two fates: further differentiation into the post-DP pool (φ_1) or death by neglect (μ_1). Post-DP thymocytes have three fates: further differentiation into the SP pool as CD4 SPs (φ_4), or CD8 SPs (φ_8), or death by apoptosis (μ_2). Finally, CD4 or CD8 SP thymocytes have three fates: maturation and exit into the periphery (ξ_4) or (ξ_8), death by apoptosis (μ_4) or (μ_8), or proliferation (λ_4) or (λ_8).

- $n_1 \xrightarrow{\mu_1} \emptyset$ – death by neglect of pre-DP thymocytes due to lack of (or weak) TCR signal,
- $n_2 \xrightarrow{\varphi_4} n_4$ – differentiation from post-DP (n_2) to CD4$^+$ SP (n_4) sustained by intermediate TCR signal,
- $n_2 \xrightarrow{\varphi_8} n_8$ – differentiation from post-DP (n_2) to CD8$^+$ SP (n_8) sustained by intermediate TCR signal,
- $n_2 \xrightarrow{\mu_2} \emptyset$ – apoptosis of post-DP (n_2) thymocytes due to strong TCR signal,
- $n_4 \xrightarrow{\xi_4}$ periphery – exit of CD4$^+$ SP thymocytes (n_4) to the periphery (thymic maturation),
- $n_8 \xrightarrow{\xi_8}$ periphery – exit of CD8$^+$ SP thymocytes (n_8) to the periphery (thymic maturation),
- $n_4 \xrightarrow{\lambda_4} 2\,n_4$ – proliferation of CD4$^+$ SP thymocytes (n_4) in the medulla,
- $n_8 \xrightarrow{\lambda_8} 2\,n_8$ – proliferation of CD8$^+$ SP thymocytes (n_8) in the medulla,
- $n_4 \xrightarrow{\mu_4} \emptyset$ – apoptosis of CD4$^+$SP (n_4) thymocytes due to strong TCR signal, and
- $n_8 \xrightarrow{\mu_8} \emptyset$ – apoptosis of CD8$^+$SP (n_8) thymocytes due to strong TCR signal.

We assume that all model parameters are positive, that is, μ_1, μ_2, μ_4, μ_8, φ_1, φ_2, φ_4, φ_8, ξ_4, ξ_8, ϕ, λ_4, $\lambda_8 > 0$, and note that the parameters and thymocyte populations of the first and second model are related by the following equations:

$$\varphi_2 = \varphi_4 + \varphi_8\,, \quad \xi_4\, n_4 + \xi_8\, n_8 = \varphi_3\, n_3\,,$$
$$\mu_4\, n_4 + \mu_8\, n_8 = \mu_3\, n_3\,, \quad \lambda_4\, n_4 + \lambda_8\, n_8 = \lambda_3\, n_3\,. \qquad (5)$$

The time evolution of the four populations can be described by the following set of ODEs:

$$\begin{cases} \frac{dn_1}{dt} = \phi - \varphi_1 n_1 - \mu_1 n_1\,, \\ \frac{dn_2}{dt} = \varphi_1 n_1 - (\varphi_4 + \varphi_8) n_2 - \mu_2 n_2\,, \\ \frac{dn_4}{dt} = \varphi_4 n_2 - \xi_4 n_4 - \mu_4 n_4 + \lambda_4 n_4\,, \\ \frac{dn_8}{dt} = \varphi_8 n_2 - \xi_8 n_8 - \mu_8 n_8 + \lambda_8 n_8\,. \end{cases} \qquad (6)$$

We are interested in studying the steady state of these populations, as the experimental data correspond to population cell numbers in the four stages (pre-DP, post-DP, CD4 SP, and CD8 SP) for a steady state thymus (26). The steady state of the system of equations [equation (6)] is given by:

$$n_1^* = \frac{\phi}{\varphi_1 + \mu_1}\,, \quad n_2^* = \frac{n_1^* \varphi_1}{\varphi_4 + \varphi_8 + \mu_2}\,,$$
$$n_4^* = \frac{n_2^* \varphi_4}{\xi_4 + \mu_4 - \lambda_4}\,, \quad n_8^* = \frac{n_2^* \varphi_8}{\xi_8 + \mu_8 - \lambda_8}\,. \qquad (7)$$

This unique steady state exists if and only if $\xi_4 + \mu_4 - \lambda_4 > 0$ and $\xi_8 + \mu_8 - \lambda_8 > 0$, so that we guarantee $n_4^* > 0$ and $n_8^* > 0$. In order to study the linear stability of the steady state, we calculate B, the Jacobian matrix of equation (6), as follows:

$$B = \begin{pmatrix} -(\varphi_1 + \mu_1) & 0 & 0 & 0 \\ \varphi_1 & -(\varphi_4 + \varphi_8 + \mu_2) & 0 & 0 \\ 0 & \varphi_4 & -(\xi_4 + \mu_4 - \lambda_4) & 0 \\ 0 & \varphi_8 & 0 & -(\xi_8 + \mu_8 - \lambda_8) \end{pmatrix}. \qquad (8)$$

B is also the Jacobian at the steady state $n^* = (n_1^*, n_2^*, n_4^*, n_8^*)$, as the system of ODEs is linear. The four eigenvalues of B are given by:

$$\beta_1 = -(\varphi_1 + \mu_1)\,, \quad \beta_2 = -(\varphi_4 + \varphi_8 + \mu_2)\,,$$
$$\beta_3 = -(\xi_4 + \mu_4 - \lambda_4)\,, \quad \beta_4 = -(\xi_8 + \mu_8 - \lambda_8)\,.$$

Therefore, the steady state equation (6) is stable if and only if $\xi_4 + \mu_4 - \lambda_4 > 0$ and $\xi_8 + \mu_8 - \lambda_8 > 0$, which is also the condition for its existence. We conclude this section with the analytical solution of the system of ODEs equation (6), given initial conditions, which provides the time evolution of the four thymocyte populations:

$$n_1(t) = n_1^* + n_1(0)\, e^{-(\varphi_1+\mu_1)t}\,,$$
$$n_2(t) = n_2^* + \frac{n_1(0)\, \varphi_1}{[(\varphi_4 + \varphi_8 + \mu_2) - (\varphi_1 + \mu_1)]}\, e^{-(\varphi_1+\mu_1)t} + n_2(0)\, e^{-(\varphi_4+\varphi_8+\mu_2)t}\,,$$

$$n_4(t) = n_4^* + \frac{n_1(0)\,\varphi_1}{[(\varphi_4+\varphi_8+\mu_2)-(\varphi_1+\mu_1)]} \times \frac{\varphi_4+\varphi_8}{[(\xi_4+\mu_4-\lambda_4)-(\varphi_1+\mu_1)]} e^{-(\varphi_1+\mu_1)t} + \frac{n_2(0)\,\xi_4}{[(\xi_4+\mu_4-\lambda_4)-(\varphi_4+\varphi_8+\mu_2)]} e^{-(\varphi_4+\varphi_8+\mu_2)t} + n_4(0)\,e^{-(\xi_4+\mu_4-\lambda_4)t},$$

$$n_8(t) = n_8^* + \frac{n_1(0)\,\varphi_1}{[(\varphi_4+\varphi_8+\mu_2)-(\varphi_1+\mu_1)]} \times \frac{\varphi_4+\varphi_8}{[(\xi_8+\mu_8-\lambda_8)-(\varphi_1+\mu_1)]} e^{-(\varphi_1+\mu_1)t} + \frac{n_2(0)\,\xi_8}{[(\xi_8+\mu_8-\lambda_8)-(\varphi_4+\varphi_8+\mu_2)]} e^{-(\varphi_4+\varphi_8+\mu_2)t} + n_8(0)\,e^{-(\xi_8+\mu_8-\lambda_8)t}, \tag{9}$$

where $n_1(0), n_2(0), n_4(0), n_8(0)$ represent the initial conditions for the thymocyte populations. Note that in the late time limit, that is, if $t \to +\infty$ and $\xi_4+\mu_4-\lambda_4 > 0$ and $\xi_8+\mu_8-\lambda_8 > 0$, then $n_1(t) \to n_1^*$, $n_2(t) \to n_2^*$, $n_4(t) \to n_4^*$, and $n_8(t) \to n_8^*$, as it is the unique stable steady state.

3. RESULTS

3.1. PARAMETER ESTIMATION FOR THE FIRST MODEL (MEANS)

In this section, we make use of previously published experimental data (26) that provide thymocyte cell counts for the three subsets considered in the first model: pre-DPs, post-DPs, and SPs. The original experiments have been carried out for two types of mice: wild type mice (Bim$^{+/-}$) and Bim deficient mice (Bim$^{-/-}$). In this paper, we will only be considering the wild type experimental results. The data will allow us to provide experimental estimates for the steady state thymocyte cell counts: n_1^*, n_2^*, n_3^*. Note that, in order to estimate rates (with units of inverse time), thymocyte cell counts are not enough. Thus, we will make use of the additional knowledge provided by experimentally determined residence times for each population, τ_i, with $i = 1, 2, 3$. If we make use of the model (see Section 2.1), the residence time in compartment i can be expressed as:

$$\tau_i = \frac{1}{\varphi_i + \mu_i}, \quad \text{for} \quad i \in \{1, 2, 3\}.$$

The experimental data (see **Table 1**) correspond to the number of cells (thymocytes) at steady state (26), in each of the thymic compartments considered in the mathematical models (see Sections 2.1 and 2.2), and for eight different mice ($j = 1, 2, \ldots, 8$).

We have made use of the following average residence times in each compartment (27–29)

$$\tau_1 = 60 \text{ h} = 2.5 \text{ days}, \quad \tau_2 = 16 \text{ h} = 0.67 \text{ days}, \quad \tau_3 = 96 \text{ h} = 4 \text{ days}.$$

In order to derive estimates for the model parameters, we have carried out the following steps:

1. We make use of the experimentally determined mature SP thymocyte flux from the medulla to the periphery, which has been estimated to be 1–4 × 10^6 cells per day (14, 26, 30). This flux corresponds to about 1% of thymocytes leaving the thymus every day (30). Given this flux, which we denote by ϕ_{out}, n_3^*, and the fact that $\phi_{\text{out}} = \varphi_3\, n_3^*$, we can obtain an estimate for φ_3. We have chosen ϕ_{out} to be 2.5 × 10^6 cells per day (14, 30).
2. Given τ_3, φ_3, and the fact that $\tau_3 = \frac{1}{\mu_3+\varphi_3}$, we can obtain an estimate for μ_3.
3. Given τ_1, n_1^*, and the fact that $n_1^* = \phi\, \tau_1$, we can obtain an estimate for ϕ.
4. We also have $n_2^* = \varphi_1\, \tau_2\, n_1^*$, which, in principle, allows us to estimate φ_1. We make use of linear regression techniques to do so (31, 32).

Let us introduce a_1 by the following equation, $a_1 = \frac{n_2^*}{n_1^*}$, and make use of the experimental data to write: $n_2^{*,i} = a\, n_1^{*,i} + \epsilon^i$, for $i = 1, 2, \ldots, 8$. Thus, the squared error is given by:

$$E(a_1) = \sum_{i=1}^{8} \left(n_2^{*,i} - a_1\, n_1^{*,i}\right)^2.$$

We minimize $E(a_1)$ with respect to a_1, that is $\frac{dE}{da_1} = 0$. Solving for a_1, we obtain:

$$a_1 = \frac{\sum_{i=1}^{8} n_1^{*,i}\, n_2^{*,i}}{\sum_{i=1}^{8} \left(n_1^{*,i}\right)^2}.$$

Table 1 | Experimental steady state thymocyte cell counts for the wild type pre-DP, post-DP, CD4 SP, and CD8 SP populations.

Mouse	n_1^* (pre-DP) (cells)	n_2^* (post-DP) (cells)	n_3^* (SP) (cells)	n_4^* (SP CD4) (cells)	n_8^* (SP CD8) (cells)
1	82.58 × 10^6	9.30 × 10^6	18.36 × 10^6	13.85 × 10^6	4.51 × 10^6
2	142.19 × 10^6	19.94 × 10^6	26.20 × 10^6	18.73 × 10^6	7.46 × 10^6
3	89.00 × 10^6	5.98 × 10^6	15.98 × 10^6	11.88 × 10^6	4.10 × 10^6
4	29.32 × 10^6	2.09 × 10^6	5.61 × 10^6	4.40 × 10^6	1.21 × 10^6
5	29.32 × 10^6	2.09 × 10^6	5.61 × 10^6	4.40 × 10^6	1.21 × 10^6
6	51.26 × 10^6	5.93 × 10^6	9.01 × 10^6	6.85 × 10^6	2.16 × 10^6
7	64.48 × 10^6	6.81 × 10^6	11.64 × 10^6	9.03 × 10^6	2.61 × 10^6
8	218.94 × 10^6	15.42 × 10^6	40.20 × 10^6	29.46 × 10^6	10.74 × 10^6
Mean	**88.39** × 10^6	**8.45** × 10^6	**16.57** × 10^6	**12.33** × 10^6	**4.25** × 10^6
Standard deviation	**60.11** × 10^6	**5.89** × 10^6	**11.05** × 10^6	**7.94** × 10^6	**3.12** × 10^6

The bold font highlights the mean and the standard deviation from the individual mice data.

Given a_1, we can then estimate φ_1 from the equation $\varphi_1 = \frac{a_1}{\tau_2}$.

5. Given τ_1, φ_1, and the fact that $\tau_1 = \frac{1}{\mu_1+\varphi_1}$, we can obtain an estimate for μ_1.
6. We are now left with three remaining parameters: φ_2, μ_2, and λ_3. Given the experimental constraints on τ_1, τ_2, and τ_3, we assume that the average time to proliferate, $1/\lambda_3$, cannot be <7 days. Therefore, we consider λ_3 to be constrained in the interval $[1/7, \tau_3^{-1}]$, with time measured in days. We sample equally spaced values for λ_3, and for each value, we compute $\varphi_2 = \frac{n_3^*(\varphi_3+\mu_3-\lambda_3)}{n_2^*}$. The ratio $a_2 = \frac{n_3^*}{n_2^*}$ is computed using the linear regression method described above (see **Figure 3**). In this way, we obtain an estimate for φ_3. We note that the p-values for a_1 and a_2 are given by 7.57×10^{-3} and 6.85×10^{-3}, respectively (both smaller than the significance level $\alpha = 0.05$).
7. Given τ_2, φ_2, and the fact that $\tau_2 = \frac{1}{\mu_2+\varphi_2}$, we can obtain an estimate for μ_2.
8. From steps 6 and 7 above, we have generated (a table of) values for φ_2 and μ_2, given a fiducial value for λ_3 in the interval $[1/7, \tau_3^{-1}]$. The mice considered in the experimental study are 5.5–17 weeks old, and their thymus is in steady state (26). Thus, we expect that the parameter values can only be accepted if the corresponding system of ODEs attains steady state by 3 weeks. Therefore, we only accept parameter values which provide thymocyte cell counts at time $t = 21$ days that are within one standard deviation from the experimentally determined values (see **Table 1**). That is, we impose for the given parameter set that the mathematically predicted value $n_i(t = 21$ days) belongs to the interval $n_i^* \pm \sigma_i$, with $i = 1, 2, 3$, and where n_i^* is the (experimental) mean number of cells in compartment i, and σ_i is the (experimental) standard deviation in compartment i, as given in **Table 1**.

We obtain the following parameter values:

$$\phi = 35.350 \times 10^6 \text{ cells/day}, \quad \mu_1 = 0.263 \text{ day}^{-1},$$
$$\mu_3 = 0.099 \text{ day}^{-1}, \quad \varphi_1 = 0.137 \text{ day}^{-1}, \quad \varphi_3 = 0.151 \text{ day}^{-1},$$

and

$$\mu_2 \in [1.295, 1.443] \text{ day}^{-1}, \quad \varphi_2 \in [0.050, 0.198] \text{ day}^{-1},$$
$$\lambda_3 \in [0.143, 0.250] \text{ day}^{-1}.$$

These parameters imply the following thymic selection rates:

3.1.1. *Death rates*

9.7×10^5 cells/h die by neglect in compartment 1 ($\mu_1\ n_1^*$), 4.8×10^5 cells/h die by negative selection in compartment 2 ($\mu_2\ n_2^*$), and 6.9×10^4 cells/h die by negative selection in compartment 3 ($\mu_3\ n_3^*$).

3.1.2. *Differentiation rates*

5.0×10^5 cells/h are positively selected in compartment 1, that is, become post-DP from pre-DP ($\varphi_1\ n_1^*$), 4.4×10^4 cells/h are positively selected in compartment 2, that is, become SP from post-DP ($\varphi_2\ n_2^*$), and 1.0×10^5 cells/h leave compartment 3 to go to the periphery ($\varphi_3\ n_3^*$).

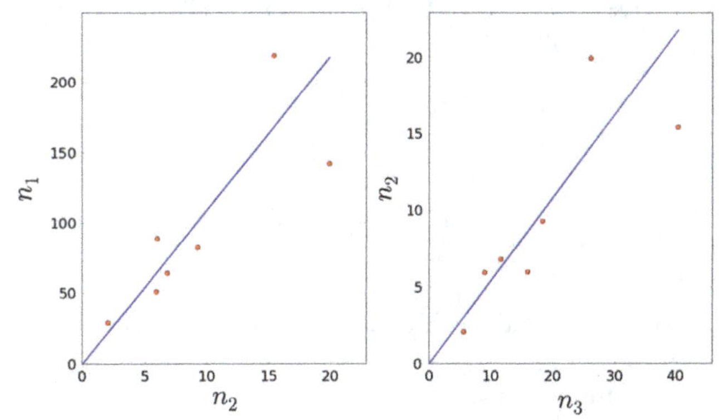

FIGURE 3 | Linear regression plots for the first model.

3.1.3. *Proliferation rate*

1.3×10^5 cells/h proliferate in compartment 3 ($\lambda_3\ n_3^*$).

We have also computed the stringency of thymic selection, which we define as given by the ratio:

$$\frac{\varphi_3\ n_3^*}{\phi} = 6.79\%.$$

Finally, we have computed the (per cell) probability to die, given that the cell is in compartment i ($i = 1, 2, 3$), as well as the (per cell) probability to proliferate in the medulla. We have obtained:

$$p_1 = \frac{\mu_1}{\mu_1 + \varphi_1} = 65.8\%, \quad p_2 = \frac{\mu_2}{\mu_2 + \varphi_2} = 91.7\%,$$
$$p_3 = \frac{\mu_3}{\mu_3 + \varphi_3 + \lambda_3} = 22.9\%, \quad q_3 = \frac{\lambda_3}{\mu_3 + \varphi_3 + \lambda_3} = 42.2\%.$$

3.2. PARAMETER ESTIMATION FOR THE SECOND MODEL (MEANS)

In this section, we make use of previously published experimental data (26) that provide thymocyte cell counts for the four subsets considered: pre-DPs, post-DPs, CD4 SPs, and CD8 SPs. We only make use of the experimental data for the wild type mice. The data will allow us to provide experimental estimates for the steady state thymocyte cell counts: $n_1^*, n_2^*, n_4^*, n_8^*$. As described in Section 3.1, we also need residence times for each population subset, τ_i, with $i = 1, 2, 4, 8$. If we make use of the model (see Section 2.2), the residence time in compartment i can be expressed as:

$$\tau_i = \frac{1}{\varphi_i + \mu_i}, \quad \text{for} \quad i \in \{1, 2\}, \quad \text{and}$$
$$\tau_i = \frac{1}{\xi_i + \mu_i}, \quad \text{for} \quad i \in \{4, 8\}.$$

Recent experimental data provide support for asymmetric death rates in the CD4 and CD8 SP compartments (21). The estimated death rates for CD4 and CD8 SP thymocytes are[1] $\mu_4 = 0.04$ day^{-1} and $\mu_8 = 0.11$ day^{-1}. We also make use of the estimates derived in Section 3.1 for ϕ, μ_1, μ_2, φ_1, and φ_2. Finally,

[1] Private communication from Ben Seddon and Andy Yates.

the average residence times in each compartment, as described in Section 3.1, are given by:

$$\tau_1 = 60\ \text{h} = 2.5\ \text{days}\,, \quad \tau_2 = 16\ \text{h} = 0.67\ \text{days}\,,$$
$$\tau_4 = 96\ \text{h} = 4\ \text{days}\,, \quad \tau_8 = 96\ \text{h} = 4\ \text{days}\,.$$

In order to derive estimates for the model parameters, we have carried out the following steps:

1. Given τ_4, μ_4, and the fact that $\tau_4 = \frac{1}{\mu_4+\xi_4}$, we can obtain an estimate for ξ_4.
2. In the same way, given τ_8, μ_8, and the fact that $\tau_8 = \frac{1}{\mu_8+\xi_8}$, we can obtain an estimate for ξ_8.
3. We are now left with four remaining parameters: $\varphi_4, \varphi_8, \lambda_4$, and λ_8. We know that $\varphi_2 = \varphi_4 + \varphi_8$. We sample φ_4 in the interval $[0, \varphi_2]$, where φ_2 is the mean value of the interval obtained in Section 2.1, and for each fiducial value for φ_4, we compute the corresponding value for φ_8.
4. Given τ_4, φ_4, and the fact that $n_4^* = \frac{n_2^*\varphi_4}{\tau_4^{-1}-\lambda_4}$, we can compute the fraction $a_3 = \frac{n_2^*}{n_4^*}$ by linear regression (see **Figure 4**), and thus obtain an estimate for λ_4. Note that we will reject values of λ_4 that imply the proliferation time is larger than 7 days (see Section 3.1).
5. In Section 3.1, we obtained an estimate for the mean of λ_3, and we know that $\lambda_4\ n_4^* + \lambda_8\ n_8^* = \lambda_3\ n_3^*$. As before, we can compute the fractions $a_4 = \frac{n_4^*}{n_8^*}$ and $a_5 = \frac{n_3^*}{n_8^*}$ by linear regression (see **Figure 4**), and thus obtain an estimate for λ_8. Note that we will reject values of λ_8 that imply the proliferation time is larger than 7 days (see Section 3.1). We note that the p-values for a_3, a_4, and a_5 are given by 8.43×10^{-3}, 3.33×10^{-7}, and 4.56×10^{-8}, respectively (smaller than the significance level).
6. From steps 3, 4, and 5 above, we have generated (a table of) values for φ_8, λ_4, and λ_8, given a fiducial value for φ_4 in the interval $[0, \varphi_2]$. As discussed in Section 3.1, we only accept parameter values which provide thymocyte cell counts at time $t = 21$ days that are within one standard deviation from the experimentally determined values (see **Table 1**).

We obtain the following parameter values:

$$\mu_4 = 0.04\ \text{day}^{-1}\,, \quad \mu_8 = 0.11\ \text{day}^{-1}\,,$$
$$\xi_4 = 0.21\ \text{day}^{-1}\,, \quad \xi_8 = 0.14\ \text{day}^{-1}\,,$$

and

$$\varphi_4 = 0.070\ \text{day}^{-1}\,, \quad \varphi_8 = 0.054\ \text{day}^{-1}\,,$$
$$\lambda_4 = 0.216\ \text{day}^{-1}\,, \quad \lambda_8 = 0.093\ \text{day}^{-1}\,.$$

These parameters imply the following thymic selection rates:

3.2.1. *Death rates*

2.05×10^4 cells/h die by negative selection in compartment 4 ($\mu_4\ n_4^*$) and 1.95×10^4 cells/h die by negative selection in compartment 8 ($\mu_8\ n_8^*$).

3.2.2. *Differentiation rates*

2.50×10^4 cells/h are CD4 positively selected in compartment 2, that is, become CD4 SP from post-DP ($\varphi_4\ n_2^*$), 1.90×10^4 cells/h are CD8 positively selected in compartment 2, that is, become CD8 SP from post-DP ($\varphi_8\ n_2^*$), 1.08×10^5 cells/h leave compartment 4 to go to the periphery ($\xi_4\ n_4^*$), and 2.48×10^4 cells/h leave compartment 8 to go to the periphery ($\xi_8\ n_8^*$).

3.2.3. *Proliferation rates*

11.10×10^4 cells/h proliferate in compartment 4 ($\lambda_4\ n_4^*$) and 1.60×10^4 cells/h proliferate in compartment 8 ($\lambda_8\ n_8^*$).

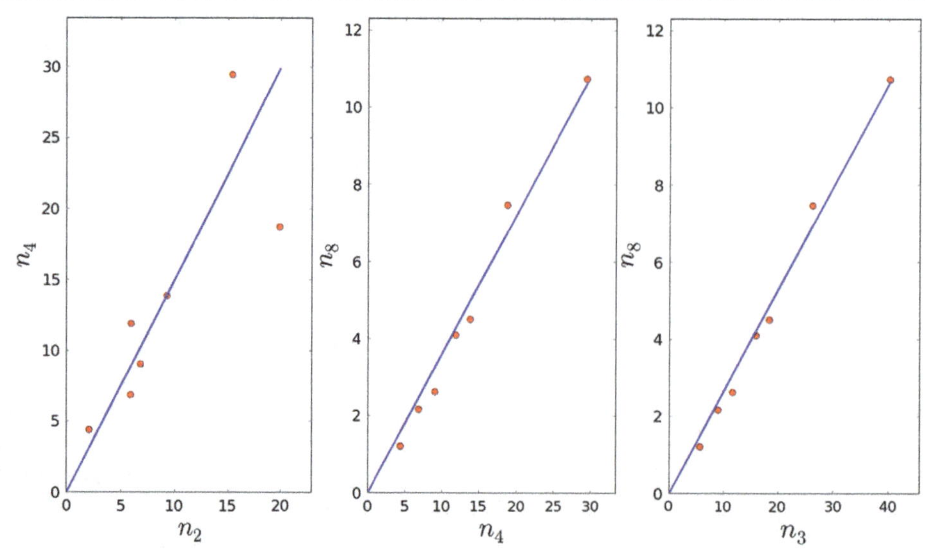

FIGURE 4 | Linear regression plots for the second model.

We can compute the stringency of thymic selection, defined by the ratio:

$$\frac{\xi_4\, n_4^* + \xi_8\, n_8^*}{\phi} = 8.96\%\,.$$

We can provide an estimate for the cortical positive selection probabilities, that is the (per post-DP cell) probability to become a CD4 SP or a CD8 SP, and the probability to be negatively selected in the cortex. We have obtained:

$$s_4 = \frac{\varphi_4}{\mu_2 + \varphi_4 + \varphi_8} = 4.7\%\,,\quad s_8 = \frac{\varphi_8}{\mu_2 + \varphi_4 + \varphi_8} = 3.6\%\,,$$
$$p_2 = \frac{\mu_2}{\mu_2 + \varphi_4 + \varphi_8} = 91.7\%\,.$$

Finally, we have computed the (per cell) probability to die, given that the cell is in compartment i, as well as the (per cell) probability to proliferate in the medulla. We obtain:

$$p_4 = \frac{\mu_4}{\mu_4 + \xi_4 + \lambda_4} = 8.6\%\,,\quad q_4 = \frac{\lambda_4}{\mu_4 + \xi_4 + \lambda_4} = 46.3\%\,,$$
$$p_8 = \frac{\mu_8}{\mu_8 + \xi_8 + \lambda_8} = 32.1\%\,,\quad q_8 = \frac{\lambda_8}{\mu_8 + \xi_8 + \lambda_8} = 27.0\%\,.$$

These probabilities imply that the probability to exit the thymus as a mature CD4 thymocyte (that has already reached the medulla) is given by $\frac{100-(8.6+46.3)}{100}$, which is 45.1%, and the probability to exit as a mature CD8 thymocyte (that has already reached the medulla) is given by $\frac{100-(32.1+27.0)}{100}$, which is 40.9%.

3.3. SENSITIVITY ANALYSIS

In this section, we explore the sensitivity of the parameters to perturbations in the experimental data. For the first model, the experimental data are given in terms of the following eight quantities:

$$\theta = (\tau_1, \tau_2, \tau_3, \phi_{\text{out}}, a_1, a_2, \bar{n}_3, \bar{n}_1)\,,$$

where a_1, a_2 are the coefficients of the linear regression of $\frac{n_2^*}{n_1^*}$ and $\frac{n_3^*}{n_2^*}$, respectively, and $\bar{n}_i$ is the experimental mean value of n_i.

We perturb each entry of the vector θ by adding and subtracting 10% of its value. Therefore, we now have two values for θ_i, equal to $\theta_i + \frac{1}{10}\theta_i$ and $\theta_i - \frac{1}{10}\theta_i$. Consequently, we have 2^8 sets of θ, which will be used to compute the corresponding model parameters as described in Section 3.1. Parameter values will only be accepted if they provide a stable solution before $t = 21$ days.

For the second model, the experimental data is given in terms of the following seven quantities:

$$\theta = (\tau_4, \tau_8, \mu_4, \mu_8, a_3, a_4, a_5)\,,$$

where a_3, a_4, a_5 are the coefficients of the linear regression of $\frac{n_2^*}{n_4^*}$, $\frac{n_4^*}{n_8^*}$, and $\frac{n_3^*}{n_8^*}$, respectively. We have made use of the means of the following parameters of the first model: $\phi, \varphi_1, \mu_1, \varphi_2, \mu_2, \lambda_3$.

Table 2 | Means, 95% trimmed and minimum–maximum intervals of the model parameters.

Parameter	Mean value	95% Trimmed interval	Minimum–maximum interval range
ϕ	35.86 × 10^6 cells/day	(35.65 × 10^6, 35.07 × 10^6) cells/day	(28.93, 43.21 × 10^6) cells/day
φ_1	0.139 day^{-1}	(0.138, 0.140) day^{-1}	(0.112, 0.167) day^{-1}
φ_2	0.136 day^{-1}	(0.134, 0.139) day^{-1}	(0.041, 0.274) day^{-1}
φ_4	0.140 day^{-1}	(0.136, 0.145) day^{-1}	(0.060, 0.264) day^{-1}
φ_8	0.134 day^{-1}	(0.129, 0.138) day^{-1}	(0.010, 0.214) day^{-1}
μ_1	0.265 day^{-1}	(0.263, 0.267) day^{-1}	(0.196, 0.333) day^{-1}
μ_2	1.372 day^{-1}	(1.365, 1.378) day^{-1}	(1.083, 1.618) day^{-1}
μ_4	0.040 day^{-1}	*n/a*	(0.036, 0.044) day^{-1}
μ_8	0.110 day^{-1}	*n/a*	(0.099, 0.121) day^{-1}
λ_4	0.181 day^{-1}	(0.179, 0.184) day^{-1}	(0.116, 0.226) day^{-1}
λ_8	0.085 day^{-1}	(0.080, 0.090) day^{-1}	(0.078, 0.092) day^{-1}
ξ_4	0.231 day^{-1}	(0.230, 0.233) day^{-1}	(0.229, 0.233) day^{-1}
ξ_8	0.152 day^{-1}	(0.150, 0.154) day^{-1}	(0.149, 0.155) day^{-1}

We perturb each entry of the vector θ as described above. Therefore, we have $2^7 n_{\varphi_4}$ sets of θ, with n_{φ_4}, the number of different values considered for φ_4 in the interval $(0, \varphi_2)$. Parameter values will only be accepted if they provide a stable solution before $t = 21$ days.

The results of the sensitivity analysis, with 95% trimmed intervals[2] and minimum–maximum interval ranges, are given in **Table 2**.

3.4. VARIABILITY IN THE SELECTION RATES

The (trimmed and minimum–maximum) intervals derived in Section 3.3 allow us to estimate the variability in the different selection rates discussed in Sections 3.1 and 3.2. For example, given variations in the parameters, the corresponding variations in the selection rates can be shown to be:

$$\Delta p_i = \frac{1}{(\mu_i + \varphi_i)^2}(\varphi_i \Delta\mu_i + \mu_i \Delta\varphi_i) \quad \text{for} \quad i = 1, 2\,, \tag{10}$$

$$\Delta p_3 = \frac{1}{(\mu_3 + \varphi_3 + \lambda_3)^2}[(\varphi_3 + \lambda_3)\Delta\mu_3 + \mu_3\Delta\varphi_3 + \mu_3\Delta\lambda_3]\,, \tag{11}$$

$$\Delta q_3 = \frac{1}{(\mu_3 + \varphi_3 + \lambda_3)^2}[\lambda_3\Delta\mu_3 + \lambda_3\Delta\varphi_3 + (\mu_3 + \varphi_3)\Delta\lambda_3]\,, \tag{12}$$

$$\Delta s_i = \frac{1}{(\mu_2 + \varphi_i + \varphi_j)^2}[\varphi_i\Delta\mu_2 + \varphi_i\Delta\varphi_j + (\mu_2 + \varphi_j)\Delta\varphi_i] \quad \text{for} \quad i = 4, j = 8 \quad \text{or} \quad i = 8, j = 4\,, \tag{13}$$

$$\Delta p_i = \frac{1}{(\mu_i + \xi_i + \lambda_i)^2}[\mu_i\Delta\xi_i + \mu_i\Delta\lambda_i + (\xi_i + \lambda_i)\Delta\mu_i] \quad \text{for} \quad i = 4, 8\,, \tag{14}$$

[2]We define the 95% trimmed interval to be the result of the sensitivity analysis after trimming the lower and upper 2.5% of values.

$$\Delta q_i = \frac{1}{(\mu_i + \xi_i + \lambda_i)^2}[\lambda_i \Delta \xi_i + \lambda_i \Delta \mu_i + (\xi_i + \mu_i)\Delta \lambda_i] \quad \text{for} \quad i = 4, 8\,. \tag{15}$$

We present in **Table 3** the variability of the selection rates.

4. DISCUSSION

We have brought together experimental data with a mathematical compartment model [similar to other progression models of CD4 and CD8 T cell development (13, 14, 18, 21, 33)] to provide estimates for the selection events that take place in the thymus. We have made use of a range of experimental data: (i) steady state thymocyte cell counts (26), mean residence times in each compartment (27–29), murine thymic export rate (14, 26, 30), and recently reported asymmetric death rates for the CD4 SP and CD8 SP thymocytes (21). Our preliminary results support the unexpectedly high death rate in the post-DP thymocyte population observed in Ref. (21). We note that our approach is unrelated to that of Sinclair et al. both experimentally and mathematically (21). This rate, μ_2, has been estimated to be at least an order of magnitude larger than any of the other death rates in the pre-DP, CD4 SP, or CD8 SP pools (see **Table 2**). In terms of selection rates, our analysis yields the following: pre-selection thymocytes (pre-DPs) have a 65.8% probability of dying by neglect in the cortex, and a 34.2% probability of becoming post-selection thymocytes (post-DPs). At the post-selection stage, post-DPs have a 91.7% probability of dying by negative selection (apoptosis) in the cortex, a 4.7% probability of becoming CD4 SPs, and a 3.6% probability of becoming CD8 SPs. In the medulla, CD4 SPs have an 8.6% probability of dying by negative selection (apoptosis), whereas CD8 SPs have a 32.1% probability of dying by negative selection. CD4 SPs have a 45.1% probability of exiting the thymus and reaching the periphery as mature thymocytes, whereas that probability for CD8 SPs is only 40.9%. Finally, the data supports some level of cellular proliferation in the medulla, with CD4 SPs having a 46.3% probability of proliferation and CD8 SPs a 27% probability.

Earlier work by Mehr and collaborators combined experimental and theoretical approaches to estimate thymic selection rates (13, 33), neglected death rates in the medulla, but considered potential feedback from mature T cells. In agreement with these authors, our results indicate that thymocyte death is highest at the post-DP stage. However, as death in the medulla had been neglected, these authors concluded that the CD4:CD8 ratio in SP thymocytes is determined by the differentiation rates. In this paper, we have made use of CD4 and CD8, or medullary, death rates, which allowed us to directly compare cortical (DP) to medullary (SP) death rates. Furthermore, our approach allowed us to conclude that medullary, or SP, death was due to negative selection, as it was rescued by Bim deficiency (26). Sinclair et al. also recently addressed the temporal dynamics of thymic selection using an unrelated approach (both experimentally and mathematically) (21). While their experimental approach did not allow them to distinguish death by negative selection from death by other mechanisms, their overall finding was consistent with ours, that thymocyte death is highest at the post-DP stage.

Table 3 | Selection rate values (initial and after perturbation) and their variability intervals.

Rate	Initial value (%)	After perturbation (%)	Δ Value (%)	Δ Min–max (%)
p_1	65.8	65.66	±0.76	±20.55
p_2	91.7	90.98	±0.49	±17.28
p_3	22.91	24.07	±0.90	±28.22
q_3	42.24	41.74	±0.99	±30.53
s_4	4.69	8.51	±0.80	±15.16
s_8	3.61	8.13	±0.79	±15.03
p_4	8.59	8.84	±0.37	±4.91
q_4	46.29	40.07	±1.29	±20.49
p_8	32.12	31.71	±2.25	±35.37
q_8	27.0	24.5	±3.58	±64.81

Further attempts to quantify thymic selection rates making use of mathematical models also include those of Faro et al. (12). The mathematical model developed by Faro and collaborators does not include time dynamics, but describes the relationship between the number of selecting ligands and the probability of selection of a given thymocyte. Thomas-Vaslin et al. (14) obtained estimates of thymic selection rates, using an experimental procedure that temporarily blocks thymic output and a mathematical model in which rates of transit from compartment to compartment depend on the number of cell divisions. Their model can capture the thymic "conveyor belt" (34, 35) scheme, but requires more differential equations and more parameters than equation (6). Despite the differences between their theoretical and experimental models and ours, similar estimates for thymic selection rates are found. For example, we estimate that 1.2 million post-DP become CD4 SP thymocytes per day and 0.5 million post-DP become CD8 SP thymocytes per day; their estimates are 0.9 and 0.2 million, respectively. Finally, we estimate that 2.6 million CD4 SP thymocytes per day and 0.6 million CD8 SP thymocytes per day exit the thymus. Their estimates are 2.4 and 0.5 million, respectively.

Our estimates of how many CD4 and CD8 SP thymocytes survive and exit the thymus reflect the skewed CD4:CD8 SP thymocyte ratio observed in C57BL/6 mice, which is approximately 4:1 (36). This ratio is similar to the reported CD4:CD8 ratio of recent thymic emigrants (37), and raises the question of what accounts for the CD4 bias. While we were able to determine death and differentiation rates for both CD4 and CD8 SP thymocytes (see **Table 2**), our experimental approach did not allow us to determine what fraction of the post-DP pool was MHC class I versus II restricted. Therefore, we could not address the issue of when and how the CD4:CD8 bias becomes established. The approach of Sinclair et al., which used MHC class I and class II deficiency, allowed them to address this question. Their data suggest that the skewed CD4:CD8 ratio reflects asymmetry in post-selection DP death rates, rather than more efficient positive selection of CD4 compared to CD8 thymocytes (21). Yet, the parameter estimation allows us to compare the following different CD4:CD8 ratios (see

Section 3.2): (i) the CD4:CD8 ratio of positive selection in the post-DP pool (differentiation from post-DP to either CD4 SP or CD8 SP) is given by $\frac{\varphi_4}{\varphi_8} \approx 5:4$, (ii) the CD4:CD8 ratio in the SP pool is given by $\frac{n_4^*}{n_8^*} \approx 3:1$, and (iii) the CD4:CD8 ratio of positive selection in the SP pool (differentiation from SP to peripheral early thymic emigrants) is given by $\frac{\xi_4 n_4^*}{\xi_8 n_8^*} \approx 4:1$. Our observations indicate that the CD4 bias is progressively established, as the thymocytes mature from the post-DP stage until the exit of the SP stage to migrate to the periphery.

Our mathematical analysis has also allowed us to estimate the stringency of thymic selection, defined by:

$$\sigma = \frac{\xi_4\, n_4^* + \xi_8\, n_8^*}{\phi} = 8.96\%\,,$$

that is, the ratio between the number of thymocytes per unit time that exit the thymus and the number of thymocytes per unit time that enter the pre-DP stage. The sensitivity analysis described in Section 3.3 allows us to provide a value of $\Delta\sigma = 0.2\%$, where we have made use of the minimum–maximum interval ranges (see fourth column of **Table 2**). A different measure of stringency could be based on the probability of a cell surviving the maturation process. In our notation, this would correspond to the following:

$$(1 - p_1) \times (1 - p_2) \times (1 - p_3) = 2.19\%\,.$$

We note that this measure of stringency is the probability of not dying in any of the three compartments considered in the model (pre-DP, post-DP, and SP). As discussed in Appendix A.1, and given that in the SP pool, thymocytes may proliferate, there is a need to consider this special case. Our estimates suggest that a population of 10^3 pre-DP thymocytes will yield 69 CD4 and 25 CD8 SP thymocytes that leave the medulla to get incorporated into the peripheral naive T cell pool (see details in Appendix A.1).

The sensitivity analysis (see Section 3.3) and the variability of the selection rates derived from it (see Section 3.4) give us the confidence to conclude, that our parameter estimation is robust. We are aware that the experimental data we have made use of [steady state thymocyte cell counts (26)] do not provide the exquisite time resolution described in Ref. (21). However, the supporting mathematical model described in Section 2.2, allows us to obtain the time evolution of the thymocyte populations, once the parameters have been estimated. In **Figure 5**, we plot the time evolution of the total number of cells in each compartment of the mathematical model: pre-DP, post-DP, CD4 SP, and CD8 SP thymocytes. We start with no cells at time zero, $n_i(t=0) = 0$ for $i = 1, 2, 4, 8$. Trajectories have been plotted for a period of 6 weeks and have been computed for every permutation of the parameter set presented in **Table 2**. The subset of parameters shared with the simple model (ϕ, φ_1, μ_1, μ_2), were fixed at their mean values. Thus, 548 distinct parameter sets were generated. The system of equations (6) was solved using a fourth order Runge–Kutta method (Python source code).

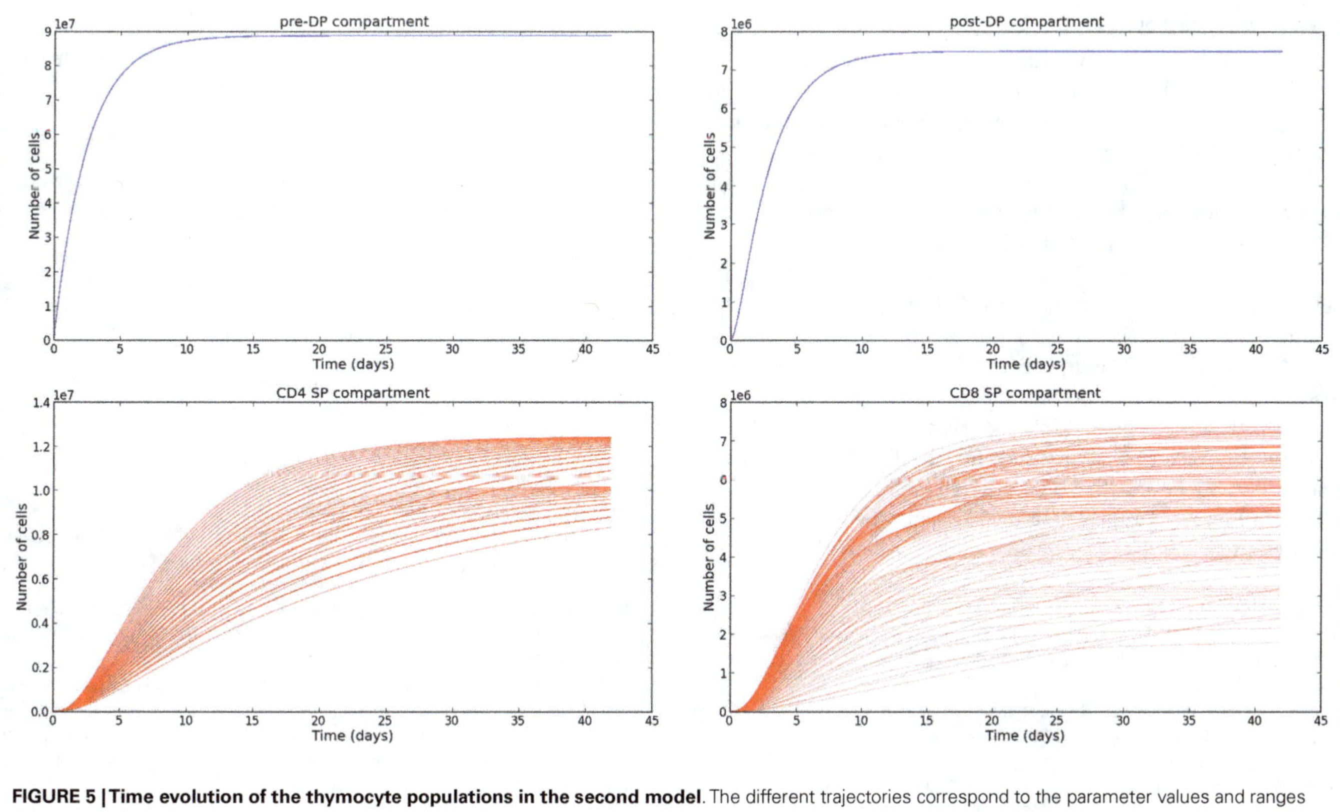

FIGURE 5 | Time evolution of the thymocyte populations in the second model. The different trajectories correspond to the parameter values and ranges described in **Table 2**.

The approaches introduced in this paper have shed some light on the probabilities and timescales that characterize cellular fate in the thymus after the DN stage. We plan to generalize the mathematical model introduced here, making use of experimental data for the strength of TCR binding in Nur77^{GFP} mice (26), to investigate issues such as the death rate in the post-DP pool and the CD4:CD8 ratio. Our model assumes that all progenitors in a particular pool behave with identical kinetics, i.e., move through the various stages of selection at the same rate. Future model refinements will come from consideration of the heterogeneity of the pools, which are known to include cells that will become iNKT cells, regulatory T cells, and intraepithelial lymphocytes (2). It is also possible that progenitors of the same general class move through the selection process with different kinetics (34). The models introduced here can serve as a first step to study human thymic selection, although comprehensive data on human thymic subsets, their sizes, and residence times are not yet available. It would be of great interest to apply the model to data on thymic subsets and cellularity in children, keeping in mind that residence times of human subsets may differ from murine ones (38). Finally, we note that we have not mentioned the relevance of cytokines, such as IL-7, during thymic development. Some differences have already been described for the role of IL-7R in human versus mouse T cell development (38, 39). We hope in the near future to combine mechanistic mathematical models of IL-7 and IL-7R (40) with the T cell development model introduced here to address these issues.

ACKNOWLEDGMENTS

We thank Ed Palmer, Robin Callard, Andy Yates, and Ben Seddon for helpful discussions, and Andy Yates and Ben Seddon for allowing us to make use of their mathematical estimates for μ_4 and μ_8. Grant Lythe and Carmen Molina-París thank Bill Hlavacek, Ruy Ribeiro, and Alan Perelson (Los Alamos National Laboratory) for their hospitality. This work was supported by a BBSRC Research Development Fellowship BB/G023395/1 (to Carmen Molina-París), an FP7 IRSES INDOEUROPEAN-MATHDS Network PIRSES-GA-2012-317893 (to Grant Lythe and Carmen Molina-París), and National Institutes of Health Grants R37 AI39560 (to Kristin A. Hogquist) and F32 AI100346 (to Gretta L. Stritesky). Maria Sawicka, Joseph Reynolds, Niloufar Abourashchi, Grant Lythe, and Carmen Molina-París acknowledge the hospitality of the Max Planck Institute for the Physics of Complex Systems, Dresden, and the International Centre for Mathematical Sciences, Edinburgh, where part of this work was discussed and presented.

REFERENCES

1. Anderson G, Lane P, Jenkinson E. Generating intrathymic microenvironments to establish T-cell tolerance. *Nat Rev Immunol* (2007) **7**(12):954–63. doi:10.1038/nri2187
2. Stritesky GL, Jameson SC, Hogquist KA. Selection of self-reactive T cells in the thymus. *Annu Rev Immunol* (2012) **30**:95. doi:10.1146/annurev-immunol-020711-075035
3. Palmer E. Negative selection: clearing out the bad apples from the T-cell repertoire. *Nat Rev Immunol* (2003) **3**(5):383–91. doi:10.1038/nri1085
4. Jameson S, Hogquist K, Bevan M. Positive selection of thymocytes. *Annu Rev Immunol* (1995) **13**(1):93–126. doi:10.1146/annurev.iy.13.040195.000521
5. Werlen G, Hausmann B, Naeher D, Palmer E. Signaling life and death in the thymus: timing is everything. *Science* (2003) **299**(5614):1859. doi:10.1126/science.1067833
6. Petrie H, Zúñiga-Pflücker J. Zoned out: functional mapping of stromal signaling microenvironments in the thymus. *Immunology* (2007) **25**(1):649. doi:10.1146/annurev.immunol.23.021704.115715
7. Zúñiga-Pflücker JC. When three negatives made a positive influence in defining four early steps in T cell development. *J Immunol* (2012) **189**(9):4201–2. doi:10.4049/jimmunol.1202553
8. Takada K, Ohigashi I, Kasai M, Nakase H, Takahama Y. Development and function of cortical thymic epithelial cells. *Curr Top Microbiol Immunol* (2013) **373**:1–17.
9. Singer A, Adoro S, Park J. Lineage fate and intense debate: myths, models and mechanisms of CD4-versus CD8-lineage choice. *Nat Rev Immunol* (2008) **8**(10):788–801. doi:10.1038/nri2416
10. Anderson MS, Su MA. Aire and T cell development. *Curr Opin Immunol* (2011) **23**(2):198–206. doi:10.1016/j.coi.2010.11.007
11. Klein L. Dead man walking: how thymocytes scan the medulla. *Nat Immunol* (2009) **10**(8):809–11. doi:10.1038/ni0809-809
12. Faro J, Velasco S, Gonzalez-Fernandez A, Bandeira A. The impact of thymic antigen diversity on the size of the selected T cell repertoire. *J Immunol* (2004) **172**(4):2247.
13. Mehr R, Globerson A, Perelson A. Modeling positive and negative selection and differentiation processes in the thymus. *J Theor Biol* (1995) **175**(1):103–26. doi:10.1006/jtbi.1995.0124
14. Thomas-Vaslin V, Altes H, de Boer R, Klatzmann D. Comprehensive assessment and mathematical modeling of T cell population dynamics and homeostasis. *J Immunol* (2008) **180**(4):2240.
15. Souza-e Silva H, Savino W, Feijóo R, Vasconcelos A. A cellular automata-based mathematical model for thymocyte development. *PLoS One* (2009) **4**(12):e8233. doi:10.1371/journal.pone.0008233
16. Efroni S, Harel D, Cohen I. Emergent dynamics of thymocyte development and lineage determination. *PLoS Comput Biol* (2007) **3**(1):e13. doi:10.1371/journal.pcbi.0030013
17. Müller V, Bonhoeffer S. Quantitative constraints on the scope of negative selection. *Trends Immunol* (2003) **24**(3):132–5. doi:10.1016/S1471-4906(03)00028-0
18. Detours V, Mehr R, Perelson A. A quantitative theory of affinity-driven T cell repertoire selection. *J Theor Biol* (1999) **200**(4):389–403. doi:10.1006/jtbi.1999.1003
19. Prasad A, Zikherman J, Das J, Roose J, Weiss A, Chakraborty A. Origin of the sharp boundary that discriminates positive and negative selection of thymocytes. *Proc Natl Acad Sci U S A* (2009) **106**(2):528. doi:10.1073/pnas.0805981105
20. Ribeiro RM, Perelson AS. Determining thymic output quantitatively: using models to interpret experimental T-cell receptor excision circle (Trec) data. *Immunol Rev* (2007) **216**(1):21–34.
21. Sinclair C, Bains I, Yates AJ, Seddon B. Asymmetric thymocyte death underlies the CD4:CD8 T-cell ratio in the adaptive immune system. *Proc Natl Acad Sci U S A* (2013) **110**(31):E2905–14. doi:10.1073/pnas.1304859110
22. Surh CD, Sprent J. T-cell apoptosis detected in situ during positive and negative selection in the thymus. *Nature* (1994) **372**(6501):100–3. doi:10.1038/372100a0
23. Laufer TM, DeKoning J, Markowitz JS, Lo D, Glimcher LH. Unopposed positive selection and autoreactivity in mice expressing class II MHC only on thymic cortex. *Nature* (1996) **383**(6595):81–5. doi:10.1038/383081a0
24. van Meerwijk JP, Marguerat S, Lees RK, Germain RN, Fowlkes B, MacDonald HR. Quantitative impact of thymic clonal deletion on the T cell repertoire. *J Exp Med* (1997) **185**(3):377–84. doi:10.1084/jem.185.3.377
25. Merkenschlager M, Graf D, Lovatt M, Bommhardt U, Zamoyska R, Fisher AG. How many thymocytes audition for selection? *J Exp Med* (1997) **186**(7):1149–58. doi:10.1084/jem.186.7.1149
26. Stritesky GL, Xing Y, Erickson JR, Kalekar LA, Wang X, Mueller DL, et al. Murine thymic selection quantified using a unique method to capture deleted T cells. *Proc Natl Acad Sci U S A* (2013) **110**(12):4679–84. doi:10.1073/pnas.1217532110
27. Egerton M, Scollay R, Shortman K. Kinetics of mature T-cell development in the thymus. *Proc Natl Acad Sci U S A* (1990) **87**(7):2579–82. doi:10.1073/pnas.87.7.2579

28. Saini M, Sinclair C, Marshall D, Tolaini M, Sakaguchi S, Seddon B. Regulation of Zap70 expression during thymocyte development enables temporal separation of CD4 and CD8 repertoire selection at different signaling thresholds. *Sci Signal* (2010) **3**(114):ra23. doi:10.1126/scisignal.2000702
29. McCaughtry TM, Wilken MS, Hogquist KA. Thymic emigration revisited. *J Exp Med* (2007) **204**(11):2513–20. doi:10.1084/jem.20070601
30. Scollay RG, Butcher EC, Weissman IL. Thymus cell migration: quantitative aspects of cellular traffic from the thymus to the periphery in mice. *Eur J Immunol* (1980) **10**(3):210–8. doi:10.1002/eji.1830100310
31. Kenney JF, Keeping ES. *Mathematics of Statistics: Part One.* Princeton: van Nostrand (1954).
32. Kenney JF, Keeping ES. *Mathematics of Statistics: Part Two.* Princeton: van Nostrand (1962).
33. Mehr R, Perelson A, Fridkis-Hareli M, Globerson A. Feedback regulation of T cell development in the thymus. *J Theor Biol* (1996) **181**(2):157–67. doi:10.1006/jtbi.1996.0122
34. Scollay R, Godfrey D. Thymic emigration: conveyor belts or lucky dips? *Immunol Today* (1995) **16**(6):268–73. doi:10.1016/0167-5699(95)80179-0
35. Tough DF, Sprent J. Thymic emigration: conveyor belts or lucky dips? *Immunol Today* (1995) **16**(6):273–4. doi:10.1016/0167-5699(95)80180-4
36. Sim B-C, Aftahi N, Reilly C, Bogen B, Schwartz RH, Gascoigne NR, et al. Thymic skewing of the CD4/CD8 ratio maps with the T-cell receptor α-chain locus. *Curr Biol* (1998) **8**(12):701–S3. doi:10.1016/S0960-9822(98)70276-3
37. Boursalian TE, Golob J, Soper DM, Cooper CJ, Fink PJ. Continued maturation of thymic emigrants in the periphery. *Nat Immunol* (2004) **5**(4):418–25. doi:10.1038/ni1049
38. Spits H. Development of $\alpha\beta$ T cells in the human thymus. *Nat Rev Immunol* (2002) **2**(10):760–72. doi:10.1038/nri913
39. Marino JH, Tan C, Taylor AA, Bentley C, Van De Wiele CJ, Ranne R, et al. Differential IL-7 responses in developing human thymocytes. *Hum Immunol* (2010) **71**(4):329–33. doi:10.1016/j.humimm.2010.01.009
40. Molina-París C, Reynolds J, Lythe G, Coles MC. Mathematical model of naive t cell division and survival il-7 thresholds. *Front Immunol* (2013) **4**:434. doi:10.3389/fimmu.2013.00434
41. Allen LJS. *An Introduction to Stochastic Processes with Applications to Biology.* New Jersey: Pearson Education (2003).

APPENDIX

A.1. STRINGENCY OF THYMIC SELECTION: A STOCHASTIC MODEL

In this section, we present the details that allow us to compute the stringency of thymic selection for the mathematical model considered in Section 2.2.

Let us assume that at time $t=0$, there exists a single T cell in a given compartment. In our case, the compartment can be the pre-DP, post-DP, or SP (either CD4 SP or CD8 SP) stages. The cell, at any time, may die (with rate, μ), divide (with rate, λ), and produce two daughter cells, or leave the compartment (with rate, ξ) to enter a different compartment. The waiting times for each event are assumed to be exponentially distributed, and daughter cells are assumed to behave identically to the initial single cell. We introduce the bivariate Markov process $\{X(t), Y(t)\}_{t\geq 0}$, where $X(t)$ is the number of cells in the compartment at time t, and $Y(t)$ is the number of cells which have left the compartment (to enter a different compartment). Our aim is to calculate the expected number of cells (and variance) that leave the compartment.

State probabilities for the Markov process are defined as follows (41)

$$p_{(x,y)}(t) = \text{Prob}\{X(t) = x, Y(t) = y | X(0) = 1, Y(0) = 0\}, \tag{A1}$$

and transition probabilities for this process are defined as follows (41)

$$\begin{aligned} p_{(w,z),(x,y)}(\Delta t) &= \text{Prob}\{X(t+\Delta t) = w, \\ &\quad Y(t+\Delta t) = z | X(t) = x, Y(t) = y\} \\ &= \begin{cases} \lambda x \Delta t + o(\Delta t), & \text{if } w = x+1, z = y, \\ \mu x \Delta t + o(\Delta t), & \text{if } w = x-1, z = y, \\ \xi x \Delta t + o(\Delta t), & \text{if } w = x-1, z = y+1, \\ 1-(\lambda+\mu+\xi)x\Delta t + o(\Delta t), & \text{if } w = x, z = y, \\ o(\Delta t), & \text{if } w, z \text{ otherwise}. \end{cases} \end{aligned} \tag{A2}$$

The Kolmogorov (or master) equation for this process is given by (41)

$$\begin{aligned} \frac{dp_{(x,y)}(t)}{dt} &= \lambda\,(x-1)p_{(x-1,y)}(t) + \mu\,(x+1)p_{(x+1,y)}(t) \\ &\quad + \xi\,(x+1)p_{(x+1,y-1)}(t) - (\lambda+\mu+\xi)\,x\,p_{(x,y)}(t). \end{aligned} \tag{A3}$$

Let $m_X(t)$ be the expected number of cells in the compartment under consideration, and $m_Y(t)$ be the expected number of cells which have left the compartment. Similarly, let $m_{XX}(t)$ be the expectation of the random variable $X(t)^2$, $m_{XY}(t)$ be the expectation of the random variable $X(t)Y(t)$, and $m_{YY}(t)$ be the expectation of the random variable $Y(t)^2$. Then, making use of the probability generating function technique (41), we derive the time evolution for the first two moments of the system:

$$\frac{dm_X(t)}{dt} = (\lambda-\mu-\xi)m_X(t), \tag{A4}$$

$$\frac{dm_Y(t)}{dt} = \xi\, m_X(t), \tag{A5}$$

$$\frac{dm_{XX}(t)}{dt} = 2(\lambda-\mu-\xi)m_{XX}(t) + (\lambda-\mu-\xi)m_X(t), \tag{A6}$$

$$\frac{dm_{XY}(t)}{dt} = (\lambda-\mu-\xi)m_{XY}(t) + \xi[m_{XX}(t) - m_X(t)], \tag{A7}$$

$$\frac{dm_{YY}(t)}{dt} = \xi[2m_{XY}(t) + m_X(t)]. \tag{A8}$$

Given that we start with a single cell, the expected number of cells at time t is given by

$$m_X(t) = e^{(\lambda-\mu-\xi)t}. \tag{A9}$$

Under the restriction $\lambda < \mu + \xi$, the expected number of cells tends to zero as $t \to +\infty$. This implies that all cells from the single T cell progenitor either die or leave the compartment for sufficiently large times. The expected number of cells which leave the compartment is given by

$$m_Y(t) = \frac{\xi}{\mu+\xi-\lambda}\left[1 - e^{(\lambda-\mu-\xi)t}\right]. \tag{A10}$$

As $t \to +\infty$, the expected number of cells to leave the compartment can be shown to be

$$\lim_{t\to+\infty} m_Y(t) = \frac{\xi}{\mu+\xi-\lambda}. \tag{A11}$$

We now solve the remaining ODEs equations (A6–A8), to find

$$\begin{aligned} m_{YY}(t) &= \frac{2\lambda\xi^2}{(\lambda-\mu-\xi)^3}\left[\frac{1}{2}e^{2(\lambda-\mu-\xi)t} - e^{(\lambda-\mu-\xi)t}\right] \\ &\quad - \frac{4\lambda\xi^2}{(\lambda-\mu-\xi)^2}\left(t - \frac{1}{\lambda-\mu-\xi}\right)e^{(\lambda-\mu-\xi)t} \\ &\quad + \frac{\xi}{\lambda-\mu-\xi}e^{(\lambda-\mu-\xi)t} - \frac{2\lambda\xi^2}{(\lambda-\mu-\xi)^3} \\ &\quad - \frac{\xi}{\lambda-\mu-\xi}. \end{aligned} \tag{A12}$$

It, therefore, follows that the random variable $Y(t)$, which represents the number of cells leaving the compartment under consideration, has the following variance (in the limit $t \to +\infty$)

$$\begin{aligned} \sigma_Y^2 = \lim_{t\to\infty}\left[m_{YY}(t) - m_Y(t)^2\right] &= \frac{2\lambda\xi^2}{(\mu+\xi-\lambda)^3} + \frac{\xi}{\mu+\xi-\lambda} \\ &\quad - \frac{\xi^2}{(\mu+\xi-\lambda)^2}. \end{aligned} \tag{A13}$$

A.2. STRINGENCY OF THYMIC SELECTION IN THE FOUR COMPARTMENT MODEL

The previous example can easily (but laboriously) be extended to the mathematical model introduced in Section 2.2.

We may evaluate the expected number of, for example, $CD4^+$ T cells produced by a single pre-DP progenitor (or more generally N pre-DP progenitors). We only present the time evolution of the moment generating function. The deterministic equations describing the mean and variance of the numbers of cells in each compartment (pre-DP, post-DP, SP CD4, and SP CD8) are left for the reader to derive. When counting the number of $CD4^+$ T cells leaving the thymus, the moment generating function satisfies the following partial differential equation

$$\begin{aligned}\frac{\partial M}{\partial t} &= \mu_1(e^{-\theta_1}-1)\frac{\partial M}{\partial \theta_1} + \varphi_1(e^{-\theta_1}e^{\theta_2}-1)\frac{\partial M}{\partial \theta_1} \\ &\quad + (\mu_2+\varphi_8)(e^{-\theta_2}-1)\frac{\partial M}{\partial \theta_2} + \varphi_4(e^{-\theta_2}e^{\theta_4}-1)\frac{\partial M}{\partial \theta_2} \\ &\quad + \mu_4(e^{-\theta_4}-1)\frac{\partial M}{\partial \theta_4} + \lambda_4(e^{\theta_4}-1)\frac{\partial M}{\partial \theta_4} \\ &\quad + \xi_4(e^{-\theta_4}e^{\theta_8}-1)\frac{\partial M}{\partial \theta_4}. \end{aligned} \tag{A14}$$

The symmetry of the mathematical model implies that an equivalent equation for the number of $CD8^+$ T cells leaving the thymus can be obtained by interchanging the indexes 4 and 8. For our derived parameter set, the previous equation allows us to conclude that the expected number of $CD4^+$ T cells, a single thymocyte in the pre-DP compartment produces, is 0.069 (standard deviation 0.96), whereas the expected number of $CD8^+$ T cells which leave the thymus is 0.025 (standard deviation 0.59).

To put this into perspective, a population of 10^3 pre-DP thymocytes is expected to produce 69 $CD4^+$ T cells which leave the thymus (standard deviation 66), and 25 $CD8^+$ T cells (standard deviation 41). More generally, a population of N pre-DP thymocytes is expected to produce $0.069N$ $CD4^+$ T cells and $0.025N$ $CD8^+$ T cells.

5

Immunotherapy for prostate cancer: lessons from responses to tumor-associated antigens

Harm Westdorp[1,2†], Annette E. Sköld[1†], Berit A. Snijer[1], Sebastian Franik[1], Sasja F. Mulder[2], Pierre P. Major[3], Ronan Foley[3], Winald R. Gerritsen[2] and I. Jolanda M. de Vries[1,2*]

[1] Department of Tumor Immunology, Radboud Institute for Molecular Life Sciences, Radboud University Medical Center, Nijmegen, Netherlands
[2] Department of Medical Oncology, Radboud University Medical Center, Nijmegen, Netherlands
[3] Juravinski Hospital and Cancer Centre, Hamilton, ON, Canada

Edited by:
Fang-Ping Huang, Imperial College London, UK

Reviewed by:
Masaaki Murakami, Osaka University, Japan
Fabio Grizzi, Humanitas Clinical and Research Center, Italy

***Correspondence:**
I. Jolanda M. de Vries, Department of Tumor Immunology, Radboud Institute for Molecular Life Sciences, Radboud University Medical Center, Geert Grooteplein 26, 6525 GA Nijmegen, Netherlands
e-mail: j.devries@ncmls.ru.nl

† Harm Westdorp and Annette E. Sköld have contributed equally to this work.

Prostate cancer (PCa) is the most common cancer in men and the second most common cause of cancer-related death in men. In recent years, novel therapeutic options for PCa have been developed and studied extensively in clinical trials. Sipuleucel-T is the first cell-based immunotherapeutic vaccine for treatment of cancer. This vaccine consists of autologous mononuclear cells stimulated and loaded with an immunostimulatory fusion protein containing the prostate tumor antigen prostate acid posphatase. The choice of antigen might be key for the efficiency of cell-based immunotherapy. Depending on the treatment strategy, target antigens should be immunogenic, abundantly expressed by tumor cells, and preferably functionally important for the tumor to prevent loss of antigen expression. Autoimmune responses have been reported against several antigens expressed in the prostate, indicating that PCa is a suitable target for immunotherapy. In this review, we will discuss PCa antigens that exhibit immunogenic features and/or have been targeted in immunotherapeutic settings with promising results, and we highlight the hurdles and opportunities for cancer immunotherapy.

Keywords: immunotherapy of cancer, prostate cancer, tumor-associated antigens, CRPC, immunotherapy

INTRODUCTION

Prostate cancer (PCa) is the most commonly diagnosed noncutaneous cancer among men in the United States and is the second leading cause of death from cancer in men (1). In Europe, PCa is also the cancer type with the highest incidence in men apart from skin cancer, while it is the third most common type of cancer after lung cancer and colorectal cancer (2). PCa is usually diagnosed in men above 65 years of age. Depending on the severity of the disease, current treatment options for PCa consist of active surveillance, prostatectomy, radiation therapy, hormonal therapy, or chemotherapy. Up to one-third of patients with a localized tumor eventually fails on local therapy and progress to advanced-stage or metastatic PCa within 10 years. For advanced PCa, androgen deprivation therapy is the standard of care. Although the majority of patients initially respond, most tumors become resistant to primary hormonal therapy within 14–30 months (3). For men with metastatic castration-resistant prostate cancer (mCRPC), the median survival in phase III studies range from 15 to 19 months. For several years, the chemotherapeutic drug docetaxel was the only treatment option for mCRPC, resulting in a median overall survival benefit of 2–3 months compared with the previous treatment regimes mitoxantrone and prednisone (4–6). However, new agents targeting the androgen signaling pathway, immunotherapeutic options, radium-223 treatment, and the new chemotherapeutic treatment modality taxane cabazitaxel are emerging therapies with the ability to improve both the survival and the quality of life.

In 2010, the first cellular immunotherapy was approved as a treatment for mCRPC by the US Food and Drug Administration (FDA). More recently, cancer immunotherapy hit a new peak, Science Magazine elected cancer immunotherapy the breakthrough of 2013 (7). Especially, modulation of T-cell checkpoints via immune checkpoint inhibiting [anti-cytotoxic T lymphocyte antigen-4 (CTLA-4) monoclonal antibodies and anti-programed death (ligand) 1 (PD-(L)1] monoclonal antibodies has been successful. Instead of tacking of the brake of the immune system, as is the case with checkpoint inhibitors, another challenge is out there: enhancement of immune responses to tumor-specific antigens. In this review, we discuss tumor antigens expressed by PCa, how they can be used to combat PCa via immunotherapy, and which hurdles need to be addressed and overcome. Other new treatment modalities are beyond the scope of this study.

INFLAMMATORY RESPONSES IN THE PROSTATE

Inflammation is an innate response to harmful stimuli, such as infections, tissue damage, or tissue malfunction (8, 9). The main goal with the inflammatory process is to clear the potential threat and restore tissue homeostasis. This normally occurs in two phases – the recognition and elimination phase and the resolution and repair phase (8, 10). If the acute response fails in eliminating the inflammatory agents, the inflammation shifts toward a chronic state. Instead of initiating the resolution phase, additional macrophages and lymphocytes are recruited and, depending on the inflammatory inducer, act to remodel the local microenvironment to adapt to an altered tissue homeostasis.

Cancer has been described as a wound that refuses to heal (11), and today many cancers have been tightly correlated with preceding inflammatory responses (12, 13). Several lines of evidence support the theory that inflammation also precedes PCa (9). Proliferative inflammatory atrophy lesions are areas in the prostate with an increased infiltration of inflammatory cells. These regions can merge with prostatic intraepithelial neoplasia, which is considered to be a risk factor for the development of PCa (14, 15). Also, a correlation with regular intake of non-steroidal anti-inflammatory drugs and reduced PCa risk has been observed (16–18).

AUTOIMMUNITY AND PCa

Inflammatory response inducers in prostate vary from infections to life style factors, such as diet or smoking (19). Symptomatic prostatitis caused by bacterial infection has been correlated with an increased risk of PCa development (20, 21). However, the causing agents of the majority of symptomatic and asymptomatic prostatitis are not well characterized and are probably multifaceted events (22).

Several studies have reported autoimmune responses against both seminal proteins (23, 24) and prostate antigens causing prostatitis to become chronic (25–27). These finding are additionally verified in animal models, where a cytotoxic cellular response seems to be driving the autoimmune reaction (28). Androgen ablation in patients with PCa is shown to induce high levels of T-cell infiltration into both benign and cancerous prostate sites, indicating that autoimmune responses against prostate antigens might be hormonally regulated (29).

ANTIGEN-BASED CANCER IMMUNOTHERAPY

The increased knowledge of how specific immune responses are evoked and the development of tools to manipulate the immune system have enabled implementation of novel immune-based cancer therapies. The rationale of these immunotherapies is to induce anti-tumor immune responses, decrease tumor-load, and change the course of the disease. Recognition of target antigens by the immune system is crucial. Several types of immunotherapeutics have been developed, such as peptide vaccines, DNA/RNA vaccines, cell-based vaccines, and T-cell modulators. Although improving overall survival is the primary endpoint of most clinical studies, a better understanding of induced T-cell responses, boosting pre-existing immune responses, and the effect of the tumor microenvironment on the T cells is needed to further improve PCa immunotherapy.

Tumor-associated antigens in PCa can be proteins that are present on prostate cells and on their malignant counterparts. Examples are prostate-specific antigen (PSA), prostate-specific membrane antigen (PSMA), and the cancer/testis antigens (CTAs). In a steady state, these antigens are not provoking strong immune responses. Immunosuppressive mechanisms in the prostate microenvironment, such as transforming growth factor (TGF)-β, regulatory T cells (Tregs), or myeloid-derived suppressor cells, will maintain prostate infiltrating lymphocytes in an inactive state (30–32). In addition, PCa cells exploit several mechanisms to enhance immune tolerance (33). Despite the immunosuppressive microenvironment, several immunotherapeutic approaches are able to induce or enhance tumor-specific immune responses. In the following section, potential tumor antigens and their application as immunotherapeutic targets will be discussed. **Table 1** provides an overview of the antigens discussed and clinical results of antigen-based immunotherapy trials.

PROSTATE CANCER ANTIGENS

PROSTATE-SPECIFIC ANTIGEN

Prostate-specific antigen is a serine protease produced primarily in the epithelial cells lining the acini and ducts of the prostate gland (51–53). Physiologically, PSA is present at high concentrations in the seminal fluid. Its function is to cleave high molecular weight proteins into smaller peptides, which results in liquification of these peptides. This allows the spermatozoa to swim freely (51). Membrane-bound PSA is expressed by most PCa cells. Upon disruption of the prostate gland tissue by cancerous growth, PSA is released into the circulation. There, PSA can interact with several inflammatory cells, including fibroblasts and macrophages, which might cause chronic inflammation (9, 54, 55). PSA serum levels correlate with the extent of disease and are therefore a useful tumor marker, accurately reflecting tumor status and prognostic for clinical outcome. In case of relapse, PSA levels correlate with tumor recurrence (51, 56). Transcription of the PSA gene is positively regulated by the androgen receptor, which can partly explain the decline in PSA levels in response to androgen deprivation therapy (52). However, high PSA levels are also observed in patients with CRPC, due to the acquired ability of the tumor cells to maintain the androgen receptor function even in the androgen-ablated environment (57).

PSA as tumor antigen

Cellular autoimmune responses against PSA have been detected in both healthy men and patients suffering from chronic prostatitis (26, 27, 58), suggesting that PSA has immunogenic properties. It has been used as a target antigen in several immunotherapeutic constructs. Hodge et al. used a vector designated TRICOM, containing three co-stimulatory molecules B7-1, ICAM-1 and LFA-3, and a PSA peptide, for T-cell stimulation (59). Using a similar approach, Kantoff et al. studied a combination of PSA-expressing recombinant viral vectors, where treatment with a vaccinia-based priming vector was followed by six booster injections of a fowlpox-based vector (PROSTVAC-VF). In the phase II, randomized controlled trial in patients with mCRPC, no significant difference in progression-free survival was detected between control group and the vaccinated group. However, vaccinated patients had a longer median overall survival, and a better 3-year survival (60). These clinically meaningful results have to be confirmed in an ongoing phase III trial (**Table 2**).

Other PSA-expressing vectors have been tested in phase I trials in patients with PCa with rising PSA levels. Vaccinations with vaccinia-based vectors expressing PSA resulted in stabilization of serum PSA levels and PSA-specific T-cell responses were observed (34). PSA-specific T cells were also detected after vaccination with a liposome-based PSA vaccine and a dendritic cell (DC)-based vaccine (35, 36). Treatment with a PSA encoding poxviral vector vaccine in combination with radiotherapy not only showed PSA-specific T-cell activation, but also T-cell responses against prostate-associated antigens not encoded by the vaccine. This is

Table 1 | Antigens and their immunogenicity in prostate cancer.

Antigen	Function	Immunogenicity in PCa	Human clinical trials in PCa	Number of patients with PCa
PSA	Serine protease which cleaves high molecular weight proteins into smaller peptides, resulting in the necessary liquification for spermatozoa to swim freely	Stimulates CTLs *in vivo*	Poxviral vaccine PROSTVAC-VF/PSA-TRICOM showed a longer median overall survival when compared to placebo (34)	82 vs. 40 controls
			A phase I trial with a recombinant vaccinia virus expressing PSA (rV-PSA) showed a stable PSA level for at least 6 months in 14 patients (35)	33
		Production of immunosuppressive cytokines	A study with JBT 1001, a recombinant PSA vaccine, showed a T-cell response in eight patients (36)	10
			A study reported a PSA decrease between 6 and 39% compared to baseline in 11 of the treated patients with PSA-loaded DCs (37)	24
PAP	Protein tyrosine phosphatase which enhances the mobility of sperm	Stimulates CTLs *in vivo*	A phase I/II study reported PAP-specific T-cell responses and an increased PSA doubling time for the plasmid DNA accine pTVG-HP PAP when compared to placebo (38)	22
		Elevated in both prostatic hyperplasia and PCa	Three phase III RCTs, of which two showed a significant increase in overall survival (39, 40), and one (41) showed a trend to increase in overall survival for sipuleucel-T compared with placebo	341 vs. 171 placebo (39) 82 vs. 45 placebo (40) 65 vs. 33 placebo (41)
PSMA	Folate hydrolase activity	Presented at the cell surface and in the endothelial lumen, the latter promotes integrin signaling	A phase I trial reported a 50% PSA reduction in four patients treated with ^{177}lutetium-labeled J591, a radiolabeled monoclonal antibody against PMSA (42)	35
		Highly overexpressed in PCa	A study using an HLA-A2 restricted PMSA peptide (LLHETDSAV) showed neither clinical nor immune responses. The authors concluded that the used PSMA epitope was poorly immunogenic compared with other HLA-A2-presented peptides (43)	12
			A phase II trial with DCs pulsed with PMSA peptides showed a 50% reduction of PSA in nine patients (44)	33
PSCA	Unknown, overexpressed by most PCas	T-cell activation and proliferation	Two vaccination studies in humans with DCs loaded with PSCA alone or in combination with PAP, PSMA, and/or PSA reported that the vaccine was well tolerated and increased both the PSA doubling time and median overall survival of the patients (45, 46)	12 (45) 6 (46)
MUC-1	Limiting the activation of inflammatory responses	T-cell proliferation	A phase I/II trial with DCs loaded with MUC-1 glycopeptide and KLH showed a reduction of PSA rise in six patients. Immune responses to KLH (6/7) and Tn-MUC-1 (5/7) have been detected (47)	7
			Radioimmunotherapy was combined with or without low-dose paclitaxel in patients with mCRPC and breast cancer. In two patients with mCRPC who received m170 (MUC-1 monoclonal antibody) linked to indium-111, a 50% decline in PSA level was shown which lasted 2 months, and two patients described a decrease in bone pain (48)	9

(Continued)

Table 1 | Continued

Antigen	Function	Immunogenicity in PCa	Human clinical trials in PCa	Number of patients with PCa
NY-ESO-1	Unknown, expressed in a variety of tumors	CTLs and antibody-mediated responses	In patients with mCRPC, NY-ESO-1 peptides vaccines were tolerable. Among nine patients, vaccinations appeared to slow PSA doubling time, and yielded antigen-specific T-cell responses in six patients (49)	14
			Immunoactivation following an NY-ESO-1 protein-based vaccine combined with CpG showed humoral and cellular immune responses specific for NY-ESO-1 in 12 and 9 of the vaccinated patients, respectively (50)	13
MAGE-A genes	Down-regulates p53 function through histone deacetylase recruitment	Stimulates CTLs *in vivo*	No human clinical trial performed in PCa	
AKAP-4	Binding protein involved in cytoskeletal regulation and organization by affecting cyclic AMP-dependent protein kinase-A	Stimulated CTLs *in vitro*	No human clinical trial performed in PCa	

indicative for tumor cell killing and subsequent epitope spreading (37). Hence, PSA-targeted immunotherapy can boost conventional treatment strategies to induce stronger and broader effects. This was also shown in a recent study combining PSA-TRICOM treatment with the T-cell checkpoint inhibitor ipilimumab, where the majority of chemo-naive patients displayed a decline in serum PSA levels (61).

Despite the fact that PSA-based immunotherapeutic approaches can stimulate cytotoxic T lymphocytes (CTLs) both *in vitro* and *in vivo*, untreated patients with PCa often fail to induce a potent immune response against this antigen (62–64). Several factors might contribute to this phenomenon: (i) PSA activates TGF-β, which can suppress immune responses in the tumor microenvironment (65, 66); (ii) PSA has a negative effect on lymphocyte proliferation and differentiation (63, 64); (iii) PSA can inhibit the maturation, function, and survival of DCs (63, 64).

In summary, the serine protease PSA is expressed at high levels by most PCa. Targeting PSA might not only elicit a tumor-specific immune response, but also counteract the negative effect of PSA on both T cells and DCs. Therefore, PSA poses as a promising target antigen in immunotherapy, and this is underscored by the results of phase II trials using PSA in vector-based peptide vaccines (60, 67). The ongoing phase III clinical trial (NCT01322490) might provide more evidence on the clinical relevance of PSA-TRICOM/PROSTVAC-VF vaccinations (**Table 2**).

PROSTATE ACID POSPHATASE

Human prostate acid posphatase (PAP) is a secreted glycoprotein enzyme synthesized in the prostate epithelium (68). Only a few substrates have so far been identified for PAP, including adenosine monophosphate, phosphotyrosine, phosphocholine, phosphocreatine, and ErbB-2 (69, 70) Since PAP can act as a protein tyrosine phosphatase, many other yet to be identified substrates might be involved in the signal transduction of this protein. PAP is secreted by the prostate gland following puberty and its expression is correlated with testosterone. It is reported to enhance the mobility of sperm (71). Serum PAP levels are low in healthy individuals and increased levels are associated with PCa. For example, it is shown that PAP is aberrantly expressed in high Gleason score PCa (72, 73). Ozu et al. showed that serum PAP levels, like serum PSA, are significantly increased within the escalating PCa disease stages. PAP is also elevated in patients with bone metastasis, compared to those without bone metastasis (74). Elevation of PAP is associated with significantly shortened survival, while its decrease is correlated with responsiveness to therapy (75–77).

PAP as tumor antigen

Due to its elevated expression in PCa, PAP has been investigated as a possible target antigen for immunotherapeutic approaches. PAP-specific cytotoxic T cells (CTLs) can be found in blood of healthy donors and in patients with chronic prostatitis (26, 78, 79). In addition, patients with PCa vaccinated with DCs loaded with murine PAP showed responses against human PAP coinciding with significant clinical anti-tumor responses (80). Specific CTLs can also be generated by culturing with antigen presenting cells pulsed with a PAP-derived HLA-A2 binding peptide. The obtained CTLs can lyse peptide-loaded target cells in an antigen-specific manner, as

Table 2 | Ongoing trials encompassing antigen-based immunotherapy.

Antigen	Study design	Trial identifier	Immunologic endpoints
PSA	Phase II trial of PROSTVAC-VF/PSA-TRICOM with docetaxel and prednisone vs. docetaxel and prednisone alone in patients with mCRPC	NCT01145508 (the study is ongoing but not recruiting new patients anymore)	Immune responses before and after docetaxel and PSA-specific immune responses Primary endpoint: overall survival
	Phase II trial with enzalutamide with or without PROSTVAC-VF/PSA-TRICOM in patients with mCRPC	NCT01867333 (ongoing and recruiting trial, estimated completion date June 2016)	Immune response (not further specified) Primary endpoint: to show increase in time to progression
	Phase III study of PROSTVAC-VF/PSA-TRICOM with or without GM-CSF in patients with mCRPC	NCT01322490 (ongoing and recruiting trial, estimated completion date August 2016)	No immunologic endpoints Primary endpoint: overall survival
PAP	Phase II trial of sipuleucel-T with a pTVG-HP DNA vaccine in patients with mCRPC	NCT01706458 (ongoing and recruiting trial, estimated completion date June 2015)	Primary endpoint: immune responses following treatment with sipuleucel-T
	Phase II trial of sipuleucel-T with concurrent or sequential abiraterone acetate plus prednisone in patients with mCRPC	NCT01487863 (active study, not recruiting, estimated completion date June 2015)	Primary endpoint: sipuleucel-T CD54 upregulation
	Phase II trial of sipuleucel-T and ipilimumab given immediately sequential vs. delayed sequential in patients with mCRPC	NCT01804465 (active study, not recruiting, estimated completion date August 2015)	Primary endpoints: safety of both treatment arms and induction of antibody responses by sipuleucel-T, the proportion of patients on each study arm who achieve an immune response to PAP and/or PA2024
	Phase I study of sipuleucel-T and ipilimumab in patients with mCRPC	NCT01832870 (ongoing and recruiting trial, estimated completion date December 2015)	Primary endpoint: antigen-specific memory T-cell response, antigen-specific proliferation and antibody responses against PAP, PA2024 and PHA
	Phase II trial of sipuleucel-T with or without anti-PD-1 monoclonal antibodies and cyclophosphamide	NCT01420965 (ongoing and recruiting trial, estimated completion date December 2017)	Primary endpoints: feasibility and the immune efficacy of sipuleucel-T alone vs. sipuleucel-T plus cyclophosphamide and anti-PD-1 monoclonal antibodies (CT011) on the change in specific immune response
PSMA	Phase I trial of adoptive T-cell transfer targeted to PSMA in patients with mCRPC	NCT01140373 (ongoing and recruiting trial, estimated completion date June 2014)	No immunologic endpoints Primary endpoint: progression-free survival
	Phase II trial of PSMA antibody drug conjugate in patients with mCRPC	NCT01695044 (ongoing and recruiting trial, estimated completion date January 2015)	Primary endpoints: changes in tumor assessments, serum PSA and circulating tumor cells
	Phase II study of prodrug chemotherapy (G-202) which is activated *in situ* by PSMA of PCa cells or within cancer blood vessels of patients with mCRPC	NCT01734681 (study is not yet open for recruitment, estimated completion date January 2015)	Changes in circulating tumor cells and humoral and cell-mediated immunity to PSMA and other known PCa antigens and to track the persistence, accumulation, and migration of genetically retargeted anti-PSMA autologous T cells Primary endpoint: safety and tolerability of immunotherapy

(Continued)

Table 2 | Continued

Antigen	Study design	Trial identifier	Immunologic endpoints
	Phase I trial of anti-PSMA designer T cells after non-myeloablative conditioning in patients with mCRPC	NCT00664196 (ongoing and recruiting trial, estimated completion date July 2016)	Pharmacokinetics and pharmacodynamics of the anti-PSMA designer T cells Primary endpoint: the safety of using modified T cells
PSCA	No active or recruiting clinical trials in patients with PCa		
NY-ESO-1	Phase I trial of IMF-001 (CHP-NY-ESO-1 complex) vaccine in NY-ESO-1 expressing malignities	NCT01234012 (active study, not recruiting, estimated completion date December 2013)	NY-ESO-1 specific cellular (specific CD4 and CD8+ T cells) and humoral immunity (NY-ESO-1 antibody titer) Primary endpoint: safety and tolerability of the vaccine
	Phase I trial of DEC-205-NY-ESO-1 fusion protein vaccine in NY-ESO-1 expressing solid tumors	NCT01522820 (ongoing and recruiting trial, estimated completion date September 2014)	NY-ESO-1 specific cellular and humoral immunity Primary endpoint: safety of the vaccine
MAGE-A genes	No active or recruiting clinical trials in patients with PCa		
AKAP-4	No active or recruiting clinical trials in patients with PCa		
MUC-1	Phase I/II study of autologous DCs loaded with Tn-MUC-1 peptide in patients with CRPC	NCT00852007 (active study, not recruiting, estimated completion date March 2014)	Induction of CD4/CD8 responses measured by CFSE or ICS assay and/or induction of humoral response measured by specific antibodies or antibody isotype switching Primary endpoint: time to radiographic progression
	Phase I study of MUC-1 vaccine in conjunction with poly-ICLC in patients with recurrent or advanced PCa	NCT00374049 (active study, not recruiting, estimated completion date July 2014)	Primary endpoint: to evaluate the efficacy of poly-ICLC in boosting the immunologic response of a MUC-1 vaccine
	Phase II study of L-BLP25 (Stimuvax) in combination with androgen deprivation therapy and radiation therapy in patients with high-risk PCa. L-BLP25 vaccination is thought to work via killing of MUC-1 overexpressing cancer cells	NCT01496131 (ongoing and recruiting trial, estimated completion date January 2016)	Change in the ELISPOT level of Mucin-1-specific T cells after radiation therapy

well as HLA-A2 positive prostate tumor cells *in vitro* (78). PAP-specific cytolytic T-cell responses have additionally been identified in HLA-A2 transgenic mice immunized with the PAP encoding DNA vaccine pTVG-HP (81). Moreover, PAP peptides with the ability to bind additional HLA-A alleles has also been described (82, 83). Also, small clinical studies using a PAP-derived peptide for different HLA-subclasses show promising results in patients with PCa (84, 85). Naturally occurring PAP-specific CD4+ T cells are only found in 7–11% of patients with PCa, but this can be augmented by immunotherapy. Overall, these data suggest that PAP-specific T-cell responses can be initiated, and that PAP is an interesting candidate to use in cancer immunotherapy (81, 83, 84).

DNA-based PAP vaccine

In a PAP-based DNA vaccine, patients with CRPC received six vaccinations with granulocyte-macrophage colony-stimulating factor (GM-CSF) biweekly. Both humoral and cellular immune responses were detected in 3 of the 22 patients, with an at least threefold increase in PAP-specific IFN-gamma secreting CD8+ T cells. Nine of 22 patients showed PAP-specific CD4+ and/or CD8+ T-cell responses, but no antibody responses were detected. Also, an increase in the PSA doubling time was observed (86). The results of two ongoing trials will shed light on the role of PAP-based DNA vaccines in PCa (**Table 2**).

APC-based PAP vaccine: sipuleucel-T

After three phase III randomized controlled trials, the PAP-targeting vaccine sipuleucel-T, became the first cellular immunotherapy ever to be approved for any malignancy by the FDA (38, 39, 41). Sipuleucel-T is a peripheral blood mononuclear cell (PBMC)-based autologous vaccine. PBMCs are cocultured with a fusion protein, consisting of GM-CSF and PAP, for *ex vivo* activation of APCs and as tumor-associated antigen, respectively. The proposed mechanism of sipuleucel-T is inducing antigen-specific immune responses and thereby destroys PCa cells (40).

Sipuleucel-T treatment consists of three injections at 2-week intervals. In three phase III randomized controlled trials, an increase in overall survival of 4 months was noticed with no difference in progression-free survival. In general, treatment was well tolerated and only rigors and pyrexia were reported as adverse events (38, 39, 41). The trial by Kantoff et al. showed a trend of superior treatment outcome of sipuleucel-T in patients in the lowest PSA-level quartile ($\leq$22.1 ng/mL). On the contrary, in the highest PSA-level quartile treatment with sipuleucel-T showed only 2.8 months overall survival benefit (41). This suggests that treatment with sipuleucel-T should be initiated directly after the diagnosis of mCRPC, when patients have a lower tumor load, hence less immune suppression.

To date, the OS benefit of sipuleucel-T cannot be fully explained by the recorded immune responses. An elevated T-cell stimulation index was observed in the sipuleucel-T treated group. Nevertheless, T-cell proliferation responses to the fusion protein (PA2024) or PAP did not show a survival difference. Increased antibody levels against PA2024 were observed in 66.2% of the sipuleucel-T treated patients and in 2.9% of the placebo-treated patients coinciding with a slight, although not significant, survival benefit ($P = 0.08$). Increased antibody levels against PAP were noticed in 28.5% of the sipuleucel-T treated patients and in 1.4% of the placebo-treated patients, not correlating with survival (41). Research is currently ongoing to define additional biomarkers that could be related to increased overall survival.

To conclude, sipuleucel-T is the first autologous cellular immunotherapy for the treatment of PCa. Three phase III trials demonstrated crucial clinical evidence for the worthiness of sipuleucel-T. However, although an increase in overall survival of 4 months is beneficial for the patients, it is not the breakthrough for immunotherapy many researchers were hoping for. Cellular immunotherapy might not be a monotherapeutic alternative for PCa. Instead, combination with standard or novel treatment modalities might be decisive. Currently ongoing trials are focusing on combination therapies with androgen deprivation therapy, chemotherapy, and immune checkpoint inhibitor antibodies (**Table 2**).

PROSTATE-SPECIFIC MEMBRANE ANTIGEN

Prostate-specific membrane antigen, also known as glutamate carboxypeptidase II, is a zinc metalloenzyme with folate hydrolase activity that is expressed in membranes of prostate epithelial cells (87, 88). Its function in the prostate is still unknown. Low expression of PSMA is also found in the kidneys, salivary glands, duodenum, and the central and peripheral nervous system.

PSMA as tumor antigen

Prostate-specific membrane antigen is highly overexpressed in PCa and increased expression correlates with advanced disease and metastasis (89–91). It has also been shown that PSMA is involved in tumor angiogenesis of many solid tumors, and it is expressed in the endothelial lumen in tumors. Normal vascular endothelium in non-cancerous tissue is PSMA negative (92, 93). PSMA displays several features that qualify it as a suitable target for immunotherapy. In addition to its specific expression in the prostate, it is also a membrane-bound antigen that is presented on the cell surface, but not released into the circulation (94). PSMA has been exploited as a possible target for PCa treatment in different pre-clinical settings and in early-stage clinical trials (42, 43, 88, 95). Wolf et al. showed that the recombinant anti-PSMA-specific single-chain immunotoxin D7-PE40 was both specific and highly toxic for PSMA-expressing PCa cells *in vitro* and *in vivo* in prostate tumor-bearing mice (88). Usage of the ^{177}lutetium radiolabeled anti-PSMA monoclonal antibody J591 induced a 50% PSA reduction in 4 of the 35 patients with mCRPC (95). A similar PSA decrease was seen in an early clinical trial with PSMA peptide-pulsed DCs, where 9 of 33 patients displayed a partial clinical response (43). However, not all studies targeting PSMA have showed encouraging results. The PMSA-derived HLA-A2-restricted peptide (LLHETDSAV) appeared to be poorly immunogenic compared with other HLA-A2-restricted peptides, both *in vitro* as well as in patients with PCa (42). This underscores the importance of pre-clinical studies before clinical testing.

In summary, based on the highly specific expression pattern of PSMA in patients with PCa, PSMA poses as a suitable target for immunotherapy. However, early clinical trials have shown varying results. Further research concerning PSMA-based immunotherapy is warranted. **Table 2** shows several ongoing clinical studies targeting PSMA as a tumor antigen.

PROSTATE STEM-CELL ANTIGEN

Prostate stem-cell antigen (PSCA) is a glycosylphosphatidylinositol (GPI)-anchored protein expressed on the cell surface of both basal and luminal cells in the normal prostate, but overexpressed by PCa cells (44, 96). It is shown that PSCA, like other GPI-anchored proteins, is involved in the survival of stem cells, in T-cell activation and proliferation, and in cytokine and growth factor responses (97, 98). Furthermore, several studies have connected the Ly-6 family of PSCA-like GPI-anchored proteins to tumor growth and metastazation (99–102).

PSCA as tumor antigen

Its distinct expression pattern and possible function in tumor-progression makes PSCA an interesting target for immunotherapy. It has already been exploited in several studies, with promising results (45, 103–105). Anti-PSCA monoclonal antibodies have been reported to inhibit tumor growth and prolong the survival of mice bearing human PCa xenografts (46, 106). Additionally, a chaperone complex vaccine made of PSCA and the heat-shock protein GRP170 was shown to enhance T-cell-mediated immune responses, inhibit tumor growth, and prolong the life span of PCa tumor-bearing mice (107). Two DC vaccination studies have been performed in humans (45, 105). In the study by Thomas-Kaskel et al., patients with mCRPC were treated with DCs loaded with PSCA and PSA peptides. Endpoints were safety and induction of antigen-specific immunity. The vaccine was well tolerated in all patients, and 6 of 12 patients showed stable disease after four vaccinations. One patient had a complete response. Interestingly, this patient displayed an increase in serum PSA levels. Positive delayed-type hypersensitivity skin reactions were seen in four patients after four vaccinations. A positive delayed-type hypersensitivity test was associated with increased overall survival. HLA tetramer analysis detected high frequencies of peptide-specific T cells in one patient, who had an overall survival of 27 months (105). In another study, vaccinations were performed in three patients with mCRPC using multi-epitope (PSCA, PSMA, PAP, and PSA) pulsed DCs. The treatment was well tolerated, and significant CTLs responses against all PSAs were observed. In addition, DC vaccination was associated with an increase in PSA doubling time (45).

To conclude, PSCA has been used as a target for antigen-based immunotherapy in several clinical studies due to its role in tumor growth and metastases. Unfortunately, the study results were less impressive than expected. This might be the reason that to date there is no ongoing clinical trial with PSCA registered.

MUCIN-1

The mucin family members include proteins that enclose tandem repeat structures with a high proportion of prolines, threonines, and serines. The family consists of secreted and transmembrane forms, designated Mucin-1 (MUC-1) to MUC-21 (108). MUC-1 is a large cell surface glycoprotein found on the apical surface of most glandular and ductal epithelial cells, such as the lungs, intestines, and the prostate (109). In chronic inflammation, MUC-1 expression is induced by inflammatory cytokines like TNF-α, IFNγ, and IL-6. Overexpression contributes to oncogenesis by activation of growth and survival pathways (Wnt-β-catenin and nuclear factor-κB pathways), promoting receptor tyrosine kinase signaling and downregulation of stress-induced death pathways (108). MUC-1 overexpression is associated with colon, breast, lung, prostate, and pancreatic cancer. Moreover, it is associated with tumor-progression and correlated with advanced disease (110–112). MUC-1 has also been shown to have immunosuppressive effects in mice, and secreted MUC-1 has been shown to block T-cell activation (113, 114). Moreover, human monocyte-derived DCs cultured *in vitro* with MUC-1 peptide displayed a decreased expression of both co-stimulatory molecules and antigen presenting molecules upon activation (115). Similarly, depletion of soluble MUC-1 in tumor cell line supernatants abolished the anti-proliferative effect of these supernatants on T cells, and MUC-1 has therefore been identified as a target in PCa (116). The inhibitory effect of MUC-1 has also been demonstrated *in vivo*, when synthetic MUC-1 decreased the immune response in patients vaccinated with an MUC-1 containing polyvalent peptide vaccine (117). In a recent phase I/II trial, an autologous DC vaccine loaded with an MUC-1 glycoproteine and KLH in patients with CRPC was studied. Patients received three injections biweekly followed by booster vaccinations at 6 and 12 months. The rate of PSA rise decreased in six of seven patients. The PSA doubling time increased from a median of 2.9 months prior to vaccination to 7.5 months during vaccination (118). Richman et al. also showed clinical benefit for some patients with mCRPC treated with the combination of radioimmunotherapy with an anti-MUC-1 monoclonal antibody and paclitaxel (47) (**Table 1**).

Taken together, MUC-1 is important in tumor-progression and therefore a very interesting tumor-associated antigen. Several trials focusing on MUC-1 as a target for cancer immunotherapy in PCa are ongoing (**Table 2**).

CANCER/TESTIS ANTIGENS

Cancer/testis antigens are normally only expressed in gametogenic tissue. However, this group of proteins is aberrantly expressed in several types of cancers, including PCa (48). CTAs have been shown to contribute to tumor formation and progression (119, 120). The CTAs NY-ESO-1, the MAGE family, and A-kinase Anchor Proteins (AKAP)-4 will be discussed here.

NY-ESO-1 is found to be expressed in a variety of malignancies. It is not expressed in normal adult tissue, with the exception of the testis. The expression of NY-ESO-1 is associated with level of disease, and higher NY-ESO mRNA and protein expression are observed in metastatic and advanced PCa, as compared to localized tumors (120–124). The function of NY-ESO-1 is unknown, but it is speculated to play a role in meiosis or in the assembly of the organelles that develops over the anterior half of the head in the spermatozoa (125, 126). The NY-ESO-1 is a promising candidate because of its tumor-restricted expression and the identification as one of the most immunogenic CTAs, eliciting spontaneous cytotoxic and antibody-mediated immune responses in patients with NY-ESO-1 + tumors (127–129). Humoral responses against NY-ESO-1 have been evoked by non-specific immune activation in patients with mCRPC treated with a combination of checkpoint inhibitor ipilimumab and GM-CSF, underscoring its immunogenicity (130). NY-ESO-1 has been used as target antigen in several clinical studies. Both MHC class I and II restricted T-cell epitopes specific for NY-ESO-1 are identified (131). MHC class I and/or II restricted NY-ESO-1 peptides were compared in a peptide-based vaccine trial in patients with mCRPC. The vaccine increased the PSA doubling time and yielded antigen-specific T-cell responses in all patients treated. The strongest results were seen in chemo-naive patients, most likely due to a lower tumor burden, thus less tumor-induced immune suppression (132). The immunogenic features of NY-ESO-1 are further supported by a study using a protein-based vaccine with CpG as an adjuvant. This vaccine was able to prime antigen-specific B-cell responses and induced NY-ESO-1 specific, tumor-reactive CTLs in patients with metastatic PCa, independently of autologous NY-ESO-1 expression (49). Vaccination against a tumor-specific protein without it being present, repositions this clinical vaccination protocol toward a preventive setting.

Second, the MAGE CTA subfamily is also expressed in PCa. Upregulation of these CTAs is found in CRPC and is associated with resistance to chemotherapeutic agents (50). MAGE-A2 downregulates p53 transactivation function through histone deacetylase recruitment, a possible explanation how MAGE-A2 expression leads to resistance to chemotherapy (50). Indeed, silencing of MAGE-A2 increased sensitivity to docetaxel chemotherapy in PCa tumor cells (120). Expression of MAGE-C2/CT10, another member of the MAGE-A subfamily, is correlated with the degree of PCa malignancy. It is an indication of higher risk for biochemical recurrence after radical prostatectomy and represents a potential target for immunotherapy (133). Members of the MAGE-A subfamily and NY-ESO-1 are often co-expressed in prostate malignancies.

Third, the CTA AKAP are a family of scaffolding proteins capable of controlling intracellular signals. AKAP is involved in cytoskeletal regulation and organization by affecting cyclic AMP-dependent protein kinase-A (134). In the prostate epithelium, the anchor proteins synthesize and secrete calcitonin. It has been shown that the calcitonin secretion from malignant prostates is several-fold higher than from benign prostates (135). The calcitonin receptor is expressed in malignant PCa, and its activation stimulates growth of PCa cells via activation of cyclic AMP as well as protein kinase C (136, 137). These mechanisms suggest a marked increase in the invasiveness of PCa cells (138). Modulation of protein kinase-A activation possibly interferes with the growth, tumor genicity, and metastatic potential of advanced tumors. First, AKAP-4 has been showed to be an immunogenic CTA in patients with multiple myeloma (139). Later, Chiriva-Internati et al. showed cytoplasmic and surface expression of AKAP-4 in the LnCAP PCa cell line. AKAP-4 expression in the prostate epithelial cells was shown in 13 of 15 patients with PCa, but not in healthy subjects. Cytotoxicity assays showed that AKAP-4-loaded DC-stimulated T cells were capable of killing autologous PCa cells *in vitro*. Neither killing of AKAP-4 negative PCa cells nor normal prostate epithelial cells was observed. This underscores the antigen specificity of the response and prevention of autoimmune reactions (140). This makes AKAP-4 a very interesting target for PCa anti-tumor vaccination.

To conclude, several CTAs, especially NY-ESO-1, the MAGE-A subfamily, and AKAP-4, could serve as therapeutic targets in the fight against PCa (120, 122, 140). Especially NY-ESO-1 is of major relevance in PCa and a target in different ongoing trials (see **Table 2**). Due to the tumor-restricted expression of CTAs, these antigens can also be used in an adjuvant or a preventive setting hindering the recurrence of CTA-positive tumors (49).

MIXTURE OF TUMOR-ASSOCIATED ANTIGENS

To date, many investigators underscore the importance of a personalized approach by selecting patient-specific mutations as target antigens for immunotherapy. The group of Noguchi took a first step in a personalized direction. They performed two phase II studies with a personalized peptide vaccine (PPV). The vaccine consisted of four peptides based on each patient's immunoreactivity profile. Peptides of a variety of tumor-associated antigens were tested, including PSA, PAP, PSMA, multidrug resistance protein, and a choice of different epithelial tumor antigens. The peptides included in the vaccine were selected on their capacity to induce CTL responses. In the first phase II trial, patients with CRPC were randomized to PPV combined with chemotherapy or chemotherapy only (141). Antibody responses were seen in 64% of the patients and cytotoxic T-cells responses in 72% of the patients. An increase in progression-free survival was observed in the PPV/chemotherapy group as compared with the patients who only received chemotherapy. However, immune responses did not correlate with clinical outcome in patients treated with PPV and chemotherapy. Interestingly, the authors found that lower levels of IL-6 before PPV vaccination were favorable for overall survival. IL-6 have been associated with more aggressive cancer progression and decreased survival in PCa (142). In this perspective, IL-6 may be seen as an indicator of prognosis and a predictor of therapy effectiveness. It is also hypothesized that inhibiting IL-6 signaling may be beneficial in patients enduring other immunotherapeutic treatment.

The results of the PPV vaccinations are promising. A randomized trial with an appropriate control group before and after chemotherapeutic treatment is needed to fully identify a clinical benefit of PPV treatment. Currently, a vaccine consisting of 20 peptides is applied to patients with CRPC in an exploratory, randomized, open-label study (UMIN000008209, **Table 2**).

PROSTATE CANCER CELL LINES

GVAX

GVAX is an allogeneic, cell-based immunotherapy consisting of the PCa cell lines LNCaP and PC-3. These cell lines are genetically modified with a recombinant GM-CSF adeno-based viral vector and irradiated before administration. Clinical results in patients with PCa are indicative for a favorable clinical outcome with no toxicities (143, 144). These results have led to phase III trials, using the most promising high-dose GVAX protocol. Unfortunately, due to an even increased mortality in the GVAX-treated group, and disappointing interim results the trials were abrogated (145, 146).

van den Eertwegh et al. combined the immune checkpoint inhibitor ipilimumab (anti-CTLA-4) with GVAX (147). More than 50% decline in PSA level was seen in 25% of the patients. All the responding patients got 3.0 or 5.0 mg/kg ipilimumab. There was dose-limiting toxicity in the 5.0 mg/kg group of patients, while the lower ipilimumab regimens were well tolerated. Markedly, all patients with immune-related adverse events showed a decrease in PSA levels. A small number of patients additionally displayed an anti-PSMA antibody response. These patients had a significant increase in median overall survival (46.5 months compared to 20.6 months for patients without this humoral response). T-cell monitoring studies were performed in 28 patients receiving the combination therapy of GVAX and ipilimumab. Compared with the control group, an increase in absolute lymphocyte counts and enhanced CD4+ and CD8+ T-cell differentiation was observed. These immune responses were associated with a significantly prolonged overall survival. In addition, an OS benefit was also seen in case of high pre-treatment levels of CD4+, CTLA-4+, CD4+/PD-1+, or non-naïve CD8+ T cells. Low pre-treatment frequencies of differentiated CD4+ or regulatory T cells resulted in a prolonged OS (148). This reveals perspectives for future biomarker research.

mRNA-TRANSFECTED DCs

An alternative approach for PCa cell lines is the use of PCa cell line-derived RNA or tumor antigen encoding mRNA. Kyte et al. transfected monocyte-derived DCs with mRNA derived from the PCa cell lines LnCAP, DU-145, and PC-3. Although the generation of mRNA-transfected DC is challenging, DC vaccination appeared feasible and safe (149, 150). Furthermore, PSA-specific T-cell responses were detected in 12 of 19 patients with PCa who underwent mRNA-DC vaccination (149). To date, patients are recruited in a phase I/II trial (NCT01197625, **Table 2**), studying the mRNA-transfected DCs in curative resected patients with PCa. More studies are needed to properly determine the strength of mRNA-transfected DCs. The usage of this immunotherapeutic modality within combination therapies might be of greater significance.

DISCUSSION

In this review, we provided overview of PCa tumor-associated antigens and how they are used to target PCa via immunotherapy (**Table 1**). PSMA and PSCA are normally expressed in the prostate gland but upregulated during cancer development and they may play a role in tumor progression (44, 89, 96, 151). Increased serum levels of secreted tumor antigens, such as PSA and PAP, can be used as biomarkers for disease and disease progression (51, 73, 74). More general tumor antigens, like MUC-1, AKAP-4, and NY-ESO-1, can also be found in PCa and might be candidates for immunotherapeutic interventions (111, 123, 140). MUC-1 is expressed in normal tissue and upregulated on several tumors, where it can exert immunosuppressive effects and attain tumor growth (110). Hence, targeting MUC-1 could have a dual role – directing the immune response toward the tumor and reducing immune suppression. This might also be valid for other immunosuppressive antigens, such as the MAGE-A subfamily or PSA (54, 120). On the other hand, the NY-ESO-1 antigen is often immunogenic *per se*, and pre-existing immune responses directed against this antigen are common in treatment-naive patients (128). Pre-existing CTL responses against PSA and PAP in healthy individuals and patients with chronic prostatitis also support the definition of PCa as an immunogenic tumor (26, 27), where tolerance against self-antigens can be broken and the immune system can be harnessed against the tumors.

Today, the only registered product for antigen-targeted immunotherapy in PCa is sipuleucel-T (38, 39, 41). Although the significance of this intervention received criticism, sipuleucel-T proves an important point: autologous cellular immunotherapy is feasible and can indeed be developed as an approved treatment modality. To date, no convincing mechanism of action has been elucidated for sipuleucel-T. Increased immune responses were observed but no correlation with clinical outcome could be established. Clinical studies aiming at identifying immunological responses and thereby hopefully providing an in-depth understanding of the mode of action of sipulecuel-T are ongoing. Unraveling the mechanism might be beneficial for further development of sipuleucel-T and other immunotherapeutic approaches.

Effective immune responses induced by immunotherapeutic treatments are still not common, and probably vary depending on tumor type, somatic differences between tumor cells, and the tumor microenvironment (66). Several recent trials have shown promising results in both clinical and immunological responses. Constructs targeting the NY-ESO-1 antigen has led to significant immunological responses, which makes NY-ESO-1 an interesting antigen to target immunotherapeutic strategies in future (49, 132). Immunological responses are also induced by several PSA-targeting vaccines, supporting the usage of PSA as an immunogenic tumor antigen (34–36).

Insight in the localization of the tumor antigen (on/in cells, normal cells vs. tumor cells, in organs) and the specificity of the antigen facilitates a precise selection of target antigens with the intention of optimizing the translation of immunotherapeutic treatments to the clinic. However, despite significant T-cell responses, tumor progression is seen most frequently in patients treated with cancer immunotherapy. This is due to the complexity of human beings and the complexity of tumors and metastases (152). The complexity of cancer is also described by Fox et al. (153). This report of the collaborating immunotherapy organizations, known as the Society for Immunotherapy of Cancer (SITC), contains the identification of nine hurdles in cancer immunotherapy that significantly delays clinical translation of promising cancer immunotherapeutics. We here discuss the hurdles relevant for this review, for a complete overview, we refer to the original article (153). The first hurdle to overcome is the complexity of cancer, tumor heterogeneity, and immune escape. The immune signature of the tumor, distinguished by genetic or histological evaluation, can predict responders to cancer immunotherapy (154, 155). The second relevant SITC hurdle for this review is the lack of definitive biomarkers for the assessment of clinical efficacy of cancer immunotherapies. Biomarkers to distinguish between patients responsive to initial treatment, patients displaying immune inhibitory features, and patients with non-immunogenic tumors, are needed. Pre-existing anti-tumor responses or the expression of inhibitory markers are examples of suggested biomarkers that could be used to predict treatment outcome and individualize the treatment regime.

A correlation of immune parameters with clinical outcome after immunotherapy is not established in patients with PCa. This can be attributed to (i) a limited number of patients per immunotherapeutic approach; (ii) a variation in clinical features of patients with PCa before treatment; and (iii) the difference in clinical signs of tumor control between conventional toxic treatments and immunotherapeutic treatments. This last argument is also one of the hurdles identified by the SITC. Effective immunotherapy does not always display initial shrinkage of the tumor, but rather a pattern of tumor growth and progression followed by shrinkage when the tumor is recognized and destroyed by the immune system (156–158). This paradox has been illustrated by the negative outcomes on progression-free survival or PSA responses in the sipuleucel-T trials and PSA-TRICOM trial. Tumor swelling, increased release of PSA due to elevated tumor cell death, and initial detrimental symptoms might be associated with a favorable clinical outcome rather than with progressive disease, as stated in the WHO and Response Evaluation Criteria In Solid Tumors (RECIST) criteria (156, 157, 159). Although clinically responding patients might have been missed, some patients do not respond, neither clinically nor immunologically. Lack of immunogenicity of the antigens used might be an explanation, but a major factor is the immunosuppressive networks within cancer patients. Infiltrating lymphocytes can be regulated by a number of inhibitory pathways within the tumor and thereby shift the direction of the ongoing immune response toward a more tolerogenic one. Other patients might have "silent" tumors that do not display an inflammatory phenotype and hence do not attract lymphocyte infiltration (66).

Novel monoclonal antibodies targeted against inhibitory receptors on T cells (anti-CTLA-4 and anti-PD-1) are able to prolong their effector functions and prevent immune inhibition. These treatment strategies are tested in combination with other immunotherapeutic approaches and showed promising results in a subset of patients (61, 147, 160). There are still ongoing combination therapy studies with ipilimumab and sipuleucel-T which will hopefully overcome the immunosuppressive signals provided by immune evading tumors (NCT01804465 and NCT 01832870). Although antigen-based immunotherapy itself seldom gives rise to severe autoimmune reactions, the combination with an immune checkpoint inhibitor likely will enhance the risk of immune-related adverse events, as recently shown in melanoma patients treated with ipilimumab (161–163).

FUTURE CHALLENGES AND OPPORTUNITIES

Until recently, patients with mCRPC had limited treatment options and a poor prognosis. With new sequential hormonal therapies, second-line chemotherapy, and new immunotherapeutic strategies, a new era has started. To date, PCa is one of the few tumor types in which immunotherapy is part of the current standard of care. Augmenting immune responses to PCa antigens is a valid therapeutic approach, and clinical responses with minimal toxic effects are observed.

In this review, we focused on commonly expressed tumor-associated antigens. Recently, patient-specific epitopes are identified as highly important to improve T-cell reactivity. Targeting these patient- and cancer-specific mutated epitopes holds promise for even better results and possibly cure of patients. By complete genome and transcriptome, sequencing and mass spectrometry-mutated HLA-binding peptides, so-called neoantigens, might be identified (164). Vaccination with individually overexpressed tumor-specific peptides could result in a unique, personalized anti-cancer vaccine (165–167). Recently, the first two demonstrations of autologous cancer exome-based T-cell responses against patient-specific neoantigens in humans were published (167, 168). This knowledge is a major step forward for both the identification of new diagnostic strategies by tumor exome analysis, as well as for the development of individualized immunotherapeutic approaches. Combination therapies harboring these patient-specific peptide vaccinations together with immune checkpoint inhibitors are likely to generate an even better immune control. There is no doubt that these are very exciting times for cancer immunotherapy.

ACKNOWLEDGMENTS

This work is supported by the Swedish Research Council and the "Koningin Wilhelmina Onderzoeksprogramma" (Queen Wilhelmina Research Program): KWF 2009-4402.

REFERENCES

1. Jemal A, Siegel R, Ward E, Hao Y, Xu J, Thun MJ. Cancer statistics, 2009. *CA Cancer J Clin* (2009) **59**(4):225–49. doi:10.3322/caac.20006
2. Ferlay J, Steliarova-Foucher E, Lortet-Tieulent J, Rosso S, Coebergh JW, Comber H, et al. Cancer incidence and mortality patterns in Europe: estimates for 40 countries in 2012. *Eur J Cancer* (2013) **49**(6):1374–403. doi:10.1016/j.ejca.2012.12.027
3. Risk M, Corman JM. The role of immunotherapy in prostate cancer: an overview of current approaches in development. *Rev Urol* (2009) **11**(1):16–27.
4. Tannock IF, de Wit R, Berry WR, Horti J, Pluzanska A, Chi KN, et al. Docetaxel plus prednisone or mitoxantrone plus prednisone for advanced prostate cancer. *N Engl J Med* (2004) **351**(15):1502–12. doi:10.1056/NEJMoa040720
5. Berthold DR, Pond GR, Soban F, de Wit R, Eisenberger M, Tannock IF. Docetaxel plus prednisone or mitoxantrone plus prednisone for advanced prostate cancer: updated survival in the TAX 327 study. *J Clin Oncol* (2008) **26**(2):242–5. doi:10.1200/JCO.2007.12.4008
6. Petrylak DP, Tangen CM, Hussain MH, Lara PN Jr, Jones JA, Taplin ME, et al. Docetaxel and estramustine compared with mitoxantrone and prednisone for advanced refractory prostate cancer. *N Engl J Med* (2004) **351**(15):1513–20. doi:10.1056/NEJMoa041318
7. Couzin-Frankel J. Breakthrough of the year 2013. Cancer immunotherapy. *Science* (2013) **342**(6165):1432–3. doi:10.1126/science.342.6165.1432
8. Medzhitov R. Origin and physiological roles of inflammation. *Nature* (2008) **454**(7203):428–35. doi:10.1038/nature07201
9. Sfanos KS, De Marzo AM. Prostate cancer and inflammation: the evidence. *Histopathology* (2012) **60**(1):199–215. doi:10.1111/j.1365-2559.2011.04033.x
10. Ortega-Gomez A, Perretti M, Soehnlein O. Resolution of inflammation: an integrated view. *EMBO Mol Med* (2013) **5**(5):661–74. doi:10.1002/emmm.201202382
11. Dvorak HF. Tumors: wounds that do not heal. Similarities between tumor stroma generation and wound healing. *N Engl J Med* (1986) **315**(26):1650–9. doi:10.1056/NEJM198612253152606
12. Coussens LM, Werb Z. Inflammation and cancer. *Nature* (2002) **420**(6917):860–7. doi:10.1038/nature01322
13. Grivennikov SI, Karin M. Inflammation and oncogenesis: a vicious connection. *Curr Opin Genet Dev* (2010) **20**(1):65–71. doi:10.1016/j.gde.2009.11.004
14. Wang W, Bergh A, Damber JE. Morphological transition of proliferative inflammatory atrophy to high-grade intraepithelial neoplasia and cancer in human prostate. *Prostate* (2009) **69**(13):1378–86. doi:10.1002/pros.20992
15. Putzi MJ, De Marzo AM. Morphologic transitions between proliferative inflammatory atrophy and high-grade prostatic intraepithelial neoplasia. *Urology* (2000) **56**(5):828–32. doi:10.1016/S0090-4295(00)00776-7
16. Salinas CA, Kwon EM, FitzGerald LM, Feng Z, Nelson PS, Ostrander EA, et al. Use of aspirin and other nonsteroidal antiinflammatory medications in relation to prostate cancer risk. *Am J Epidemiol* (2010) **172**(5):578–90. doi:10.1093/aje/kwq175
17. Jafari S, Etminan M, Afshar K. Nonsteroidal anti-inflammatory drugs and prostate cancer: a systematic review of the literature and meta-analysis. *Can Urol Assoc J* (2009) **3**(4):323–30.
18. Liu X, Plummer SJ, Nock NL, Casey G, Witte JS. Nonsteroidal antiinflammatory drugs and decreased risk of advanced prostate cancer: modification by lymphotoxin alpha. *Am J Epidemiol* (2006) **164**(10):984–9. doi:10.1093/aje/kwj294
19. Aggarwal BB, Vijayalekshmi RV, Sung B. Targeting inflammatory pathways for prevention and therapy of cancer: short-term friend, long-term foe. *Clin Cancer Res* (2009) **15**(2):425–30. doi:10.1158/1078-0432.CCR-08-0149
20. Brede CM, Shoskes DA. The etiology and management of acute prostatitis. *Nat Rev Urol* (2011) **8**(4):207–12. doi:10.1038/nrurol.2011.22
21. Roberts RO, Bergstralh EJ, Bass SE, Lieber MM, Jacobsen SJ. Prostatitis as a risk factor for prostate cancer. *Epidemiology* (2004) **15**(1):93–9. doi:10.1097/01.ede.0000101022.38330.7c
22. Krieger JN, Nyberg L Jr, Nickel JC. NIH consensus definition and classification of prostatitis. *JAMA* (1999) **282**(3):236–7. doi:10.1001/jama.282.3.236
23. Alexander RB, Brady F, Ponniah S. Autoimmune prostatitis: evidence of T cell reactivity with normal prostatic proteins. *Urology* (1997) **50**(6):893–9. doi:10.1016/S0090-4295(97)00456-1
24. Batstone GR, Doble A, Gaston JS. Autoimmune T cell responses to seminal plasma in chronic pelvic pain syndrome (CPPS). *Clin Exp Immunol* (2002) **128**(2):302–7. doi:10.1046/j.1365-2249.2002.01853.x
25. Penna G, Fibbi B, Maggi M, Adorini L. Prostate autoimmunity: from experimental models to clinical counterparts. *Expert Rev Clin Immunol* (2009) **5**(5):577–86. doi:10.1586/eci.09.37
26. Motrich RD, Maccioni M, Molina R, Tissera A, Olmedo J, Riera CM, et al. Presence of INFgamma-secreting lymphocytes specific to prostate antigens in a group of chronic prostatitis patients. *Clin Immunol* (2005) **116**(2):149–57. doi:10.1016/j.clim.2005.03.011
27. Ponniah S, Arah I, Alexander RB. PSA is a candidate self-antigen in autoimmune chronic prostatitis/chronic pelvic pain syndrome. *Prostate* (2000)

44(1):49–54. doi:10.1002/1097-0045(20000615)44:1<49::AID-PROS7>3.3.CO;2-Z

28. Motrich RD, Maccioni M, Riera CM, Rivero VE. Autoimmune prostatitis: state of the art. *Scand J Immunol* (2007) **66**(2–3):217–27. doi:10.1111/j.1365-3083.2007.01971.x
29. Mercader M, Bodner BK, Moser MT, Kwon PS, Park ES, Manecke RG, et al. T cell infiltration of the prostate induced by androgen withdrawal in patients with prostate cancer. *Proc Natl Acad Sci U S A* (2001) **98**(25):14565–70. doi:10.1073/pnas.251140998
30. Nagaraj S, Gabrilovich DI. Tumor escape mechanism governed by myeloid-derived suppressor cells. *Cancer Res* (2008) **68**(8):2561–3. doi:10.1158/0008-5472.CAN-07-6229
31. Talmadge JE. Pathways mediating the expansion and immunosuppressive activity of myeloid-derived suppressor cells and their relevance to cancer therapy. *Clin Cancer Res* (2007) **13**(18 Pt 1):5243–8. doi:10.1158/1078-0432.CCR-07-0182
32. Ostrand-Rosenberg S, Sinha P. Myeloid-derived suppressor cells: linking inflammation and cancer. *J Immunol* (2009) **182**(8):4499–506. doi:10.4049/jimmunol.0802740
33. Cha E, Fong L. Immunotherapy for prostate cancer: biology and therapeutic approaches. *J Clin Oncol* (2011) **29**(27):3677–85. doi:10.1200/JCO.2010.34.5025
34. Eder J, Kantoff PW, Roper K, Xu GX, Bubley GJ, Boyden J, et al. A phase I trial of a recombinant vaccinia virus expressing prostate-specific antigen in advanced prostate cancer. *Clin Cancer Res* (2000) **6**(5):1632–8.
35. Meidenbauer N, Harris DT, Spitler LE, Whiteside TL. Generation of PSA-reactive effector cells after vaccination with a PSA-based vaccine in patients with prostate cancer. *Prostate* (2000) **43**(2):88–100. doi:10.1002/(SICI)1097-0045(20000501)43:2<88::AID-PROS3>3.0.CO;2-G
36. Barrou B, Benoît G, Ouldkaci M, Cussenot O, Salcedo M, Agrawal S, et al. Vaccination of prostatectomized prostate cancer patients in biochemical relapse, with autologous dendritic cells pulsed with recombinant human PSA. *Cancer Immunol Immunother* (2004) **53**(5):453–60. doi:10.1007/s00262-003-0451-2
37. Gulley JL, Arlen PM, Bastian A, Morin S, Marte J, Beetham P, et al. Combining a recombinant cancer vaccine with standard definitive radiotherapy in patients with localized prostate cancer. *Clin Cancer Res* (2005) **11**(9):3353–62. doi:10.1158/1078-0432.CCR-04-2062
38. Higano CS, Schellhammer PF, Small EJ, Burch PA, Nemunaitis J, Yuh L, et al. Integrated data from 2 randomized, double-blind, placebo-controlled, phase 3 trials of active cellular immunotherapy with sipuleucel-T in advanced prostate cancer. *Cancer* (2009) **115**(16):3670–9. doi:10.1002/cncr.24429
39. Small EJ, Schellhammer PF, Higano CS, Redfern CH, Nemunaitis JJ, Valone FH, et al. Placebo-controlled phase III trial of immunologic therapy with sipuleucel-T (APC8015) in patients with metastatic, asymptomatic hormone refractory prostate cancer. *J Clin Oncol* (2006) **24**(19):3089–94. doi:10.1200/JCO.2005.04.5252
40. Sheikh NA, Petrylak D, Kantoff PW, Dela Rosa C, Stewart FP, Kuan LY, et al. Sipuleucel-T immune parameters correlate with survival: an analysis of the randomized phase 3 clinical trials in men with castration-resistant prostate cancer. *Cancer Immunol Immunother* (2013) **62**(1):137–47. doi:10.1007/s00262-012-1317-2
41. Kantoff P, Higano CS, Shore ND, Berger ER, Small EJ, Penson DF, et al. Sipuleucel-T immunotherapy for castration-resistant prostate cancer. *N Engl J Med* (2010) **363**(5):411–22. doi:10.1056/NEJMoa1001294
42. Knight D, Peterson AC, Rini BI, Harlin H, Gajewski TF, Stadler WM. The HLA-A2-restricted PSMA peptide LLHETDSAV is poorly immunogenic in patients with metastatic prostate cancer. *Prostate* (2009) **69**(2):142–8. doi:10.1002/pros.20864
43. Tjoa BA, Simmons SJ, Bowes VA, Ragde H, Rogers M, Elgamal A, et al. Evaluation of phase I/II clinical trials in prostate cancer with dendritic cells and PSMA peptides. *Prostate* (1998) **36**(1):39–44. doi:10.1002/(SICI)1097-0045(19980615)36:1<39::AID-PROS6>3.0.CO;2-6
44. Gu Z, Thomas G, Yamashiro J, Shintaku IP, Dorey F, Raitano A, et al. Prostate stem cell antigen (PSCA) expression increases with high gleason score, advanced stage and bone metastasis in prostate cancer. *Oncogene* (2000) **19**(10):1288–96. doi:10.1038/sj.onc.1203426
45. Waeckerle-Men Y, Uetz-von Allmen E, Fopp M, von Moos R, Böhme C, Schmid HP, et al. Dendritic cell-based multi-epitope immunotherapy of hormone-refractory prostate carcinoma. *Cancer Immunol Immunother* (2006) **55**(12):1524–33. doi:10.1007/s00262-006-0157-3
46. Ross S, Spencer SD, Holcomb I, Tan C, Hongo J, Devaux B, et al. Prostate stem cell antigen as therapy target: tissue expression and in vivo efficacy of an immunoconjugate. *Cancer Res* (2002) **62**(9):2546–53.
47. Richman CM, Denardo SJ, O'Donnell RT, Yuan A, Shen S, Goldstein DS, et al. High-dose radioimmunotherapy combined with fixed, low-dose paclitaxel in metastatic prostate and breast cancer by using a MUC-1 monoclonal antibody, m170, linked to indium-111/yttrium-90 via a cathepsin cleavable linker with cyclosporine to prevent human anti-mouse antibody. *Clin Cancer Res* (2005) **11**(16):5920–7. doi:10.1158/1078-0432.ccr-05-0211
48. Scanlan MJ, Gure AO, Jungbluth AA, Old LJ, Chen YT. Cancer/testis antigens: an expanding family of targets for cancer immunotherapy. *Immunol Rev* (2002) **188**:22–32. doi:10.1034/j.1600-065X.2002.18803.x
49. Karbach J, Neumann A, Atmaca A, Wahle C, Brand K, von Boehmer L, et al. Efficient in vivo priming by vaccination with recombinant NY-ESO-1 protein and CpG in antigen naive prostate cancer patients. *Clin Cancer Res* (2011) **17**(4):861–70. doi:10.1158/1078-0432.CCR-10-1811
50. Monte M, Simonatto M, Peche LY, Bublik DR, Gobessi S, Pierotti MA, et al. MAGE-A tumor antigens target p53 transactivation function through histone deacetylase recruitment and confer resistance to chemotherapeutic agents. *Proc Natl Acad Sci U S A* (2006) **103**(30):11160–5. doi:10.1073/pnas.0510834103
51. Oesterling JE. Prostate specific antigen: a critical assessment of the most useful tumor marker for adenocarcinoma of the prostate. *J Urol* (1991) **145**(5):907–23.
52. Balk SP, Ko YJ, Bubley GJ. Biology of prostate-specific antigen. *J Clin Oncol* (2003) **21**(2):383–91. doi:10.1200/JCO.2003.02.083
53. Watt KW, Lee PJ, M'Timkulu T, Chan WP, Loor R. Human prostate-specific antigen: structural and functional similarity with serine proteases. *Proc Natl Acad Sci U S A* (1986) **83**(10):3166–70. doi:10.1073/pnas.83.10.3166
54. Williams SA, Jelinek CA, Litvinov I, Cotter RJ, Isaacs JT, Denmeade SR. Enzymatically active prostate-specific antigen promotes growth of human prostate cancers. *Prostate* (2011) **71**(15):1595–607. doi:10.1002/pros.21375
55. Williams SA, Singh P, Isaacs JT, Denmeade SR. Does PSA play a role as a promoting agent during the initiation and/or progression of prostate cancer? *Prostate* (2007) **67**(3):312–29. doi:10.1002/pros.20531
56. Aalamian M, Tourkova IL, Chatta GS, Lilja H, Huland E, Huland H, et al. Inhibition of dendropoiesis by tumor derived and purified prostate specific antigen. *J Urol* (2003) **170**(5):2026–30. doi:10.1097/01.ju.0000091264.46134.b7
57. Isaacs JT, Isaacs WB. Androgen receptor outwits prostate cancer drugs. *Nat Med* (2004) **10**(1):26–7. doi:10.1038/nm0104-26
58. Corman JM, Sercarz EE, Nanda NK. Recognition of prostate-specific antigenic peptide determinants by human CD4 and CD8 T cells. *Clin Exp Immunol* (1998) **114**(2):166–72. doi:10.1046/j.1365-2249.1998.00678.x
59. Hodge JW, Sabzevari H, Yafal AG, Gritz L, Lorenz MG, Schlom J. A triad of costimulatory molecules synergize to amplify T-cell activation. *Cancer Res* (1999) **59**(22):5800–7.
60. Kantoff P, Schuetz TJ, Blumenstein BA, Glode LM, Bilhartz DL, Wyand M, et al. Overall survival analysis of a phase II randomized controlled trial of a Poxviral-based PSA-targeted immunotherapy in metastatic castration-resistant prostate cancer. *J Clin Oncol* (2010) **28**(7):1099–105. doi:10.1200/JCO.2009.25.0597
61. Madan R, Mohebtash M, Arlen PM, Vergati M, Rauckhorst M, Steinberg SM, et al. Ipilimumab and a poxviral vaccine targeting prostate-specific antigen in metastatic castration-resistant prostate cancer: a phase 1 dose-escalation trial. *Lancet Oncol* (2012) **13**(5):501–8. doi:10.1016/S1470-2045(12)70006-2
62. Correale P, Walmsley K, Nieroda C, Zaremba S, Zhu M, Schlom J, et al. In vitro generation of human cytotoxic T lymphocytes specific for peptides derived from prostate-specific antigen. *J Natl Cancer Inst* (1997) **89**(4):293–300. doi:10.1093/jnci/89.4.293
63. Kennedy-Smith AG, McKenzie JL, Owen MC, Davidson PJ, Vuckovic S, Hart DN. Prostate specific antigen inhibits immune responses in vitro: a potential role in prostate cancer. *J Urol* (2002) **168**(2):741–7. doi:10.1097/00005392-200208000-00092
64. Miller A, Pisa P. Tumor escape mechanisms in prostate cancer. *Cancer Immunol Immunother* (2007) **56**(1):81–7. doi:10.1007/s00262-005-0110-x
65. Dallas SL, Zhao S, Cramer SD, Chen Z, Peehl DM, Bonewald LF. Preferential production of latent transforming growth factor beta-2 by primary prostatic

epithelial cells and its activation by prostate-specific antigen. *J Cell Physiol* (2005) **202**(2):361–70. doi:10.1002/jcp.20147

66. Gajewski T, Schreiber H, Fu Y-X. Innate and adaptive immune cells in the tumor microenvironment. *Nat Immunol* (2013) **14**(10):1014–22. doi:10.1038/ni.2703
67. Gulley JL, Arlen PM, Madan RA, Tsang KY, Pazdur MP, Skarupa L, et al. Immunologic and prognostic factors associated with overall survival employing a poxviral-based PSA vaccine in metastatic castrate-resistant prostate cancer. *Cancer Immunol Immunother* (2010) **59**(5):663–74. doi:10.1007/s00262-009-0782-8
68. Kong H, Byun J. Emerging roles of human prostatic acid phosphatase. *Biomol Ther (Seoul)* (2013) **21**(1):10–20. doi:10.4062/biomolther.2012.095
69. Hassan MI, Aijaz A, Ahmad F. Structural and functional analysis of human prostatic acid phosphatase. *Expert Rev Anticancer Ther* (2010) **10**(7):1055–68. doi:10.1586/era.10.46
70. Dave BN, Rindani TH. Acid phosphatase activity in human semen. *Int J Fertil* (1988) **33**(1):45–7.
71. Afzal S, Ahmad M, Mushtaq S, Mubarik A, Qureshi AH, Khan SA. Morphological features correlation with serum tumour markers in prostatic carcinoma. *J Coll Physicians Surg Pak* (2003) **13**(9):511–4.
72. Gunia S, Koch S, May M, Dietel M, Erbersdobler A. Expression of prostatic acid phosphatase (PSAP) in transurethral resection specimens of the prostate is predictive of histopathologic tumor stage in subsequent radical prostatectomies. *Virchows Arch* (2009) **454**(5):573–9. doi:10.1007/s00428-009-0759-1
73. Oesterling JE, Brendler CB, Epstein JI, Kimball AW Jr, Walsh PC. Correlation of clinical stage, serum prostatic acid phosphatase and preoperative Gleason grade with final pathological stage in 275 patients with clinically localized adenocarcinoma of the prostate. *J Urol* (1987) **138**(1):92–8.
74. Ozu C, Nakashima J, Horiguchi Y, Oya M, Ohigashi T, Murai M. Prediction of bone metastases by combination of tartrate-resistant acid phosphatase, alkaline phosphatase and prostate specific antigen in patients with prostate cancer. *Int J Urol* (2008) **15**(5):419–22. doi:10.1111/j.1442-2042.2008.02029.x
75. Graddis TJ, McMahan CJ, Tamman J, Page KJ, Trager JB. Prostatic acid phosphatase expression in human tissues. *Int J Clin Exp Pathol* (2011) **4**(3):295–306.
76. Jacobs EL, Haskell CM. Clinical use of tumor markers in oncology. *Curr Probl Cancer* (1991) **15**(6):299–360. doi:10.1016/0147-0272(91)90005-U
77. Matera L. The choice of the antigen in the dendritic cell-based vaccine therapy for prostate cancer. *Cancer Treat Rev* (2010) **36**(2):131–41. doi:10.1016/j.ctrv.2009.11.002
78. Peshwa MV, Shi JD, Ruegg C, Laus R, van Schooten WC. Induction of prostate tumor-specific CD8+ cytotoxic T-lymphocytes in vitro using antigen-presenting cells pulsed with prostatic acid phosphatase peptide. *Prostate* (1998) **36**(2):129–38. doi:10.1002/(SICI)1097-0045(19980701)36:2<129::AID-PROS8>3.0.CO;2-D
79. Olson BM, Frye TP, Johnson LE, Fong L, Knutson KL, Disis ML, et al. HLA-A2-restricted T-cell epitopes specific for prostatic acid phosphatase. *Cancer Immunol Immunother* (2010) **59**(6):943–53. doi:10.1007/s00262-010-0820-6
80. Fong L, Brockstedt D, Benike C, Breen JK, Strang G, Ruegg CL, et al. Dendritic cell-based xenoantigen vaccination for prostate cancer immunotherapy. *J Immunol* (2001) **167**(12):7150–6. doi:10.4049/jimmunol.167.12.7150
81. Johnson L, McNeel D. Identification of prostatic acid phosphatase (PAP) specific HLA-DR1-restricted T-cell epitopes. *Prostate* (2012) **72**(7):730–40. doi:10.1002/pros.21477
82. Mohamed ER, Naito M, Terasaki Y, Niu Y, Gohara S, Komatsu N, et al. Capability of SART3(109-118) peptide to induce cytotoxic T lymphocytes from prostate cancer patients with HLA class I-A11, -A31 and -A33 alleles. *Int J Oncol* (2009) **34**(2):529–36. doi:10.3892/ijo_00000178
83. Terasaki Y, Shichijo S, Niu Y, Komatsu N, Noguchi M, Todo S, et al. An HLA-A3-binding prostate acid phosphatase-derived peptide can induce CTLs restricted to HLA-A2 and -A24 alleles. *Cancer Immunol Immunother* (2009) **58**(11):1877–85. doi:10.1007/s00262-009-0699-2
84. Becker JT, Olson BM, Johnson LE, Davies JG, Dunphy EJ, McNeel DG. DNA vaccine encoding prostatic acid phosphatase (PAP) elicits long-term T-cell responses in patients with recurrent prostate cancer. *J Immunother* (2010) **33**(6):639–47. doi:10.1097/CJI.0b013e3181dda23e
85. McNeel DG, Nguyen LD, Ellis WJ, Higano CS, Lange PH, Disis ML. Naturally occurring prostate cancer antigen-specific T cell responses of a Th1 phenotype can be detected in patients with prostate cancer. *Prostate* (2001) **47**(3):222–9. doi:10.1002/pros.1066
86. McNeel DG, Dunphy EJ, Davies JG, Frye TP, Johnson LE, Staab MJ, et al. Safety and immunological efficacy of a DNA vaccine encoding prostatic acid phosphatase in patients with stage D0 prostate cancer. *J Clin Oncol* (2009) **27**(25):4047–54. doi:10.1200/JCO.2008.19.9968
87. Mesters JR, Barinka C, Li W, Tsukamoto T, Majer P, Slusher BS, et al. Structure of glutamate carboxypeptidase II, a drug target in neuronal damage and prostate cancer. *EMBO J* (2006) **25**(6):1375–84. doi:10.1038/sj.emboj.7600969
88. Wolf P, Alt K, Wetterauer D, Bühler P, Gierschner D, Katzenwadel A, et al. Preclinical evaluation of a recombinant anti-prostate specific membrane antigen single-chain immunotoxin against prostate cancer. *J Immunother* (2010) **33**(3):262–71. doi:10.1097/CJI.0b013e3181c5495c
89. O'Keefe D, Bacich D, Heston W. Comparative analysis of prostate-specific membrane antigen (PSMA) versus a prostate-specific membrane antigen-like gene. *Prostate* (2004) **58**(2):200–10. doi:10.1002/pros.10319
90. Lapidus RG, Tiffany CW, Isaacs JT, Slusher BS. Prostate-specific membrane antigen (PSMA) enzyme activity is elevated in prostate cancer cells. *Prostate* (2000) **45**(4):350–4. doi:10.1002/1097-0045(20001201)45:4<350::AID-PROS10>3.0.CO;2-U
91. Murphy GP, Elgamal AA, Su SL, Bostwick DG, Holmes EH. Current evaluation of the tissue localization and diagnostic utility of prostate specific membrane antigen. *Cancer* (1998) **83**(11):2259–69. doi:10.1002/(SICI)1097-0142(19981201)83:11<2259::AID-CNCR5>3.3.CO;2-K
92. Chang SS, O'Keefe DS, Bacich DJ, Reuter VE, Heston WD, Gaudin PB. Prostate-specific membrane antigen is produced in tumor-associated neovasculature. *Clin Cancer Res* (1999) **5**(10):2674–81.
93. Milowsky MI, Nanus DM, Kostakoglu L, Sheehan CE, Vallabhajosula S, Goldsmith SJ, et al. Vascular targeted therapy with anti-prostate-specific membrane antigen monoclonal antibody J591 in advanced solid tumors. *J Clin Oncol* (2007) **25**(5):540–7. doi:10.1200/JCO.2006.07.8097
94. Ghosh A, Heston W. Tumor target prostate specific membrane antigen (PSMA) and its regulation in prostate cancer. *J Cell Biochem* (2004) **91**(3):528–39. doi:10.1002/jcb.10661
95. Bander NH, Milowsky MI, Nanus DM, Kostakoglu L, Vallabhajosula S, Goldsmith SJ. Phase I trial of 177lutetium-labeled J591, a monoclonal antibody to prostate-specific membrane antigen, in patients with androgen-independent prostate cancer. *J Clin Oncol* (2005) **23**(21):4591–601. doi:10.1200/JCO.2005.05.160
96. Reiter RE, Gu Z, Watabe T, Thomas G, Szigeti K, Davis E, et al. Prostate stem cell antigen: a cell surface marker overexpressed in prostate cancer. *Proc Natl Acad Sci U S A* (1998) **95**(4):1735–40. doi:10.1073/pnas.95.4.1735
97. Presky DH, Low MG, Shevach EM. Role of phosphatidylinositol-anchored proteins in T cell activation. *J Immunol* (1990) **144**(3):860–8.
98. Rege TA, Hagood JS. Thy-1, a versatile modulator of signaling affecting cellular adhesion, proliferation, survival, and cytokine/growth factor responses. *Biochim Biophys Acta* (2006) **1763**(10):991–9. doi:10.1016/j.bbamcr.2006.08.008
99. Eshel R, Zanin A, Sagi-Assif O, Meshel T, Smorodinsky NI, Dwir O, et al. The GPI-linked Ly-6 antigen E48 regulates expression levels of the FX enzyme and of E-selectin ligands on head and neck squamous carcinoma cells. *J Biol Chem* (2000) **275**(17):12833–40. doi:10.1074/jbc.275.17.12833
100. Malek T, Ortega G, Chan C, Kroczek RA, Shevach EM. Role of Ly-6 in lymphocyte activation. II. Induction of T cell activation by monoclonal anti-Ly-6 antibodies. *J Exp Med* (1986) **164**:709–22.
101. Treister A, Sagi-Assif O, Meer M, Smorodinsky NI, Anavi R, Golan I, et al. Expression of Ly-6, a marker for highly malignant murine tumor cells, is regulated by growth conditions and stress. *Int J Cancer* (1998) **77**(2):306–13. doi:10.1002/(SICI)1097-0215(19980717)77:2<306::AID-IJC22>3.0.CO;2-7
102. Witz IP. Differential expression of genes by tumor cells of a low or a high malignancy phenotype: the case of murine and human Ly-6 proteins. *J Cell Biochem Suppl* (2000) **34**:61–6. doi:10.1002/(SICI)1097-4644(2000)77:34+<61::AID-JCB11>3.3.CO;2-J
103. Garcia-Hernandez Mde L, Gray A, Hubby B, Klinger OJ, Kast WM. Prostate stem cell antigen vaccination induces a long-term protective immune response against prostate cancer in the absence of autoimmunity. *Cancer Res* (2008) **68**(3):861–9. doi:10.1158/0008-5472.CAN-07-0445
104. Morgenroth A, Cartellieri M, Schmitz M, Günes S, Weigle B, Bachmann M, et al. Targeting of tumor cells expressing the prostate stem cell antigen (PSCA) using genetically engineered T-cells. *Prostate* (2007) **67**(10):1121–31. doi:10.1002/pros.20608

105. Thomas-Kaskel AK, Zeiser R, Jochim R, Robbel C, Schultze-Seemann W, Waller CF, et al. Vaccination of advanced prostate cancer patients with PSCA and PSA peptide-loaded dendritic cells induces DTH responses that correlate with superior overall survival. *Int J Cancer* (2006) **119**(10):2428–34. doi:10.1002/ijc.22097
106. Saffran DC, Raitano AB, Hubert RS, Witte ON, Reiter RE, Jakobovits A. Anti-PSCA mAbs inhibit tumor growth and metastasis formation and prolong the survival of mice bearing human prostate cancer xenografts. *Proc Natl Acad Sci U S A* (2001) **98**(5):2658–63. doi:10.1073/pnas.051624698
107. Huo W, Ye J, Liu R, Chen J, Li Q. Vaccination with a chaperone complex based on PSCA and GRP170 adjuvant enhances the CTL response and inhibits the tumor growth in mice. *Vaccine* (2010) **28**(38):6333–7. doi:10.1016/j.vaccine.2010.06.093
108. Kufe DW. Mucins in cancer: function, prognosis and therapy. *Nat Rev Cancer* (2009) **9**(12):874–85. doi:10.1038/nrc2761
109. Hollingsworth MA, Swanson BJ. Mucins in cancer: protection and control of the cell surface. *Nat Rev Cancer* (2004) **4**(1):45–60. doi:10.1038/nrc1251
110. Andrén O, Fall K, Andersson SO, Rubin MA, Bismar TA, Karlsson M, et al. MUC-1 gene is associated with prostate cancer death: a 20-year follow-up of a population-based study in Sweden. *Br J Cancer* (2007) **97**(6):730–4. doi:10.1038/sj.bjc.6603944
111. Cozzi PJ, Wang J, Delprado W, Perkins AC, Allen BJ, Russell PJ, et al. MUC1, MUC2, MUC4, MUC5AC and MUC6 expression in the progression of prostate cancer. *Clin Exp Metastasis* (2005) **22**(7):565–73. doi:10.1007/s10585-005-5376-z
112. Gendler SJ. MUC1, the renaissance molecule. *J Mammary Gland Biol Neoplasia* (2001) **6**(3):339–53. doi:10.1023/A:1011379725811
113. Agrawal B, Krantz MJ, Parker J, Longenecker BM. Expression of MUC1 mucin on activated human T cells: implications for a role of MUC1 in normal immune regulation. *Cancer Res* (1998) **58**(18):4079–81.
114. Tempero RM, VanLith ML, Morikane K, Rowse GJ, Gendler SJ, Hollingsworth MA. CD4+ lymphocytes provide MUC1-specific tumor immunity in vivo that is undetectable in vitro and is absent in MUC1 transgenic mice. *J Immunol* (1998) **161**(10):5500–6.
115. Rughetti A, Pellicciotta I, Biffoni M, Bäckström M, Link T, Bennet EP, et al. Recombinant tumor-associated MUC1 glycoprotein impairs the differentiation and function of dendritic cells. *J Immunol* (2005) **174**(12):7764–72. doi:10.4049/jimmunol.174.12.7764
116. Chan AK, Lockhart DC, von Bernstorff W, Spanjaard RA, Joo HG, Eberlein TJ, et al. Soluble MUC1 secreted by human epithelial cancer cells mediates immune suppression by blocking T-cell activation. *Int J Cancer* (1999) **82**(5):721–6. doi:10.1002/(SICI)1097-0215(19990827)82:5<721::AID-IJC16>3.3.CO;2-E
117. Slovin SF, Ragupathi G, Fernandez C, Diani M, Jefferson MP, Wilton A, et al. A polyvalent vaccine for high-risk prostate patients: "are more antigens better?". *Cancer Immunol Immunother* (2007) **56**(12):1921–30. doi:10.1007/s00262-007-0335-y
118. Major P, Lacombe L, Fradet Y, Foley R, Scheid E, Bergeron A, et al. Abstract A16: a phase I/II clinical trial of a MUC1-glycopeptide dendritic cell vaccine in castrate resistant non-metastatic prostate cancer patients. *Cancer Res* (2012) **72**(4 Suppl):A16. doi:10.1158/1538-7445.PRCA2012-A16
119. Simpson AJ, Caballero OL, Jungbluth A, Chen YT, Old LJ. Cancer/testis antigens, gametogenesis and cancer. *Nat Rev Cancer* (2005) **5**(8):615–25. doi:10.1038/nrc1669
120. Suyama T, Shiraishi T, Zeng Y, Yu W, Parekh N, Vessella RL, et al. Expression of cancer/testis antigens in prostate cancer is associated with disease progression. *Prostate* (2010) **70**(16):1778–87. doi:10.1002/pros.21214
121. Fosså A, Berner A, Fosså SD, Hernes E, Gaudernack G, Smeland EB. NY-ESO-1 protein expression and humoral immune responses in prostate cancer. *Prostate* (2004) **59**(4):440–7. doi:10.1002/pros.20025
122. Hudolin T, Juretic A, Spagnoli GC, Pasini J, Bandic D, Heberer M, et al. Immunohistochemical expression of tumor antigens MAGE-A1, MAGE-A3/4, and NY-ESO-1 in cancerous and benign prostatic tissue. *Prostate* (2006) **66**(1):13–8. doi:10.1002/pros.20312
123. Nakada T, Noguchi Y, Satoh S, Ono T, Saika T, Kurashige T, et al. NY-ESO-1 mRNA expression and immunogenicity in advanced prostate cancer. *Cancer Immun* (2003) **3**:10.
124. Caballero OL, Chen YT. Cancer/testis (CT) antigens: potential targets for immunotherapy. *Cancer Sci* (2009) **100**(11):2014–21. doi:10.1111/j.1349-7006.2009.01303.x
125. Ono T, Kurashige T, Harada N, Noguchi Y, Saika T, Niikawa N, et al. Identification of proacrosin binding protein sp32 precursor as a human cancer/testis antigen. *Proc Natl Acad Sci U S A* (2001) **98**(6):3282–7. doi:10.1073/pnas.041625098
126. Türeci O, Sahin U, Zwick C, Koslowski M, Seitz G, Pfreundschuh M. Identification of a meiosis-specific protein as a member of the class of cancer/testis antigens. *Proc Natl Acad Sci U S A* (1998) **95**(9):5211–6. doi:10.1073/pnas.95.9.5211
127. Zeng G, Wang X, Robbins PF, Rosenberg SA, Wang RF. CD4(+) T cell recognition of MHC class II-restricted epitopes from NY-ESO-1 presented by a prevalent HLA DP4 allele: association with NY-ESO-1 antibody production. *Proc Natl Acad Sci U S A* (2001) **98**(7):3964–9. doi:10.1073/pnas.061507398
128. Gati A, Lajmi N, Derouiche A, Marrakchi R, Chebil M, Benammar-Elgaaied A. NY-ESO-1 expression and immunogenicity in prostate cancer patients. *Tunis Med* (2011) **89**(10):779–83.
129. Gnjatic S, Nishikawa H, Jungbluth AA, Güre AO, Ritter G, Jäger E, et al. NY-ESO-1: review of an immunogenic tumor antigen. *Adv Cancer Res* (2006) **95**:1–30. doi:10.1016/S0065-230X(06)95001-5
130. Fong L, Kwek SS, O'Brien S, Kavanagh B, McNeel DG, Weinberg V, et al. Potentiating endogenous antitumor immunity to prostate cancer through combination immunotherapy with CTLA4 blockade and GM-CSF. *Cancer Res* (2009) **69**(2):609–15. doi:10.1158/0008-5472.CAN-08-3529
131. Zeng G, Touloukian CE, Wang X, Restifo NP, Rosenberg SA, Wang RF. Identification of CD4+ T cell epitopes from NY-ESO-1 presented by HLA-DR molecules. *J Immunol* (2000) **165**(2):1153–9. doi:10.4049/jimmunol.165.2.1153
132. Sonpavde G, Wang M, Peterson LE, Wang HY, Joe T, Mims MP, et al. HLA-restricted NY-ESO-1 peptide immunotherapy for metastatic castration resistant prostate cancer. *Invest New Drugs* (2013) **32**(2):235–42. doi:10.1007/s10637-013-9960-9
133. von Boehmer L, Keller L, Mortezavi A, Provenzano M, Sais G, Hermanns T, et al. MAGE-C2/CT10 protein expression is an independent predictor of recurrence in prostate cancer. *PLoS One* (2011) **6**(7):e21366. doi:10.1371/journal.pone.0021366
134. Jin J, Smith FD, Stark C, Wells CD, Fawcett JP, Kulkarni S, et al. Proteomic, functional, and domain-based analysis of in vivo 14-3-3 binding proteins involved in cytoskeletal regulation and cellular organization. *Curr Biol* (2004) **14**(16):1436–50. doi:10.1016/j.cub.2004.07.051
135. Shah GV, Noble MJ, Austenfeld M, Weigel J, Deftos LJ, Mebust WK. Presence of calcitonin-like immunoreactivity (iCT) in human prostate gland: evidence for iCT secretion by cultured prostate cells. *Prostate* (1992) **21**(2):87–97. doi:10.1002/pros.2990210202
136. Shah GV, Rayford W, Noble MJ, Austenfeld M, Weigel J, Vamos S, et al. Calcitonin stimulates growth of human prostate-cancer cells through receptor-mediated increase in cyclic adenosine 3′,5′-monophosphates and cytoplasmic Ca2+ transients. *Endocrinology* (1994) **134**(2):596–602. doi:10.1210/en.134.2.596
137. Chien J, Shah GV. Role of stimulatory guanine nucleotide binding protein (GSalpha) in proliferation of PC-3M prostate cancer cells. *Int J Cancer* (2001) **91**(1):46–54. doi:10.1002/1097-0215(20010101)91:1<46::AID-IJC1008>3.0.CO;2-0
138. Sabbisetti VS, Chirugupati S, Thomas S, Vaidya KS, Reardon D, Chiriva-Internati M, et al. Calcitonin increases invasiveness of prostate cancer cells: role for cyclic AMP-dependent protein kinase A in calcitonin action. *Int J Cancer* (2005) **117**(4):551–60. doi:10.1002/ijc.21158
139. Chiriva-Internati M, Ferrari R, Yu Y, Hamrick C, Gagliano N, Grizzi F, et al. AKAP-4: a novel cancer testis antigen for multiple myeloma. *Br J Haematol* (2008) **140**(4):465–8. doi:10.1111/j.1365-2141.2007.06940.x
140. Chiriva-Internati M, Yu Y, Mirandola L, D'Cunha N, Hardwicke F, Cannon MJ, et al. Identification of AKAP-4 as a new cancer/testis antigen for detection and immunotherapy of prostate cancer. *Prostate* (2012) **72**(1):12–23. doi:10.1002/pros.21400
141. Noguchi M, Kakuma T, Uemura H, Nasu Y, Kumon H, Hirao Y, et al. A randomized phase II trial of personalized peptide vaccine plus low dose estramustine phosphate (EMP) versus standard dose EMP in patients with castration resistant prostate cancer. *Cancer Immunol Immunother* (2010) **59**(7):1001–9. doi:10.1007/s00262-010-0822-4

142. Shariat SF, Andrews B, Kattan MW, Kim J, Wheeler TM, Slawin KM. Plasma levels of interleukin-6 and its soluble receptor are associated with prostate cancer progression and metastasis. *Urology* (2001) **58**(6):1008–15. doi:10.1016/S0090-4295(01)01405-4
143. Small EJ, Sacks N, Nemunaitis J, Urba WJ, Dula E, Centeno AS, et al. Granulocyte macrophage colony-stimulating factor – secreting allogeneic cellular immunotherapy for hormone-refractory prostate cancer. *Clin Cancer Res* (2007) **13**(13):3883–91. doi:10.1158/1078-0432.CCR-06-2937
144. Higano CS, Corman JM, Smith DC, Centeno AS, Steidle CP, Gittleman M, et al. Phase 1/2 dose-escalation study of a GM-CSF-secreting, allogeneic, cellular immunotherapy for metastatic hormone-refractory prostate cancer. *Cancer* (2008) **113**(5):975–84. doi:10.1002/cncr.23669
145. Higano C, Somer B, Curti B, Petrylak D, Drake CG, Schnell F, et al. *A Phase III Trial of GVAX Immunotherapy for Prostate Cancer Versus Docetaxel Plus Prednisone in Asymptomatic, Castration-Resistant Prostate Cancer (CRPC)*, in *2009 Genitourinary Cancers Symposium*, Orlando, FL (2009).
146. Small E, Demkow T, Gerritsen WR, Rolland F, Hoskin P, Smith DC, et al. *A Phase III trial of GVAX Immunotherapy for Prostate Cancer in Combination with Docetaxel Versus Docetaxel Plus Prednisone in Symptomatic, Castration-Resistant Prostate Cancer (CRPC)*, in *2009 Genitourinary Cancers Symposium*, Orlando, FL (2009).
147. van den Eertwegh A, Versluis J, van den Berg HP, Santegoets SJ, van Moorselaar RJ, van der Sluis TM, et al. Combined immunotherapy with granulocyte-macrophage colony-stimulating factor-transduced allogeneic prostate cancer cells and ipilimumab in patients with metastatic castration-resistant prostate cancer: a phase 1 dose-escalation trial. *Lancet Oncol* (2012) **13**(5):509–17. doi:10.1016/S1470-2045(12)70007-4
148. Santegoets SJ, Stam AG, Lougheed SM, Gall H, Scholten PE, Reijm M, et al. T cell profiling reveals high CD4+CTLA-4 + T cell frequency as dominant predictor for survival after prostate GVAX/ipilimumab treatment. *Cancer Immunol Immunother* (2013) **62**(2):245–56. doi:10.1007/s00262-012-1330-5
149. Kyte JA, Gaudernack G. Immuno-gene therapy of cancer with tumour-mRNA transfected dendritic cells. *Cancer Immunol Immunother* (2006) **55**(11):1432–42. doi:10.1007/s00262-006-0161-7
150. Mu LJ, Kyte JA, Kvalheim G, Aamdal S, Dueland S, Hauser M, et al. Immunotherapy with allotumour mRNA-transfected dendritic cells in androgen-resistant prostate cancer patients. *Br J Cancer* (2005) **93**(7):749–56. doi:10.1038/sj.bjc.6602761
151. Conway RE, Joiner K, Patterson A, Bourgeois D, Rampp R, Hannah BC, et al. Prostate specific membrane antigen produces pro-angiogenic laminin peptides downstream of matrix metalloprotease-2. *Angiogenesis* (2013) **16**(4):847–60. doi:10.1007/s10456-013-9360-y
152. Chiriva-Internati M, Grizzi F, Bright RK, Martin Kast W. Cancer immunotherapy: avoiding the road to perdition. *J Transl Med* (2004) **2**(1):26. doi:10.1186/1479-5876-2-26
153. Fox BA, Schendel DJ, Butterfield LH, Aamdal S, Allison JP, Ascierto PA, et al. Defining the critical hurdles in cancer immunotherapy. *J Transl Med* (2011) **9**(1):214. doi:10.1186/1479-5876-9-214
154. Galon J, Costes A, Sanchez-Cabo F, Kirilovsky A, Mlecnik B, Lagorce-Pagès C, et al. Type, density, and location of immune cells within human colorectal tumors predict clinical outcome. *Science* (2006) **313**(5795):1960–4. doi:10.1126/science.1129139
155. Gajewski TF, Louahed J, Brichard VG. Gene signature in melanoma associated with clinical activity: a potential clue to unlock cancer immunotherapy. *Cancer J* (2010) **16**(4):399–403. doi:10.1097/PPO.0b013e3181eacbd8
156. Hoos A. Evolution of end points for cancer immunotherapy trials. *Ann Oncol* (2012) **23**(Suppl 8):viii47–52. doi:10.1093/annonc/mds263
157. Hoos A, Eggermont AM, Janetzki S, Hodi FS, Ibrahim R, Anderson A, et al. Improved endpoints for cancer immunotherapy trials. *J Natl Cancer Inst* (2010) **102**(18):1388–97. doi:10.1093/jnci/djq310
158. Hoos A, Parmiani G, Hege K, Sznol M, Loibner H, Eggermont A, et al. A clinical development paradigm for cancer vaccines and related biologics. *J Immunother* (2007) **30**(1):1–15. doi:10.1097/01.cji.0000211341.88835.ae
159. Eisenhauer EA, Therasse P, Bogaerts J, Schwartz LH, Sargent D, Ford R, et al. New response evaluation criteria in solid tumours: revised RECIST guideline (version 1.1). *Eur J Cancer* (2009) **45**(2):228–47. doi:10.1016/j.ejca.2008.10.026
160. Vasaturo A, Di Blasio S, Peeters DG, de Koning CC, de Vries JM, Figdor CG, et al. Clinical implications of co-inhibitory molecule expression in the Tumor microenvironment for DC vaccination: a game of stop and go. *Front Immunol* (2013) **4**:417. doi:10.3389/fimmu.2013.00417
161. Hodi FS, O'Day SJ, McDermott DF, Weber RW, Sosman JA, Haanen JB, et al. Improved survival with ipilimumab in patients with metastatic melanoma. *N Engl J Med* (2010) **363**(8):711–23. doi:10.1056/NEJMoa1003466
162. Robert C, Thomas L, Bondarenko I, O'Day S, Weber J, Garbe C, et al. Ipilimumab plus dacarbazine for previously untreated metastatic melanoma. *N Engl J Med* (2011) **364**(26):2517–26. doi:10.1056/NEJMoa1104621
163. Wolchok JD, Kluger H, Callahan MK, Postow MA, Rizvi NA, Lesokhin AM, et al. Nivolumab plus ipilimumab in advanced melanoma. *N Engl J Med* (2013) **369**(2):122–33. doi:10.1056/NEJMoa1302369
164. Rammensee HG, Singh-Jasuja H. HLA ligandome tumor antigen discovery for personalized vaccine approach. *Expert Rev Vaccines* (2013) **12**(10):1211–7. doi:10.1586/14760584.2013.836911
165. Castle JC, Kreiter S, Diekmann J, Löwer M, van deRoemer N, de Graaf J, et al. Exploiting the mutanome for tumor vaccination. *Cancer Res* (2012) **72**(5):1081–91. doi:10.1158/0008-5472.CAN-11-3722
166. Matsushita H, Vesely MD, Koboldt DC, Rickert CG, Uppaluri R, Magrini VJ, et al. Cancer exome analysis reveals a T-cell-dependent mechanism of cancer immunoediting. *Nature* (2012) **482**(7385):400–U149. doi:10.1038/nature10755
167. van Rooij N, van Buuren MM, Philips D, Velds A, Toebes M, Heemskerk B, et al. Tumor exome analysis reveals neoantigen-specific T-cell reactivity in an ipilimumab-responsive melanoma. *J Clin Oncol* (2013) **31**(32):e439–42. doi:10.1200/JCO.2012.47.7521
168. Robbins PF, Lu YC, El-Gamil M, Li YF, Gross C, Gartner J, et al. Mining exomic sequencing data to identify mutated antigens recognized by adoptively transferred tumor-reactive T cells. *Nat Med* (2013) **19**(6):747–52. doi:10.1038/nm.3161

Conflict of Interest Statement: Harm Westdorp, Annette E. Sköld, Berit A. Snijer, Sebastian Franik, Sasja F. Mulder, Pierre P. Major, Ronan Foley, and I. Jolanda M. de Vries declare no disclosures of potential conflicts of interest. Winald R. Gerritsen is a consult for Aglaia Biomedical Ventures, is on the supervisory board for PsytoBe, has received speakers fee from J&J and BMS, and is on the advisory boards for Amgen, BMS, Janssen-Cilag, Sanofi, Astellas, Bayer, and Merck.

6

An updated view of the intracellular mechanisms regulating cross-presentation

Priyanka Nair-Gupta[1] and J. Magarian Blander[1,2]*

[1] Department of Medicine, Immunology Institute, Graduate School of Biological Sciences, Icahn School of Medicine at Mount Sinai, New York, NY, USA
[2] Tisch Cancer Institute, Icahn School of Medicine at Mount Sinai, New York, NY, USA

Edited by:
Penelope Anne Morel, University of Pittsburgh, USA

Reviewed by:
Juan J. Garcia-Vallejo, VU University Medical Center, Netherlands
Florent Ginhoux, Singapore Immunology Network, Singapore
Guillaume Hoeffel, Singapore Immunology Network, Singapore

***Correspondence:**
J. Magarian Blander, Department of Medicine, Immunology Institute, Tisch Cancer Institute, and the Graduate School of Biological Sciences, Icahn School of Medicine at Mount Sinai, 1425 Madison Avenue, 12-20D, New York, NY 10029, USA
e-mail: julie.blander@mssm.edu

Cross-presentation involves the presentation of peptides derived from internalized cargo on major histocompatibility complex class I molecules by dendritic cells, a process critical for tolerance and immunity. Detailed studies of the pathways mediating cross-presentation have revealed that this process takes place in a specialized subcellular compartment with a unique set of proteins. In this review, we focus on the recently appreciated role for intracellular vesicular traffic, which serves to equip compartments such as endosomes and phagosomes with the necessary apparatus for conducting the various steps of cross-presentation. We also consider how these pathways may integrate with inflammatory signals particularly from pattern recognition receptors that detect the presence of microbial components during infection. We discuss the consequences of such signals on initiating cross-presentation to stimulate adaptive CD8 T cell responses.

Keywords: cross-presentation, major histocompatibility complex class I, pattern recognition receptor, Toll-like receptor, vesicular traffic, phagosomes, endosomes, dendritic cells

INTRODUCTION

Classically, endogenous antigens such as proteins synthesized by virally infected cells or tumor cells, are presented on major histocompatibility class I (MHC I) molecules for detection by CD8 T cells. However, a seminal study by Bevan (1) showed that in animals immunized with fully allogeneic cells, cytotoxic CD8 T cell responses were seen specific for minor antigens from the graft that were presented on MHC I molecules of the host (1). This finding indicated that antigens from the transplanted cells could be internalized by antigen presenting cells (APC) of the host and presented on the host MHC I molecules. Bevan termed the activation of CD8 T cells to this process of antigen transfer as "cross-priming," and later the actual process of antigen transfer was called "cross-presentation" (2). A once poorly defined phenomenon, cross-presentation is now considered to be a critical mechanism to mediate immune responses against infectious agents and tumors as well as to induce peripheral tolerance (3).

The importance of cross-presentation becomes apparent given the existence of several viruses that exhibit strict tissue tropisms such as papilloma virus where infection is mainly confined to epithelial cells in the skin barrier (4). Other examples for viruses that do not infect APC include encephalomyocarditis virus (EMCV) and semliki forest virus (SFV) (5). Additionally, some viruses such as herpes simplex virus (HSV), measles, retrovirus, canarypox virus, vaccinia virus, and lymphocytic choriomeningitis virus infect APC, but impair direct presentation of antigen (6–13). Additionally, cross-presentation has been demonstrated to play a critical role in mediating CD8 T cell immune responses against parasitic infections such as *Toxoplasma gondii* (14). Cross-priming has also been studied in the context of bacterial infections such as *Listeria monocytogenes* and *Mycobacterium tuberculosis*. In these infections, host defense is primarily mediated by dendritic cells (DC) that phagocytose infected apoptotic cells and mediate cross-priming, thus allowing for effective cytotoxic T lymphocytes (CTL) responses against the pathogens (15–17). Hence, cross-presentation allows for a mechanism through which the antigen can be presented by the APC without the need for direct infection.

Although other phagocytes have been reported to cross-present antigen, DC are considered to be the primary cross-presenting cell. The superior ability of DC to cross-present is largely attributed to their antigen processing capacity. Endocytic pathways in DC preserve and retain antigen epitopes via low lysosomal proteolysis and expression of protease inhibitors (18). This aspect makes sense when one considers that DC pick up antigen in the peripheral tissue and migrate for several hours-days (12–24 h for dermal DC and 3 days for Langerhans cells) reaching the lymph nodes (19). Thus, instead of being processed and degraded prematurely, retention of antigen would allow optimal cross-presentation for subsequent recognition by lymph node resident naïve CD8 T cells. However, DC subsets are heterogeneous in their ability to cross-present antigens. Subsets such as conventional splenic and lymph node resident CD8α$^+$ DC, migratory DC populations such as lung and dermal CD103$^+$ DC as well as monocyte-derived inflammatory DC excel at cross-presentation (20–24). It is still unclear why these DC subsets are specialized for cross-presentation. Interestingly, conventional CD8α$^+$ DC as well migratory CD103$^+$ DC populations appear to rely exclusively on Batf3 and IRF8 transcription factors for their development (25–28). Therefore, it is curious to ask if the ability to cross-present is developmentally controlled by the Batf3/IRF8 transcription programs that enable these subsets to have unique and specialized compartments geared toward cross-presentation. On the other hand, *in vitro* studies argue that the ability of splenic CD8α$^+$ DC to cross-present antigen is induced as a subsequent step in maturation aided by cytokines such as granulocyte-macrophage colony-stimulating factor (GMCSF) or exposure to microbial products (29).

Recent studies in human DC have proposed the lymphoid and non-lymphoid resident BDCA3$^+$ (CD141$^+$) DC to be the human counterparts of the cross-presenting murine lymphoid CD8α$^+$ DC and non-lymphoid CD103$^+$ DC (30–34). The BDCA3$^+$ DC subset is indeed an attractive candidate for the human homolog as it shares with the murine CD8α$^+$ and CD103$^+$ DC several cell surface markers, including DNGR1 and XCR1, transcription factors such as Batf3 and IRF8, along with excelling at *in vitro* cross-presentation assays. However, evidence also exists contradicting the superiority of the BDCA3$^+$ DC subset at cross-presentation (35–37). Furthermore, patients harboring an autosomal dominant mutation in *IRF8* selectively lose BDCA-1$^+$ DCs but not BDCA3$^+$ DCs in the peripheral blood, indicating that BDCA3$^+$ DC is at least not developmentally regulated in the same manner as murine cross-presenting subsets (38). Additionally although Batf3 deficiency impairs development of BDCA3$^+$ DC *in vitro*, humanized mice reconstituted with Batf3 deficient progenitors still display sufficient and comparable numbers of BDCA3$^+$ DCs (39). Thus, even though the human BDCA3$^+$ DC subset appears to be functionally related to the murine CD8α$^+$ and CD103$^+$ DC, further studies are warranted to determine their developmental program and subsequent specialization for cross-presentation.

Several groups have also focused their efforts on revealing the intracellular pathways and molecular mechanisms mediating cross-presentation at steady state. Three major mechanisms have been determined. The phagosome-to-cytosol pathway involves escape of the antigen into the cytosol, possibly mediated by Sec61, followed by degradation by the proteasome and transport of peptides into the endoplasmic reticulum (ER) by the transporter associated with antigen presentation (TAP) to be loaded onto MHC I molecules (40, 41). The ER-phagosome fusion pathway involves fusion of the ER-Golgi intermediate compartment (ERGIC) with the phagosome, leading to the formation of a so called "ERgosome," where ERGIC components such as TAP and components of the peptide loading complex are recruited directly to the phagosome. This recruitment is mediated through pairing of the ER SNARE Sec22b with the plasma membrane SNARE syntaxin-4, which is also found on phagosomes (42). In this model, the antigen still requires escape into the cytosol for proteasomal degradation and is then imported back to the "ERgosome" by TAP to be loaded onto MHC I molecules (43, 44). In contrast to the cytosolic pathways, the vacuolar pathway involves direct processing of the antigen within the phagosome by endocytic proteases such as cathepsins and subsequent loading of peptides onto MHC I molecules (45).

Some of the above pathways suggest that cross-presentation takes place in a specialized intracellular compartment. This compartment could be endosomes or phagosomes depending on the size of the exogenous antigen and mode of internalization. For instance, in the ERgosome model, cross-presentation takes place in a subcellular compartment bearing characteristics of both the ERGIC and the endosome/phagosome. In this review, we elaborate on the vesicular pathways that serve to bring various components of the cross-presentation machinery to such specialized intracellular compartments. We discuss the unique combination of proteins in these compartments that make it attractive for cross-presentation at steady state and how this compartment might be modified and further optimized for efficient cross-presentation in the scenario of infection. We also review evidence for regulation of cross-presentation during microbial stimulation and discuss if this process can still take place at steady state.

NATURE OF THE CROSS-PRESENTING COMPARTMENT AT STEADY STATE

In recent years, several groups have elucidated the architecture of the "cross-presenting" compartment at steady state. This compartment contains several identified proteins brought in by distinct vesicular pathways. These proteins may all be present in the compartment. Alternatively, these vesicular pathways may be mutually exclusive of one another, culminating in the presence of only some of these identified proteins. Regardless, these proteins serve as important players in executing different steps of the cross-presentation response (**Figure 1**).

MAINTENANCE OF OPTIMAL ALKALINE pH

As antigens are internalized by endocytosis or phagocytosis, they undergo gradual proteolytic degradation along their journey from early endosomes and phagosomes to lysosomes (**Figure 1A**). Once in lysosomes, antigens are degraded by lysosomal proteases, which could destroy potential peptide epitopes crucial for T cell activation. DC circumvent this problem by expressing low levels of lysosomal proteases (18). Additionally, since most of these proteases function optimally at acidic pH (46), maintenance of a strongly alkaline pH in the cross-presentation compartment would inhibit protease activity, thus preventing overt and premature degradation of antigens. To this end, DC were reported to have high phagosomal pH, reaching values of 7.5–8 in contrast to macrophages which rapidly acidified their phagosomes, reaching values of 4.5–5 following phagocytosis of inert latex beads (47). Alkalinization of phagosomes in DC was attributed to selective recruitment, assembly and functioning of nicotinamide adenine dinucleotide phosphate (NADPH) oxidase NOX2. Finally, NOX2 activity was shown to be crucial for cross-presentation as genetic deletion of NOX2 subunit gp91phox led to abrogation of cross-presentation.

How does NOX2 reach the cross-presenting compartment? Recruitment of NOX2 is facilitated by Rab27a (48), a small guanosine tri-phosphatase (GTPase), which was initially characterized to mediate regulatory exocytosis of secretory vesicles in hematopoietic and non-hematopoietic cells (49). In a separate study, the Rac2 GTPase was demonstrated to also control the recruitment and assembly of phagosomal NOX2 in splenic CD8α$^+$ DC as well as in *in vitro* derived bone-marrow derived DC (50). Additionally, VAMP-8, a SNARE protein which interacts with plasma membrane and phagosomal SNAREs syntaxin-4 and SNAP-23 (51), has also been recently reported to play a role in NOX2 recruitment and in mediating cross-presentation of phagocytic antigen (52). Interestingly, the protozoan *Leishmania* specifically cleaves VAMP-8

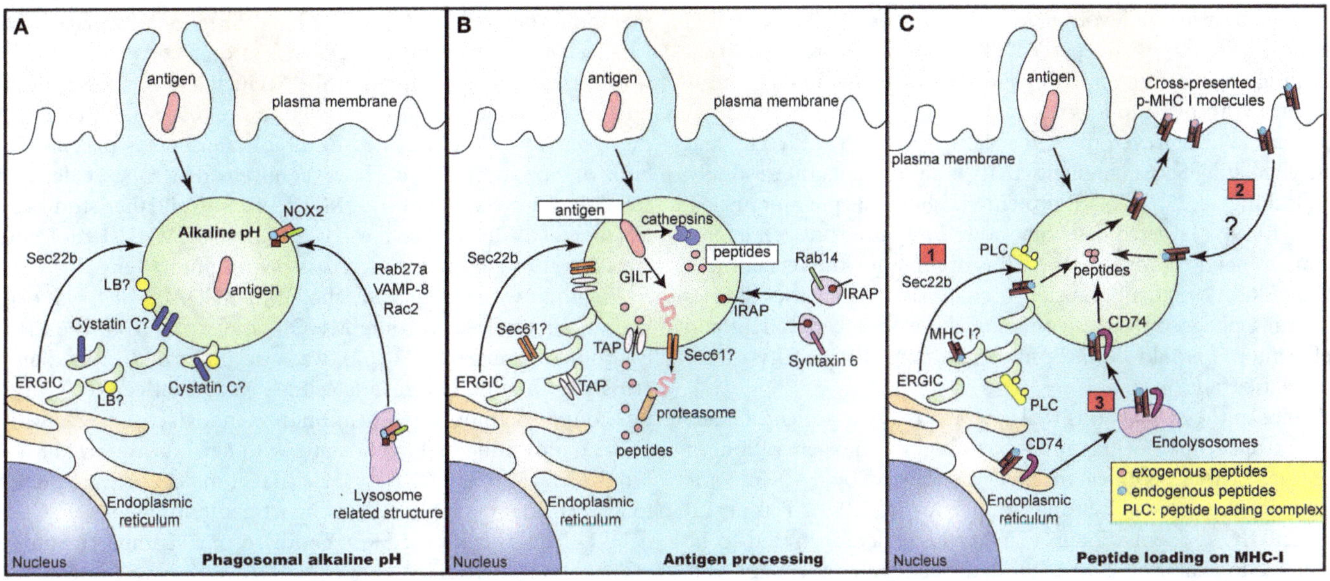

FIGURE 1 | The cross-presentation compartment at steady state. Several vesicular pathways have been proposed to mediate delivery of key proteins that play an integral role in the crucial steps of cross-presentation including maintenance of alkaline pH **(A)**, processing of antigen to peptides **(B)** and subsequent loading of peptides onto MHC I molecules **(C)**. **(A)** Delivery of NOX2 via Rab27a, VAMP-8, and Rac2 is critical for maintaining an alkaline pH in intracellular cross-presenting compartments. Alternatively, recruitment of ERGIC via Sec22b also regulates pH and proteolytic activity in phagosomes. The ERGIC may contain protease inhibitors such as Cystatin C and lipid bodies (LB) that could directly alter phagosomal pH and enzymatic activity of proteases. **(B)** In the vacuolar pathway, antigen is directly processed into peptides by phagosome resident proteases such as cathepsins. In the cytosolic pathway, the antigen may need to be first unfolded by GILT prior to exit into the cytosol via a channel. This mystery translocon may be Sec61 and could be present in ERGIC, thereby recruited to the cross-presenting compartment via Sec22b. Once in the cytosol, antigen is then degraded into peptides and shuttled back into the phagosome via phagosomal TAP. TAP is dependent on Sec22b for its recruitment from ERGIC to endocytic compartments. Finally, IRAP, which is present on Rab14$^+$ and Syntaxin 6$^+$ endosomes, is recruited to phagosomes and mediates trimming of imported peptides that are further optimized for cross-presentation. **(C)** Lastly, processed and trimmed peptides have to now be loaded onto MHC I molecules. Source of MHC I in such compartments is unclear and could either be recruited from (1) ERGIC via Sec22b or (2) recycling from plasma membrane or (3) recruitment from endolysosomal compartments via CD74. In all cases, the peptide loading complex (PLC) is recruited from ERGIC via Sec22b to the compartment and can chaperone loading of exogenous foreign peptides to create "cross-presentable" peptide-MHC complexes.

in phagocytes to prevent NOX2 assembly, thereby acidifying the phagosomes, in order to evade the cross-presentation response. However, it is still unclear if these GTPases and SNARE proteins act in concert or independently of one another to mediate recruitment of NOX2 and in turn to control cross-presentation. Given that VAMP-8 also participates in trafficking of secretory vesicles (53, 54), it is tempting to speculate that VAMP-8 and Rab27a might be present in similar secretory granules and are routed to the cross-presenting compartment upon entry of antigen.

In a second pathway, Sec22b mediated recruitment of ERGIC components has additionally been implicated in the maintenance of an alkaline pH (42). Sec22b silenced DC phagosomes have higher levels of mature cathepsin D, increased proteolytic activity, leading to accelerated degradation of antigen. These results therefore suggest that the ERGIC contains protease inhibitors. Which protease inhibitors could be involved? The cystatin family of protease inhibitors has been implicated to play a role in antigen presentation. Cystatin C was demonstrated to inhibit degradation of CD74, leading to enhanced accumulation of MHC II in endolysosomal compartments (31). Interestingly, cystatin C is abundantly expressed by CD8α^+ DC compared to CD8α^- DC from the spleen (32), and only partially colocalizes with endolysosomal compartments (31, 32). Given that the cellular localization of cystatin C as well as its role in cross-presentation is still unclear, a feasible possibility is that cystatin C could perhaps colocalize with ERGIC and play a role in cross-presentation.

Another explanation for why recruitment of ERGIC would delay phagosome maturation is that the ERGIC may contain lipid bodies (LB) that have been implicated in regulating phagosomal alkalinization and antigen cross-presentation (55). These LB accumulate in the cytosol and on DC phagosomes in an interferon (IFN)-inducible ER-resident GTPase (Igtp) dependent manner. Specifically, Igtp was shown to interact with LB resident adipose differentiation related protein (ADFP) to mediate formation of LB, which were crucial for cross presentation (55).

ANTIGEN PROCESSING

The cytosolic pathway model of cross-presentation stipulates that once antigen is internalized, it has to make its way out of the endosome/phagosome and into the cytosol for proteasomal degradation (**Figure 1B**). It is generally thought that prior to export into the cytosol, antigens may need to be unfolded. For certain antigens, this is a challenge owing to specific di-sulfide bonds holding the structure of the antigen together. In this case, gamma-interferon-inducible lysosomal thiolreductase (GILT) has been shown to be critical for cross-presentation of di-sulfide bonds containing antigen derived from HSV infected cells (56). Once unfolded, antigen is then routed to the cytosol through a channel, the identity of which still remains enigmatic and controversial. Sec61, a translocon involved in the ER associated degradation pathway (ERAD) was regarded as a top candidate given that blocking Sec61 activity by using *Pseudomonas aeruginosa* bacteria exotoxin A resulted in loss of cross-presentation of soluble OVA antigen (41). However, the evidence for exotoxin A directly and solely blocking Sec61 channel activity is still lacking. Interestingly, DC lacking Sec22b SNARE protein via short hairpin ribonucleic acid (shRNA) targeted deletion, showed impaired antigen export from endocytic compartments, thus arguing for the recruitment of an ERGIC resident translocon channel (42). Further studies analyzing phagosomal proteomics of these Sec22b sufficient and deficient DC would be integral to revealing the identity of the enigmatic translocon.

Once in the cytosol, it is well accepted that the antigen undergoes proteasomal degradation resulting in the generation of peptides. These peptides are then reimported by TAP into the lumen of the cross-presenting compartment (57). TAP is an ER and ERGIC resident protein that has been demonstrated to be recruited to phagosomes in a Sec22b dependent manner (42). Several groups have confirmed the dependence of cross-presentation on TAP, although in the case of certain bacterial antigens, cross-presentation can take place even in the absence of TAP via the vacuolar pathway where antigens are processed within endosomes and phagosomes by resident proteases (3).

Upon internalization of exogenous antigens, newly generated peptides can be trimmed by endosomal insulin-regulated aminopeptidase (IRAP) to be further optimized for cross-presentation (58). IRAP$^{-/-}$ DC are impaired in their ability to cross-present soluble and particulate antigen, thus implicating the importance of IRAP in cross-presentation. IRAP colocalizes with Rab14^{+} and syntaxin 6^{+} endosomes at steady state, and is recruited to phagosomes after antigen uptake (58, 59). Whether IRAP depends on Rab14 GTPase and syntaxin 6 SNARE proteins for its delivery to the phagosomes remains to be studied.

PEPTIDE LOADING ON MHC I

Processed and trimmed peptides are now faced with the possibility of being loaded on MHC I molecules that are present within endosomes and phagosomes (**Figure 1C**). A question that remains is where these MHC I molecules are recruited from. An attractive possibility is that MHC I molecules are present in the ERGIC and that perhaps Sec22b can deliver MHC I along with its chaperone proteins such as calreticulin and tapasin to the cross-presenting compartment. However, analysis of MHC I molecules in cell lines has revealed that MHC I molecules are transiently trafficked through the ERGIC at steady state. In fact, MHC I accumulated in ERGIC only in conditions where these molecules are not bound to high affinity peptides which could occur in the absence of TAP or calreticulin or when traffic out of the ERGIC is blocked (60–64). Whether MHC I trafficking in APC occurs similarly is still unclear.

An alternative possibility is that MHC I may be derived from the plasma membrane. Indeed, endocytosis and subsequent recycling of MHC I has been extensively documented in several cell lines where internalized MHC I are delivered to endosomal recycling compartments (ERC) in a step prior to being re-routed to the plasma membrane (63). Trafficking patterns of MHC I in APC are less clear. Some studies in APC confirm the reliance on plasma membrane derived MHC I, where internalization of surface MHC I molecules was shown to be dependent on a conserved tyrosine within the cytosolic domain of the MHC I, and to a lesser extent on a conserved serine phosphorylation site (65, 66). Mutations in these conserved sites resulted in inhibition of cross-presentation both *in vitro* and *in vivo*. However, given the strong evidence in cell lines for accumulation of MHC I in ERC, further studies are warranted to determine the contribution of MHC I molecules recycling through the ERC to cross-presentation.

Finally, it was also recently shown that CD74, which was originally characterized to route MHC II molecules from the ER to lysosomal compartments (67), was also important in mediating cross-presentation of viral and cell-associated antigen (68). CD74 was found in complex with immature endoglycosidase sensitive MHC I, indicating that it associates with newly synthesized MHC I in the ER (69). In CD74$^{-/-}$ DC, MHC I molecules were present to a lesser extent in LAMP-1^{+} compartments, implying that CD74 delivers MHC I from the ER to endolysosomal compartments.

NATURE OF THE CROSS-PRESENTING COMPARTMENT DURING INFECTION

In spite of these studies detailing the molecular and cellular makeup of cross-presenting compartments at steady state, the mechanisms underlying regulation and remodeling of this compartment during infection remain largely undefined. Upon uptake of microbial or infected cellular cargo, the phagosomal or endosomal compartment can be substantially modified by the acquisition of pattern recognition receptors (PRRs) (16). PRRs are evolutionarily conserved receptors that recognize and respond to conserved pathogen-associated molecular patterns (PAMPs) which are unique to microbes (70). Upon PRR engagement, intracellular signal transduction pathways are initiated such as those mediated by nuclear factor-κB (NF-κB), mitogen-activated protein kinases (MAPKs), and IFN-regulatory factors (IRFs) (71). These pathways are critical for providing immunity against several pathogen infections.

Several families of mammalian PRRs have been identified, namely Toll-like receptors (TLRs), nucleotide-binding oligomerization domain-like (NOD-like) receptors (NLRs), RIG-I like receptors (RLRs), and C-type lectin receptors (CLRs) (72). Indeed, TLRs were the first family of PRRs to be studied in detail (73–75). We focus here on recent developments in the biology of TLR that enable the recruitment of these receptors and assembly of their signaling machinery. This recruitment aids in the transduction of responses from the compartment itself, allowing localized phagosomal or endosomal specific control of responses, including presentation of exogenous antigen on MHC I and MHC II molecules. To signal and regulate presentation of exogenous antigen from endosomal compartments, TLRs first need to be recruited to the relevant compartment.

TLR4

TLR4 is a plasma membrane resident "surface" TLR that can be endocytosed and also signal from intracellular compartments upon interaction with its ligand lipopolysaccharide (LPS). TLR4 initially engages toll-interleukin 1 receptor (TIR) domain-containing adaptor protein (TIRAP) and myeloid differentiation primary-response protein (MyD88) to initiate signal transduction from the plasma membrane (76). Subsequently, TLR4 is internalized into endocytic compartments and engages TRIF-related adaptor molecule (TRAM) and TIR-domain-containing adaptor inducing IFN-β (TRIF) (76). In fact, blocking TLR4 endocytosis using dynamin inhibitors selectively inhibits TRIF-TRAM mediated IRF3 dependent type I IFN responses without affecting TIRAP-MyD88 dependent signaling (77).

Recently, CD14 was shown to regulate the endocytosis of TLR4 from the plasma membrane during stimulation with LPS (78). TLR4 acts as a cargo for CD14, which transports the receptor and LPS to endosomes in a Syk and PLCγ2 dependent process where TRIF signaling leads to IFN-β production. While CD14 is critical for TLR4 endocytosis and IFN-β production in response to soluble LPS, TLR4 endocytosis in DC can proceed in the absence of CD14 during phagocytosis of *E. coli* or LPS-coated beads, although a lower percent of TLR4 is internalized compared to soluble LPS. Notably, despite lower percent TLR4 internalization in response to these particles, IFN-β production, which relies on TLR4 signaling from endocytic compartments, was unaffected in the absence of CD14. This result suggests that in the case of phagocytosed cargo, TLR4 can accumulate on phagosomes from another source independently of the plasma membrane.

Indeed, the small GTPase Rab11a was shown to play a crucial role in trafficking TLR4 from ERC to phagosomes containing gram-negative and not gram-positive bacteria, leading to IRF3 activation and IFN-β transcription (79). Additionally, adaptor protein 3 (AP-3) also plays a role in recruiting TLR4 and MyD88 from intracellular stores to phagosomes containing TLR4 ligands (80). Interestingly, AP-3 dependent recruitment of TLR4 and MyD88 was crucial for mediating production of pro-inflammatory cytokines selectively in response to phagocytic cargo and not to soluble LPS. Hence, the mode of uptake can dictate the pathway of delivery of TLR4.

It is curious to ask if the recruitment of TLR4 via these regulatory transport proteins contributes toward antigen presentation and adaptive immunity. For MHC II presentation, phagosome autonomous TLR4 signaling led to accelerated phagosome maturation and subsequent degradation of CD74 specifically in phagosomes bearing TLR ligands and not other phagosomes in the same DC (81, 82). Additionally, impaired recruitment of TLR4 to phagosomes in AP-3 deficient mice also led to decreased MHC II presentation (80). However, whether any of these proteins regulate cross-presentation of antigen internalized via endocytosis or phagocytosis remains to be investigated.

TLR9

TLR9 is an endosomal receptor and begins its journey in the ER, where it associates with the chaperone protein Unc-93 homolog B (UNC93B), which mediates its transport to endosomes (83). Recently, recruitment of TLR9 and UNC93B was demonstrated selectively to phagosomes that contained DNA and anti-DNA immunoglobulin (Ig) complexes (84). Importantly, phagosomal TLR9 recruitment did not depend on its ability to sense the presence of TLR9 ligand DNA but instead relied on Fc receptor γ (FcRγ) mediated engagement by Ig complexes. These data suggest that Ig mediated FcRγ signaling leads to recruitment of TLR9 to phagosomes. When these phagosomes also contain the TLR9 ligand DNA, TLR9 signaling is engaged, resulting in IFN-α secretion. Given that engagement of FcRγ prepares phagosomes for optimal TLR9 signaling, it is tempting to speculate that this synergy between FcRγ and TLR9 may also impact subsequent cross-presentation responses of antigen complexed with DNA-Ig aggregates.

TLR2

TLR2 is a cell surface TLR that synergizes with other surface TLRs such as TLR1 and TLR6 to mediate MyD88 dependent signal transduction responses. Similar to TLR4, there are reports showing TLR2 localization to endosomal compartments specifically early endosomes, lysosomes, and Rab11a^{+} vesicles in monocytes (85). Some studies also indicate TLR2 dependent induction of type I IFN signaling from endocytic compartments (86, 87). How TLR2 is directed to such compartments is still unclear.

PRR REGULATION OF CROSS-PRESENTATION

Studies looking at the role of PRRs in cross-presentation have been largely limited to TLRs and CLRs. These receptors are well suited to regulate cross-presentation as they are present at the plasma membrane as well as along the endocytic pathway, where they encounter microbial antigen and initiate signaling to regulate adaptive immune responses such as cross-presentation. Here, we present evidence supporting regulation by these receptors.

TOLL-LIKE RECEPTORS

There are several studies that show that TLR signaling enhances cross-priming of CD8 T cells (88). The *in vivo* contribution of TLR3 to cross-priming became clear after an elegant study demonstrated that signaling via TLR3 leads to maturation of DC and therefore promotes virus-specific CD8 T cell responses (5). Another study showed that injecting mice with apoptotic vesicles derived from *M. tuberculosis* infected macrophages, activates DC via TLR2 in a MyD88 dependent manner and can cross-prime CD8 T cells, thereby protecting mice from developing tuberculosis infection (17). Moreover, by employing biodegradable microspheres for the delivery of phagocytic cargo to DC, Schlosser et al. were able to demonstrate that the presence of both TLR ligand and antigen within the same phagosome yielded efficient CTL responses as compared to when the ligand and antigen are located in separate phagosomes (89).

One caveat of the studies above is the inability to distinguish the effects of TLR signaling on cross-presentation versus cross-priming. For example, a couple of studies revealed that TLR3 and TLR9 ligands could both induce cross-presentation of OVA by DC (90, 91). This induction of cross-presentation was found to be dependent on TLR signaling as DC from *Tlr9*$^{-/-}$ and *Myd88*$^{-/-}$ mice were unable to cross-present antigen after exposure to TLR ligands. However, the authors of these studies relied exclusively on T cell activation as a measure of displayed peptide-MHC I complexes. Given that TLR signaling also controls DC maturation and expression of co-stimulatory molecules that are pivotal for T cell activation, it is difficult to rule out the confounding factor of impaired co-stimulation and decreased DC maturation seen with TLR deficient DC. In fact, the inability of *Myd88*$^{-/-}$ DC to activate CD8 T cells after phagocytosis of virally infected cells was fully restored by treatment with a CD40 cross-linking antibody suggesting that defective cross-priming was due to impaired TLR induced co-stimulation rather than cross-presentation *per se* in this particular case (92).

The most direct way to assess cross-presentation is to use a conformation dependent antibody directly against preformed peptide-MHC I complexes on the surface of the APC. However, these antibodies are quite insensitive and work successfully only when DC were pulsed with large amounts of antigen. Nevertheless, Christian Kurts' group successfully used 25D1.16 antibody to detect SIINFEKL-MHC I complexes and thus demonstrated increased cross-presentation with TLR signaling after uptake of soluble OVA in the presence of LPS (93). This increase in cross-presentation was mediated by TLR4, MyD88 and not TRIF signaling. However, this study was focused on the cross-presentation of soluble antigen and hence whether TLR signaling enhances cross-presentation of phagocytosed particulate antigen remains to be determined.

C-TYPE LECTIN RECEPTORS

C-type lectin receptors contain at least one carbohydrate recognition domain via which they bind to sugar moieties on self or microbial derived antigens. CLRs can regulate cross-presentation, although most of them do so by regulating antigen uptake. For example, CD209 and mannose receptor have been reported to increase internalization of cargo and target antigens to early endosomes for cross-presentation (94, 95). DNGR1 was also reported to enhance cross-presentation of cellular antigens derived from necrotic dying cells (96). Interestingly, despite intact maturation phenotypes and maintenance of signals to relay co-stimulation in DNGR1 deficient DC, these DC were impaired in cross-presentation, suggesting specific regulation of cross-presentation rather than cross-priming (97). DNGR1 is also expressed at high levels in subsets of DC specialized for cross-presentation including murine CD8α^+ DCs and tissue-resident CD103$^+$ CD11b$^-$ DCs as well as in human counterparts BDCA3$^+$ DC (39).

CAN CROSS-PRESENTATION STILL TAKE PLACE AT STEADY STATE?

In the absence of inflammation or infection, cross-presentation of self-antigens at steady state can take place, leading to tolerance to host antigens and deletion of potentially auto-reactive CD8 T cells. Indeed, generation and activity of CTL must be tightly controlled to avoid auto-reactivity to self, given the potency of CTL in killing infected target host cells (98, 99). Here, we review existing evidence for the role of cross-presentation in both central and peripheral tolerance mechanisms.

PERIPHERAL TOLERANCE

Peripheral tolerance constitutes mechanisms of tolerance that take place after mature lymphocytes enter into the periphery. There are several studies that argue for the constitutive TLR or PRR-independent nature of cross-presentation for the induction of peripheral cross-tolerance to non-inflammatory self-antigens, leading to deletion of self-reactive CTL. Many of these models employed the expression of neo-self-antigens under the control of tissue-specific promoters like the rat insulin promoter (RIP). These models ensure that the antigens are expressed outside of the thymus, allowing researchers to specifically study peripheral tolerance.

Cross-tolerance was first demonstrated when OVA specific OT-I CD8 T cells were efficiently deleted after being adoptively transferred into a mouse expressing OVA under control of the RIP (RIP-mOVA) (100). Cross-tolerance was also shown to be important for the control of endogenous auto-reactive CD8 T cells specific for naturally expressed self-antigen (101). In this study, the authors bred the RIP-mOVA mice with mice lacking GTPase Rac1 in CD11c$^+$ cells to generate Rac1-RIP mice. Conveniently, deficiency in Rac1 GTPase selectively affected the ability of CD8α^+ DC to internalize antigen (33), resulting in impaired cross-presentation while leaving the classical MHC II and MHC I pathways of antigen presentation unaffected (101). Consequently, they were able to demonstrate that DC in Rac1-RIP mice failed to cross-present transgenic self-antigen and hence failed to delete transferred OT-I T cells. Moreover these mice developed symptoms of diabetes. Interestingly, mice that just had Rac1 deleted in CD11c$^+$ cells also had higher numbers of endogenous CD8 T cells, although the mice seemed healthy and did not develop autoimmunity. However, when CD25 depleted T cells from these mice were transferred into lymphopenic hosts, the hosts developed several signs of autoimmunity as a result of homeostatic T cell proliferation. Hence, the above studies clearly demonstrate the role of cross-presentation under steady state to induce peripheral tolerance.

An interesting study by Christian Kurts' group looked to see if tolerogenic DC could be converted into autoimmunogenic DC after exposure to stimulating conditions such as TLR ligands (102). TLR ligands were able to induce CTL mediated autoimmunity only in cases where antigen specific CD4 T cell help was provided concomitantly. These results demonstrated that the mere presence of TLR ligands, such as those present in commensal bacteria or those derived from the use of vaccine adjuvants, is not sufficient to break cross-tolerance mechanisms.

CENTRAL TOLERANCE

In addition to peripheral tolerance, cross-presentation was also implicated in the induction of central tolerance (103). Central tolerance is induced in the thymus where developing thymocytes that recognize peptide-MHC complexes are positively selected to express either CD4 or CD8 molecules. Subsequently, thymocytes that are able to recognize self-peptide-MHC complexes with high affinity are efficiently deleted via negative selection. Medullary thymic epithelial cells (mTECs) and DC play a critical role in mediating negative selection. mTECs exclusively express a broad range of tissue-specific antigens (TSA) (104, 105). In spite of expressing both MHC II and MHC I molecules, mTECs are poor APC. Bevan's group was the first to show that bone-marrow derived cells in the thymus were capable of cross-presenting antigen captured from mTECs (103). However, this study also showed that mTECs, by themselves, were capable of direct presentation on MHC I molecules and were sufficient to induce CD8 T cell deletion, thus diminishing the importance of cross-presentation in central tolerance. A recent report does point to the relevance of cross-presentation by human thymic DC. Upon analyzing peptides eluted from both MHC I and MHC II molecules of human thymic DC, the authors observed that around 22% of the MHC I ligands were derived from proteins present in the vesicular/extracellular compartment the presentation of which would typically be associated with the classical MHC II pathway (30).

CONCLUSION

The studies we reviewed here certainly point to the constitutive nature of cross-presentation, however, an increasingly large body of work now provides strong evidence for the capacity to enhance cross-presentation by signals from inflammatory PRRs. Having mechanisms of regulation in place allows for the generation of robust CTL responses during an infection while maintaining induction of tolerance at steady state. Further insight into these regulatory mechanisms may potentially help in tailoring better therapeutic strategies to combat infectious agents as well as tumors, while preventing autoimmunity. Hence, elucidating the mechanistic differences in vesicular trafficking between steady state and inflammatory cross-presentation would be important for developing new rationales in the design of safe and effective vaccines for anti-viral, anti-bacterial as well as anti-tumor immunity.

REFERENCES

1. Bevan MJ. Minor H antigens introduced on H-2 different stimulating cells cross-react at the cytotoxic T cell level during in vivo priming. *J Immunol* (1976) **117**:2233–8.
2. Carbone FR, Kurts C, Bennett SR, Miller JF, Heath WR. Cross-presentation: a general mechanism for CTL immunity and tolerance. *Immunol Today* (1998) **19**:368–73. doi:10.1016/S0167-5699(98)01301-2
3. Joffre OP, Segura E, Savina A, Amigorena S. Cross-presentation by dendritic cells. *Nat Rev Immunol* (2012) **12**:557–69. doi:10.1038/nri3254
4. Tindle RW, Frazer IH. Immune response to human papillomaviruses and the prospects for human papillomavirus-specific immunisation. *Curr Top Microbiol Immunol* (1994) **186**:217–53. doi:10.1007/978-3-642-78487-3_12
5. Schulz O, Diebold SS, Chen M, Naslund TI, Nolte MA, Alexopoulou L, et al. Toll-like receptor 3 promotes cross-priming to virus-infected cells. *Nature* (2005) **433**:887–92. doi:10.1038/nature03326
6. Gabrilovich DI, Patterson S, Harvey JJ, Woods GM, Elsley W, Knight SC. Murine retrovirus induces defects in the function of dendritic cells at early stages of infection. *Cell Immunol* (1994) **158**:167–81. doi:10.1006/cimm.1994.1265
7. Fugier-Vivier I, Servet-Delprat C, Rivailler P, Rissoan MC, Liu YJ, Rabourdin-Combe C. Measles virus suppresses cell-mediated immunity by interfering with the survival and functions of dendritic and T cells. *J Exp Med* (1997) **186**:813–23. doi:10.1084/jem.186.6.813
8. Engelmayer J, Larsson M, Subklewe M, Chahroudi A, Cox WI, Steinman RM, et al. Vaccinia virus inhibits the maturation of human dendritic cells: a novel mechanism of immune evasion. *J Immunol* (1999) **163**:6762–8.
9. Salio M, Cella M, Suter M, Lanzavecchia A. Inhibition of dendritic cell maturation by herpes simplex virus. *Eur J Immunol* (1999) **29**:3245–53. doi:10.1002/(SICI)1521-4141(199910)29:10<3245::AID-IMMU3245>3.3.CO;2-O
10. Sigal LJ, Crotty S, Andino R, Rock KL. Cytotoxic T-cell immunity to virus-infected non-haematopoietic cells requires presentation of exogenous antigen. *Nature* (1999) **398**:77–80. doi:10.1038/18038
11. Ignatius R, Marovich M, Mehlhop E, Villamide L, Mahnke K, Cox WI, et al. Canarypox virus-induced maturation of dendritic cells is mediated by apoptotic cell death and tumor necrosis factor alpha secretion. *J Virol* (2000) **74**:11329–38. doi:10.1128/JVI.74.23.11329-11338.2000
12. Servet-Delprat C, Vidalain PO, Bausinger H, Manie S, Le Deist F, Azocar O, et al. Measles virus induces abnormal differentiation of CD40 ligand-activated human dendritic cells. *J Immunol* (2000) **164**:1753–60.
13. Sevilla N, Kunz S, Holz A, Lewicki H, Homann D, Yamada H, et al. Immunosuppression and resultant viral persistence by specific viral targeting of dendritic cells. *J Exp Med* (2000) **192**:1249–60. doi:10.1084/jem.192.9.1249
14. John B, Harris TH, Tait ED, Wilson EH, Gregg B, Ng LG, et al. Dynamic Imaging of CD8(+) T cells and dendritic cells during infection with *Toxoplasma gondii*. *PLoS Pathog* (2009) **5**:e1000505. doi:10.1371/journal.ppat.1000505
15. Jung S, Unutmaz D, Wong P, Sano G, De Los Santos K, Sparwasser T, et al. In vivo depletion of CD11c+ dendritic cells abrogates priming of CD8+ T cells by exogenous cell-associated antigens. *Immunity* (2002) **17**:211–20. doi:10.1016/S1074-7613(02)00365-5
16. Schaible UE, Winau F, Sieling PA, Fischer K, Collins HL, Hagens K, et al. Apoptosis facilitates antigen presentation to T lymphocytes through MHC-I and CD1 in tuberculosis. *Nat Med* (2003) **9**:1039–46. doi:10.1038/nm906
17. Winau F, Weber S, Sad S, De Diego J, Hoops SL, Breiden B, et al. Apoptotic vesicles crossprime CD8 T cells and protect against tuberculosis. *Immunity* (2006) **24**:105–17. doi:10.1016/j.immuni.2005.12.001
18. Delamarre L, Pack M, Chang H, Mellman I, Trombetta ES. Differential lysosomal proteolysis in antigen-presenting cells determines antigen fate. *Science* (2005) **307**:1630–4. doi:10.1126/science.1108003
19. Kamath AT, Henri S, Battye F, Tough DF, Shortman K. Developmental kinetics and lifespan of dendritic cells in mouse lymphoid organs. *Blood* (2002) **100**:1734–41.
20. Bedoui S, Whitney PG, Waithman J, Eidsmo L, Wakim L, Caminschi I, et al. Cross-presentation of viral and self antigens by skin-derived CD103+ dendritic cells. *Nat Immunol* (2009) **10**:488–95. doi:10.1038/ni.1724
21. Segura E, Villadangos JA. Antigen presentation by dendritic cells in vivo. *Curr Opin Immunol* (2009) **21**:105–10. doi:10.1016/j.coi.2009.03.011
22. Cheong C, Matos I, Choi JH, Dandamudi DB, Shrestha E, Longhi MP, et al. Microbial stimulation fully differentiates monocytes to DC-SIGN/CD209(+) dendritic cells for immune T cell areas. *Cell* (2010) **143**:416–29. doi:10.1016/j.cell.2010.09.039
23. Henri S, Poulin LF, Tamoutounour S, Ardouin L, Guilliams M, De Bovis B, et al. CD207+ CD103+ dermal dendritic cells cross-present keratinocyte-derived antigens irrespective of the presence of Langerhans cells. *J Exp Med* (2010) **207**:189–206. doi:10.1084/jem.20091964
24. Shortman K, Heath WR. The CD8+ dendritic cell subset. *Immunol Rev* (2010) **234**:18–31. doi:10.1111/j.0105-2896.2009.00870.x
25. Aliberti J, Schulz O, Pennington DJ, Tsujimura H, Reis E, Sousa C, et al. Essential role for ICSBP in the in vivo development of murine CD8alpha + dendritic cells. *Blood* (2003) **101**:305–10. doi:10.1182/blood-2002-04-1088
26. Hildner K, Edelson BT, Purtha WE, Diamond M, Matsushita H, Kohyama M, et al. Batf3 deficiency reveals a critical role for CD8alpha+ dendritic cells in cytotoxic T cell immunity. *Science* (2008) **322**:1097–100. doi:10.1126/science.1164206
27. Ginhoux F, Liu K, Helft J, Bogunovic M, Greter M, Hashimoto D, et al. The origin and development of nonlymphoid tissue CD103+ DCs. *J Exp Med* (2009) **206**:3115–30. doi:10.1084/jem.20091756
28. Edelson BT, Kc W, Juang R, Kohyama M, Benoit LA, Klekotka PA, et al. Peripheral CD103+ dendritic cells form a unified subset developmentally related to CD8alpha+ conventional dendritic cells. *J Exp Med* (2010) **207**:823–36. doi:10.1084/jem.20091627
29. Sathe P, Pooley J, Vremec D, Mintern J, Jin JO, Wu L, et al. The acquisition of antigen cross-presentation function by newly formed dendritic cells. *J Immunol* (2011) **186**:5184–92. doi:10.4049/jimmunol.1002683
30. Bachem A, Guttler S, Hartung E, Ebstein F, Schaefer M, Tannert A, et al. Superior antigen cross-presentation and XCR1 expression define human CD11c+CD141+ cells as homologues of mouse CD8+ dendritic cells. *J Exp Med* (2010) **207**:1273–81. doi:10.1084/jem.20100348
31. Crozat K, Guiton R, Contreras V, Feuillet V, Dutertre CA, Ventre E, et al. The XC chemokine receptor 1 is a conserved selective marker of mammalian cells homologous to mouse CD8alpha+ dendritic cells. *J Exp Med* (2010) **207**:1283–92. doi:10.1084/jem.20100223
32. Jongbloed SL, Kassianos AJ, Mcdonald KJ, Clark GJ, Ju X, Angel CE, et al. Human CD141+ (BDCA-3)+ dendritic cells (DCs) represent a unique myeloid DC subset that cross-presents necrotic cell antigens. *J Exp Med* (2010) **207**:1247–60. doi:10.1084/jem.20092140

33. Poulin LF, Salio M, Griessinger E, Anjos-Afonso F, Craciun L, Chen JL, et al. Characterization of human DNGR-1+ BDCA3+ leukocytes as putative equivalents of mouse CD8alpha+ dendritic cells. *J Exp Med* (2010) **207**:1261–71. doi:10.1084/jem.20092618
34. Haniffa M, Shin A, Bigley V, Mcgovern N, Teo P, See P, et al. Human tissues contain CD141hi cross-presenting dendritic cells with functional homology to mouse CD103+ nonlymphoid dendritic cells. *Immunity* (2012) **37**:60–73. doi:10.1016/j.immuni.2012.04.012
35. Mittag D, Proietto AI, Loudovaris T, Mannering SI, Vremec D, Shortman K, et al. Human dendritic cell subsets from spleen and blood are similar in phenotype and function but modified by donor health status. *J Immunol* (2011) **186**:6207–17. doi:10.4049/jimmunol.1002632
36. Cohn L, Chatterjee B, Esselborn F, Smed-Sorensen A, Nakamura N, Chalouni C, et al. Antigen delivery to early endosomes eliminates the superiority of human blood BDCA3+ dendritic cells at cross presentation. *J Exp Med* (2013) **210**:1049–63. doi:10.1084/jem.20121251
37. Segura E, Durand M, Amigorena S. Similar antigen cross-presentation capacity and phagocytic functions in all freshly isolated human lymphoid organ-resident dendritic cells. *J Exp Med* (2013) **210**:1035–47. doi:10.1084/jem.20121103
38. Hambleton S, Salem S, Bustamante J, Bigley V, Boisson-Dupuis S, Azevedo J, et al. IRF8 mutations and human dendritic-cell immunodeficiency. *N Engl J Med* (2011) **365**:127–38. doi:10.1056/NEJMoa1100066
39. Poulin LF, Reyal Y, Uronen-Hansson H, Schraml BU, Sancho D, Murphy KM, et al. DNGR-1 is a specific and universal marker of mouse and human Batf3-dependent dendritic cells in lymphoid and nonlymphoid tissues. *Blood* (2012) **119**:6052–62. doi:10.1182/blood-2012-01-406967
40. Kovacsovics-Bankowski M, Rock KL. A phagosome-to-cytosol pathway for exogenous antigens presented on MHC class I molecules. *Science* (1995) **267**:243–6. doi:10.1126/science.7809629
41. Ackerman AL, Giodini A, Cresswell P. A role for the endoplasmic reticulum protein retrotranslocation machinery during crosspresentation by dendritic cells. *Immunity* (2006) **25**:607–17. doi:10.1016/j.immuni.2006.08.017
42. Cebrian I, Visentin G, Blanchard N, Jouve M, Bobard A, Moita C, et al. Sec22b regulates phagosomal maturation and antigen crosspresentation by dendritic cells. *Cell* (2011) **147**:1355–68. doi:10.1016/j.cell.2011.11.021
43. Guermonprez P, Saveanu L, Kleijmeer M, Davoust J, Van Endert P, Amigorena S. ER-phagosome fusion defines an MHC class I cross-presentation compartment in dendritic cells. *Nature* (2003) **425**:397–402. doi:10.1038/nature01911
44. Houde M, Bertholet S, Gagnon E, Brunet S, Goyette G, Laplante A, et al. Phagosomes are competent organelles for antigen cross-presentation. *Nature* (2003) **425**:402–6. doi:10.1038/nature01912
45. Shen L, Sigal LJ, Boes M, Rock KL. Important role of cathepsin S in generating peptides for TAP-independent MHC class I crosspresentation in vivo. *Immunity* (2004) **21**:155–65. doi:10.1016/j.immuni.2004.07.004
46. Claus V, Jahraus A, Tjelle T, Berg T, Kirschke H, Faulstich H, et al. Lysosomal enzyme trafficking between phagosomes, endosomes, and lysosomes in J774 macrophages. Enrichment of cathepsin H in early endosomes. *J Biol Chem* (1998) **273**:9842–51. doi:10.1074/jbc.273.16.9842
47. Savina A, Jancic C, Hugues S, Guermonprez P, Vargas P, Moura IC, et al. NOX2 controls phagosomal pH to regulate antigen processing during crosspresentation by dendritic cells. *Cell* (2006) **126**:205–18. doi:10.1016/j.cell.2006.05.035
48. Jancic C, Savina A, Wasmeier C, Tolmachova T, El-Benna J, Dang PM, et al. Rab27a regulates phagosomal pH and NADPH oxidase recruitment to dendritic cell phagosomes. *Nat Cell Biol* (2007) **9**:367–78. doi:10.1038/ncb1552
49. Tolmachova T, Anders R, Stinchcombe J, Bossi G, Griffiths GM, Huxley C, et al. A general role for Rab27a in secretory cells. *Mol Biol Cell* (2004) **15**:332–44. doi:10.1091/mbc.E03-07-0452
50. Savina A, Peres A, Cebrian I, Carmo N, Moita C, Hacohen N, et al. The small GTPase Rac2 controls phagosomal alkalinization and antigen crosspresentation selectively in CD8(+) dendritic cells. *Immunity* (2009) **30**:544–55. doi:10.1016/j.immuni.2009.01.013
51. Stow JL, Murray RZ. Intracellular trafficking and secretion of inflammatory cytokines. *Cytokine Growth Factor Rev* (2013) **24**:227–39. doi:10.1016/j.cytogfr.2013.04.001
52. Matheoud D, Moradin N, Bellemare-Pelletier A, Shio MT, Hong WJ, Olivier M, et al. Leishmania evades host immunity by inhibiting antigen cross-presentation through direct cleavage of the SNARE VAMP8. *Cell Host Microbe* (2013) **14**:15–25. doi:10.1016/j.chom.2013.06.003
53. Puri N, Roche PA. Mast cells possess distinct secretory granule subsets whose exocytosis is regulated by different SNARE isoforms. *Proc Natl Acad Sci U S A* (2008) **105**:2580–5. doi:10.1073/pnas.0707854105
54. Tiwari N, Wang CC, Brochetta C, Ke G, Vita F, Qi Z, et al. VAMP-8 segregates mast cell-preformed mediator exocytosis from cytokine trafficking pathways. *Blood* (2008) **111**:3665–74. doi:10.1182/blood-2007-07-103309
55. Bougneres L, Helft J, Tiwari S, Vargas P, Chang BH, Chan L, et al. A role for lipid bodies in the cross-presentation of phagocytosed antigens by MHC class I in dendritic cells. *Immunity* (2009) **31**:232–44. doi:10.1016/j.immuni.2009.06.022
56. Singh R, Cresswell P. Defective cross-presentation of viral antigens in GILT-free mice. *Science* (2010) **328**:1394–8. doi:10.1126/science.1189176
57. Blum JS, Wearsch PA, Cresswell P. Pathways of antigen processing. *Annu Rev Immunol* (2013) **31**:443–73. doi:10.1146/annurev-immunol-032712-095910
58. Saveanu L, Carroll O, Weimershaus M, Guermonprez P, Firat E, Lindo V, et al. IRAP identifies an endosomal compartment required for MHC class I cross-presentation. *Science* (2009) **325**:213–7. doi:10.1126/science.1172845
59. Weimershaus M, Maschalidi S, Sepulveda F, Manoury B, Van Endert P, Saveanu L. Conventional dendritic cells require IRAP-Rab14 endosomes for efficient cross-presentation. *J Immunol* (2012) **188**:1840–6. doi:10.4049/jimmunol.1101504
60. Raposo G, Van Santen HM, Leijendekker R, Geuze HJ, Ploegh HL. Misfolded major histocompatibility complex class I molecules accumulate in an expanded ER-Golgi intermediate compartment. *J Cell Biol* (1995) **131**:1403–19. doi:10.1083/jcb.131.6.1403
61. Spiliotis ET, Pentcheva T, Edidin M. Probing for membrane domains in the endoplasmic reticulum: retention and degradation of unassembled MHC class I molecules. *Mol Biol Cell* (2002) **13**:1566–81. doi:10.1091/mbc.01-07-0322
62. Garstka M, Borchert B, Al-Balushi M, Praveen PV, Kuhl N, Majoul I, et al. Peptide-receptive major histocompatibility complex class I molecules cycle between endoplasmic reticulum and cis-Golgi in wild-type lymphocytes. *J Biol Chem* (2007) **282**:30680–90. doi:10.1074/jbc.M701721200
63. Donaldson JG, Williams DB. Intracellular assembly and trafficking of MHC class I molecules. *Traffic* (2009) **10**:1745–52. doi:10.1111/j.1600-0854.2009.00979.x
64. Van Hateren A, James E, Bailey A, Phillips A, Dalchau N, Elliott T. The cell biology of major histocompatibility complex class I assembly: towards a molecular understanding. *Tissue Antigens* (2010) **76**:259–75. doi:10.1111/j.1399-0039.2010.01550.x
65. Lizee G, Basha G, Tiong J, Julien JP, Tian M, Biron KE, et al. Control of dendritic cell cross-presentation by the major histocompatibility complex class I cytoplasmic domain. *Nat Immunol* (2003) **4**:1065–73. doi:10.1038/ni989
66. Basha G, Lizee G, Reinicke AT, Seipp RP, Omilusik KD, Jefferies WA. MHC class I endosomal and lysosomal trafficking coincides with exogenous antigen loading in dendritic cells. *PLoS One* (2008) **3**:e3247. doi:10.1371/journal.pone.0003247
67. Bakke O, Dobberstein B. MHC class II-associated invariant chain contains a sorting signal for endosomal compartments. *Cell* (1990) **63**:707–16. doi:10.1016/0092-8674(90)90137-4
68. Basha G, Omilusik K, Chavez-Steenbock A, Reinicke AT, Lack N, Choi KB, et al. A CD74-dependent MHC class I endolysosomal cross-presentation pathway. *Nat Immunol* (2012) **13**:237–45. doi:10.1038/ni.2225
69. Kornfeld R, Kornfeld S. Assembly of asparagine-linked oligosaccharides. *Annu Rev Biochem* (1985) **54**:631–64. doi:10.1146/annurev.bi.54.070185.003215
70. Blander JM, Sander LE. Beyond pattern recognition: five immune checkpoints for scaling the microbial threat. *Nat Rev Immunol* (2012) **12**:215–25. doi:10.1038/nri3167
71. Takeuchi O, Akira S. Pattern recognition receptors and inflammation. *Cell* (2010) **140**:805–20. doi:10.1016/j.cell.2010.01.022
72. Kumar H, Kawai T, Akira S. Pathogen recognition by the innate immune system. *Int Rev Immunol* (2011) **30**:16–34. doi:10.3109/08830185.2010.529976
73. Lemaitre B, Nicolas E, Michaut L, Reichhart JM, Hoffmann JA. The dorsoventral regulatory gene cassette spatzle/Toll/cactus controls the potent antifungal response in *Drosophila* adults. *Cell* (1996) **86**:973–83. doi:10.1016/S0092-8674(00)80172-5
74. Medzhitov R, Preston-Hurlburt P, Janeway CA Jr. A human homologue of the *Drosophila* Toll protein signals activation of adaptive immunity. *Nature* (1997) **388**:394–7. doi:10.1038/41131

75. Poltorak A, He X, Smirnova I, Liu MY, Van Huffel C, Du X, et al. Defective LPS signaling in C3H/HeJ and C57BL/10ScCr mice: mutations in Tlr4 gene. *Science* (1998) **282**:2085–8. doi:10.1126/science.282.5396.2085
76. Kanzler H, Barrat FJ, Hessel EM, Coffman RL. Therapeutic targeting of innate immunity with Toll-like receptor agonists and antagonists. *Nat Med* (2007) **13**:552–9. doi:10.1038/nm1589
77. Kagan JC, Su T, Horng T, Chow A, Akira S, Medzhitov R. TRAM couples endocytosis of Toll-like receptor 4 to the induction of interferon-beta. *Nat Immunol* (2008) **9**:361–8. doi:10.1038/ni1569
78. Zanoni I, Ostuni R, Marek LR, Barresi S, Barbalat R, Barton GM, et al. CD14 controls the LPS-induced endocytosis of Toll-like receptor 4. *Cell* (2011) **147**:868–80. doi:10.1016/j.cell.2011.09.051
79. Husebye H, Aune MH, Stenvik J, Samstad E, Skjeldal F, Halaas O, et al. The Rab11a GTPase controls Toll-like receptor 4-induced activation of interferon regulatory factor-3 on phagosomes. *Immunity* (2010) **33**:583–96. doi:10.1016/j.immuni.2010.09.010
80. Mantegazza AR, Guttentag SH, El-Benna J, Sasai M, Iwasaki A, Shen H, et al. Adaptor protein-3 in dendritic cells facilitates phagosomal toll-like receptor signaling and antigen presentation to CD4(+) T cells. *Immunity* (2012) **36**:782–94. doi:10.1016/j.immuni.2012.02.018
81. Blander JM, Medzhitov R. Regulation of phagosome maturation by signals from toll-like receptors. *Science* (2004) **304**:1014–8. doi:10.1126/science.1096158
82. Blander JM, Medzhitov R. Toll-dependent selection of microbial antigens for presentation by dendritic cells. *Nature* (2006) **440**:808–12. doi:10.1038/nature04596
83. Kim YM, Brinkmann MM, Paquet ME, Ploegh HL. UNC93B1 delivers nucleotide-sensing toll-like receptors to endolysosomes. *Nature* (2008) **452**:234–8. doi:10.1038/nature06726
84. Henault J, Martinez J, Riggs JM, Tian J, Mehta P, Clarke L, et al. Noncanonical autophagy is required for type I interferon secretion in response to DNA-immune complexes. *Immunity* (2012) **37**:986–97. doi:10.1016/j.immuni.2012.09.014
85. Nilsen NJ, Deininger S, Nonstad U, Skjeldal F, Husebye H, Rodionov D, et al. Cellular trafficking of lipoteichoic acid and Toll-like receptor 2 in relation to signaling: role of CD14 and CD36. *J Leukoc Biol* (2008) **84**:280–91. doi:10.1189/jlb.0907656
86. Ip WK, Takahashi K, Moore KJ, Stuart LM, Ezekowitz RA. Mannose-binding lectin enhances Toll-like receptors 2 and 6 signaling from the phagosome. *J Exp Med* (2008) **205**:169–81. doi:10.1084/jem.20071164
87. Barbalat R, Lau L, Locksley RM, Barton GM. Toll-like receptor 2 on inflammatory monocytes induces type I interferon in response to viral but not bacterial ligands. *Nat Immunol* (2009) **10**:1200–7. doi:10.1038/ni.1792
88. Kurts C, Robinson BW, Knolle PA. Cross-priming in health and disease. *Nat Rev Immunol* (2010) **10**:403–14. doi:10.1038/nri2780
89. Schlosser E, Mueller M, Fischer S, Basta S, Busch DH, Gander B, et al. TLR ligands and antigen need to be coencapsulated into the same biodegradable microsphere for the generation of potent cytotoxic T lymphocyte responses. *Vaccine* (2008) **26**:1626–37. doi:10.1016/j.vaccine.2008.01.030
90. Maurer T, Heit A, Hochrein H, Ampenberger F, O'Keeffe M, Bauer S, et al. CpG-DNA aided cross-presentation of soluble antigens by dendritic cells. *Eur J Immunol* (2002) **32**:2356–64. doi:10.1002/1521-4141(200208)32:8<2356::AID-IMMU2356>3.0.CO;2-Z
91. Datta SK, Redecke V, Prilliman KR, Takabayashi K, Corr M, Tallant T, et al. A subset of Toll-like receptor ligands induces cross-presentation by bone marrow-derived dendritic cells. *J Immunol* (2003) **170**:4102–10.
92. Chen M, Barnfield C, Naslund TI, Fleeton MN, Liljestrom P. MyD88 expression is required for efficient cross-presentation of viral antigens from infected cells. *J Virol* (2005) **79**:2964–72. doi:10.1128/JVI.79.5.2964-2972.2005
93. Burgdorf S, Scholz C, Kautz A, Tampe R, Kurts C. Spatial and mechanistic separation of cross-presentation and endogenous antigen presentation. *Nat Immunol* (2008) **9**:558–66. doi:10.1038/ni.1601
94. Burgdorf S, Kautz A, Bohnert V, Knolle PA, Kurts C. Distinct pathways of antigen uptake and intracellular routing in CD4 and CD8 T cell activation. *Science* (2007) **316**:612–6. doi:10.1126/science.1137971
95. Tacken PJ, Ginter W, Berod L, Cruz LJ, Joosten B, Sparwasser T, et al. Targeting DC-SIGN via its neck region leads to prolonged antigen residence in early endosomes, delayed lysosomal degradation, and cross-presentation. *Blood* (2011) **118**:4111–9. doi:10.1182/blood-2011-04-346957
96. Sancho D, Joffre OP, Keller AM, Rogers NC, Martinez D, Hernanz-Falcon P, et al. Identification of a dendritic cell receptor that couples sensing of necrosis to immunity. *Nature* (2009) **458**:899–903. doi:10.1038/nature07750
97. Zelenay S, Keller AM, Whitney PG, Schraml BU, Deddouche S, Rogers NC, et al. The dendritic cell receptor DNGR-1 controls endocytic handling of necrotic cell antigens to favor cross-priming of CTLs in virus-infected mice. *J Clin Invest* (2012) **122**:1615–27. doi:10.1172/JCI60644
98. Bendelac A, Carnaud C, Boitard C, Bach JF. Syngeneic transfer of autoimmune diabetes from diabetic NOD mice to healthy neonates. Requirement for both L3T4+ and Lyt-2+ T cells. *J Exp Med* (1987) **166**:823–32. doi:10.1084/jem.166.4.823
99. Miller BJ, Appel MC, O'Neil JJ, Wicker LS. Both the Lyt-2+ and L3T4+ T cell subsets are required for the transfer of diabetes in nonobese diabetic mice. *J Immunol* (1988) **140**:52–8.
100. Kurts C, Kosaka H, Carbone FR, Miller JF, Heath WR. Class I-restricted cross-presentation of exogenous self-antigens leads to deletion of autoreactive CD8(+) T cells. *J Exp Med* (1997) **186**:239–45. doi:10.1084/jem.186.2.239
101. Luckashenak N, Schroeder S, Endt K, Schmidt D, Mahnke K, Bachmann MF, et al. Constitutive crosspresentation of tissue antigens by dendritic cells controls CD8+ T cell tolerance in vivo. *Immunity* (2008) **28**:521–32. doi:10.1016/j.immuni.2008.02.018
102. Hamilton-Williams EE, Lang A, Benke D, Davey GM, Wiesmuller KH, Kurts C. Cutting edge: TLR ligands are not sufficient to break cross-tolerance to self-antigens. *J Immunol* (2005) **174**:1159–63.
103. Gallegos AM, Bevan MJ. Central tolerance to tissue-specific antigens mediated by direct and indirect antigen presentation. *J Exp Med* (2004) **200**:1039–49. doi:10.1084/jem.20041457
104. Derbinski J, Schulte A, Kyewski B, Klein L. Promiscuous gene expression in medullary thymic epithelial cells mirrors the peripheral self. *Nat Immunol* (2001) **2**:1032–9. doi:10.1038/ni723
105. Anderson MS, Venanzi ES, Klein L, Chen Z, Berzins SP, Turley SJ, et al. Projection of an immunological self shadow within the thymus by the aire protein. *Science* (2002) **298**:1395–401. doi:10.1126/science.1075958

7

Models of somatic hypermutation targeting and substitution based on synonymous mutations from high-throughput immunoglobulin sequencing data

Gur Yaari[1,2], Jason A. Vander Heiden[3], Mohamed Uduman[2], Daniel Gadala-Maria[3], Namita Gupta[3], Joel N. H. Stern[4,5], Kevin C. O'Connor[4,6], David A. Hafler[4,7], Uri Laserson[8], Francois Vigneault[9] and Steven H. Kleinstein[2,3] *

[1] Bioengineering Program, Faculty of Engineering, Bar Ilan University, Ramat Gan, Israel
[2] Department of Pathology, Yale School of Medicine, New Haven, CT, USA
[3] Interdepartmental Program in Computational Biology and Bioinformatics, Yale University, New Haven, CT, USA
[4] Department of Neurology, Yale School of Medicine, New Haven, CT, USA
[5] Department of Science Education, Hofstra North Shore-LIJ School of Medicine, Hempstead, NY, USA
[6] Human and Translational Immunology Program, Yale School of Medicine, New Haven, CT, USA
[7] Department of Immunobiology, Yale School of Medicine, New Haven, CT, USA
[8] Department of Genetics, Harvard Medical School, Boston, MA, USA
[9] AbVitro, Inc., Boston, MA, USA

Edited by:
Ramit Mehr, Bar-Ilan University, Israel

Reviewed by:
Ronald B. Corley, Boston University School of Medicine, USA
Masaki Hikida, Kyoto University, Japan

****Correspondence:***
Steven H. Kleinstein, Department of Pathology, Yale School of Medicine, Suite 505, 300 George Street, New Haven, CT 06511, USA
e-mail: steven.kleinstein@yale.edu

Analyses of somatic hypermutation (SHM) patterns in B cell immunoglobulin (Ig) sequences contribute to our basic understanding of adaptive immunity, and have broad applications not only for understanding the immune response to pathogens, but also to determining the role of SHM in autoimmunity and B cell cancers. Although stochastic, SHM displays intrinsic biases that can confound statistical analysis, especially when combined with the particular codon usage and base composition in Ig sequences. Analysis of B cell clonal expansion, diversification, and selection processes thus critically depends on an accurate background model for SHM micro-sequence targeting (i.e., hot/cold-spots) and nucleotide substitution. Existing models are based on small numbers of sequences/mutations, in part because they depend on data from non-coding regions or non-functional sequences to remove the confounding influences of selection. Here, we combine high-throughput Ig sequencing with new computational analysis methods to produce improved models of SHM targeting and substitution that are based only on synonymous mutations, and are thus independent of selection. The resulting "S5F" models are based on 806,860 Synonymous mutations in 5-mer motifs from 1,145,182 Functional sequences and account for dependencies on the adjacent four nucleotides (two bases upstream and downstream of the mutation). The estimated profiles can explain almost half of the variance in observed mutation patterns, and clearly show that both mutation targeting and substitution are significantly influenced by neighboring bases. While mutability and substitution profiles were highly conserved across individuals, the variability across motifs was found to be much larger than previously estimated. The model and method source code are made available at http://clip.med.yale.edu/SHM

Keywords: immunoglobulin, B cell, somatic hypermutation, mutability, substitution, targeting, AID, affinity maturation

1. INTRODUCTION

During the course of an immune response, B cells that initially bind antigen with low affinity through their immunoglobulin (Ig) receptor are modified through cycles of proliferation, somatic hypermutation (SHM), and affinity-dependent selection to produce high-affinity memory and plasma cells. Current models of SHM recognize activation-induced deaminase (AID), along with several DNA repair pathways, as critical to the mutation process (1). AID initiates SHM by converting cytosines (Cs) to uracils (Us), thus creating U:G mismatches in the Ig V(D)J sequence. If not repaired before cell replication, these mismatches produce C → T (thymine) transition mutations (2). The AID-induced mismatches can alternatively be recognized by UNG or MSH2/MSH6 to initiate base excision or mismatch repair pathways, respectively. These pathways operate in an error-prone manner to introduce the full spectrum of mutations at the initial lesion, as well as spreading mutations to the surrounding bases. Overall, SHM introduces point mutations into the Ig locus at a rate of $\sim 10^{-3}$ per base-pair per division (3, 4). While the process of SHM appears to be stochastic, there are clear intrinsic biases, both in the bases that are targeted (5, 6) as well as the substitutions that are introduced (7, 8). Accurate background models for SHM micro-sequence targeting (i.e., hot/cold-spots) and nucleotide substitution would greatly aid the analysis of B cell clonal expansion, diversification, and selection processes. In addition, targeting and substitution models could provide important insights into the relative contributions of the various error-prone DNA repair pathways that mediate SHM.

Computational models and analyses of SHM have separated the process into two independent components (7–11): (1) a targeting model that defines where mutations occur (by specifying the relative rates at which positions in the Ig sequence are mutated), and (2) a nucleotide substitution model that defines the resulting mutation (by specifying the probability of each base mutating to each of the other three possibilities). In experimentally derived Ig sequences, observed mutation patterns are influenced by selection. The affinity maturation process selects for affinity-increasing mutations, while many mutations at structurally important positions in the framework regions are selected against (12). To avoid the confounding influences of selection, most existing models are built using mutation data from intronic regions flanking the V gene (13) and non-productively rearranged Ig genes (6–10, 14). These works have identified several specific motifs as being "hot" or "cold" spots of SHM. Hot-spots include WR$\underline{C}$Y/R$\underline{G}$YW and W$\underline{A}$/$\underline{T}$W (where W = {A, T}, Y = {C, T} R = {G, A}, and the mutated position is underlined, see for example (5, 6)). Although it has been argued that WR$\underline{C}$H/D$\underline{G}$YW (where H = {A, C, T} and D = {A, G, T}) is a better predictor of mutability at C:G bases (15). A single cold-spot motif has also been recognized: SY$\underline{C}$/$\underline{G}$RS (where S = {C, G}) (16). Despite the wide recognition of these specific hot-spot and cold-spot motifs, it is clear that a hierarchy of mutabilities exists that is highly dependent on the surrounding bases (7, 10). More recently, it has been recognized that the profile of nucleotide substitutions may also be dependent on the surrounding bases (8, 17). Modeling SHM targeting and substitution is important for the analysis of mutation patterns since these intrinsic biases can give the appearance of selection due to the particular codon usage and base composition in Ig sequences (17, 18). Moreover, having such a model could shed light on the molecular mechanisms underlying SHM, which are not fully understood.

Previous work has attempted to model the dependencies on surrounding bases, but has been limited to (at most) the targeted base and three surrounding bases (19), mainly due to the relatively small data sets available. The use of intronic regions has also limited the number of motifs that can be modeled (because of the limited diversity of these regions), and non-productively rearranged Ig genes may still be influenced by selection (e.g., if the event rendering the sequence non-productive happened in the course of affinity maturation). In this study, we take advantage of the wealth of data available from high-throughput Ig sequencing technologies to build improved targeting and substitution models for SHM. To avoid the biasing effects of selection, we have developed a new methodology for constructing models from synonymous mutations only, thus avoiding the need to limit analysis to non-productive Ig sequences. The increased data set size allows modeling of dependencies on the surrounding four bases (two bases upstream and downstream of the mutation). These "S5F" (Synonymous, 5-mer, Functional) models confirm the existence of proposed hot- and cold-spots of SHM, but also show much more extreme difference between hot- and cold-spots compared with previous models. We also find that the nucleotide substitution profiles at all bases are dependent on the surrounding nucleotides. The S5F targeting and substitution models can be employed as background distributions for mutation analysis, such as the detection and quantification of affinity-dependent selection in Ig sequences (11, 20). These models improve dramatically the ability to analyze mutation patterns in Ig sequences, and provide insights into the SHM process.

2. RESULTS

To develop models for SHM targeting and substitution preferences, we curated a large database of mutations from high-throughput sequencing studies (**Table 1**). These data were derived from 7 human blood and lymph node samples, and Ig sequencing was carried out using both Roche 454 and Illumina MiSeq next-generation sequencing technologies. In total, the data contained 42,122,509 raw reads, which were processed (see Materials and Methods) to arrive at 1,145,182 "high-fidelity" Ig sequences, which were each supported by a minimum of two independent reads in a sample. These high-fidelity sequences were clustered to identify clones (sequences related by a common ancestor) and one effective sequence was constructed per clone so that each observed mutation corresponded to an independent event. Overall, this process produced a set of 806,860 synonymous mutations that were used to model somatic hypermutation targeting and substitution.

2.1. THE NUCLEOTIDE SUBSTITUTION SPECTRUM IS AFFECTED BY ADJACENT NUCLEOTIDES

A nucleotide substitution model specifies the probability of each base (A, T, G, or C) mutating to each of the other three possibilities. For example, when a C is mutated, we might find that 50% of the time it is replaced by T, while 30% of the substitutions are to G, and the remaining 20% lead to A. These probabilities may depend on the surrounding bases (i.e., the micro-sequence context), as was previously suggested for mutations at A (17) and more generally (8). To derive a nucleotide substitution model, the set of mutations was filtered to include only those that occurred in positions where none of the possible base substitutions lead to amino acid exchanges. Focusing on positions where only synonymous mutations were possible removes the confounding influence of selection. The resulting 408,422 mutations were analyzed and grouped into "5-mers" according to the germline sequence of the mutated position and surrounding bases (two base-pairs upstream and two base-pairs downstream of the mutated position). For each of the 1024 possible 5-mers (M), a substitution model was derived by calculating S_B^M, the probability that the central base in the 5-mer motif (M) mutates to base B. For example, in the 5-mer CCATC mutations at A are always synonymous whenever this motif starts a reading frame, in which case it codes for a Proline (CCA) followed by a Serine (TCN). In this case, the number of observed mutations that led to each of the other three possible nucleotides (C, G, or T) was recorded: N_C^{CCATC}, N_G^{CCATC}, N_T^{CCATC}. The maximum likelihood value for the probability that A is substituted by base B is then calculated as:

$$S_B^{CCATC} = \frac{N_B^{CCATC}}{N_C^{CCATC} + N_G^{CCATC} + N_T^{CCATC}}$$

Table 1 | Next-generation sequencing data sets used to construct the "S5F" targeting and substitution models.

Study	Sample	Subject	Tissue	Tech.	Raw reads	Processed reads	Clones	# Mutations (substitution)	# Mutations (targeting)
1	3931LN	1	LN	MiSeq	3,641,633	79,777	16,272	25,307	53,840
1	4014LN	2	LN	MiSeq	3,714,152	106,006	32,972	57,215	106,265
1	4106LN	3	LN	MiSeq	10,917,517	231,387	54,400	108,591	208,338
1	3928LN	4	LN	MiSeq	7,691,509	99,519	76,375	68,051	132,795
2	PGP1-1	5	PBMC	MiSeq	3,851,658	55,606	50,514	23,939	48,558
2	PGP1-2	5	PBMC	MiSeq	3,946,514	59,611	54,374	24,971	50,117
2	PGP1-3	5	PBMC	MiSeq	4,543,353	48,971	45,788	20,865	42,737
2	PGP1-4	5	PBMC	MiSeq	3,121,884	52,844	49,054	23,243	47,049
3	hu420143	6	PBMC	454	178,584	92,055	14,956	23,260	48,838
3	420IV	7	PBMC	454	398,517	248,363	39,047	24,771	50,899
3	PGP1-5	5	PBMC	454	117,188	71,043	12,275	8,209	17,424
Total	–	–	–	–	42,122,509	1,145,182	446,027	408,422	806,860

Tissue types are lymph node (LN) or peripheral blood mononuclear cell (PBMC). The different filters applied to arrive at the number of (synonymous) mutations used for the targeting and substitution models are described in the text. All three studies relate to manuscripts in preparation.

A bootstrapping procedure was used to estimate 95% confidence intervals (21).

Comparison of the substitution profiles for different 5-mer motifs with the same central base clearly showed the significant influence of surrounding bases. As an example, **Figure 1A** shows how the profile of substitutions at G changes for several different 5-mers (AC<u>G</u>AT, GC<u>G</u>AG, GT<u>G</u>TA, and GG<u>G</u>AA). Such dependencies were identified for every base (A, T, G, and C) (**Figure 1B** and Figure S1 in Supplementary Material). The importance of including two bases upstream and downstream was confirmed by comparing these profiles with analogous profiles that only account for the immediately adjacent bases (3-mer motifs) (**Figure 1A**). For the 3-mer C<u>G</u>A, G → C and G → A substitutions were equally likely (45% and 43% of substitutions, respectively), while G → C substitutions were significantly more likely than G → A in the context of the GC<u>G</u>AG motif (51% and 35% of substitutions, respectively). If one ignores neighboring nucleotides, the substitution profiles were qualitatively similar to previous estimates (7), although significant quantitative differences were apparent (presumably due to the much larger size of the dataset compiled here). Thus, nucleotide substitution profiles at every base are significantly affected by adjacent nucleotides, including at least two bases on either side of the mutating base.

2.1.1. *The complete substitution model for somatic hypermutation is not strand-symmetric*

It is not possible to estimate substitution profiles for all 5-mer motifs using the above methodology because: (1) not all 5-mers appear within the set of Ig sequences, and (2) some 5-mers (such as NA<u>N</u>NN) can never appear in a context where all substitutions at the central (underlined) base are synonymous. Among the 11 datasets used here, these issues prevent estimation of the substitution profiles for 717 of the 1024 5-mers. For the profiles that could be directly estimated, there was a high correlation (on average Pearson $R = 0.63$) between different individuals (Figures S2 and S3 in Supplementary Material), and so all the samples were combined to estimate a single substitution model. To infer values for the missing motifs, four methods were evaluated. In the first method ("inner 3-mer"), the substitution profile for each missing 5-mer was inferred by averaging over profiles for all 5-mers with the same 3-mer core (i.e., for which the middle three bases were shared). In the second and third methods, missing values were replaced by averaging over motifs sharing the two bases upstream and downstream of the mutated base, respectively. In the fourth method ("hot-spot"), the missing substitution profile was inferred by averaging over 5-mers sharing the two upstream bases when the mutated position was "C" or "A," and two downstream bases when the mutated position was "G" or "T." This final option was motivated by the dependencies of known "hot" and "cold" spots for SHM targeting (5, 6). To choose between these four methods, we compared their performance on 5-mers that could be directly estimated from the data. Specifically, we calculated the correlation between the inferred and directly estimated ratios for the parameter *R*, which was defined as the ratio between the highest substitution probability with the next highest one for a given 5-mer (**Table 2**). Pearson and Spearman coefficients were both used in order to be robust to the linear dependency assumption, and they yielded comparable results. While the "hot-spot" method clearly had the worst performance, the other three methods resulted in very similar models. The "inner 3-mer" method produced the highest Pearson correlation (0.4, see **Table 2**) and was chosen as the basis to infer missing values. We refer to the resulting substitution model as a "S5F" model since it is based on Synonymous mutations at 5-mers in Functional Ig sequences. In contrast to previous studies (8), there was no significant correlation between substitution values of 5-mers and their reverse complements (Pearson correlation of 0.005, Spearman correlation of 0.087), suggesting that at least one component of the substitution mechanism is not strand-symmetric.

2.2. THE HIERARCHY OF MOTIF MUTABILITIES IS CONSERVED ACROSS INDIVIDUALS

The mutability of a motif is defined here as the (non-normalized) probability of the central base in the motif being targeted for SHM relative to all other motifs. Similar to the substitution model, the targeting model was based on 5-mer motifs, including the

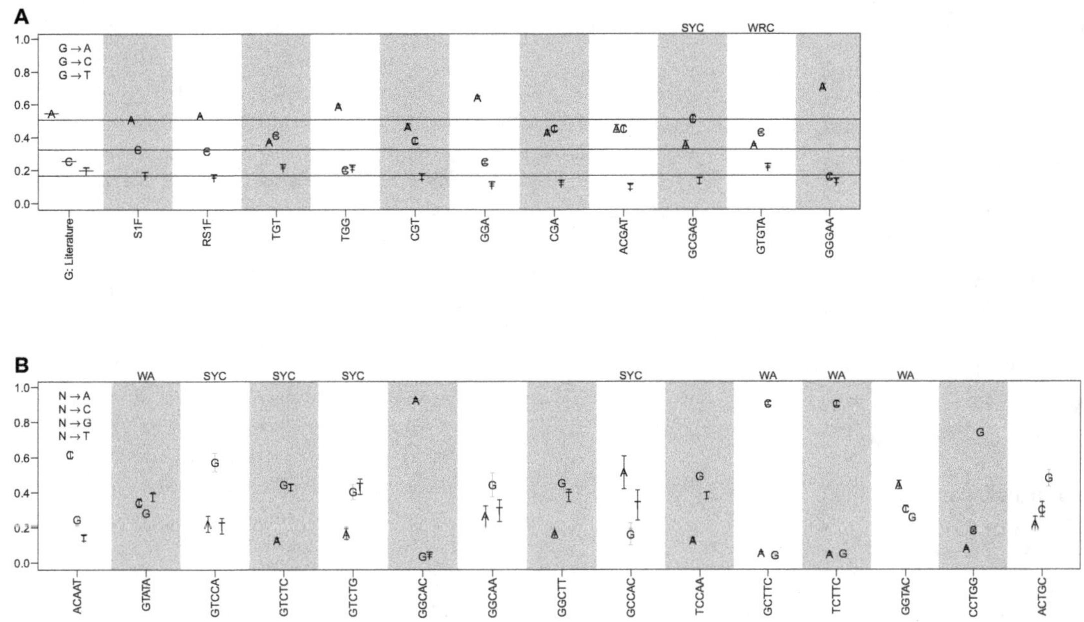

FIGURE 1 | The substitution profile is significantly influenced by surrounding bases. Substitution profiles for various micro-sequence contexts are shown for substitutions at **(A)** guanine and **(B)** adenosine, cytidine, and thymidine. G: literature indicates values estimated by Smith et al. (7), while S1F and RS1F refer to models estimated using the methods proposed here using all (replacement and silent) or only silent mutations, respectively, and averaging over surrounding bases. 3-mer motifs were estimated using silent mutations and dependencies on the immediately adjacent bases (S3F), while 5-mer motifs refer to the complete S5F model. Horizontal lines in **(A)** indicate the substitution values for the S1F model following the color scheme shown in the legend. Motifs that fall into one of the standard hot or cold-spots categories are indicated by the motif above the column.

Table 2 | Correlation coefficients for inferring missing mutability/substitution values.

Model	Correlation	Middle	Upstream	Downstream	Hot spots
Substitution	Pearson	0.40	0.37	0.15	0.04
	Spearman	0.20	0.24	0.23	0.09
Mutability	Pearson	0.58	0.57	0.61	0.73
	Spearman	0.61	0.58	0.64	0.79

two nucleotides immediately upstream and downstream of the mutated base. The use of a 5-mer model is motivated by the well-known WRC̲Y hot-spot (where the underlined C is targeted for mutation), and its reverse-complement (RG̲YW) which, when taken together, create dependencies with the two bases on either side of the mutating base.

When estimating the mutability (μ) for a motif (M), it is critical to account for the background frequency of M. To see why this is the case, consider the extreme example of a sequence composed of all C nucleotides. Since all mutations will occur at CCC̲CC motifs, one might consider this motif a hot-spot, except that its background frequency is 100% so it is actually targeted at the expected frequency. When calculating mutabilities it is also important to avoid statistical artifacts due to heterogeneity (e.g., the Simpson paradox (22)). Thus, Ig sequences were first analyzed individually since each has a different background 5-mer distribution. These individual-sequence targeting models were then combined into a single aggregated targeting model for each data set. Estimating the relative mutabilities of 5-mer motifs for an individual Ig sequence involves two steps: (1) Calculating the background frequency of the different 5-mers based on the germline (unmutated) version of the sequence, and (2) creating a table of the 5-mers that were mutated in the sequence. To avoid the confounding influence of selection, only mutations that were synonymous (i.e., that do not produce an amino acid exchange in the germline context) were included in the analysis. Note that these criteria are slightly different from those used in the substitution model. In the substitution model, mutations were used only where all possible mutations at that position had to be synonymous, while all synonymous mutations were considered for mutabilities (see **Table 1**).

For each of the 1024 possible 5-mers motifs (M) in each Ig sequence, the background frequency (B_M) was calculated as follows:

$$B_{\mathrm{M}} = \sum_i \sum_b S_b^{\mathrm{M}} I_{\overrightarrow{GL}}(i, \mathrm{M}, b) \qquad (1)$$

where i is summed over all (non-N) positions in the Ig sequence, M is the 5-mer nucleotide sequence centered at position i and b includes all possible nucleotides ({A, C, T, G}). In this equation GL is a vector containing the nucleic content of each position in the germline sequence, S_b^{M} is the relative rate at which the center nucleotide in M ($GL[i]$) mutates to b (as estimated in the previous section, and where $S_{GL[i]}^{\mathrm{M}} = 0$) and $I_{\overrightarrow{GL}}(i, M, b)$ is an indicator function that is 1 in cases where the 5-mer surrounding $GL[i]$

is M and a mutation in position i from $GL[i]$ to b results in a synonymous mutation (and 0 otherwise). A similar array was also calculated for the mutated positions:

$$C_M = \sum_i I_{\overrightarrow{GL},\overrightarrow{OS}}(i, M) \quad (2)$$

where i is summed over all (non-N) positions in the observed Ig sequence (OS), and the indicator function $I_{\overrightarrow{GL},\overrightarrow{OS}}$ (i, M) is 1 in cases where the 5-mer surrounding $GL[i]$ is M and a mutation in position i from $GL[i]$ to $OS[i]$ is synonymous and 0 otherwise. After calculating the arrays $\vec{C}$ and $\vec{B}$, a mutability score, μ, was defined for each motif M in the vector (for sequence j) as:

$$\mu_M^j = C_M^j / B_M^j \quad (3)$$

which was then normalized to one:

$$\bar{\mu}_M^j = \mu_M^j / \sum_m \mu_m^j \quad (4)$$

where m is an index spanning all positions in $\vec{\mu}^j$. Note that μ_M^j is not defined wherever $B_M^j = 0$ (i.e., the motif M does not appear in the Ig sequence, or can not admit any synonymous mutations). Finally, a single mutability score is generated for each 5-mer motif (M) as the weighted average of the mutabilities scores for each sequence j ($\bar{\mu}_M^j$), where weights correspond to the number of synonymous mutations in the sequence ($\sum_M C_M^j$). This process resulted in an array of (relative) mutabilities, μ_M for each of the 5-mers observed in the dataset. The resulting vector was renormalized so that the mean mutability was one.

2.2.1. *Inference of missing values to complete targeting model*

It was not possible to estimate mutabilities for 468 of the 1024 possible 5-mer motifs because not all 5-mers appeared within the set of Ig sequences. The same four methods tested for inferring missing values in the substitution model were also tested to infer these mutabilities (see 2.1.1 and **Table 2**). The "inner 3-mer" method produced a Pearson correlation of 0.58 (0.61 for Spearman), while the "hot-spot" method had a correlation of 0.73 (0.79 for Spearman). Thus, in contrast to the nucleotide substitution model, mutabilities were best predicted by averaging over 5-mers which shared the two upstream bases when the mutated position was "C" or "A," and two downstream bases when the mutated position was "G" or "T." This result is consistent with the expected influence of the classic SHM hot-spot (WRCY/RGYW).

2.2.2. *Targeting is conserved across individuals*

To test whether the micro-sequence specificity of SHM was conserved across individuals, separate targeting models were constructed for each of the 11 samples in our study (**Table 1**). Comparison of the motif mutabilities between pairs of samples showed that the models were highly consistent, with Pearson correlation ~0.9 (**Figure 2** and Figure S4 in Supplementary Material). Thus, we combined the data from all of the samples and generated a single targeting model, with confidence intervals based on the middle 50% quantiles of the mutability across samples. As with the substitution model, we refer to this targeting model as a "S5F" model. In order to visualize this model, we created "hedgehog" plots to display the directly estimated mutability values and the complete S5F model (**Figures 3A,B**, respectively).

2.2.3. *The true "hotness" of SHM hot-spots*

Visual inspection of the "hedgehog" plots (**Figure 3B**) shows clearly that the S5F model is consistent with known micro-sequence preferences for SHM (5, 6). WRC/GYW and WA/TW hot-spot motifs are generally more mutable, while SYC/GRS cold-spot motifs generally show the lowest mutability. However, the mutability of "hot-spot" motifs was observed to be highly variable. There is a 62.7-fold difference between the most mutable (GGGCA, mutability = 9.56) and least mutable (TGCGA, mutability = 0.15) WRC/GYW hot-spot motif. Indeed, ~10% of so-called "hot-spots" had mutabilities that were lower than the mean mutability for "neutral" motifs (**Figure 4A**). This high variance was especially obvious when looking at the subset of WRCA/TGYW hot-spot motifs, and may help explain why WRCH/DGYW has been proposed to be a better predictor of mutation at C:G compared with WRCY/RGYW (15). The mutabilities estimated by the S5F approach paint a qualitatively different picture of SHM when compared with those estimated by the existing tri-nucleotide model of Shapiro et al. (10). In the S5F model, the average mutability of motifs that correspond to the WRC/GYW SHM hot-spot was 3.2-fold higher than neutral motifs, and 9.6-fold higher than the mutability of motifs corresponding to the cold-spot SYC/GRS (**Figure 4A**). Using the tri-nucleotide model, hot-spots were only 1.3-fold and 1.6-fold more mutable than neutral and cold-spots, respectively (**Figure 4B**). In addition, in direct opposition to the S5F model, the tri-nucleotide method predicted that A/T hot-spots (WA/TW) were more mutable than C/G hot-spots (WRC/GYW). The mutabilities estimated by the S5F model better predicted the positional-distribution of *in vivo* mutations. The Pearson correlation between the expected mutability and observed mutation frequency calculated over IMGT-numbered positions in 12,000 sequences derived from a variety of germline segments was 0.67 and 0.47 for the S5F and tri-nucleotide models, respectively (**Figure 5** and Figure S5 in Supplementary Material). In both methods, deviations from the expected frequencies that likely reflect both positive and negative selection were observed (**Figure 5**). The observation of position-specific signals suggests that there is something generic about the Ig structure at these positions, and may help refine traditional definitions of the complementarity determining regions (CDR) and framework regions (FWR) (see also (23)). Consistent with previous studies (24), the S5F model displayed significant strand-bias at A/T hot-spots, but not C/G hot-spots (**Figure 6**). Overall, the S5F targeting model provides a new view of SHM with hot-spots being significantly more targeted (and significantly more variable) than previously thought.

3. MATERIALS AND METHODS

3.1. HIGH-THROUGHPUT IG SEQUENCING DATA SETS

A total of 11 human Ig repertoires were sequenced from blood and lymph node samples from 7 different individuals. Next-generation sequencing was carried out using Illumina MiSeq 250

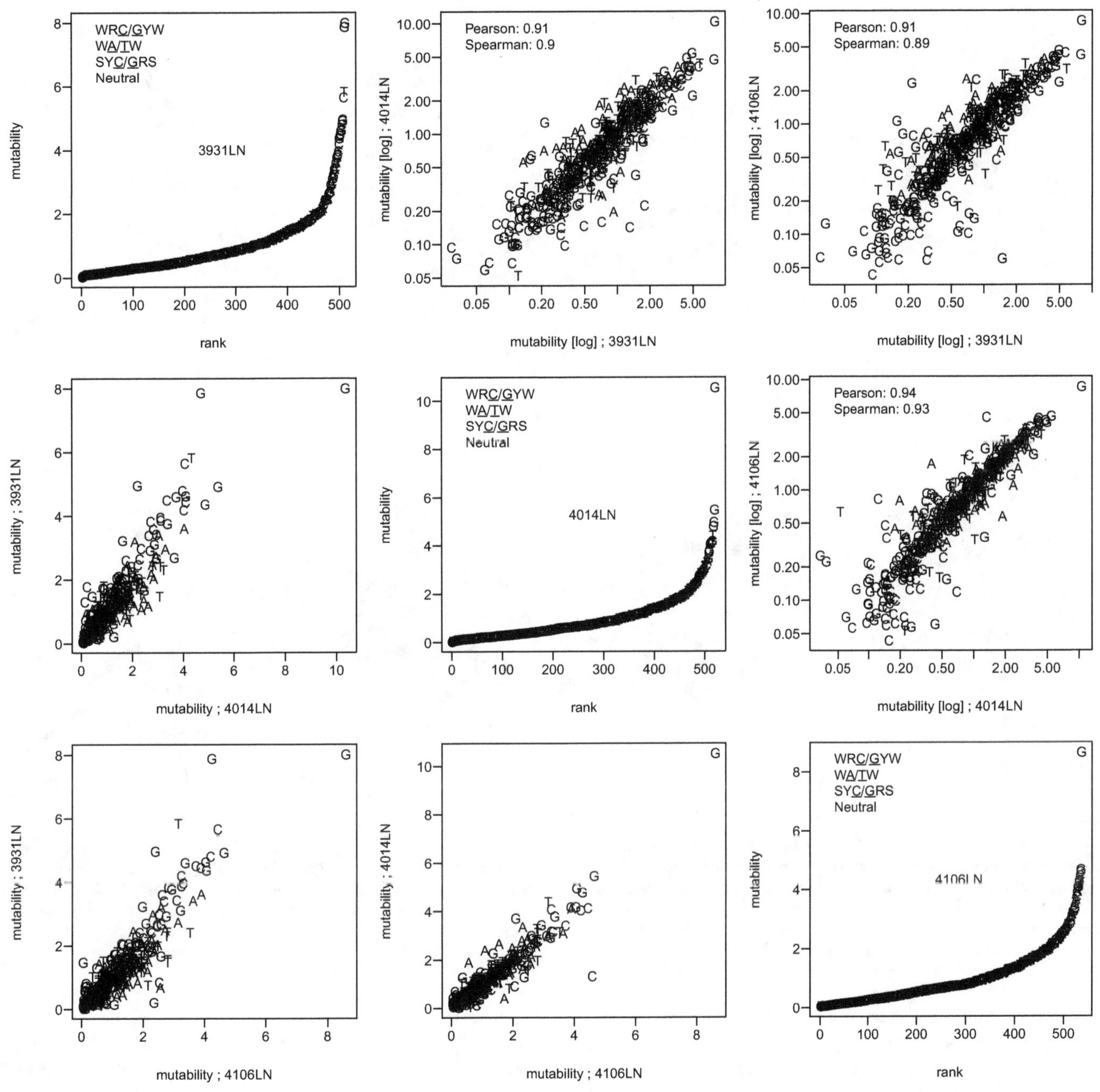

FIGURE 2 | The S5F targeting model is consistent across individuals. Targeting models were constructed independently for each of the samples listed in **Table 1**. Estimated values for all 5-mer motifs derived using lymph node samples from three individuals (3931LN, 4014LN, and 4106LN) are shown along the diagonal. Mutability values are ranked (from lowest to highest) and color coded by their category (WRC/GYW are red, SYC/GRS are blue, WA/TW are green, and the rest are gray). Symbols indicate the mutated nucleotide (in the center of the 5-mer). Correlations between the mutabilities for all 5-mer motifs across individuals are shown in the upper (log-log scale) and lower (linear scale) triangles.

base-pair paired-end reads (8 samples) and Roche/454 GS FLX (3 samples). Details are provided in **Table 1**. These samples were originally collected and sequenced as part of three ongoing studies (manuscripts in preparation).

3.1.1. Illumina MiSeq data

Human lymph node specimens were collected under an exempt protocol approved by the Human Research Protection Program at Yale School of Medicine. Tissues were processed and RNA isolated as previously described (25). Blood samples were collected under the approval of the Personal Genome Project (26). Total RNA was immediately extracted from each blood sample and stored at −80°C until use. To carry out sequencing, mRNA was reverse transcribed into cDNA using gene-specific primers mapping to the constant region of the Ig heavy chain. Resultant cDNA was tagged with 17 nucleotide single-molecule barcodes and amplified

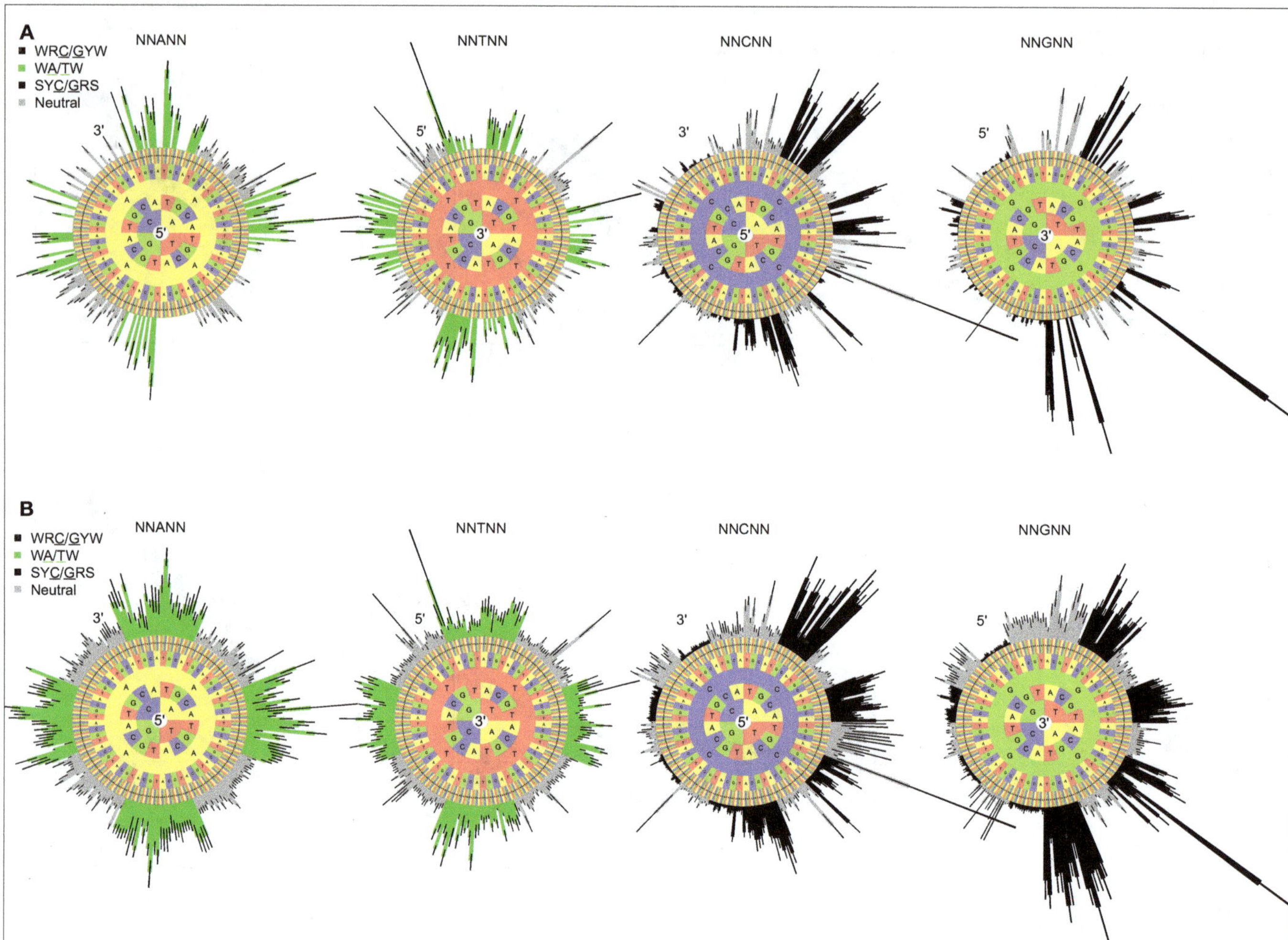

FIGURE 3 | "Hedgehog" plots for the S5F targeting model for somatic hypermutation targeting A, T, C, and G nucleotides (individual circles). **(A)** 5-mer mutabilities estimated directly from the Ig sequencing data. **(B)** The complete S5F targeting model after inferring values for missing 5-mer motifs. Bars radiating from each circle depict the mutability as a function of surrounding bases. The inner-most ring in the circle corresponds to two positions upstream (5′) of the mutated base for A and C, and two positions downstream (3′) of the mutated base for T and G. Bar colors indicate known hot/cold-spot motifs (WRC/GYW are red, WA/TW are green, SYC/GRS are blue, and "neutral" are gray). Each plot corresponds to a different mutated nucleotide. Error bars indicate confidence intervals based on the middle 50% quantiles of the mutability value distribution across the set of samples.

by PCR in a multiplex reaction using primer sets for all possible V-regions ($n = 45$) and isotype/J-regions ($n = 6$) to generate heavy chain transcripts. The amplified library was tagged with barcodes for sample multiplexing, PCR enriched, and annealed to the required Illumina clustering adapters. High-throughput 250 base-pair paired-end sequencing was performed using the Illumina MiSeq platform. Raw reads were exported without the sample barcodes and Illumina clustering adapters.

3.1.2. Roche/454 GS FLX data

Blood samples were collected under the approval of the Personal Genome Project (26). Total RNA was immediately extracted from each blood sample and stored at −80°C until use. Ig heavy chain mRNA were reverse-transcribed using a pool of 6 primers specific to the Ig constant regions and cDNA was amplified using 16 cycles of PCR with a pool of 46 V-region-specific primers and 6 nested constant region primers. Following ligation of 454-compatible sequencing adapters, the expected heavy chain V gene fragments were purified using PAGE. Each sample was uniquely barcoded during the ligation process, allowing subsequent mixing of all the samples into one common reaction sample (performed independently for each replicate run). Emulsion PCR and 454 GS FLX sequencing were performed directly at the 454 Life Sciences facility according to the manufacturer's standard protocols.

3.2. SEQUENCING DATA PRE-PROCESSING

Raw sequencing reads were filtered in several steps to identify and remove low-quality sequences. Conservative thresholds were applied in all cases to increase the reliability of the resulting mutation calls, at the potential expense of excluding some real mutations. Pre-processing was carried out using the Repertoire

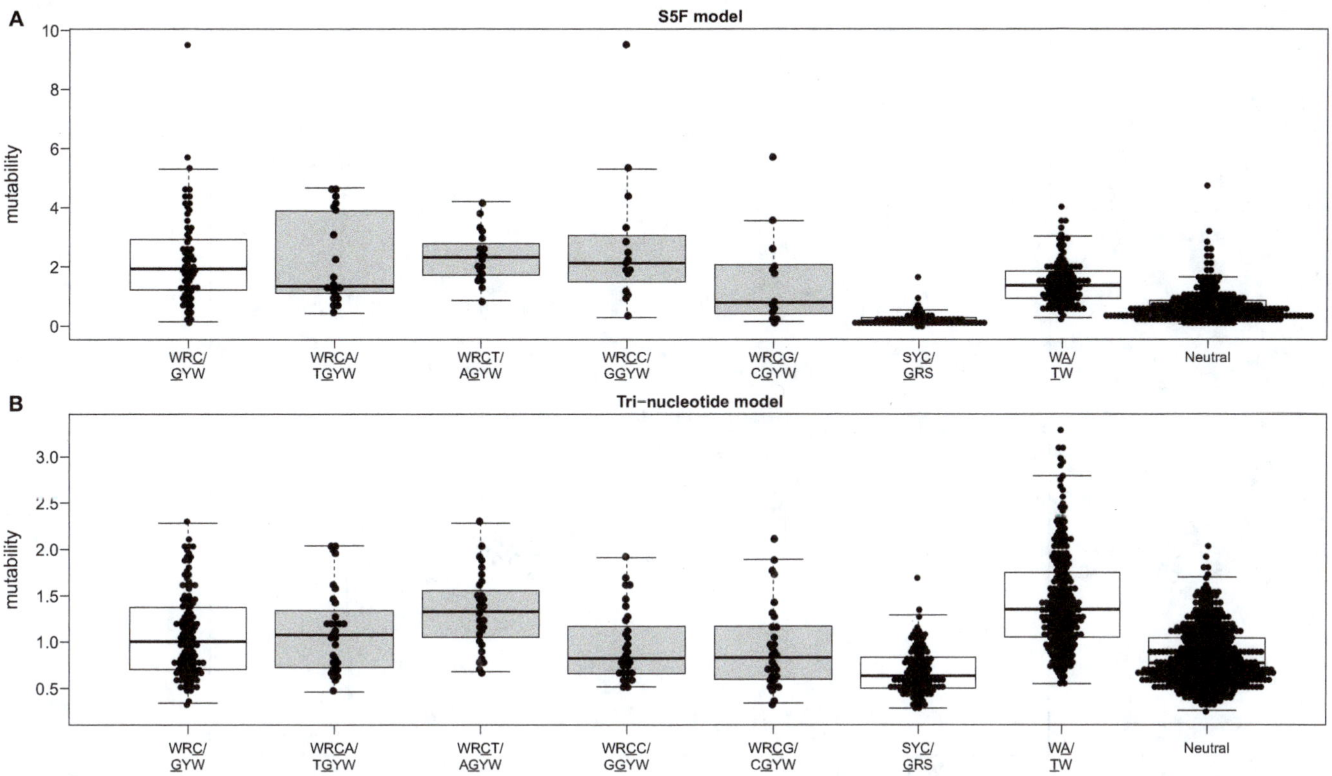

FIGURE 4 | The hierarchy of hot/cold-spot motifs. Mutability values predicted by the **(A)** S5F model or **(B)** the tri-nucleotide model of Shapiro et al. were grouped by the type of motif. Boxes borders correspond to the first and fourth quartiles while the horizontal bar inside the box corresponds to the median of the distribution. Hot/cold spot motif groups are plotted using the same colors as in **Figure 3B** with open boxes. WRCN/NGYW motifs are plotted using filled boxes.

Sequencing Toolkit (pRESTO) (http://clip.med.yale.edu/pRESTO, manuscript in preparation), and involved:

- Quality control
  1. Removal of low-quality reads (mean Phred quality score <20).
  2. Removal of reads where the primer could not be identified or had a poor alignment score (mismatch rate greater than 0.1).
  3. For the MiSeq data, sets of sequences with identical molecular IDs (corresponding to the same mRNA molecule) were identified. Sets were collapsed into one consensus sequence per set, after discarding those having a mean mismatch rate across all positions >0.2.
  4. For the MiSeq data, the two paired-end reads were assembled into a complete Ig sequence.
  5. Removal of sequences that do not appear in a single sample at least twice.
- Assignment of germline V(D)J segments for each of the Ig sequences: initial V(D)J assignments for each sequence were obtained using IMGT/HighV-QUEST (27). Using these assignments, non-mutated sequences were identified and a V segment germline repertoire for each individual was determined as the set of: (1) V genes that composed at least 0.1% of the sequences, and (2) V gene alleles that composed at least 10% of the assignments to that V gene. Ig sequences that were initially assigned V segments not included in this germline repertoire were then re-assigned to the closest present V segment based on the Hamming distance.
- Removal of non-functional sequences due to the occurrence of a stop codon or/and a reading frame shift between the V gene and the J gene.
- Removal of sequences with more than 30 mutations and masking (replacement with Ns) of positions with Phred quality scores <20.
- Removal of mutations in codons that had more than one mutation, as it is usually not possible to infer the order in which the mutations occurred (and thus the micro-sequence context of the mutations is unknown).
- Identification of clonally related sequences: a two-step approach was applied to identify sequences that were part of a B cell clone (i.e., related through descent from a common ancestor). First, the sequences were divided into groups based on equivalence of their V-gene assignment, J-gene assignment, and the number of nucleotides in their junction. Second, clones were defined within each of these groups as the collection of sequences with junction regions that differed from one sequence to any of the others by no more than three point mutations.

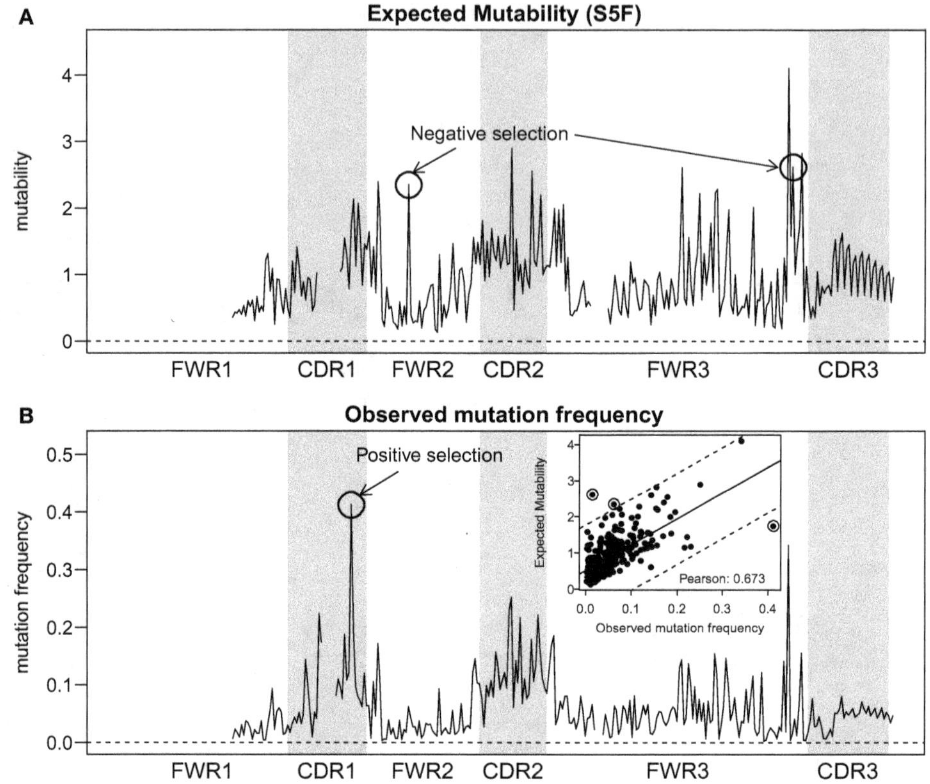

FIGURE 5 | Comparison between expected and observed somatic hypermutation targeting. **(A)** The predicted mutability from the S5F model and **(B)** the observed mutation frequency from sample 3931LN (averaged over all clones) for each position in the Ig sequence (IMGT-aligned along the *x*-axis). The correlation across positions (points) is shown in the inset of **(B)**. Two positions with evidence of negative selection (red circles) and one position with positive selection (blue circles) are indicated. The threshold for calling a position with significant selection was set to 3 SD away from the linear regression line (shown as a solid line in the inset, with thresholds plotted as dashed lines).

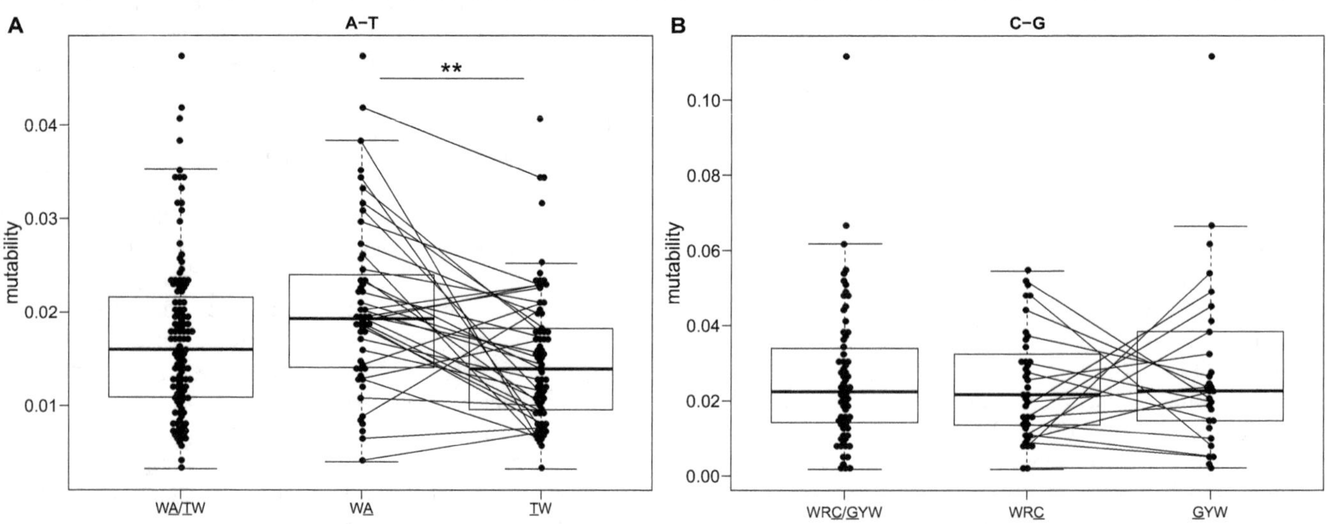

FIGURE 6 | Somatic hypermutation targeting at C/G, but not A/T, hot-spots is strand symmetric. Mutability values directly estimated by the S5F model (**Figure 3**) for **(A)** WA and **(B)** WRC "hot-spot" motifs are compared between different strands. Lines connect reverse-complement motifs for cases where both could be directly estimated from the data. $^{**}P < 5 \times 10^{-4}$ by a paired Mann–Whitney–Wilcoxon test.

The threshold of three was determined after manual inspection of the mutation patterns in resulting clones identified through building lineage trees.

4. DISCUSSION

We have constructed new SHM targeting and substitution models using a collection of more than 800,000 synonymous mutations from next-generation Ig sequencing studies. The exclusive use of synonymous mutations allowed us to include mutations from functional Ig sequences without the biasing influence of selection. The large size of the resulting mutation data set allowed us to model targeting and substitution dependencies on the mutating base as well as on two bases upstream and downstream of the mutation. The resulting "S5F" models validate, and also help refine, previously defined SHM hot and cold spots. **Figure 4** shows how the classic WRCY/RGYW hot-spot excludes some highly mutable WRCA/TGYW motifs, implying that, as proposed by Rogozin and Diaz (15), WRCH/DGYW could be a better predictor of mutation. However, while the most mutable WRCA/TGYW motifs are even hotter than WRCY/RGYW, others are comparable to neutral motifs. This high variance demonstrates the importance of including higher order dependencies, as we have done.

It has been suggested that nucleotide substitution profiles are also dependent on the micro-sequence context of the mutating base (8, 17). We confirm that the substitution profiles at all nucleotides are highly dependent on neighboring bases and these dependencies are conserved across individuals. Interestingly, the fact that substitution rates depend on surrounding bases may resemble the situation in meiotic mutations as was suggested in the past (9). The ability of the S5F models to estimate mutability and substitution at each of the 1024 DNA 5-mer motifs will allow for detailed, quantitative comparison of SHM with other mutation processes.

A potential source of error in the approach taken here is the existence of novel polymorphisms among the seven individuals studied (**Table 1**). Since mutation detection depends on comparison with known V and J segments that are part of the IMGT repertoire, undetected polymorphisms will look like mutations. However, any effect on the S5F model is expected to be small relative to the estimated confidence intervals. Based on a new statistical tool to detect novel germline alleles from high-throughput sequencing data (manuscript in preparation), the magnitude of this effect was estimated to be less than ~1% of the sequences and less than ~0.1% of the mutations used for the current analysis. The S5F mutability and substitution models presented here were developed using human heavy chain data, and thus may not be valid for light chains or mouse sequences. Given the large amount of sequencing data becoming available, it may be possible to extend the proposed approach to model 7-mers instead of 5-mers. However, even with 5-mers, the values for some motifs had to be inferred because of the limited diversity in germline repertoires. It will be important to estimate the quality of these inferences experimentally. Future experiments might be designed to enrich for non-productively rearranged Ig sequences which could then be sequenced using high-throughput technologies. Since mutations in these sequences are (presumably) not subject to selection, they provide a way to independently estimate substitution profiles and mutabilities for at least some of the motifs inferred in the S5F model. It will be important to confirm that the mutation process operating on these non-productive sequences is equivalent to the process at the productive alleles. This uncertainty is one reason why only productively rearranged Ig sequences were included in the current model.

The targeting and substitution models developed here provide a quantitative description of SHM in the absence of selection, and thus provide an important background for statistical analysis of SHM patterns in experimental data. For example, such models play an important role in quantifying antigen-driven selection in Ig sequences (11, 20), and we have now made the S5F model available as an option on our website for quantifying selection (http://clip.med.yale.edu/baseline). When combined with high-throughput sequencing, it should now be possible to quantify selection for each position of the Ig sequence independently and link these values back to the physical structure of the protein. Following the approach of Brard and Guguen (28), these models could also be incorporated into methods for building lineage trees of B cell clones (29), thus helping to provide insight into the underlying population dynamics of adaptive immunity. The model and method source code are made available at http://clip.med.yale.edu/SHM.

ACKNOWLEDGMENTS

We thank the Yale High Performance Computing Center (funded by NIH grant: RR19895) for use of their computing resources. Funding: this work was partially supported by NIH R03AI092379. The work of Jason A. Vander Heiden, Daniel Gadala-Maria and Namita Gupta were supported in part by NIH Grant T15 LM07056 from the National Library of Medicine.

REFERENCES

1. Chahwan R, Edelmann W, Scharff MD, Roa S. AIDing antibody diversity by error-prone mismatch repair. *Semin Immunol* (2012) **24**(4):293–300. doi:10.1016/j.smim.2012.05.005
2. Peled JU, Kuang FL, Iglesias-Ussel MD, Roa S, Kalis SL, Goodman MF, et al. The biochemistry of somatic hypermutation. *Annu Rev Immunol* (2008) **26**(1):481–511. doi:10.1146/annurev.immunol.26.021607.090236
3. McKean D, Huppi K, Bell M, Staudt L, Gerhard W, Weigert M. Generation of antibody diversity in the immune response of BALB/c mice to influenza virus hemagglutinin. *Proc Natl Acad Sci U S A* (1984) **81**(10):3180–4. doi:10.1073/pnas.81.10.3180
4. Kleinstein SH, Louzoun Y, Shlomchik MJ. Estimating hypermutation rates from clonal tree data. *J Immunol* (2003) **171**(9):4639–49.
5. Betz AG, Rada C, Pannell R, Milstein C, Neuberger MS. Passenger transgenes reveal intrinsic specificity of the antibody hypermutation mechanism: clustering, polarity, and specific hot spots. *Proc Natl Acad Sci U S A* (1993) **90**(6):2385–8. doi:10.1073/pnas.90.6.2385
6. Shapiro GS, Aviszus K, Ikle D, Wysocki LJ. Predicting regional mutability in antibody v genes based solely on di- and trinucleotide sequence composition. *J Immunol* (1999) **163**(1):259–68.
7. Smith DS, Creadon G, Jena PK, Portanova JP, Kotzin BL, Wysocki LJ. Di- and trinucleotide target preferences of somatic mutagenesis in normal and autoreactive b cells. *J Immunol* (1996) **156**:2642–52.
8. Cowell LG, Kepler TB. The nucleotide-replacement spectrum under somatic hypermutation exhibits microsequence dependence that is strand-symmetric

and distinct from that under germline mutation. *J Immunol* (2000) **164**(4):1971–6.
9. Oprea M, Cowell LG, Kepler TB. The targeting of somatic hypermutation closely resembles that of meiotic mutation. *J Immunol* (2001) **166**(2):892–9.
10. Shapiro GS, Ellison MC, Wysocki LJ. Sequence-specific targeting of two bases on both DNA strands by the somatic hypermutation mechanism. *Mol Immunol* (2003) **40**(5):287–95. doi:10.1016/S0161-5890(03)00101-9
11. Uduman M, Yaari G, Hershberg U, Stern JA, Shlomchik MJ, Kleinstein SH. Detecting selection in immunoglobulin sequences. *Nucleic Acids Res* (2011) **39**(Suppl 2):W499–504. doi:10.1093/nar/gkr413
12. Shlomchik MJ, Watts P, Weigert MG, Litwin S. Clone: a Monte-Carlo computer simulation of b cell clonal expansion, somatic mutation, and antigen-driven selection. *Curr Top Microbiol Immunol* (1998) **229**:173–97. doi:10.1007/978-3-642-71984-4_13
13. MacCarthy T, Kalis SL, Roa S, Pham P, Goodman MF, Scharff MD, et al. V-region mutation in vitro, in vivo, and in silico reveal the importance of the enzymatic properties of AID and the sequence environment. *Proc Natl Acad Sci U S A* (2009) **106**(21):8629–34. doi:10.1073/pnas.0903803106
14. Spencer J, Dunn M, Dunn-Walters DK. Characteristics of sequences around individual nucleotide substitutions in IgVH genes suggest different GC and AT mutators. *J Immunol* (1999) **162**(11):6596–601.
15. Rogozin IB, Diaz M. Cutting edge: DGYW/WRCH is a better predictor of mutability at G:C bases in ig hypermutation than the widely accepted RGYW/WRCY motif and probably reflects a two-step activation-induced cytidine deaminase-triggered process. *J Immunol* (2004) **172**(6):3382–4.
16. Bransteitter R, Pham P, Calabrese P, Goodman MF. Biochemical analysis of hypermutational targeting by wild type and mutant activation-induced cytidine deaminase. *J Biol Chem* (2004) **279**(49):51612–21. doi:10.1074/jbc.M408135200
17. Spencer J, Dunn-Walters DK. Hypermutation at A-T base pairs: the A nucleotide replacement spectrum is affected by adjacent nucleotides and there is no reverse complementarity of sequences flanking mutated A and T nucleotides. *J Immunol* (2005) **175**(8):5170–7.
18. Bose B, Sinha S. Problems in using statistical analysis of replacement and silent mutations in antibody genes for determining antigen-driven affinity selection. *Immunology* (2005) **116**(2):172–83. doi:10.1111/j.1365-2567.2005.02208.x
19. Cohen RM, Kleinstein SH, Louzoun Y. Somatic hypermutation targeting is influenced by location within the immunoglobulin Z region. *Mol Immunol* (2011) **48**(12-13):1477–83. doi:10.1016/j.molimm.2011.04.002
20. Yaari G, Uduman M, Kleinstein SH. Quantifying selection in high-throughput immunoglobulin sequencing data sets. *Nucleic Acids Res* (2012) **40**(17):e134. doi:10.1093/nar/gks457
21. Correa J. *Interval Estimation of the Parameters of the Multinomial Distribution.* Statistics on the Internet (2001). Available from: interstat.statjournals.net.
22. Simpson EH. The interpretation of interaction in contingency tables. *J R Stat Soc B* (1951) **13**(2):238–41.
23. Kunik V, Ashkenazi S, Ofran Y. Paratome: an online tool for systematic identification of antigen-binding regions in antibodies based on sequence or structure. *Nucleic Acids Res* (2012) **40**:W521–4. doi:10.1093/nar/gks480
24. Rogozin IB, Pavlov YI, Bebenek K, Matsuda T, Kunkel TA. Somatic mutation hotspots correlate with DNA polymerase error spectrum. *Nat Immunol* (2001) **2**(6):530–6. doi:10.1038/88732
25. Willis SN, Mallozzi SS, Rodig SJ, Cronk KM, McArdel SL, Caron T, et al. The microenvironment of germ cell tumors harbors a prominent antigen-driven humoral response. *J Immunol* (2009) **182**(5):3310–7. doi:10.4049/jimmunol.0803424
26. Nirantar SR, Ghadessy FJ. Compartmentalized linkage of genes encoding interacting protein pairs. *Proteomics* (2011) **11**(7):1335–9. doi:10.1002/pmic.201000643
27. Lefranc M-P, Pommi C, Ruiz M, Giudicelli V, Foulquier E, Truong L, et al. IMGT unique numbering for immunoglobulin and t cell receptor variable domains and ig superfamily v-like domains. *Dev Comp Immunol* (2003) **27**(1):55–77. doi:10.1016/S0145-305X(02)00039-3
28. Brard J, Guguen L. Accurate estimation of substitution rates with neighbor-dependent models in a phylogenetic context. *Syst Biol* (2012) **61**(3):510–21. doi:10.1093/sysbio/sys024
29. Barak M, Zuckerman NS, Edelman H, Unger R, Mehr R. IgTree: creating immunoglobulin variable region gene lineage trees. *J Immunol Methods* (2008) **338**(12):67–74. doi:10.1016/j.jim.2008.06.006

8

Opportunistic autoimmune disorders potentiated by immune-checkpoint inhibitors anti-CTLA-4 and anti-PD-1

Yi-chi M. Kong[1]* and Jeffrey C. Flynn[2]

[1] Department of Immunology and Microbiology, Wayne State University School of Medicine, Detroit, MI, USA
[2] Department of Orthopaedic Surgery, Providence Hospital and Medical Centers, Southfield, MI, USA

Edited by:
Fang-Ping Huang, Imperial College London, UK

Reviewed by:
Christopher E. Rudd, University of Cambridge, UK
José Mordoh, Fundación Instituto Leloir, Argentina
Julian Pardo, Fundación Agencia Aragonesa para la Investigación y el Desarrollo, Spain

***Correspondence:**
Yi-chi M. Kong, Department of Immunology and Microbiology, Wayne State University School of Medicine, 540 E. Canfield Avenue, Detroit, MI 48201, USA
e-mail: ykong@med.wayne.edu

To improve the efficacy of immunotherapy for cancer and autoimmune diseases, recent ongoing and completed clinical trials have focused on specific targets to redirect the immune network toward eradicating a variety of tumors and ameliorating the self-destructive process. In a previous review, both systemic immunomodulators and monoclonal antibodies (mAbs), anti-CTLA-4, and anti-CD52, were discussed regarding therapeutics and autoimmune sequelae, as well as predisposing factors known to exacerbate immune-related adverse events (irAEs). This review will focus on immune-checkpoint inhibitors, and the data from most clinical trials involve blockade with anti-CTLA-4 such as ipilimumab. However, despite the mild to severe irAEs observed with ipilimumab in ~60% of patients, overall survival (OS) averaged ~22–25% at 3–5 years. To boost OS, other mAbs targeting programed death-1 and its ligand are undergoing clinical trials as monotherapy or dual therapy with anti-CTLA-4. Therapeutic combinations may generate different spectrum of opportunistic autoimmune disorders. To simulate clinical scenarios, we have applied regulatory T cell perturbation to murine models combined to examine the balance between thyroid autoimmunity and tumor-specific immunity.

Keywords: anti-CTLA-4, anti-PD-1, autoimmune disease, tumor immunity, immune-checkpoint inhibitor

INTRODUCTION

In recent decades, cancer therapy has focused on amplifying the immune system to bolster the host's anti-tumor response. Utilizing systemic immunomodulators, monoclonal antibodies (mAbs), and stem cell transplantation, progress has been rapid in prolonging survival. However, targeted immunotherapy has come with a price; altered immunoregulation provoking immune dysfunction has opened the door to opportunistic autoimmune disorders. Previously, both systemic immunomodulators and mAbs, anti-CTLA-4 and anti-CD52, were discussed in terms of therapeutic usage, autoimmune sequelae, and important predisposing factors, e.g., *HLA* class II genes and gender predilection, known to influence immune-related adverse events (irAEs) (1). Similar and additional immunotherapeutic modalities associated with autoimmunity, particularly thyroid dysfunction, were likewise highlighted by others (2, 3). In addition to CTLA-4, a number of immune-checkpoints are also being targeted in cancer immunotherapy. Thus far, the most information has come from longer and larger clinical trials with anti-CTLA-4 (ipilimumab and tremelimumab), accompanied by mild to severe irAEs (4–6). In early trials, it was hoped that irAEs could serve as a predictor of improving anti-CTLA-4 immunotherapy (7, 8). However, analysis of 139 metastatic melanoma patients given ipilimumab revealed that the frequency of irAEs after a 2–4 year follow-up was 81% with a total response rate of 17% (23 of 139) (7); of the 86 patients with irAEs, 74% (64 of 86) showed no objective improvement (1).

Thus, targeting CTLA-4, a T cell regulatory molecule, impacts on its two primary functions in the immune network: (1) Its upregulation during a T cell-mediated response serves as a negative regulator by engaging the B7 family costimulatory molecules on antigen-presenting cells with higher avidity than CD28 (9); and (2) Its constitutive expression on regulatory T cells (Tregs) is critical to the Foxp3 function in suppressing autoreactive T cell activation (10, 11). *ctla4*$^{-/-}$ mice develop severe multiorgan autoimmunity, indicative of deficiency in both these functions (12, 13). When humanized CTLA-4 mAbs were first used to treat advanced melanoma a decade ago, the major goal was to interfere with the negative signaling of an ongoing anti-tumor response discernible in many patients (4, 6). However, since a key role of CTLA-4 is to enable Treg suppression of autoreactive T cell activation at the costimulatory level of DC (10, 11), it was no surprise that opportunistic autoimmune disorders surfaced as prominent irAEs from CTLA-4 blockade. The variety stems from the ever-present autoantigens and autoreactive T cells unleashed from self tolerance regulation (1). For example, in our tolerance induction study in murine experimental autoimmune thyroiditis (EAT), a model for the prevalent Hashimoto's thyroiditis (14), co-injection of anti-CTLA-4 with the autoantigen, thyroglobulin (Tg), interfered with activation of naturally existing CD4$^+$CD25$^+$Foxp3$^+$ Tregs (nTregs); the mice developed thyroiditis, mimicking a major clinical autoimmune sequela (15).

Using revised assessment criteria including overall survival (OS) in phase II/III trials to take into account the longer survival kinetics for ipilimumab (16), recent compilation of ipilimumab phase I/II trial results showed a range of 12–36% OS at 3–5 years, with variables including the dose, patient number, prior, or adjunct treatment (4). Pooling phase II/III trials showed irAEs approximating 60% with less severe grade 3–4 in the phase III trials, likely due to earlier recognition and management of autoimmune sequelae (4, 17). While the percentages of irAEs varied, most included skin rashes, colitis, thyroid dysfunction, hypophysitis, hepatitis, and pancreatitis (4, 17), as also reported in western Europe (5). Treatment-related deaths continued to occur and severe morbidity required stringent life-long treatment and hormonal supplementation (4, 5). The second mAb, tremelimumab, likewise underwent phase I/II trials [see Ref. (1)] and phase III trials with similar irAEs but less durable OS than with ipilimumab; in fact, survival was not much longer than after standard chemotherapy with temozolomide or dacarbazine (6). To boost OS, mAbs that blockade the function of another immune-checkpoint, programed death-1 (PD-1), or its ligand (PD-L1), have been undergoing clinical trials as monotherapy or dual therapy with anti-CTLA-4.

MODELS TO PROBE THE BALANCE BETWEEN AUTOIMMUNITY AND TUMOR IMMUNITY UPON Treg PERTURBATION

The high percentages of irAEs from anti-CTLA-4 therapy clearly show that maintenance of Treg function and self tolerance constitutes a premier CTLA-4 function. Autoimmune thyroid disease, including Hashimoto's thyroiditis and Graves' disease, represents the most prevalent autoimmune condition (18), and CTLA-4 blockade has joined other systemic immunomodulators [e.g., interferon-α, -β, interleukin (IL)-2] and leukocyte-target agents (e.g., anti-CD52) in triggering thyroid dysfunction (1, 3, 19, 20). As EAT has long served as a model to study Treg function in self tolerance to mouse Tg (14, 21, 22), we developed in recent years four murine models combining EAT and breast cancer vaccine protocols under Treg perturbation and MHC class II gene influence, using autoimmune thyroiditis as a sequela indicator (23).

The first three utilized well-established tumor models in wild type mice or mice transgenic for Her-2/neu breast cancer antigen, which harbor class II-linked, EAT-resistant haplotype ($H2^d$ or $H2^b$). In the first model, we induced EAT concurrently with anti-tumor immunity in wild type mice at the time of Treg depletion with mAb to CD25 (24). Treg depletion enhanced tumor regression and thyroiditis. Immune responses to neu and mouse Tg were greater than control groups given tumor or Tg alone, indicating that ongoing tumor regression and autoimmune response provided additional mutual stimuli. In the second model, we used rat neu-transgenic mice, which required both Treg depletion and neu DNA vaccination to develop resistance to tumor challenge and spontaneous tumorigenesis (25). Mutual stimulation during responses to neu and mouse Tg was again observed. In tumor-regressing mice, there were significant increases in interferon-γ-producing T cells and greater thyroid destruction even in the EAT-resistant strain. Lastly, in the third model, we introduced the HLA-DR3 transgene, an EAT-susceptible allele (26), and an Her-2 transgene into EAT-resistant $H2A^b$ mice to determine if anti-tumor response was independent of EAT susceptibility. (A^b-Her-2xDR3)F_1 mice expressed both A^b and DR3 and were tolerant to both Tg and Her-2 (27). After Treg depletion followed by Her-2 DNA and mouse Tg injections, tumor rejection was similar in Her-2 transgenic mice expressing either A^b or A^b/DR3, but thyroiditis was augmented only in (A^b/DR3)F_1 mice, showing that Her-2 immunity, unlike autoimmunity, was independent of DR3 expression.

In the fourth combined model, we used an EAT-susceptible CBA/J ($H2^k$) haplotype with demonstrated antigen-specific nTreg-mediated tolerance. Depleting pre-existing nTregs markedly enhanced thyroiditis development with soluble mouse Tg even without adjuvant (15). Control mice with nTregs, which had been activated/expanded after exposure to mouse Tg by either injection or physiologic release (via thyroid-stimulating hormone infusion in an osmotic pump), withstood EAT induction with mouse Tg plus adjuvant (22, 28). In contrast, nTreg-depleted mice were incapable of establishing this strong and long-lasting tolerance (14, 15, 22). For the cancer portion, CBA/J tumor was derived from a spontaneous mammary adenocarcinoma line, and resistance to lethal challenge was instilled by prior Treg depletion and vaccination with irradiated tumor cells (23). To simulate patients with MHC class II-associated predisposition to autoimmunity and subjected to immune targeting, mouse Tg was also given. Treg depletion not only augmented tumor immunity but also thyroidal infiltration (29). Furthermore, to simulate the scenario in some cancer patients with pre-existing autoimmunity and given immunotherapy, mice were pretreated with mouse Tg + low doses of IL-1 to establish a subclinical, mild thyroiditis condition. Treg depletion, tumor vaccination, and mouse Tg injections then followed. While anti-tumor immunity remained unchanged, thyroiditis was exacerbated (29). Thus, this recent model takes into account genetically predisposed patients who have no underlying thyroid dysfunction or have pre-existing, undiagnosed disease.

TARGETING CTLA-4 LED TO UNUSUAL SPECTRUM OF AUTOIMMUNE SEQUELAE

In murine EAT, tolerance induction with the known autoantigen, mouse Tg, and its blockade of nTreg activation by anti-CTLA-4 to allow thyroiditis development can be followed with timed co-administration (15). However, in cancer patients, there are multiple self antigens for which the maintenance mechanisms of self tolerance can be disrupted with anti-CTLA-4 therapy at varying doses and intervals, resulting in unpredictable manifestations of 20–60% of irAEs with grade 1–4 severity. In addition to advanced melanoma, both ipilimumab and tremelimumab have been used to treat other solid tumors and hematologic cancers and the frequent irAEs have included dermatitis, enterocolitis, hepatitis, thyroid dysfunction, and hypophysitis with widespread endocrinopathies, irrespective of cancer types (3–6, 19, 20). Although these autoimmune diseases are primarily organ-specific, T cell-mediated, and with mononuclear cell infiltration of the specific organ, plasma cells may be seen with time. Moreover, when several organs are involved with attendant proinflammatory cytokines, irAEs may become exacerbated and more widespread. Thus, different irAEs often occur throughout the treatment period and beyond.

There is agreement that the extent of severe irAEs is dose-dependent, but OS improvement generally does not correspond linearly with dosage (5), nor correlates with severity of irAEs (1, 19). Torino et al. (19) undertook an in-depth analysis of endocrine dysfunction for 21 phase I–III trials with ipilimumab treatment of melanoma and several other solid tumors. The primary emphasis was on hypophysitis of grades 3–4, but the involvement of other endocrine dysfunctions (hypothyroidism, adrenal insufficiency) and other common irAEs (e.g., diarrhea, colitis/enterocolitis, dermatitis, hepatitis, and arthritis) was also included. A more recent report by some of the same authors, Corsello et al. (20), extended the analysis to 28 trials, subcategorizing classifiable endocrine disorders and other common irAEs, which may or may not be autoimmune in origin. As mentioned above, since irAEs generally involved up to 60% of patients, at 2–3× the OS, a direct correlation of OS with irAE would be difficult at this time (4).

As discussed earlier (1), while the increase in thyroid dysfunction could have been anticipated, given the high prevalence in the general population, the most unusual and distinct association with anti-CTLA-4 therapy is autoimmune hypophysitis, with an incidence of 3–9% in early trials far exceeding its rare occurrence (~1 in 0.5 million) (19, 30). Another early melanoma trial with ipilimumab reported 17% (8 of 46) (31). The analyses of clinical trials with ipilimumab and tremelimumab gave an average of ~4% hypophysitis, closely rivaling hypothyroidism (19, 20). While hypothyroidism is 5–6× more prevalent in females in Caucasians (18), thus far hypophysitis from anti-CTLA-4 therapy has occurred mostly in males, in part influenced by the ratio of female:male of ~1:2 in melanoma patients. Other genetic (HLA, CTLA-4 gene polymorphism, mutations) and environmental factors may also take part (1, 4, 32). The high incidence of hypophysitis, its need for early corticosteroid intervention and life-long hormonal replacement prompted the advocacy of early recognition and management, together with thyroid function tests (17, 19, 20). Searches for specific pituitary antigens for early antibody detection to replace immunofluorescence on pituitary sections are ongoing (33–35).

Although autoimmune sequelae (e.g., hypophysitis, thyroid dysfunction, and hormonal imbalance) are gaining recognition, the high incidences of colitis and dermatitis have not been investigated as to culprit antigens, which could be self, commensally microbial, or tumor-associated. A recent survey of anti-CTLA-4 therapy in 752 melanoma patients at 19 skin centers in western Europe excluded colitis and dermatitis from the usually observed 60% irAEs (4, 5), and concentrated on raising awareness to rare yet severe toxicities, some of which may be related to prior chemo- or radio-therapy. A total of 88 irAEs from 82 of 752 (11%) patients were tabulated, 12 with hypophysitis (5). With melanoma patients, the side effects of vitiligo and uveitis were often noted because of shared melanocyte antigens, often aggravated by vaccination (1, 5). The 15 rarer cases included gastric problems, ischemia and bowel perforations, fatal hepatitis, hypophysitis with brain edema, and inflammation of the central nervous system. There were also respiratory and cardiac problems. Thus, the untoward autoimmune disorders are opportunistic and unpredictable, as well as far-reaching.

SPECIFIC ANTIGENS TO BOOST TUMOR IMMUNITY AND MONITOR Treg ACTIVITY

As seen above, the weakly immunogenic, tumor-associated antigens, which can be overexpressed self, altered self, or neoantigens, are further interwoven with unexpected pathogenic autoantigens during CTLA-4 blockade. Examination of tumor infiltrates after tremelimumab therapy revealed an increase in activated $CD8^+$ T cells in many melanoma patients; while not Tregs, this non-specific increase was observed in a greater proportion of patients than patients deriving any clinical benefit and showed no correlation with either tumor progression or regression (36). In phase II trials of melanoma patients with ipilimumab, a peripheral increase in the $\%CD4^+$ and $\%CD8^+$ activated T cells, but not those with a Treg phenotype, was noted (37). Of interest was the greater serologic reactivity to several melanoma antigens and a cancer-testis antigen NY-ESO-1. Because NY-ESO-1 is expressed in a number of solid tumors and 30–40% of advanced melanoma patients, it has been examined as a specific biomarker for increased T and B cell reactivity after CTLA-4 blockade, and if such reactivities could be associated with positive clinical outcome (37–40). While an increase in anti-NY-ESO-1 has often been detected, its association with positive benefit is still controversial (38–40). However, it appeared that clinical benefit could be associated with NY-ESO-1 reactivity if both antibody and $CD8^+$ T cells were considered in concert (10 of 13 or 77%) (39). More such studies will be needed to determine if specific reactivity to NY-ESO-1 as well as other melanoma peptides has a predictive value. Meanwhile, to increase the efficacy of CTLA-4 blockade and detect changes in tumor-specific effector T cells, therapeutic vaccines are being incorporated. In a large phase III trial (41), a gp100 peptide vaccine was given with ipilimumab (403 patients), compared to ipilimumab (137) or gp100 (136) alone. However, there was no significant increase in OS provided by including gp100 vaccination, compared to ipilimumab alone.

Detecting antigen-specific effector T cells is complicated by the presence of Tregs. In the tumor microenvironment, induced Tregs (iTregs) represent a major component of suppressor cell subsets and, as opposed to nTregs, usually arise or are converted from naive T cells in response to antigenic stimulus plus local TGF-β and IL-10 production (42). Intratumoral iTregs often exist in greater percentages than in the periphery. Although in murine melanoma studies Fc-dependent ADCC-like depletion of Tregs was demonstrable upon anti-CTLA treatment (43), the frequent detection of intratumoral iTregs in the human suggests that this kind of depletion might be an adjunct to improved clinical benefit. But the challenge remains to identify whether the effect was on tumor-specific iTregs, so as to monitor and inhibit their suppressor role (44). Following therapeutic vaccination, multiple peptides have been used to monitor iTreg activity. In one phase II trial in renal cell cancer patients, cyclophosphamide, known to deplete Tregs (22), was given before the IMA901 vaccine, consisting of multiple tumor-associated peptides used to demonstrate heightened T cell responses (45). In another study, synthetic peptides were used to compare the repertoire of tumor-specific iTregs and effector T cells in colorectal carcinoma patients (46). While differences were noted between the two populations, the suppressor activity was shown to stem from iTregs that shared the same repertoire as effector T cells. Additional studies have made use of class II tetramers to monitor antigen specificity. After vaccination of melanoma patients with HLA-A2-restricted Melan-A peptide, monitoring with HLA-DQ6-restricted Melan-A peptide multimers revealed a downshift in specific Tregs with increased effector T cell responses (47). In breast cancer patients, tetramers from HLA-DR4-, DR7-restricted mammaglobin peptides were used to detect iTregs in the periphery (48). After their depletion *in vitro*, effector T cell responses to several mammaglobin peptides increased. Thus, antigenic specificity, if known, could aid assessment of immunotherapeutic efficacy.

PD-1 AND PD-L1 BLOCKADE TO AUGMENT TUMOR IMMUNITY

Recent reviews have discussed in depth the phenomenon of T cell exhaustion, where activated T cells highly expressing PD-1, as exemplified by virus-specific $CD8^+$ cells, exhibited exhaustion phenotypes and failed to combat chronic infections (49–51). In the tumor microenvironment, PD-1 expression was found on impaired infiltrating lymphocytes (52) and Tregs (53). Its major ligand, PD-L1, has been found on multiple epithelial carcinomas, compared to PD-L2 on lymphoid tumors associated with its expression pattern (49–51). There is no clear consensus on whether PD-L1 expression by tumors is associated with greater objective response from PD-1 blockade; more specific staining reagents have led to reports of positive association (54, 55). PD-1 is also expressed on activated B, NK, and NKT cells and is involved in down-regulating autoimmunity. PD-1-deficient C57BL/6 mice exhibited lupus-like arthritis and glomerulonephritis (56), and PD-1-deficient BALB/c mice developed cardiomyopathy from an autoantibody to cardiac troponin 1 (57). Thus, these autoimmune syndromes have a strong pathogenic autoantibody component. While preclinical tumor models have shown clinical benefit with PD-1 blockade, it is uncertain if only activated $CD8^+$ cells participated in the OS (50).

Two phase I, ongoing dose-escalation trials have been reported with two IgG4 mAbs to PD-1. Lambrolizumab (MK-3475), which has recently been designated by the FDA as a "breakthrough therapy" drug to treat advanced melanoma (58), was used to treat 135 melanoma patients, who were evaluated for up to 70 weeks (59). The confirmed response rate was 38% (44 of 117), irrespective of prior ipilimumab treatment, and appeared dose-dependent. Biopsies of regressing lesions revealed densely infiltrated $CD8^+$ T cells. irAEs were 79% (107 of 135); 17 of the 107 had grade 3–4. Beside skin and gastrointestinal problems, hypothyroidism was 8%. The second phase I trial with nivolumab (BMS-936558) included 296 patients with melanoma, non-small cell lung cancer, prostate cancer, renal cell, or colorectal cancer. The first report in 2012 was after ~1 year and the objective response averaged ~20–25% (55). Grade 3–4 irAEs were observed in 14% (41 of 296), of which 11% were considered serious; 15 patients discontinued the study and 3 deaths (1%) were attributed to pneumonitis. The spectrum of irAEs was mostly similar to lambrolizumab therapy (59). But with twice the number of patients, the variety of irAEs resembled those seen with ipilimumab, albeit at lower overall percentages. The spectrum was dose-dependent and included rash, pruritus, and diarrhea (all at ~27%), with hyperthyroidism and hypothyroidism at 3–7% (55). An exception to the ipilimumab treatment was the prominent pulmonary toxicities seen in 2–4% of patients (55, 59). In addition to fatalities (55), the 2–4% in phase I trials were of grade 3–4 (55, 59). A recent report about ongoing phase II/III trials also listed pneumonitis as a notable side effect (60). Whether it is autoimmune in origin is undetermined. An updated analysis on 107 melanoma patients treated with nivolumab showed 40% OS at 3 years (61).

Another multicenter phase I trial enrolled 207 patients without prior experience with CTLA-4, PD-1, or PD-L1 mAb, who were given anti-PD-L1 (IgG4, BMS-936559) for a number of solid tumors for up to 2 years (62). The durable response rate was 6–17%. Treatment-related adverse events were noted in 61% (126 of 207), and 39% (81 of 207) were considered irAEs; these patients have a somewhat different spectrum and a lower percentage of irAEs compared to patients in the anti-PD-1 trials. Because these investigators were also conducting the phase I trial with nivolumab (55), their initial clinical impression was that anti-PD-L1 blockade was inferior to anti-PD-1 in achieving objective responses (62).

Interestingly, pneumonitis was not a noted side effect in the anti-PD-L1 phase I trials (60, 62), but the 39% irAEs showed a distinct autoimmune-related trend: rash, hypothyroidism, hepatitis, plus isolated cases of diabetes mellitus, and myasthenia gravis, all mostly of grade 1–2 (62). PD-1 binds to both PD-L1 (broad tissue distribution) and PD-L2 (limited primarily to DCs) (63, 64). Since lung tissues express PD-L1 and contain activated alveolar macrophages, it is possible that anti-PD-1 blockade removes the inhibitory signals that control tissue proliferation and cytokine production more so in the lung, resulting in pneumonitis, whereas anti-PD-L1 blockade does not block the immune-checkpoint between PD-1 and PD-L2. Another possibility is that, since self tolerance is maintained by the continuing interaction between PD-1 and PD-L1 to prevent TCR-driven signaling (65), upon anti-PD-L1 blockade, autoreactive T cells could become activated resulting in the autoimmune syndromes reported.

COMBINING IMMUNE-CHECKPOINT INHIBITORS COULD POTENTIATE AUTOIMMUNE SEQUELAE

There are multiple national clinical trials planned or ongoing with ipilimumab plus chemo- or radio-therapeutic agents, cytokines (e.g., GM-CSF, IL-2, IL-21), and other systemic immunomodulators, most with the goal of stimulating the effector T cell arm with some targeting dendritic and B cells also [see Ref. (51)]. Because anti-CTLA inhibited Treg function and potentiated irAEs, the use of low dose cyclophosphamide could further target nTregs (22, 45) and increase autoimmune sequelae, similar to Treg-depleting anti-CD52 (1). In murine models of B16 melanoma tumors (66) and CT26 colon and ID8-VEGF ovarian carcinomas (67), dual blockade of CTLA-4 and PD-1 enhanced greater tumor rejection than each alone. It should be noted that, unlike in clinical trials, these tumors were manipulated to express GM-CSF, as was

Table 1 | Function of CTLA-4 and PD-1 in the immune network and the impact of immune-checkpoint inhibitors anti-CTLA-4 and/or anti-PD-1 on examples of tumor immunity and autoimmunity.

Functions	Consequences	Examples of anti-CTLA-4 and/or anti-PD-1 blockade on	
		Tumor immunity	**Autoimmunity**
CTLA-4 upregulation on APCs/peptide-stimulated Tregs downmodulates B7-1/B7-2 on APCs	Suppresses priming of naive/autoreactive T cells and maintains peripheral tolerance		Morris et al. (15): EAT Read et al. (70): colitis Ansari et al. (72): type I diabetes
CTLA-4 binding to B7-1 and B7-2 causes reverse signaling through B7-1/B7-2	Activation of the tryptophan-catabolizing enzyme indoleamine 2,3-dioxygenase inhibits T cell priming and proliferation	Holmgaard et al. (68): melanoma	Kwidzinski et al. (73): EAE
CTLA-4 signaling stimulates production of cytokines TGF-β and/or IL-10 by Tregs	Inhibits function of APCs and T cells		Liu et al. (75): colitis
CTLA-4 upregulation on activated T cells binds to B7-1/B7-2 at high affinity	Negative feedback signaling inhibits continued T cell proliferation	Leach et al. (69): colon carcinoma Hurwitz et al. (71): prostate cancer	Oaks and Hallett (76): AITD Hurwitz et al. (71): prostatitis Choi et al. (77): CIA Hurwitz et al. (78): EAE Torino et al. (19): clinical hypophysitis
	Fc-dependent depletion of iTregs	Simpson et al. (43) melanoma	
CTLA-4 signaling alters motility and inhibits T cell receptor-mediated "stop" signal	Reduces efficiency of effector T cell killing and APC interaction	Ruocco et al. (74): breast cancer	
PD-1 signaling enhances Treg function	Inhibits T cell priming and maintains self tolerance		Ansari et al. (72): type I diabetes
PD-1 signaling inhibits motility and T cell receptor-mediated "stop" signal	Inhibits autoreactive T cell activation and reduces effector T cell function	Holmgaard et al. (68): melanoma	Fife et al. (65): type I diabetes
PD-1 upregulation on activated T cells	Inhibits effector T cell function (anergy or exhaustion)	Holmgaard et al. (68): melanoma Ahmadzadeh et al. (52): melanoma patients Wang et al. (53): melanoma patients	Ansari et al. (72) type I diabetes
Dual blockade		Duraiswamy et al. (67): colon and ovarian cancers Curran et al. (66): melanoma	

AITD, human autoimmune thyroid disease; APC, antigen-presenting cell; CIA, collagen-induced arthritis; EAE, experimental autoimmune encephalomyelitis; EAT, experimental autoimmune thyroiditis; iTreg, induced regulatory T cell; Treg, regulatory T cell.

whole cell vaccination included in some experiments. The presence of GM-CSF could influence the expression pattern reported for tumor-infiltrating lymphocytes (67). **Table 1** lists the important functions of CTLA-4 and PD-1 molecules in maintaining homeostasis of the immune network, and provides examples of the impact of anti-CTLA-4 and/or anti-PD-1 blockade on tumor immunity and autoimmunity.

Since CTLA-4 blockade interferes with peripheral tolerance induction/maintenance and affects primarily the early stages of the immune response, and PD-1 blockade acts toward the late stages at the tissue sites (79) and each can augment OS, dual therapy could further enhance OS, provided that the irAEs are not unreasonably additive. In melanoma patients, a phase I trial combining ipilimumab and nivolumab has begun (80). The need to test different regimens resulted in small patient sizes of 33–53. While the spectrum of irAEs was essentially similar to monotherapy, OS was higher at 24 weeks, based on previous experience.

Longer follow-ups and additional trials will be necessary to assess various parameters affecting irAEs: HLA genotype, environmental and gender influences, and antigen specificities for both Tregs and effector T cells. As seen in our EAT-anti-tumor models, subclinical autoimmune conditions (29), and mutual stimulation arising from anti-tumor and autoimmune inflammation also contribute to the overall response enhancing tumor immunity and autoimmunity (24, 25). Importantly, there appears to be different pathogenic pathways to autoimmune manifestations, with PD-1-deficiency favoring a pathogenic autoantibody profile and CTLA-4 blockade favoring T cell-mediated organ damage.

REFERENCES

1. Kong YM, Wei W-Z, Tomer Y. Opportunistic autoimmune disorders: from immunotherapy to immune dysregulation. *Ann N Y Acad Sci* (2010) **1183**:222–36. doi:10.1111/j.1749-6632.2009.05138.x
2. Amos SM, Duong CP, Westwood JA, Ritchie DS, Junghans RP, Darcy PK, et al. Autoimmunity associated with immunotherapy of cancer. *Blood* (2011) **118**:499–509. doi:10.1182/blood-2011-01-325266
3. Hamnvik OP, Larsen PR, Marqusee E. Thyroid dysfunction from antineoplastic agents. *J Natl Cancer Inst* (2011) **103**:1572–87. doi:10.1093/jnci/djr373
4. Wolchok JD, Hodi FS, Weber JS, Allison JP, Urba WJ, Robert C, et al. Development of ipilimumab: a novel immunotherapeutic approach for the treatment of advanced melanoma. *Ann N Y Acad Sci* (2013) **1291**:1–13. doi:10.1111/nyas.12180
5. Voskens CJ, Goldinger SM, Loquai C, Robert C, Kaehler KC, Berking C, et al. The price of tumor control: an analysis of rare side effects of anti-CTLA-4 therapy in metastatic melanoma from the ipilimumab network. *PLoS One* (2013) **8**:e53745. doi:10.1371/journal.pone.0053745
6. Ribas A, Kefford R, Marshall MA, Punt CJ, Haanen JB, Marmol M, et al. Phase III randomized clinical trial comparing tremelimumab with standard-of-care chemotherapy in patients with advanced melanoma. *J Clin Oncol* (2013) **31**:616–22. doi:10.1200/JCO.2012.44.6112
7. Downey SG, Klapper JA, Smith FO, Yang JC, Sherry RM, Royal RE, et al. Prognostic factors related to clinical response in patients with metastatic melanoma treated by CTL-associated antigen-4 blockade. *Clin Cancer Res* (2007) **13**:6681–8. doi:10.1158/1078-0432.ccr-07-0187
8. Beck KE, Blansfield JA, Tran KQ, Feldman AL, Hughes MS, Royal RE, et al. Enterocolitis in patients with cancer after antibody blockade of cytotoxic T-lymphocyte-associated antigen 4. *J Clin Oncol* (2006) **24**:2283–9. doi:10.1200/jco.2005.04.5716
9. Krummel MF, Allison JP. CD28 and CTLA-4 have opposing effects on the response of T cells to stimulation. *J Exp Med* (1995) **182**:459–65. doi:10.1084/jem.182.2.459
10. Wing K, Onishi Y, Prieto-Martin P, Yamaguchi T, Miyara M, Fehervari Z, et al. CTLA-4 control over Foxp3$^+$ regulatory T cell function. *Science* (2008) **322**:271–5. doi:10.1126/science.1160062
11. Sakaguchi S, Miyara M, Constantino CM, Hafler DA. FOXP3+ regulatory T cells in the human immune system. *Nat Rev Immunol* (2010) **10**:490–500. doi:10.1038/nri2785
12. Waterhouse P, Penninger JM, Timms E, Wakeham A, Shahinian A, Lee KP, et al. Lymphoproliferative disorders with early lethality in mice deficient in *Ctla-4. Science* (1995) **270**:985–8. doi:10.1126/science.270.5238.985
13. Tivol EA, Borriello F, Schweitzer AN, Lynch WP, Bluestone JA, Sharpe AH. Loss of CTLA-4 leads to massive lymphoproliferation and fatal multiorgan tissue destruction, revealing a critical negative regulatory role of CTLA-4. *Immunity* (1995) **3**:541–7. doi:10.1016/1074-7613(95)90125-6
14. Kong YM, Morris GP, Brown NK, Yan Y, Flynn JC, David CS. Autoimmune thyroiditis: a model uniquely suited to probe regulatory T cell function. *J Autoimmun* (2009) **33**:239–46. doi:10.1016/j.jaut.2009.09.004
15. Morris GP, Brown NK, Kong YM. Naturally-existing CD4$^+$CD25$^+$Foxp3$^+$ regulatory T cells are required for tolerance to experimental autoimmune thyroiditis induced by either exogenous or endogenous autoantigen. *J Autoimmun* (2009) **33**:68–76. doi:10.1016/j.jaut.2009.03.010
16. Hoos A, Eggermont AM, Janetzki S, Hodi FS, Ibrahim R, Anderson A, et al. Improved endpoints for cancer immunotherapy trials. *J Natl Cancer Inst* (2010) **102**:1388–97. doi:10.1093/jnci/djq310
17. Weber JS, Kahler KC, Hauschild A. Management of immune-related adverse events and kinetics of response with ipilimumab. *J Clin Oncol* (2012) **30**:2691–7. doi:10.1200/JCO.2012.41.6750
18. Jacobson DL, Gange SJ, Rose NR, Graham NMH. Epidemiology and estimated population burden of selected autoimmune diseases in the United States. *Clin Immunol Immunopathol* (1997) **84**:223–43. doi:10.1006/clin.1997.4412
19. Torino F, Barnabei A, De VL, Salvatori R, Corsello SM. Hypophysitis induced by monoclonal antibodies to cytotoxic T lymphocyte antigen 4: challenges from a new cause of a rare disease. *Oncologist* (2012) **17**:525–35. doi:10.1634/theoncologist.2011-0404
20. Corsello SM, Barnabei A, Marchetti P, De VL, Salvatori R, Torino F. Endocrine side effects induced by immune checkpoint inhibitors. *J Clin Endocrinol Metab* (2013) **98**:1361–75. doi:10.1210/jc.2012-4075
21. Kong YM, Okayasu I, Giraldo AA, Beisel KW, Sundick RS, Rose NR, et al. Tolerance to thyroglobulin by activating suppressor mechanisms. *Ann N Y Acad Sci* (1982) **392**:191–209. doi:10.1111/j.1749-6632.1982.tb36108.x
22. Kong YM, Giraldo AA, Waldmann H, Cobbold SP, Fuller BE. Resistance to experimental autoimmune thyroiditis: L3T4$^+$ cells as mediators of both thyroglobulin-activated and TSH-induced suppression. *Clin Immunol Immunopathol* (1989) **51**:38–54. doi:10.1016/0090-1229(89)90204-3
23. Kong YM, Jacob JB, Flynn JC, Elliott BE, Wei W-Z. Autoimmune thyroiditis as an indicator of autoimmune sequelae during cancer immunotherapy. *Autoimmun Rev* (2009) **9**:28–33. doi:10.1016/j.autrev.2009.02.034
24. Wei W-Z, Jacob JB, Zielinski JF, Flynn JC, Shim KD, Alsharabi G, et al. Concurrent induction of antitumor immunity and autoimmune thyroiditis in CD4$^+$CD25$^+$ regulatory T cell-depleted mice. *Cancer Res* (2005) **65**:8471–8. doi:10.1158/0008-5472.CAN-05-0934
25. Jacob JB, Kong YM, Nalbantoglu I, Snower DP, Wei W-Z. Tumor regression following DNA vaccination and regulatory T cell depletion in neu transgenic mice leads to an increased risk for autoimmunity. *J Immunol* (2009) **182**:5873–81. doi:10.4049/jimmunol.0804074
26. Kong YM, Lomo LC, Motte RW, Giraldo AA, Baisch J, Strauss G, et al. HLA-DRB1 polymorphism determines susceptibility to autoimmune thyroiditis in transgenic mice: definitive association with HLA-DRB1*0301 (DR3) gene. *J Exp Med* (1996) **184**:1167–72. doi:10.1084/jem.184.3.1167
27. Jacob JB, Kong YM, Meroueh C, Snower DP, David CS, Ho Y-S, et al. Control of Her-2 tumor immunity and thyroid autoimmunity by MHC and regulatory T cells. *Cancer Res* (2007) **67**:7020–7. doi:10.1158/0008-5472.CAN-06-4755
28. Lewis M, Giraldo AA, Kong YM. Resistance to experimental autoimmune thyroiditis induced by physiologic manipulation of thyroglobulin level. *Clin Immunol Immunopathol* (1987) **45**:92–104. doi:10.1016/0090-1229(87)90115-2
29. Kari S, Flynn JC, Zulfiqar M, Snower DP, Elliott BE, Kong YM. Enhanced autoimmunity associated with induction of tumor immunity in thyroiditis-susceptible mice. *Thyroid* (2013) **23**:1590–9. doi:10.1089/thy.2013.0064
30. Caturegli P, Lupi I, Landek-Salgado M, Kimura H, Rose NR. Pituitary autoimmunity: 30 years later. *Autoimmun Rev* (2008) **7**:631–7. doi:10.1016/j.autrev.2008.04.016
31. Maker AV, Yang JC, Sherry RM, Topalian SL, Kammula US, Royal RE, et al. Intrapatient dose escalation of anti-CTLA-4 antibody in patients with metastatic melanoma. *J Immunother* (2006) **29**:455–63. doi:10.1097/01.cji.0000208259.73167.58
32. Eggermont AM, Spatz A, Robert C. Cutaneous melanoma. *Lancet* (2014) **383**:816–27. doi:10.1016/S0140-6736(13)60802-8
33. Landek-Salgado MA, Leporati P, Lupi I, Geis A, Caturegli P. Growth hormone and proopiomelanocortin are targeted by autoantibodies in a patient with biopsy-proven IgG4-related hypophysitis. *Pituitary* (2012) **15**:412–9. doi:10.1007/s11102-011-0338-8
34. Smith CJ, Bensing S, Burns C, Robinson PJ, Kasperlik-Zaluska AA, Scott RJ, et al. Identification of TPIT and other novel autoantigens in lymphocytic hypophysitis: immunoscreening of a pituitary cDNA library and development of immunoprecipitation assays. *Eur J Endocrinol* (2012) **166**:391–8. doi:10.1530/EJE-11-1015
35. Lupi I, Raffaelli V, Di Cianni G, Caturegli P, Manetti L, Ciccarone AM, et al. Pituitary autoimmunity in patients with diabetes mellitus and other endocrine disorders. *J Endocrinol Invest* (2013) **36**:127–31. doi:10.1007/BF03346747
36. Huang RR, Jalil J, Economou JS, Chmielowski B, Koya RC, Mok S, et al. CTLA4 blockade induces frequent tumor infiltration by activated lymphocytes regardless of clinical responses in humans. *Clin Cancer Res* (2011) **17**:4101–9. doi:10.1158/1078-0432.CCR-11-0407

37. Weber JS, Hamid O, Chasalow SD, Wu DY, Parker SM, Galbraith S, et al. Ipilimumab increases activated T cells and enhances humoral immunity in patients with advanced melanoma. *J Immunother* (2012) **35**:89–97. doi:10.1097/CJI.0b013e31823aa41c
38. Yuan J, Gnjatic S, Li H, Powel S, Gallardo HF, Ritter E, et al. CTLA-4 blockade enhances polyfunctional NY-ESO-1 specific T cell responses in metastatic melanoma patients with clinical benefit. *Proc Natl Acad Sci U S A* (2008) **105**:20410–5. doi:10.1073/pnas.0810114105
39. Yuan J, Adamow M, Ginsberg BA, Rasalan TS, Ritter E, Gallardo HF, et al. Integrated NY-ESO-1 antibody and $CD8^+$ T-cell responses correlate with clinical benefit in advanced melanoma patients treated with ipilimumab. *Proc Natl Acad Sci U S A* (2011) **108**:16723–8. doi:10.1073/pnas.1110814108
40. Goff SL, Robbins PF, El-Gamil M, Rosenberg SA. No correlation between clinical response to CTLA-4 blockade and presence of NY-ESO-1 antibody in patients with metastatic melanoma. *J Immunother* (2009) **32**:884–5. doi:10.1097/CJI.0b013e3181affbf0
41. Hodi FS, O'Day SJ, McDermott DF, Weber RW, Sosman JA, Haanen JB, et al. Improved survival with ipilimumab in patients with metastatic melanoma. *N Engl J Med* (2010) **363**:711–23. doi:10.1056/NEJMoa1003466
42. Venuprasad K, Kong YM, Farrar MA. Control of Th2-mediated inflammation by regulatory T cells. *Am J Pathol* (2010) **177**:525–31. doi:10.2353/ajpath.2010.090936
43. Simpson TR, Li F, Montalvo-Ortiz W, Sepulveda MA, Bergerhoff K, Arce F, et al. Fc-dependent depletion of tumor-infiltrating regulatory T cells co-defines the efficacy of anti-CTLA-4 therapy against melanoma. *J Exp Med* (2013) **210**:1695–710. doi:10.1084/jem.20130579
44. Zitvogel L, Tanchot C, Granier C, Tartour E. Following up tumor-specific regulatory T cells in cancer patients. *Oncoimmunology* (2013) **2**:e25444. doi:10.4161/onci.25444
45. Walter S, Weinschenk T, Stenzl A, Zdrojowy R, Pluzanska A, Szczylik C, et al. Multipeptide immune response to cancer vaccine IMA901 after single-dose cyclophosphamide associates with longer patient survival. *Nat Med* (2012) **18**:1254–61. doi:10.1038/nm.2883
46. Bonertz A, Weitz J, Pietsch DH, Rahbari NN, Schlude C, Ge Y, et al. Antigen-specific Tregs control T cell responses against a limited repertoire of tumor antigens in patients with colorectal carcinoma. *J Clin Invest* (2009) **119**:3311–21. doi:10.1172/JCI39608
47. Jandus C, Bioley G, Dojcinovic D, Derre L, Baitsch L, Wieckowski S, et al. Tumor antigen-specific FOXP3+ CD4 T cells identified in human metastatic melanoma: peptide vaccination results in selective expansion of Th1-like counterparts. *Cancer Res* (2009) **69**:8085–93. doi:10.1158/0008-5472.CAN-09-2226
48. Schmidt HH, Ge Y, Hartmann FJ, Conrad H, Klug F, Nittel S, et al. HLA Class II tetramers reveal tissue-specific regulatory T cells that suppress T-cell responses in breast carcinoma patients. *Oncoimmunology* (2013) **2**:e24962. doi:10.4161/onci.24962
49. Wherry EJ. T cell exhaustion. *Nat Immunol* (2011) **12**:492–9. doi:10.1038/ni.2035
50. Intlekofer AM, Thompson CB. At the bench: preclinical rationale for CTLA-4 and PD-1 blockade as cancer immunotherapy. *J Leukoc Biol* (2013) **94**:25–39. doi:10.1189/jlb.1212621
51. Callahan MK, Wolchok JD. At the bedside: CTLA-4- and PD-1-blocking antibodies in cancer immunotherapy. *J Leukoc Biol* (2013) **94**:41–53. doi:10.1189/jlb.1212631
52. Ahmadzadeh M, Johnson LA, Heemskerk B, Wunderlich JR, Dudley ME, White DE, et al. Tumor antigen-specific CD8 T cells infiltrating the tumor express high levels of PD-1 and are functionally impaired. *Blood* (2009) **114**:1537–44. doi:10.1182/blood-2008-12-195792
53. Wang W, Lau R, Yu D, Zhu W, Korman A, Weber J. PD1 blockade reverses the suppression of melanoma antigen-specific CTL by $CD4^+CD25^{Hi}$ regulatory T cells. *Int Immunol* (2009) **21**:1065–77. doi:10.1093/intimm/dxp072
54. Velcheti V, Schalper KA, Carvajal DE, Anagnostou VK, Syrigos KN, Sznol M, et al. Programmed death ligand-1 expression in non-small cell lung cancer. *Lab Invest* (2014) **94**:107–16. doi:10.1038/labinvest.2013.130
55. Topalian SL, Hodi FS, Brahmer JR, Gettinger SN, Smith DC, McDermott DF, et al. Safety, activity, and immune correlates of anti-PD-1 antibody in cancer. *N Engl J Med* (2012) **366**:2443–54. doi:10.1056/NEJMoa1200690
56. Nishimura H, Nose M, Hiai H, Minato N, Honjo T. Development of lupus-like autoimmune diseases by disruption of the PD-1 gene encoding an ITIM motif-carrying immunoreceptor. *Immunity* (1999) **11**:141–51. doi:10.1016/S1074-7613(00)80089-8
57. Okazaki T, Tanaka Y, Nishio R, Mitsuiye T, Mizoguchi A, Wang J, et al. Autoantibodies against cardiac troponin I are responsible for dilated cardiomyopathy in PD-1-deficient mice. *Nat Med* (2003) **9**:1477–83. doi:10.1038/nm955
58. PD-1 inhibitor becomes "breakthrough therapy". *Cancer Discov* (2013) **3**:OF14. doi:10.1158/2159-8290.CD-NB2013-074
59. Hamid O, Robert C, Daud A, Hodi FS, Hwu WJ, Kefford R, et al. Safety and tumor responses with lambrolizumab (anti-PD-1) in melanoma. *N Engl J Med* (2013) **369**:134–44. doi:10.1056/NEJMoa1305133
60. Kyi C, Postow MA. Checkpoint blocking antibodies in cancer immunotherapy. *FEBS Lett* (2014) **588**:368–76. doi:10.1016/j.febslet.2013.10.015
61. Topalian SL, Sznol M, McDermott DF, Kluger HM, Carvajal RD, Sharfman WH, et al. Survival, durable tumor remission, and long-term safety in patients with advanced melanoma receiving nivolumab. *J Clin Oncol* (2014) **32**:1020–30. doi:10.1200/JCO.2013.53.0105
62. Brahmer JR, Tykodi SS, Chow LQ, Hwu WJ, Topalian SL, Hwu P, et al. Safety and activity of anti-PD-L1 antibody in patients with advanced cancer. *N Engl J Med* (2012) **366**:2455–65. doi:10.1056/NEJMoa1200694
63. Latchman Y, Wood CR, Chernova T, Chaudhary D, Borde M, Chernova I, et al. PD-L2 is a second ligand for PD-1 and inhibits T cell activation. *Nat Immunol* (2001) **2**:261–8. doi:10.1038/85330
64. Tseng SY, Otsuji M, Gorski K, Huang X, Slansky JE, Pai SI, et al. B7-DC, a new dendritic cell molecule with potent costimulatory properties for T cells. *J Exp Med* (2001) **193**:839–46. doi:10.1084/jem.193.7.839
65. Fife BT, Pauken KE, Eagar TN, Obu T, Wu J, Tang Q, et al. Interactions between PD-1 and PD-L1 promote tolerance by blocking the TCR-induced stop signal. *Nat Immunol* (2009) **10**:1185–92. doi:10.1038/ni.1790
66. Curran MA, Montalvo W, Yagita H, Allison JP. PD-1 and CTLA-4 combination blockade expands infiltrating T cells and reduces regulatory T and myeloid cells within B16 melanoma tumors. *Proc Natl Acad Sci U S A* (2010) **107**:4275–80. doi:10.1073/pnas.0915174107
67. Duraiswamy J, Kaluza KM, Freeman GJ, Coukos G. Dual blockade of PD-1 and CTLA-4 combined with tumor vaccine effectively restores T-cell rejection function in tumors. *Cancer Res* (2013) **73**:3591–603. doi:10.1158/0008-5472.CAN-12-4100
68. Holmgaard RB, Zamarin D, Munn DH, Wolchok JD, Allison JP. Indoleamine 2,3-dioxygenase is a critical resistance mechanism in antitumor T cell immunotherapy targeting CTLA-4. *J Exp Med* (2013) **210**:1389–402. doi:10.1084/jem.20130066
69. Leach DR, Krummel MF, Allison JP. Enhancement of antitumor immunity by CTLA-4 blockade. *Science* (1996) **271**:1734–6. doi:10.1126/science.271.5256.1734
70. Read S, Malmström V, Powrie F. Cytotoxic T lymphocyte-associated antigen 4 plays an essential role in the function of $CD25^+CD4^+$ regulatory cells that control intestinal inflammation. *J Exp Med* (2000) **192**:295–302. doi:10.1084/jem.192.2.295
71. Hurwitz AA, Foster BA, Kwon ED, Truong T, Choi EM, Greenberg NM, et al. Combination immunotherapy of primary prostate cancer in a transgenic mouse model using CTLA-4 blockade. *Cancer Res* (2000) **60**:2444–8.
72. Ansari MJI, Salama AD, Chitnis T, Smith RN, Yagita H, Akiba H, et al. The programmed death-1 (PD-1) pathway regulates autoimmune diabetes in nonobese diabetic (NOD) mice. *J Exp Med* (2003) **198**:63–9. doi:10.1084/jem.20022125
73. Kwidzinski E, Bunse J, Aktas O, Richter D, Mutlu L, Zipp F, et al. Indolamine 2,3-dioxygenase is expressed in the CNS and down-regulates autoimmune inflammation. *FASEB J* (2005) **19**:1347–9. doi:10.1096/fj.04-3228fje
74. Ruocco MG, Pilones KA, Kawashima N, Cammer M, Huang J, Babb JS, et al. Suppressing T cell motility induced by anti-CTLA-4 monotherapy improves antitumor effects. *J Clin Invest* (2012) **122**:3718–30. doi:10.1172/JCI61931
75. Liu H, Hu B, Xu D, Liew FY. $CD4^+CD25^+$ regulatory T cells cure murine colitis: the role of IL-10, TGF-β, and CTLA4. *J Immunol* (2003) **171**:5012–7. doi:10.4049/jimmunol.171.10.5012

76. Oaks MK, Hallett KM. Cutting edge: a soluble form of CTLA-4 in patients with autoimmune thyroid disease. *J Immunol* (2000) **164**:5015–8. doi:10.4049/jimmunol.164.10.5015
77. Choi JM, Kim SH, Shin JH, Gibson T, Yoon BS, Lee DH, et al. Transduction of the cytoplasmic domain of CTLA-4 inhibits TcR-specific activation signals and prevents collagen-induced arthritis. *Proc Natl Acad Sci U S A* (2008) **105**:19875–80. doi:10.1073/pnas.0805198105
78. Hurwitz AA, Sullivan TJ, Krummel MF, Sobel RA, Allison JP. Specific blockade of CTLA-4/B7 interactions results in exacerbated clinical and histologic disease in an actively-induced model of experimental allergic encephalomyelitis. *J Neuroimmunol* (1997) **73**:57–62.
79. Fife BT, Bluestone JA. Control of peripheral T-cell tolerance and autoimmunity via the CTLA-4 and PD-1 pathways. *Immunol Rev* (2008) **224**:166–82. doi:10.1111/j.1600-065X.2008.00662.x
80. Wolchok JD, Kluger H, Callahan MK, Postow MA, Rizvi NA, Lesokhin AM, et al. Nivolumab plus ipilimumab in advanced melanoma. *N Engl J Med* (2013) **369**:122–33. doi:10.1056/NEJMoa1302369

Conflict of Interest Statement: The authors declare that the research was conducted in the absence of any commercial or financial relationships that could be construed as a potential conflict of interest.

Global inhibition of DC priming capacity in the spleen of self-antigen vaccinated mice requires IL-10

Douglas M. Marvel and Olivera J. Finn*

Department of Immunology, University of Pittsburgh School of Medicine, Pittsburgh, PA, USA

Edited by:
Penelope Anne Morel, University of Pittsburgh, USA

Reviewed by:
Luisa Martinez-Pomares, The University of Nottingham, UK
Benjamin M. J. Owens, University of Oxford, UK

Correspondence:
Olivera J. Finn, Department of Immunology, University of Pittsburgh School of Medicine, 200 Lothrop Street, BST E1044, Pittsburgh, PA 15261, USA
e-mail: ojfinn@pitt.edu

Dendritic cells (DC) in the spleen are highly activated following intravenous vaccination with a foreign-antigen, promoting expansion of effector T cells, but remain phenotypically and functionally immature after vaccination with a self-antigen. Up-regulation or suppression of expression of a cohort of pancreatic enzymes 24–72 h post-vaccination can be used as a biomarker of stimulatory versus tolerogenic DC, respectively. Here we show, using MUC1 transgenic mice and a vaccine based on the MUC1 peptide, which these mice perceive as a self-antigen, that the difference in enzyme expression that predicts whether DC will promote immune response or immune tolerance is seen as early as 4–8 h following vaccination. We also identify early production of IL-10 as a predominant factor that both correlates with this early-time point and controls DC function. Pre-treating mice with an antibody against the IL-10 receptor prior to vaccination results in DC that up-regulate CD40, CD80, and CD86 and promote stronger IFNγ+ T cell responses. This study suggests that transient inhibition of IL-10 prior to vaccination could improve responses to cancer vaccines that utilize self-tumor antigens.

Keywords: IL-10, dendritic cells, cancer vaccine, MUC1, T cell response

INTRODUCTION

The impact of IL-10 on the cells of the immune system is well studied and varied. Originally identified as cytokine synthesis inhibitory factor, IL-10 can play a role in the development and maturation of almost all immune cells (1, 2). Signaling through the IL-10 receptor (IL-10R) occurs through a STAT3 intermediate and is known to induce SOCS-3 expression, to suppress IFN signaling by blocking STAT1 phosphorylation, and to inhibit NF-κB signaling by preventing its nuclear translocation as well as inhibiting its binding to DNA (2, 3). In dendritic cells (DC), known for being the most important professional antigen presenting cells, IL-10 can reduce expression of MHC Class II and the costimulatory molecules CD80/86 and CD40, as well as reduce IL-12 secretion (3–6). This is true even for DC previously activated with IFNγ. IL-10 can also prevent monocyte differentiation into DC (2).

IL-10 has a profound effect on T cells as well. For example, reduced IL-12 production by DC affected by IL-10 antagonizes the development of T helper type 1 (Th1) responses while reduced MHC II levels on DC result in presentation of low density antigen that preferentially stimulates differentiation of regulatory CD4 T cells (7, 8). IL-10 can also act directly on T cells to inhibit synthesis of cytokines like IL-2 and IFNγ in CD4 T cells or to inhibit their proliferation (3). The effect of IL-10 on CD8 T cells is less clear although some studies have shown that IL-10 can favor activation of CD8 T cells (9–11).

Recently, our group implicated IL-10 in controlling in part the function of DCs post-vaccination with antigens derived from self-proteins. Using the MUC1 transgenic (MUC1.Tg) mouse model and a peptide derived from the extracellular domain of the tumor antigen MUC1, we showed that 24 h following vaccination, there is an IL-10 dependent suppression of DC activation that is detectable via suppression of expression of a newly discovered biomarker: a cohort of pancreatic enzymes. These enzymes, expressed in the spleen only by DC and represented by trypsin 1 and carboxypeptidase B1 (CPB1), are up-regulated post-vaccination with a foreign but not a self-antigen and identified a DC population that has higher MHC Class II, higher costimulatory molecule expression, and a higher T cell stimulatory capacity (12).

In this study, we present new evidence of an important role for IL-10 in the suppression of splenic DC following intravenous vaccination with a self-antigen. We show an early (4–8 h) up-regulation in IL-10 levels in spleens of self-antigen vaccinated mice that is not seen in mice that see that same antigen as foreign and coincides with the time when we also see differences in biomarker enzyme expression. Furthermore, DC in the spleens of self-antigen vaccinated mice have an increased sensitivity to IL-10. When the effect of IL-10 is blocked by pre-vaccination treatment of mice with an anti-IL-10R blocking antibody, there is a significant increase in the activation level and stimulatory capacity of DC at 24 h post-vaccination and a significant increase in CD4 T cell responses 7 days post-vaccination. These data implicate IL-10 in the regulation of antigen-specific immunity versus tolerance at a previously underappreciated early time post-vaccination, and suggest that manipulating its function at the time of vaccination might overcome tolerance and improve responses to cancer vaccines that utilize self-antigens.

MATERIALS AND METHODS

MICE

Human MUC1.Tg mice (13) on the C57Bl/6 background were a generous gift from Dr. Sandra Gendler (Mayo Clinic) and were bred and maintained in the University of Pittsburgh Animal

Facility. C57Bl/6 (WT) mice were purchased from The Jackson Laboratory. All experiments were approved by the Institutional Animal Care and Use Committee of the University of Pittsburgh.

MUC1 VACCINATION

A 100-aa peptide containing five repeats of the MUC1 VNTR sequence HGVTSAPDTRPAPGSTAPPA, was synthesized as previously described (14) by the University of Pittsburgh Genomics and Proteomics Core Laboratories. For soluble peptide vaccinations, 100 μg of this 100mer peptide admixed with 50 μg polyinosinic–polycytidylic acid and poly-L-lysine (Poly-ICLC; Hiltonol) was brought up to 100 μL with PBS and injected via tail vein. For DC-based vaccinations, DC were prepared as previously described (15). Briefly, RBC lysed bone marrow cells were put into culture for 6 days in AIM-V supplemented with 10 ng/mL GM-CSF (Miltenyi), feeding once on day 3. On day 6, semi-adherent cells were collected by gentle agitation and put into culture overnight in AIM-V containing 33 μg/mL MUC1 100mer peptide and 25 μg/mL Poly-ICLC. The next day, mature DC were collected and resuspended in PBS at a final concentration of $0.5^{-1} \times 10^6$ cells/mL. One hundred microliters of this solution was then injected intravenously via tail vein.

IL-10R BLOCKADE

Where indicated, mice were given 250 μg of an antibody against the IL-10R (Bio X Cell, Clone 1B1.3A) or an isotype-matched control antibody (Bio X Cell, Clone HPRN), intraperitoneally. Twenty-four to forty-eight hours following treatment, mice were vaccinated as described in "MUC1 vaccination" above and analyzed as described.

QUANTITATIVE RT-PCR

RNA was extracted from whole spleen using TRIzol (Invitrogen) according to the manufacturer's protocol. Following extraction, cDNA was generated using oligo(dT) primers and SuperScript III reverse transcriptase (Invitrogen). qPCR was performed using QuantiTect SYBR Green PCR kit (Qiagen) according to the manufacturer's protocol. Reactions were run on a StepOnePlus instrument (Applied Biosystems). The following primer pairs were used: trypsin 1 (forward: 5′ACTGTGGCTCTGCCCAGCTC3′; reverse: 5′AGCAGGTCTGGTTCAATGACTGT3′), CPB1 (forward: 5′GCCCTGGTGAAAGGTGCAGCAAAGG3′; reverse: 5′AGCCCAGTCGTCAGATCCCCCAGCA3′), IL-10 (forward: 5′CTTCCCAGTCGGCCAGAGCCA3′; reverse: 5′ CTCAGCCGCATCCTGAGGGTCT3′), and HPRT (forward: 5′TGAGCCATTGCTGAGGCGGCGA3′; reverse: 5′CGGCTCGCGGCAAAAAGCGGTC3′).

INTRACELLULAR CYTOKINE STAINING/FLOW CYTOMETRY

For *ex vivo* T cells assays, 7–9 days post MUC1 vaccination, mice were sacrificed and spleens were removed. Single-cell suspensions were made by mashing the spleens through a 40-μm filter. Total T cells were then bead isolated (Pan T Cell Isolation Kit II, Miltenyi) and cultured with day 6 MUC1-loaded BMDC (prepared as described in "MUC1 vaccination") for 4–6 h in the presence of GolgiStop (BD biosciences). Cells were then stained with the indicated antibodies using the BD Cytofix/Cytoperm™ kit (BD Bioscience) according to the manufacturer's protocol. All samples were run on a Fortessa (BD bioscience) flow cytometer and analyzed using FACSDiva (BD Bioscineces) and FlowJo software (Tree Star Inc.). Antibodies used: CD3-PerCP, CD11c-BV421, CD80-FITC, CD86-APC/Cy7, CD40-APC, CD3-PeCy5, CD4-V450, CD8-AF700, IFNγ-PeCy7, TNFα-PE, IL-2-APC, CD44-FITC, CD3-APC/Cy7, and CD8 PerCP.

PHOSPHOFLOW

Twenty-four hours following MUC1 vaccination, splenocytes were harvested as above. Post isolation, cells were put into AIM-V with or without 30 ng/mL IL-10 (PeproTech) for 20 min. At the end of culture, cells were immediately fixed in 1.6% PFA for 10 min at room temperature. After 10 min, four volumes of ice-cold methanol were added and samples were stored at −80°C. At the time of staining cells were put at room temp for 10 min and then immediately spun down and resuspended in flow buffer (PBS containing 1% BSA, 0.02% sodium azide, and 2 nM EDTA). After 10 min incubation at room temperature, cells were spun down and washed with flow buffer twice. Samples were then stained with antibodies against cell surface antigens CD11c, NK1.1, and CD3 and phospho-specific anti-pSAT3 antibody for 1 h at room temperature and prepared for analysis via standard protocol and as described above. Antibodies used: CD11c-Pacific Blue, pSTAT3-AF647, NK1.1-PE, and CD3-APC/Cy7.

EX VIVO DC STIMULATORY CAPACITY ANALYSIS

MUC1 transgenic mice were pretreated with antibodies and vaccinated as in "IL-10R Blockade." Post-vaccination, DC were bead isolated (CD11c MicroBeads, Miltenyi) from the spleens of the vaccinated animals. These DC were put into culture with bead isolated (CD4 T cell Isolation Kit II, Miltenyi) CFSE stained MUC1 specific VFT CD4 T cells (15) at a ratio of 1 DC to 5 VFT cells in complete DMEM. Twenty-four hours after the start of culture half of the media was removed and saved for cytokine analysis. IL-2 was analyzed by ELISA (BD OptEIA Mouse IL-2 ELISA set, BD) according to the manufacturer's protocol. The media was replaced with fresh cDMEM and the cultures were allowed to incubate for three more days. T cell proliferation was then analyzed by CFSE dilution.

ELISPOT

Millipore MultiScreen® Filter Plates (Millipore) were pretreated according to the manufacturer's instructions using the Mouse IFNg ELISPOT kit (Mabtech). Bead isolated CD4 and CD8 T cells (CD4 T cell Isolation Kit II and CD8α Isolation Kit II, Miltenyi) were cultured as above (see Intracellular Cytokine Staining/Flow Cytometry) with MUC1 pulsed BMDC and analyzed according to the established protocol. DC alone, media alone, and T cells alone were used to establish background cytokine production.

STATISTICAL ANALYSIS

Where appropriate, statistical significance was determined by performing an unpaired Student's t-test. *Denotes a p-value <0.05 and **denotes a p-value of <0.01. When indicated, to allow for pooling of data from multiple experiments, values have been transformed to account for minor variations in instrument settings and other potential sources of variation (i.e., minor batch to batch variance in DC vaccine prep, etc.). Briefly, all experimental values were

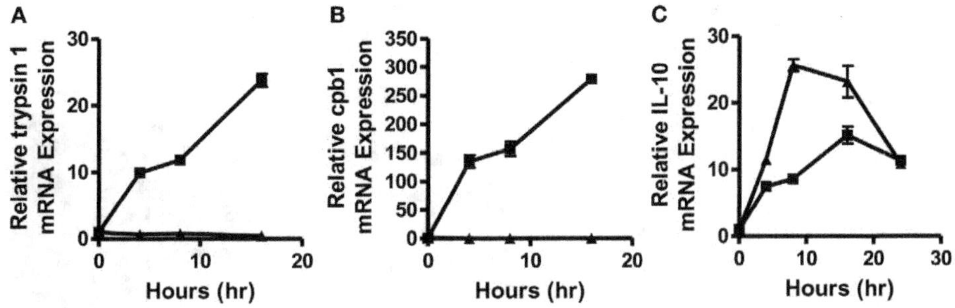

FIGURE 1 | Splenic DC activation is suppressed as early as 4–8 h post-vaccination with a self-, but not a foreign-antigen and correlated with early IL-10 production in the spleens of these animals. WT (squares) and MUC1.Tg mice (triangles) were vaccinated with MUC1p plus Poly-ICLC via tail vein. Spleens were removed at indicated hours post-vaccination and total splenic mRNA levels of trypsin 1 **(A)**, carboxypeptidase B1 (CPB1) **(B)**, and IL-10 **(C)** were determined relative to the control gene HPRT. Values shown represent expression relative to the baseline expression in mice of that genotype (WT and MUC1.Tg) at 0 h post-vaccination. Data are representative of three pooled mice were group per time point shown. Data points show mean ± SEM of three technical replicates and are representative of two independent experiments.

divided by the mean value of the control group from the experiment in which they were run. "Relative" values therefore represent a standardized deviance from control.

RESULTS

IL-10 EXPRESSION IN THE SPLEEN IS INCREASED 4–8H POST-VACCINATION WITH MUC1p AS SELF-ANTIGEN AND CORRELATES WITH DC SUPPRESSION

In order to determine how quickly post-vaccination with a self- versus a foreign-antigen DC phenotype and function begin to diverge and to obtain a more accurate picture of what factors might be responsible for supporting this divergence, we vaccinated intravenously WT and MUC1.Tg mice with the MUC1 100mer peptide (MUC1p) admixed with the Poly-ICLC adjuvant. MUC1.Tg mice express the human tumor antigen MUC1 under the control of its endogenous promoter and therefore MUC1p is seen as a self-antigen in these mice, whereas it is seen as a foreign-antigen in WT animals. Mice were sacrificed 4, 6, 8, and 16 h post-vaccination and the spleens removed for mRNA isolation and analysis. As early as 4 h post-vaccination, two newly discovered biomarkers of DC activation, trypsin 1 and CPB1 (12), were up-regulated in the spleens of WT mice but suppressed in MUC1.Tg mice (**Figures 1A,B**). In addition to differences in the levels of these enzymes, which our previous study showed to be expressed only in DC and representative of a larger cohort of "pancreatic" enzymes that robustly activated DC expression, we also detected at this early-time point higher levels of IL-10 mRNA in the spleens of vaccinated MUC1.Tg mice compared to WT mice. At 24 h post-vaccination and later, IL-10 production was at equal levels in self- and foreign-antigen vaccinated mice (**Figure 1C** and data not shown).

DC FROM SPLEENS OF MUC1p (SELF-ANTIGEN)-VACCINATED MUC1.Tg MICE ARE MORE SENSITIVE TO IL-10 THAN MUC1p (FOREIGN-ANTIGEN)-VACCINATED WT MICE

The above data showing differences in IL-10 levels early post-vaccination but no difference at 24 h and later would indicate a modest and transient effect by IL-10 on DC. This was, however, inconsistent with our previous observations that functional differences between DC post self-antigen versus foreign-antigen vaccine were evident as late as 72 h post-vaccination (12). We considered the possibility that the early action of IL-10 on DC, along with other factors, might increase their sensitivity to IL-10 at the later-time points. To query this, DC were removed from the spleens of WT and MUC1.Tg mice 24 h post MUC1p vaccination and exposed to IL-10. As signaling through the IL-10R is known to occur through a STAT3 intermediate, the sensitivity of DC to IL-10 was assessed by phosphoflow, measuring phospho-STAT3 levels post *ex vivo* exposure to IL-10. As hypothesized, there was a significant increase in the number of DC showing STAT3 phosphorylation as well as higher levels of pSTAT3 in the spleens of MUC1p-vaccinated MUC1.Tg mice (**Figures 2A–C**) indicating that DC in the spleens of MUC1.Tg mice are not only exposed to more IL-10 early on, but are also more sensitive to it at the later-time points.

IL-10R BLOCKADE INCREASES COSTIMULATORY MOLECULE EXPRESSION ON DC FOLLOWING VACCINATION WITH MUC1p AS SELF-ANTIGEN

Given the inverse correlation between IL-10 production and DC pancreatic enzyme expression in the first 24 h following vaccination and previously published data showing that IL-10 is necessary for suppression of trypsin 1 and CPB1 following vaccination with a self-antigen (12), we hypothesized that blocking IL-10 signaling in self-antigen vaccinated mice would improve DC activation and costimulatory molecule expression. We injected MUC1.Tg mice with an antibody against IL-10R and vaccinated intravenously 24–48 h later with MUC1p plus Poly-ICLC. At 24 h post-vaccination, the surface phenotype of splenic DC was analyzed by flow cytometry. As hypothesized, there was an increase in the level of cell surface expression of CD40, CD80, and CD86 in DC from mice pretreated with the antibody to IL-10R, but not from mice treated with the isotype control antibody (**Figures 3A–C**). Increases in CD40 and CD86 were statistically significant, which is of interest because these two molecules were shown previously to be specifically inhibited in mice vaccinated with a self- but not a foreign-antigen (12). In addition to being less active as measured by surface marker expression, these DC are also less capable of stimulating MUC1 specific CD4 T cells *in vitro*. DC isolated from MUC1.Tg mice

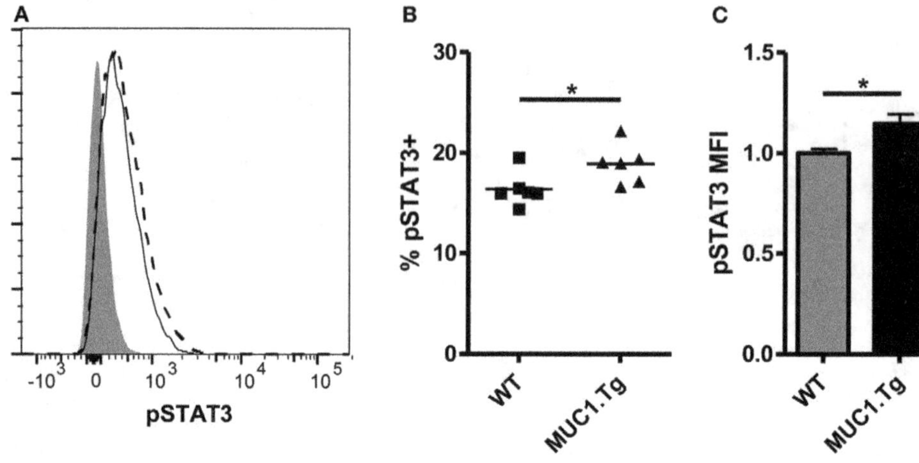

FIGURE 2 | Dendritic cell from spleens of mice vaccinated with self-antigen have higher levels of phosphorylated STAT3 after IL-10 treatment than DC from spleens of mice vaccinated with foreign-antigen. WT (solid line) and MUC1.Tg (dashed line) mice were vaccinated with MUC1p via the tail vein. Twenty-four hours post-vaccination splenocytes were removed and treated with 30 ng/mL of IL-10 for 20 min. Following incubation, cells were fixed and phospho-STAT3 expression in CD11c+NK1.1− splenocytes was analyzed via phoshpoflow. **(A)** A representative flow plot is shown. The shaded histogram represents the fluorescence level when cells are treated with standard surface markers and an isotype-matched control instead of the phosphospecific antibody. pSTAT3 positivity **(B)** and MFI **(C)** were analyzed. In **(B)** symbols correspond to individual animals and are representative of two independent experiments. **(C)** Values shown have been normalized to the expression level of the control group (WT) in order to allow for pooling of data from separate experiments run on multiple days. Bars are representative of nine mice from two combined experiments and show the mean ± SEM. *Indicates a *p*-value of <0.05.

pretreated with an antibody against the IL-10R prior to MUC1 vaccination and put into culture with MUC1 specific CD4 T cells induce higher levels of IL-2 (**Figure 4A**) and CD4 T cell proliferation (**Figures 4B,C**) compared to DC from MUC1.Tg mice pretreated with an isotype-matched control antibody.

BLOCKING IL-10 SIGNALING PRIOR TO VACCINATION WITH MUC1p AS SELF-ANTIGEN IMPROVES CD4 T CELL RESPONSE

The increase of costimulatory molecule expression when IL-10 signaling was blocked just prior to vaccination suggested that there would be a resultant increase in the T cell response. To test this, we again pretreated mice with an anti-IL-10R antibody or an isotype-matched control and injected with a vaccine composed of DC loaded with MUC1p. We chose the DC-based vaccine expecting that it would optimally stimulate both CD4 and CD8 T cells, as has been previously shown (16). Seven to nine days post-vaccination, splenic T cells were isolated and their production of relevant cytokines analyzed by ELISPOT and intracellular flow cytometry. In MUC1.Tg mice treated with anti-IL-10R, there was a significant increase in MUC1p specific, IFNγ+ CD4 T cells when compared to mice treated with an isotype-matched control antibody (**Figures 5A,C**). The level of the response was equivalent to the response of WT mice pretreated with the isotype control antibody (**Figure 5A**). There was no increase over the isotype control of the T cell response in WT mice pretreated with the anti-IL-10R antibody (**Figures 5A,C**), indicating that the effect of IL-10 we saw in MUC1.Tg mice was specific for controlling responses to self- but not foreign-antigens. There was a small but not significant increase in the CD8 response that was detectable only by the more sensitive ELISPOT (**Figures 5B,D**).

DISCUSSION

Vaccines against cancer have garnered a lot of attention in recent years. Much of this was sparked by the relatively recent approval of Sipuleucel-T, the first vaccine to show survival benefit in a solid metastatic tumor (17, 18). Implementation of Gardasil®, a quadrivalent human papilloma virus specific vaccination intended to prevent cervical cancer in women (19, 20) has also sparked new efforts in designing prophylactic cancer vaccines not just for viral cancers but for many tumor types (21–24). Most non-viral tumor antigens fall into the category of self- or altered self-antigens. Mounting an effective immune response against them represents a unique challenge. One must design vaccines that overcome the natural tolerizing forces acting on responses to self-antigens, while minimizing adverse autoimmune effects.

Our work with the MUC1 tumor antigen in the MUC1.Tg mouse model system has shown that hyporesponsiveness to the MUC1 peptide vaccines in these mice is neither due to the elimination of MUC1 peptide-specific T cells by central tolerance, nor solely to their conditioning in the periphery, but rather by the control of their activation (15). Indeed, even when unconditioned MUC1 specific T cells are transferred into MUC1.Tg hosts, they are hyporesponsive to MUC1 peptide vaccination but respond vigorously in WT hosts. Most recently, we determined that the major reason for the lack of T cell response is profound, albeit transient, tolerization of DC in MUC1p-vaccinated MUC1.Tg mice early post-vaccination (12). Here, we show that this is likely due to the very early and exaggerated effect of IL-10 on these DC in the first 4–24 h post-vaccination. IL-10 is known to reduce MHC Class II and costimulatory molecule expression on DC (4–6), DC motility (25, 26), and overall T cell stimulatory capacity (27, 28), all

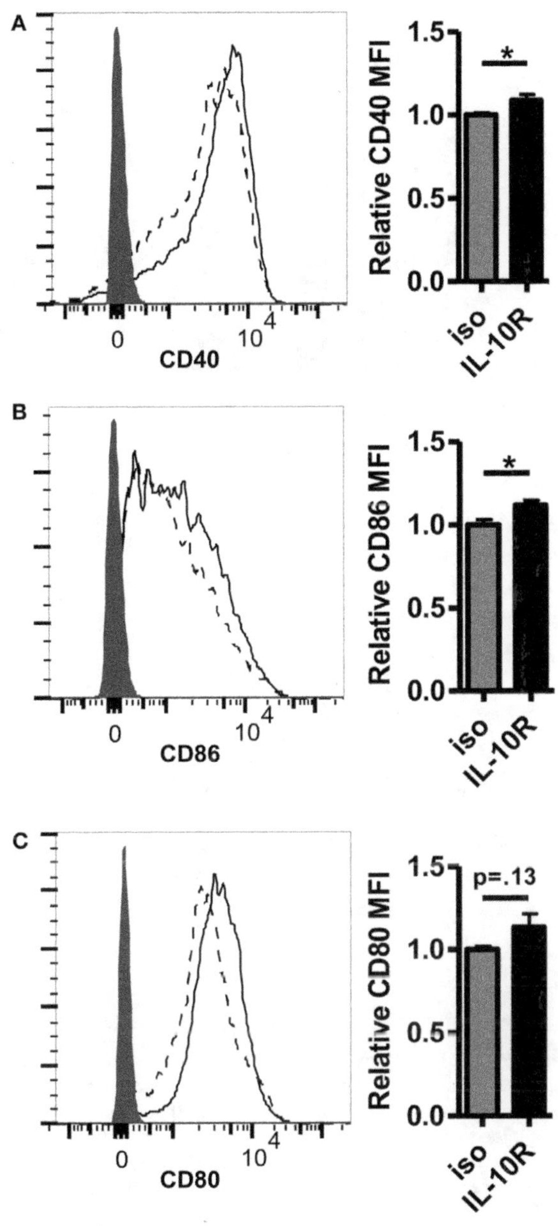

FIGURE 3 | Pretreatment with an antibody against the IL-10 receptor increases the level of costimulatory molecule expression on DC in the spleens of self antigen vaccinated mice. MUC1.Tg mice were pretreated with an antibody against the IL-10 receptor (IL-10R, solid lines) or were given a non-specific isotype control (iso, dashed lines). One to two days later they were vaccinated as in **Figure 1** and 24 h post-vaccination, splenocytes were removed and analyzed via flow cytometry. The expression level of CD40 **(A)**, CD86 **(B)**, and CD80 **(C)** on splenic DC (CD11C+, MHC Class II+) was determined. Shaded histograms represent fluorescence in samples stained with isotype alone. Bar graph values shown have been normalized to the expression level of the control group (iso) in order to allow for pooling of data from separate experiments run on multiple days. **(A,C)** Data are combined from two independent experiments and representative of six mice. **(B)** Data are combined from three independent experiments and are representative of 10 mice. Bars represent mean ± SEM. *p*-Values are as stated unless designated by a *, which indicates a *p*-value of <0.05.

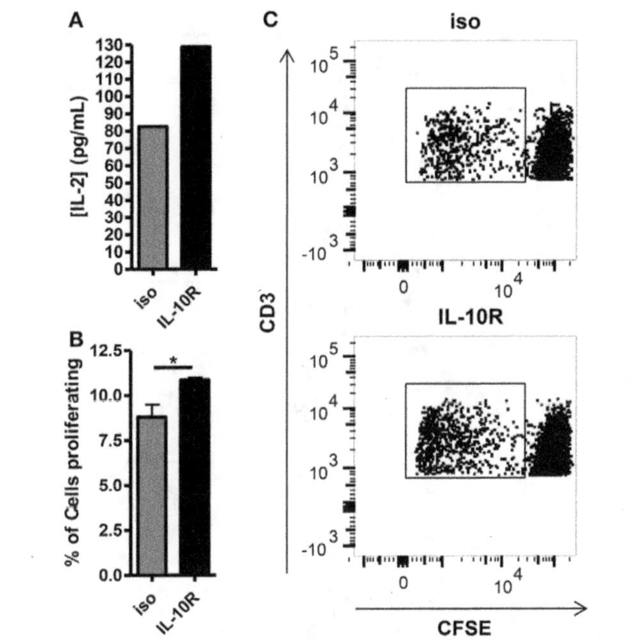

FIGURE 4 | Blocking of the IL-10 receptor prior to intravenous MUC1 peptide vaccination increases the ability of splenic DC from MUC1.Tg mice to stimulate MUC1 specific CD4T cells *ex vivo*. MUC1.tg mice were treated as in **Figure 3**. Twenty-four hours post MUC1 vaccination, splenocytes from three to four mice per treatment group were pooled and bead isolated DC from these pooled splenocytes were put into culture with CFSE labeled MUC1 specific CD4 T cells (VFT cells) at a ratio 1DC:5VFT. Twenty-four hours after the start of culture, half of the culture media was removed and the concentration of IL-2 was measured by ELISA **(A)**. Cultures were allowed to incubate three more days for a total of four and VFT proliferation was analyzed by CFSE dilution **(B,C)**. **(B)** Bars represent the mean percentage of CD3+CD4+ T cells that had proliferated at 4 days of three technical replicates ±SEM. **(C)** A representative flow plot is shown. Data are representative of two to three independent experiments. *Indicates a *p*-value of <0.05.

of which are characteristics of DC in the spleens of MUC1p-vaccinated MUC1.Tg mice (12).

The effects of IL-10 on vaccines have been observed previously. In the therapeutic setting, IL-10R blockade alone or along with vaccination can improve Th1 responses and enhance pathogen clearance (29–31). In a prophylactic setting, mice given the BCG vaccination for prevention of *Mycobacterium tuberculosis* show improved Th1 responses and enhanced resistance to pathogen challenge when IL-10R is blocked at the time of vaccination (32). In this paper, we describe a distinct new role for IL-10 in impacting vaccine outcome that is unique in its specificity for self-antigen. The same MUC1 peptide, given as a self-antigen to MUC1.Tg mice but as a foreign-antigen to WT mice, causes only low levels IL-10 production in WT mice and increased production in MUC1.Tg mice. In previously published studies showing improvement in immune responses after IL-10R blockade, IL-10 was produced in response to acute or persistent pathogen infections, whereas in this case it was specifically triggered in response to the presence of a self-antigen or specifically inhibited in the presence of a foreign-antigen.

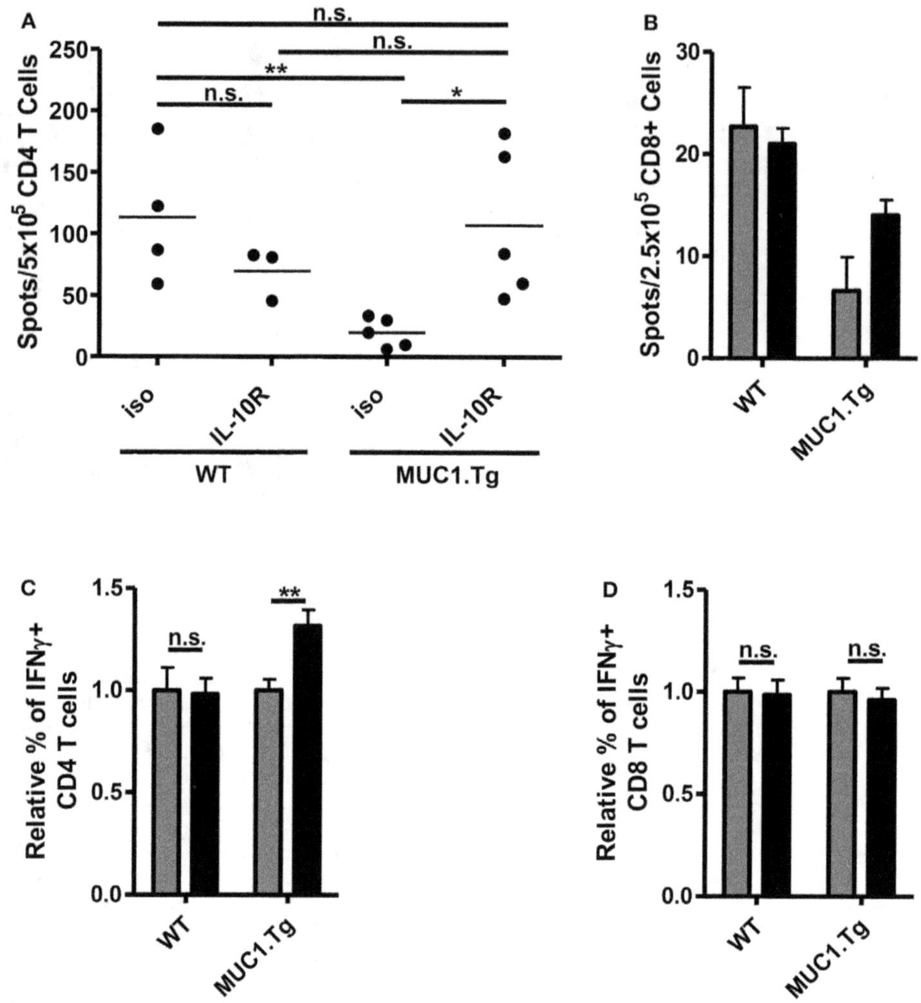

FIGURE 5 | Treatment with anti-IL-10R antibody at the time of vaccination increases the number of MUC1p specific, IFNγ+ CD4 T cells without an effect on CD8 T cells. WT and MUC1.Tg mice were pretreated with an antibody against the IL-10 receptor (IL-10R, black bars) or a non-specific isotype control (iso, gray bars). One to two days following antibody treatment, mice were vaccinated with DC loaded with MUC1p. Seven to nine days post-vaccination, spleens were removed and bead isolated CD4 **(A,C)** and CD8 T cells **(B,D)** were cultured with MUC1p loaded bone marrow derived DC overnight and analyzed by ELISPOT **(A,B)**, or were cultured for 6–8 h in the presence of brefeldin-A and analyzed by intracellular flow cytometry **(C,D)**. **(A)** Data are combined from two independent experiments with each spot indicating an individual animal. Data are representative of three independent experiments. **(B)** Bars indicate the average of three technical replicates pooled from three individual animals per group. Data are representative of two independent experiments. **(C,D)** Values shown are normalized to the response of mice of that genotype (WT versus MUC1.Tg) given the control treatment (iso). Data are combined from two independent experiments and are representative of five to six mice per group. Bars represent mean ± SEM. *Indicates a *p*-value of <0.05; **indicates a *p*-value of <0.005.

We have yet to identify the source in the spleen of this early IL-10 production in self-antigen vaccinated mice. Every cell of the immune system can produce IL-10 given proper stimulation. However the kinetics and pattern of IL-10 production in MUC1p-vaccinated MUC1.Tg mice limits the possibilities considerably. The fact that IL-10 production was antigen dependent suggests a cell of the adaptive immune system. Regulatory T cells have previously been shown to be important in preventing MUC1p specific immune responses in MUC1.Tg mice (12, 33). However, preliminary experiments have been unable to identify IL-10 producing regulatory T cells in MUC1.Tg mice at rest or immediately following vaccination (data not shown), as has been shown in some models after self-peptide administration (34). Given that regulatory T cells can modulate the function of a wide variety of innate cells, including NK cells (35, 36) and DCs (37, 38), it is possible that through secretion of another cytokine or through direct interactions, they induce IL-10 production either directly or indirectly in another cell population.

Irrespective of the source, the self-antigen specific role of IL-10 reported in this paper supports IL-10 inhibition as a way of improving the efficacy of vaccines against self-antigens that are candidate tumor antigens. While our major success in this study was in improving CD4 T cell responses, we would hypothesize that CD8 T cell responses generated upon boosting would be improved as well in these animals as a consequence of generation of a larger population of helper CD4 T cells that are required for effective CD8 T cell memory differentiation (39, 40). The concern remains that any manipulation leading to enhanced responses to self/tumor antigens might cause adverse autoimmune reactions. However, current research has shown this concern can be addressed by proper antigen selection. For example, vaccines against self/tumor antigens MUC1 and α-lactalbumin have shown clinical and preclinical efficacy with no induction of autoimmunity (23, 41, 42). And vitiligo, caused by successful anti-melanoma vaccines is an autoimmune event that can be easily tolerated (43–45). Furthermore, while long term IL-10 deficiency can cause adverse autoimmune effects (46, 47), our data suggest that in order to improve the vaccine response, IL-10 would need to be blocked only transiently at the time of initial vaccination.

AUTHOR CONTRIBUTIONS

The research reported in this article was conducted by Douglas M. Marvel. Douglas M. Marvel and Olivera J. Finn jointly designed the experiments and prepared the manuscript.

ACKNOWLEDGMENTS

The authors would like to acknowledge Jia Xue for her expert assistance with the animal husbandry necessary for this work and Dr. Adam Farkas for stimulating discussions. This work was supported by the National Institutes of Health Grants R01 CA168392 and R01 CA56103 (to Olivera J. Finn), T32 CA082084 (Douglas M. Marvel), and the University of Pittsburgh Cancer Center Core Support Grant 2P30 CA47904.

REFERENCES

1. Moore KW, O'garra A, Malefyt RW, Vieira P, Mosmann TR. Interleukin-10. *Annu Rev Immunol* (1993) **11**:165–90. doi:10.1146/annurev.iy.11.040193.001121
2. Moore KW, De Waal Malefyt R, Coffman RL, O'garra A. Interleukin-10 and the interleukin-10 receptor. *Annu Rev Immunol* (2001) **19**:683–765. doi:10.1146/annurev.immunol.19.1.683
3. Asadullah K, Sterry W, Volk HD. Interleukin-10 therapy – review of a new approach. *Pharmacol Rev* (2003) **55**:241–69. doi:10.1124/pr.55.2.4
4. De Smedt T, Van Mechelen M, De Becker G, Urbain J, Leo O, Moser M. Effect of interleukin-10 on dendritic cell maturation and function. *Eur J Immunol* (1997) **27**:1229–35. doi:10.1002/eji.1830270526
5. Steinbrink K, Wolfl M, Jonuleit H, Knop J, Enk AH. Induction of tolerance by IL-10-treated dendritic cells. *J Immunol* (1997) **159**:4772–80.
6. Brossart P, Zobywalski A, Grünebach F, Behnke L, Stuhler G, Reichardt VL, et al. Tumor necrosis factor α and CD40 ligand antagonize the inhibitory effects of interleukin 10 on T-cell stimulatory capacity of dendritic cells. *Cancer Res* (2000) **60**:4485–92.
7. Turner MS, Kane LP, Morel PA. Dominant role of antigen dose in CD4+Foxp3+ regulatory T cell induction and expansion. *J Immunol* (2009) **183**:4895–903. doi:10.4049/jimmunol.0901459
8. Gottschalk RA, Corse E, Allison JP. TCR ligand density and affinity determine peripheral induction of Foxp3 in vivo. *J Exp Med* (2010) **207**:1701–11. doi:10.1084/jem.20091999
9. Mocellin S, Marincola FM, Young HA. Interleukin-10 and the immune response against cancer: a counterpoint. *J Leukoc Biol* (2005) **78**:1043–51. doi:10.1189/jlb.0705358
10. Brooks DG, Walsh KB, Elsaesser H, Oldstone MBA. IL-10 directly suppresses CD4 but not CD8 T cell effector and memory responses following acute viral infection. *Proc Natl Acad Sci U S A* (2010) **107**:3018–23. doi:10.1073/pnas.0914500107
11. Emmerich J, Mumm JB, Chan IH, Laface D, Truong H, Mcclanahan T, et al. IL-10 directly activates and expands tumor-resident CD8+ T cells without de novo infiltration from secondary lymphoid organs. *Cancer Res* (2012) **72**:3570–81. doi:10.1158/0008-5472.CAN-12-0721
12. Farkas AM, Marvel DM, Finn OJ. Antigen choice determines vaccine-induced generation of immunogenic versus tolerogenic dendritic cells that are marked by differential expression of pancreatic enzymes. *J Immunol* (2013) **190**:3319–27. doi:10.4049/jimmunol.1203321
13. Rowse GJ, Tempero RM, Vanlith ML, Hollingsworth MA, Gendler SJ. Tolerance and immunity to MUC1 in a human MUC1 transgenic murine model. *Cancer Res* (1998) **58**:315–21.
14. Turner MS, Cohen PA, Finn OJ. Lack of effective MUC1 tumor antigen-specific immunity in MUC1-transgenic mice results from a Th/T regulatory cell imbalance that can be corrected by adoptive transfer of wild-type Th cells. *J Immunol* (2007) **178**:2787–93.
15. Ryan SO, Turner MS, Gariepy J, Finn OJ. Tumor antigen epitopes interpreted by the immune system as self or abnormal-self differentially affect cancer vaccine responses. *Cancer Res* (2010) **70**:5788–96. doi:10.1158/0008-5472.CAN-09-4519
16. Soares MM, Mehta V, Finn OJ. Three different vaccines based on the 140-amino acid MUC1 peptide with seven tandemly repeated tumor-specific epitopes elicit distinct immune effector mechanisms in wild-type versus MUC1-transgenic mice with different potential for tumor rejection. *J Immunol* (2001) **166**:6555–63.
17. Kantoff PW, Higano CS, Shore ND, Berger ER, Small EJ, Penson DF, et al. Sipuleucel-T immunotherapy for castration-resistant prostate cancer. *N Engl J Med* (2010) **363**:411–22. doi:10.1056/NEJMoa1001294
18. Boikos SA, Antonarakis ES. Immunotherapy for prostate cancer enters its golden age. *Clin Med Insights Oncol* (2012) **6**:263–73. doi:10.4137/CMO.S7475
19. McCormack PL, Joura EA. Quadrivalent human papillomavirus (types 6, 11, 16, 18) recombinant vaccine (Gardasil(R)): a review of its use in the prevention of premalignant genital lesions, genital cancer and genital warts in women. *Drugs* (2010) **70**:2449–74. doi:10.2165/11204920-000000000-00000
20. McCormack PL, Joura EA. Spotlight on quadrivalent human papillomavirus (types 6, 11, 16, 18) recombinant vaccine (Gardasil(R)) in the prevention of premalignant genital lesions, genital cancer, and genital warts in women. *BioDrugs* (2011) **25**:339–43. doi:10.2165/11205060-000000000-00000
21. Czerniecki BJ, Roses RE, Koski GK. Development of vaccines for high-risk ductal carcinoma in situ of the breast. *Cancer Res* (2007) **67**:6531–4. doi:10.1158/0008-5472.CAN-07-0878
22. Kimura T, Finn OJ. MUC1 immunotherapy is here to stay. *Expert Opin Biol Ther* (2013) **13**:35–49. doi:10.1517/14712598.2012.725719
23. Kimura T, Mckolanis JR, Dzubinski LA, Islam K, Potter DM, Salazar AM, et al. MUC1 vaccine for individuals with advanced adenoma of the colon: a cancer immunoprevention feasibility study. *Cancer Prev Res* (2013) **6**:18–26. doi:10.1158/1940-6207.CAPR-12-0275
24. Liao JB, Disis ML. Therapeutic vaccines for ovarian cancer. *Gynecol Oncol* (2013) **130**:667–73. doi:10.1016/j.ygyno.2013.06.023
25. Wang B, Amerio P, Sauder DN. Role of cytokines in epidermal Langerhans cell migration. *J Leukoc Biol* (1999) **66**:33–9.
26. Demangel C, Bertolino P, Britton WJ. Autocrine IL-10 impairs dendritic cell (DC)-derived immune responses to mycobacterial infection by suppressing DC trafficking to draining lymph nodes and local IL-12 production. *Eur J Immunol* (2002) **32**:994–1002. doi:10.1002/1521-4141(200204)32:43.3.CO;2-Y
27. Macatonia SE, Doherty TM, Knight SC, O'garra A. Differential effect of IL-10 on dendritic cell-induced T cell proliferation and IFN-gamma production. *J Immunol* (1993) **150**:3755–65.
28. Commeren DL, Van Soest PL, Karimi K, Löwenberg B, Cornelissen JJ, Braakman E. Paradoxical effects of interleukin-10 on the maturation of murine myeloid dendritic cells. *Immunology* (2003) **110**:188–96. doi:10.1046/j.1365-2567.2003.01730.x
29. Murray HW, Lu CM, Mauze S, Freeman S, Moreira AL, Kaplan G, et al. Interleukin-10 (IL-10) in experimental visceral leishmaniasis and IL-10 receptor blockade as immunotherapy. *Infect Immun* (2002) **70**:6284–93. doi:10.1128/IAI.70.11.6284-6293.2002
30. Murray HW, Moreira AL, Lu CM, DeVecchio JL, Matsuhashi M, Ma X, et al. Determinants of response to interleukin-10 receptor blockade immunotherapy in experimental visceral leishmaniasis. *J Infect Dis* (2003) **188**:458–64. doi:10.1086/376510
31. Brooks DG, Lee AM, Elsaesser H, Mcgavern DB, Oldstone MBA. IL-10 blockade facilitates DNA vaccine-induced T cell responses and enhances clearance

of persistent virus infection. *J Exp Med* (2008) **205**:533–41. doi:10.1084/jem.20071948

32. Pitt JM, Stavropoulos E, Redford PS, Beebe AM, Bancroft GJ, Young DB, et al. Blockade of IL-10 signaling during Bacillus Calmette-Guérin vaccination enhances and sustains Th1, Th17, and innate lymphoid IFN-γ and IL-17 responses and increases protection to mycobacterium tuberculosis infection. *J Immunol* (2012) **189**:4079–87. doi:10.4049/jimmunol.1201061
33. Sugiura D, Denda-Nagai K, Takashima M, Murakami R, Nagai S, Takeda K, et al. Local effects of regulatory T cells in MUC1 transgenic mice potentiate growth of MUC1 expressing tumor cells in vivo. *PLoS One* (2012) **7**:e44770. doi:10.1371/journal.pone.0044770
34. Burkhart C, Liu GY, Anderton SM, Metzler B, Wraith DC. Peptide-induced T cell regulation of experimental autoimmune encephalomyelitis: a role for IL-10. *Int Immunol* (1999) **11**:1625–34. doi:10.1093/intimm/11.10.1625
35. Kerdiles Y, Ugolini S, Vivier E. T cell regulation of natural killer cells. *J Exp Med* (2013) **210**:1065–8. doi:10.1084/jem.20130960
36. Pedroza-Pacheco I, Madrigal A, Saudemont A. Interaction between natural killer cells and regulatory T cells: perspectives for immunotherapy. *Cell Mol Immunol* (2013) **10**:222–9. doi:10.1038/cmi.2013.2
37. Houot R, Perrot I, Garcia E, Durand I, Lebecque S. Human CD4+CD25 high regulatory T cells modulate myeloid but not plasmacytoid dendritic cells activation. *J Immunol* (2006) **176**:5293–8.
38. Veldhoen M, Moncrieffe H, Hocking RJ, Atkins CJ, Stockinger B. Modulation of dendritic cell function by naive and regulatory CD4+ T cells. *J Immunol* (2006) **176**:6202–10.
39. Sun JC, Bevan MJ. Defective CD8 T cell memory following acute infection without CD4 T cell help. *Science* (2003) **300**:339–42. doi:10.1126/science.1083317
40. Williams MA, Bevan MJ. Effector and memory CTL differentiation. *Annu Rev Immunol* (2007) **25**:171–92. doi:10.1146/annurev.immunol.25.022106.141548
41. Finn OJ, Forni G. Prophylactic cancer vaccines. *Curr Opin Immunol* (2002) **14**:172–7. doi:10.1016/S0952-7915(02)00317-5
42. Flemming A. Cancer: steps towards a prophylactic breast cancer vaccine. *Nat Rev Drug Discov* (2010) **9**:594–5. doi:10.1038/nrd3233
43. Overwijk WW, Lee DS, Surman DR, Irvine KR, Touloukian CE, Chan C-C, et al. Vaccination with a recombinant vaccinia virus encoding a "self" antigen induces autoimmune vitiligo and tumor cell destruction in mice: requirement for CD4+ T lymphocytes. *Proc Natl Acad Sci U S A* (1999) **96**:2982–7. doi:10.1073/pnas.96.6.2982
44. van Elsas A, Hurwitz AA, Allison JP. Combination immunotherapy of B16 melanoma using anti-cytotoxic T lymphocyte-associated antigen 4 (Ctla-4) and granulocyte/macrophage colony-stimulating factor (Gm-Csf)-producing vaccines induces rejection of subcutaneous and metastatic tumors accompanied by autoimmune depigmentation. *J Exp Med* (1999) **190**:355–66.
45. Byrne KT, Côté AL, Zhang P, Steinberg SM, Guo Y, Allie R, et al. Autoimmune melanocyte destruction is required for robust CD8+ memory T cell responses to mouse melanoma. *J Clin Invest* (2011) **121**:1797–809. doi:10.1172/JCI44849
46. Kotlarz D, Beier R, Murugan D, Diestelhorst J, Jensen O, Boztug K, et al. Loss of interleukin-10 signaling and infantile inflammatory bowel disease: implications for diagnosis and therapy. *Gastroenterology* (2012) **143**:347–55. doi:10.1053/j.gastro.2012.04.045
47. Shah N, Kammermeier J, Elawad M, Glocker E-O. Interleukin-10 and interleukin-10-receptor defects in inflammatory bowel disease. *Curr Allergy Asthma Rep* (2012) **12**:373–9. doi:10.1007/s11882-012-0286-z

10

CD4$^+$ T cell-receptor repertoire diversity is compromised in the spleen but not in the bone marrow of aged mice due to private and sporadic clonal expansions

Eric Shifrut[1], Kuti Baruch[2], Hilah Gal[1], Wilfred Ndifon[1], Aleksandra Deczkowska[2], Michal Schwartz[2] and Nir Friedman[1]*

[1] Department of Immunology, Weizmann Institute of Science, Rehovot, Israel
[2] Department of Neurobiology, Weizmann Institute of Science, Rehovot, Israel

Edited by:
Carmen Molina-Paris, University of Leeds, UK

Reviewed by:
António Gil Castro, University of Minho, Portugal
Maria L. Toribio, Spanish Research Council (CSIC), Spain

***Correspondence:**
Nir Friedman, Department of Immunology, Weizmann Institute of Science, 76100 Rehovot, Israel
e-mail: nir.friedman@weizmann.ac.il

Reduction in T cell receptor (TCR) diversity in old age is considered as a major cause for immune complications in the elderly population. Here, we explored the consequences of aging on the TCR repertoire in mice using high-throughput sequencing (TCR-seq). We mapped the TCRβ repertoire of CD4+ T cells isolated from bone marrow (BM) and spleen of young and old mice. We found that TCRβ diversity is reduced in spleens of aged mice but not in their BM. Splenic CD4+ T cells were also skewed toward an effector memory phenotype in old mice, while BM cells preserved their memory phenotype with age. Analysis of Vβ and Jβ gene usage across samples, as well as comparison of CDR3 length distributions, showed no significant age dependent changes. However, comparison of the frequencies of amino-acid (AA) TCRβ sequences between samples revealed repertoire changes that occurred at a more refined scale. The BM-derived TCRβ repertoire was found to be similar among individual mice regardless of their age. In contrast, the splenic repertoire of old mice was not similar to those of young mice, but showed an increased similarity with the BM repertoire. Each old-mouse had a private set of expanded TCRβ sequences. Interestingly, a fraction of these sequences was found also in the BM of the same individual, sharing the same nucleotide sequence. Together, these findings show that the composition and phenotype of the CD4+ T cell BM repertoire are relatively stable with age, while diversity of the splenic repertoire is severely reduced. This reduction is caused by idiosyncratic expansions of tens to hundreds of T cell clonotypes, which dominate the repertoire of each individual. We suggest that these private and abundant clonotypes are generated by sporadic clonal expansions, some of which correspond to pre-existing BM clonotypes. These organ- and age-specific changes of the TCRβ repertoire have implications for understanding and manipulating age-associated immune decline.

Keywords: TCR repertoire, aging, immune niche, clonal dominance, high throughput sequencing, TCR-seq, CD4+ T cells

INTRODUCTION

Effective T cell immunity is founded on a diverse T cell-receptor (TCR) repertoire. This diversity, generated by the V(D)J recombination mechanism in the thymus (1), is essential for coping with the plethora of invading and fast evolving pathogens. Loss of diversity, whether naturally occurring with age (2) or induced (3), is associated with increased susceptibility to infections, as well as reduced responses to vaccination (4, 5). One of the most dramatic manifestations of aging on the immune system is thymus involution. Toward old age, both in human and mice (6), the thymic epithelial tissue is replaced by connective and adipose tissue (7), causing reduction in *de novo* production of naive T cells through differentiation of precursor cells. Without thymic activity, naïve T cells are thought to be generated only through homeostatic proliferation of existing single-positive T cells (CD4$^+$ and CD8$^+$ T cells). In adult humans, this is the main mechanism for maintenance of the naïve T cell pool, while in mice there is evidence of lingering thymic output of naïve T cells (8).

Although both the phenotypic balance between memory and naïve T cells as well as the ratio of CD4$^+$ to CD8$^+$ T cells do not alter drastically with age (9), this does not indicate that the TCR repertoire is static (10). By using spectratyping to measure the distributions of TCR lengths across Vβ chains, studies have shown that both the CD8$^+$ and CD4$^+$ TCR repertoires in old mice were skewed compared to young mice (11). Moreover, the perturbations in CDR3 lengths were idiosyncratic to each individual. Deviations from the normal distribution for CDR3 lengths are assumed to be caused by massive T cell expansions during aging both in mice and humans (12). These changes in the composition of the TCR repertoire with aging can create vulnerability to pathogens, such as influenza (13), by providing incomplete clonal coverage.

The bone marrow (BM) is considered as the principal immune niche for both CD4$^+$ and CD8$^+$ memory T cells (14). Following massive clonal expansion during primary immune response against a pathogen, the contraction phase leaves only a small fraction of antigen-specific memory T cells. These long-lived cells reside mainly in the BM and represent the main T cell reservoir for secondary responses. In line with these observations, the BM was proposed as a "nest" for memory T cells (15), which can be expanded by homeostasis-driven proliferation for fighting viral infections (16), tumor (17), and even age-related cognitive loss (18, 19). It was demonstrated that antigen-specific CD4$^+$ T lymphocytes which relocate throughout life to the BM have a slow turnover, but can fast react as professional memory CD4$^+$ T cells, when stimulated (14).

Although effects of aging on TCR diversity have been evaluated in antigen-specific clones (10), it is still unclear what global changes the TCR repertoire undergoes during lifespan. These large-scale changes have been studied mostly using spectratyping (20, 21), a technique that maps the repertoire with very low resolution. Furthermore, the differences between immune niches, such as the BM and spleen (SPL), in terms of their distinct TCR repertoires and their development with age remain to be explored.

Here we show that the TCRβ repertoire of CD4$^+$ T cells is shaped both by their immunological niche and by age. We used high throughput sequencing to map the murine TCRβ repertoire, of both splenic and BM-derived CD4$^+$ T cells. Aged mice display a marked reduction in diversity of splenic T cells, while diversity of BM-derived T cells is relatively constant with age. Moreover, the TCRβ repertoire of splenic T cells in aged mice becomes more similar to the repertoire of BM-derived T cells. The loss of diversity in old mice is associated with expansion of tens to hundreds T cell clones, and occurs in parallel to segregation of the repertoires of different mice, creating distinct and private immune signatures in each aged individual. Finally, we evaluated clonal expansion and convergent recombination (22) in aging in order to find evidence for the mechanism that creates private repertoires in old age. We show multiple occurrences of sharing at the nucleotide (nt) level between TCR sequences derived from BM T cells and from massively expanded SPL T cell clones of the same aged animal. These results suggest that the degenerate repertoire in old age is shaped by rare events of massive clonal expansions which allow distinctive T cell clones to dominate the immune repertoire of individuals.

MATERIALS AND METHODS

ANIMALS

Inbred male 6- to 8-week-old C57BL/6 mice were supplied by the Animal Breeding Center of The Weizmann Institute of Science. Inbred male 17- to 20-months-old C57BL/6 mice were supplied by the National Institute on Aging (NIA). Aged mice were allowed 1 month adaptation period following shipment from the NIA to our laboratory. All animals were handled according to regulations formulated by The Weizmann Institute's Animal Care and Use Committee and maintained in a pathogen-free environment.

SAMPLE PREPARATION AND CD4+ T CELLS ISOLATION

Prior to tissue collection, mice were intracardially perfused with PBS. Spleens were mashed with a syringe plunger and treated with ammonium-chloride potassium (ACK) lysing buffer to remove erythrocytes. BM was extracted from the femur and tibiae of the mice. Single-cell suspensions of the samples were loaded on MACS column (Miltenyi Biotec) and CD4$^+$ T cells were isolated according to manufacturer's protocol.

FLOW CYTOMETRY AND ANALYSIS

The following fluorochrome-labeled mAbs were used according to the manufacturers' protocols: PercpCy5.5-conjugated anti-TCRβ, PE-conjugated anti-CD4, FITC-conjugated anti-CD44, and APC-conjugated anti-CD62L (BD Pharmingen and eBioscience). Cells were analyzed on an LSRII cytometer (BD Biosciences) using FACSDiva (BD Biosciences) and FlowJo (Tree Star) softwares. In each experiment, relevant negative-control groups and single-stained samples for each tissue were used to identify the populations of interest and to exclude others.

LIBRARY PREPARATION FOR TCR-SEQ

All libraries in this work were prepared and pre-processed as published (23). Briefly, we extracted total RNA from CD4$^+$ T cells (from spleen or BM) of C57BL/6 mice using RNeasy Mini Kit (Qiagen). The RNA was reverse transcribed using SuperScript II reverse transcriptase (Invitrogen) and a TCR Cβ-specific primer linked to the 3′-end Illumina sequencing adapter. The resulting cDNA was then amplified using PCR (Phusion; Finnzymes) with a Cβ-3′adp primer and a set of 23 Vβ-specific 5′ primers, each of which was anchored to a restriction site sequence for the ACUI restriction enzyme. PCR products were then cleaned using QIAquick PCR purification kit (Qiagen), followed by enzymatic digestion with ACUI (New England BioLabs). The ACUI enzyme was used to cleave the amplicons such that sequencing starts closer to the V-D junction region. This allows for good coverage of CDR3β with a single Illumina read. This was followed by ligation of a 5′ Illumina adaptor (T4 ligase; Fermentas), which also contained a 3-nt tag for sample multiplexing. A second round of PCR amplification was performed, using primers for the 5′ and 3′ Illumina adapters. Final PCR products were run on a 2% agarose gel, cut at the desired length, and purified using Wizard SV Gel and PCR Clean-Up System (Promega) to produce the final library. The libraries were sequenced using Genome Analyzer II (Illumina).

PRE-PROCESSING AND ERROR CORRECTION FOR RAW READS

We filtered out raw reads containing bases with Q-value $\leq$30, and then separated the remaining reads according to their barcodes. Then, we aligned the reads to each of the germline Vβ/Jβ gene segments from IMGT (24) using the Smith–Waterman algorithm. Each read was assigned its best-aligning Vβ/Jβ if the number of matching nt (alignment length) was above a threshold: 11 nt for Vβ, 9 nt for Jβ. To reduce the effect of sequencing errors, we clustered (hierarchically) reads assigned the same Vβ and Jβ genes to correct up to 2 nt misincorporation errors. Then, we annotated the sequences by matching the Dβ to the junction, identifying deleted/inserted nt and elongated the read to its full CDR3β length (by IMGT convention). Finally, we translated the nt sequences into amino acid (AA) CDR3β. For the entire analysis here, we used only sequences that are fully annotated (V, J segments assigned), are in-frame (i.e., they encode for a functional peptide, without stop codons), have a cluster size of at least two and have less than 2 bp enzyme cleavage error. We also corrected the copy-number, to adjust for PCR and sub-sampling bias, as published (23).

STATISTICAL ANALYSIS

All statistical analysis was performed using R Statistical Software (R (25)). We also used ShortRead package (26) for the pre-processing pipeline, "ineq" package (27) to calculate the Gini coefficient and "ggplot2" (28) for generating figures. Statistical tests performed are stated in the text.

RESULTS

DIVERSITY OF THE SPLENIC TCRβ REPERTOIRE IS COMPROMISED IN OLD MICE

We aimed to explore the changes in the repertoire landscape at old age, with emphasis on evaluating the diversity of the TCR repertoire. To accomplish this, we measured using TCR-seq the TCRβ repertoire in mice from two age groups: 6–8 weeks old (termed "young," $n = 3$) and 17–20 months old ("old," $n = 3$). In addition, to evaluate the differences between immune organs, we isolated CD4$^+$ T cells from the SPL and BM of each mouse. Properties of all samples are detailed in **Table 1**. On average, we have ~2e6 sequence reads that have passed the quality threshold (see Materials and Methods), for each sample. These quality-filtered reads produced an average of ~2.8e5 reads that could be annotated with full CDR3β sequence properties (see Materials and Methods), including translation to an in-frame AA sequence. BM samples resulted in about 10-fold less annotated reads compared with SPL samples. In total, we have found 108,124 distinct CDR3β AA sequences in these 12 samples.

To evaluate the diversity of TCR sequences in the samples, we first checked the cumulative frequencies of clonotypes, ordered by their rank. Hence, we sorted all of the AA clonotypes by their frequency in ascending order. To adjust for varying sample size, we normalized the rank between 0 (the rarest clone) to 1 (the most abundant clone). We then calculated the mean cumulative frequency for increasing rank bins across mice belonging to the same group (**Figure 1A**). In this representation, also known as a Lorenz curve, a repertoire that has maximal diversity (i.e., all clonotypes are present in equal frequency), will be plotted as a straight line across the diagonal. In contrast, a skewed repertoire (i.e., few and very abundant clonotypes dominate the sample) will deviate below the diagonal with a sharp incline only toward the higher ranks. We observe that the most skewed repertoire belongs to the old SPL, while BM from young mice is the most diverse of the repertoires studied here. The old SPL repertoire had a decreased diversity compared with that of the young SPL, while the BM repertoire showed only a slight decrease in diversity with age.

As another measure for repertoire skewness, we applied the Gini coefficient for inequality, used to measure evenness of wealth distribution in economics, which was applied recently for evaluation of TCR repertoire diversity (29). High values of the Gini coefficient, which ranges from 0 to 1, are indicative of a skewed repertoire. We calculated the Gini coefficient for each of the samples and grouped the results by organ and age (**Figure 1B**). The Gini coefficient is highest for the old SPL group, consistent with the Lorenz curve. The decline in clonal equality with age is evident in the spleen ($p < 0.05$, Student's t test), but not in the BM ($p = 0.42$).

We used an additional metric for measuring diversity in TCR samples, the Simpson's diversity index (30, 31). This metric takes into account both the number of unique clonotypes and their relative frequency. The Simpson's diversity index represents the probability that any two clonotypes randomly drawn from the sample will have different sequences. The Simpson index ranges from 0 to 1, with 1 representing maximal diversity, i.e., all clonotypes are present in equal sizes. For each sample, we calculated the mean Simpson's diversity index for 500 randomly sampled clones in 1,000 iterations (**Figure 1C**). Consistent with our observation for the skewness of the repertoire in old mice, the old SPL group has a significantly lower diversity compared with the young SPL [$p < 0.001$, permutations test, see Ref. (30)]. To conclude, we find that the diversity of the splenic TCRβ repertoire is significantly reduced at old age, based on the three analysis methods. Reduction in the diversity of the BM repertoire is minimal and not statistically significant with current sample sizes.

Table 1 | Sample properties.

Sample name	Age group	Organ	Raw reads	Total annotated	Unique reads
ySP1	Young	Spleen	2,653,822	1,075,670	77,991
ySP2	Young	Spleen	804,529	134,372	12,298
ySP3	Young	Spleen	1,426,160	470,363	32,293
yBM1	Young	BM	1,538,612	84,111	6,167
yBM2	Young	BM	1,211,410	4,492	722
yBM3	Young	BM	2,857,600	65,879	6,183
oSP1	Old	Spleen	4,325,524	459,288	18,363
oSP2	Old	Spleen	2,790,495	384,664	17,004
oSP3	Old	Spleen	2,226,719	579,364	9,594
oBM1	Old	BM	1,747,231	16,653	1,443
oBM2	Old	BM	2,036,502	87,758	8,964
oBM3	Old	BM	1,533,444	52,905	4,076

SPLENIC CD4$^+$ T CELLS ARE SKEWED TOWARD AN EFFECTOR MEMORY PHENOTYPE

Next, we wished to determine whether these two immunological compartments, SPL and BM, age differently in terms of the memory phenotype of CD4$^+$ T cells. Using flow cytometry, we measured the proportions of effector memory (T_{EM}) and central memory (T_{CM}) phenotypes in the CD4$^+$ memory T cell compartment (**Figure 1D**). We found that T_{EM} CD4$^+$ T cells are significantly more abundant in spleens of old mice (93.5 ± 2.7%) compared to young mice (76.7 ± 1.8%). Increase in the effector phenotype could point to expansion driven by antigen-specific responses and suggests that these CD4$^+$ T_{EM} cells contribute to the skewed repertoire we observe in old spleen. No significant change in T_{EM}/T_{CM} balance was observed in BM samples between age groups (**Figure 1D**), suggesting maintenance of the phenotypic balance in the BM niche.

ORGAN SPECIFIC PATTERNS OF Vβ AND Jβ SEGMENT USAGE ARE CONSTANT WITH AGE

We next examined how the gene segment usage changes with aging (**Figures 2A,B**). Qualitatively, the Jβ distributions look similar in all samples, with few segments that differ in frequency between spleen and BM. For example, Jβ1.3 is over-expressed

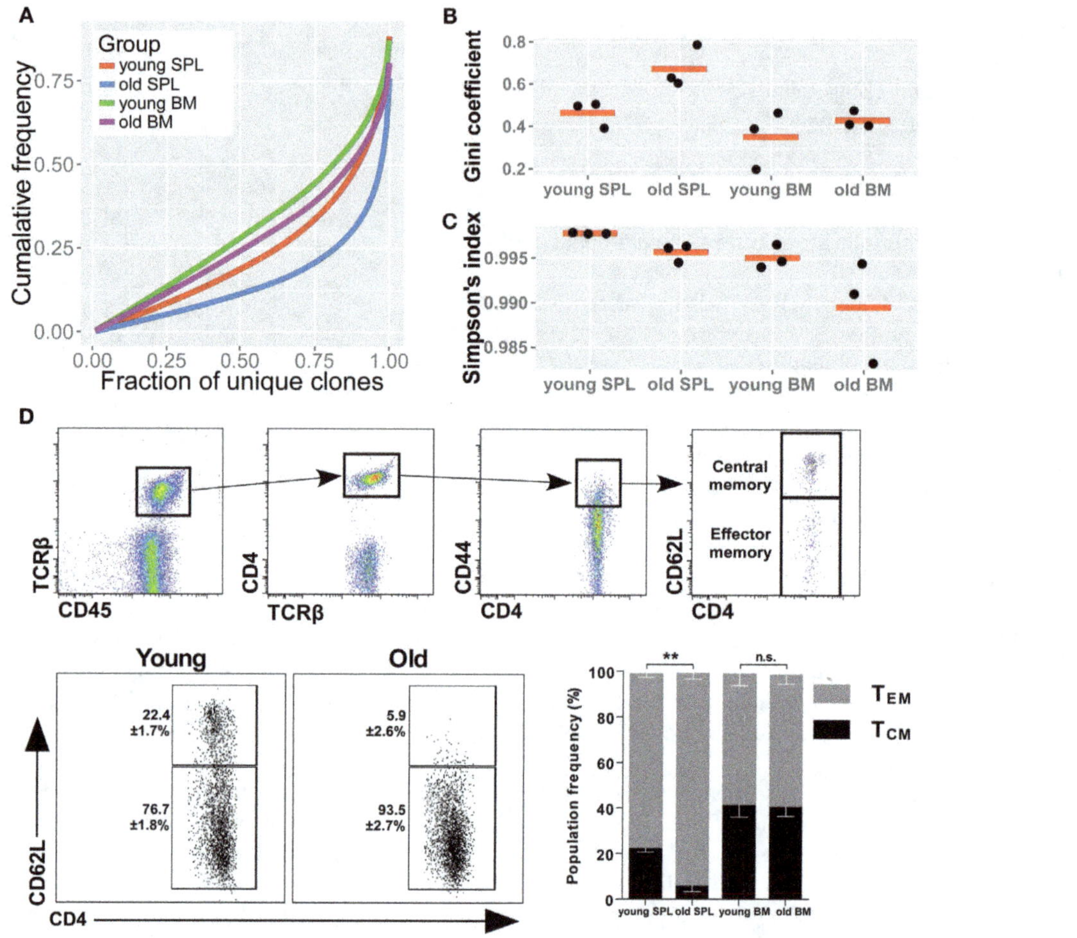

FIGURE 1 | TCRβ repertoire is less diverse in the spleens of old mice. **(A)** Skewness of the TCRβ repertoire for CD4+ T cells from spleen and BM of young and aged mice. For each mouse, clonotypes were ordered by frequency. We then compared the cumulative frequency at each rank (normalized to sample size). From the curves, which represent the mean for each group, we observe that old SPL has the most skewed repertoire. **(B)** Gini coefficient per group. Horizontal lines represent the mean for each group and dots are individual samples. Old SPL group has the highest values, thus it is the most skewed. **(C)** Simpson's diversity index calculated for each mouse (dots). Horizontal lines represent the mean for each group. The old SPL group has a significantly lower diversity than the young SPL group. **(D)** Phenotypic changes of CD4+ memory T cells in aging. Top panels show flow cytometric gating strategy. Old spleen samples have significantly higher percentage of effector memory T cells compared to young spleen samples (bottom panels and bar graph). BM samples have similar central/effector memory ratios across age groups (mean ± SE of each group ($n = 4$–5 per group; $^{**}P < 0.01$; Student's t test).

in SPL samples (both young and old) compared to BM samples, whereas Jβ2.7 is under-expressed in SPL samples. The Vβ distributions vary between samples to a larger extent, evidenced also by the overall lower correlation scores (**Figure 2C**). Inter-group correlations in gene segment usage (**Figure 2D**) show similarity between organ specific repertoires across age, which is higher than between repertoires of different organs within age groups. Thus, gene segment usage is more similar between young and old BM samples, and between young and old SPL samples; it is less similar between BM and SPL samples, both in young and aged mice. This suggests that the tissue microenvironment plays a major factor in shaping of the TCRβ repertoire.

Spectratyping analysis is often used to test for skewness and clonal dominance in TCR repertoires. Thus, we generated virtual spectratypes of CDR3 length distributions for sequences grouped by their Vβ segment. Specifically, as our analysis detected skewness in old SPL samples, we aimed to test if a particular CDR3 length was dominant in that age group (see **Figure 2E** for representative plots). This analysis revealed length distributions that are largely homogenous across samples, with neither significant changes in skewness nor enrichment of a specific CDR3 length. Thus, coarse analysis of the CD4$^+$ TCR repertoire, comparing gene segment usage as well as spectratyping analysis, could not explain the measured loss in diversity in aged mice.

BM TCR REPERTOIRES ARE SIMILAR BETWEEN MICE AND AGE GROUPS, WHILE SPL TCR REPERTOIRES CHANGE AND BECOME PRIVATE WITH AGE

TCR-seq allows for comparison of repertoires at a higher resolution, beyond gene segment usage or CDR3 length distributions,

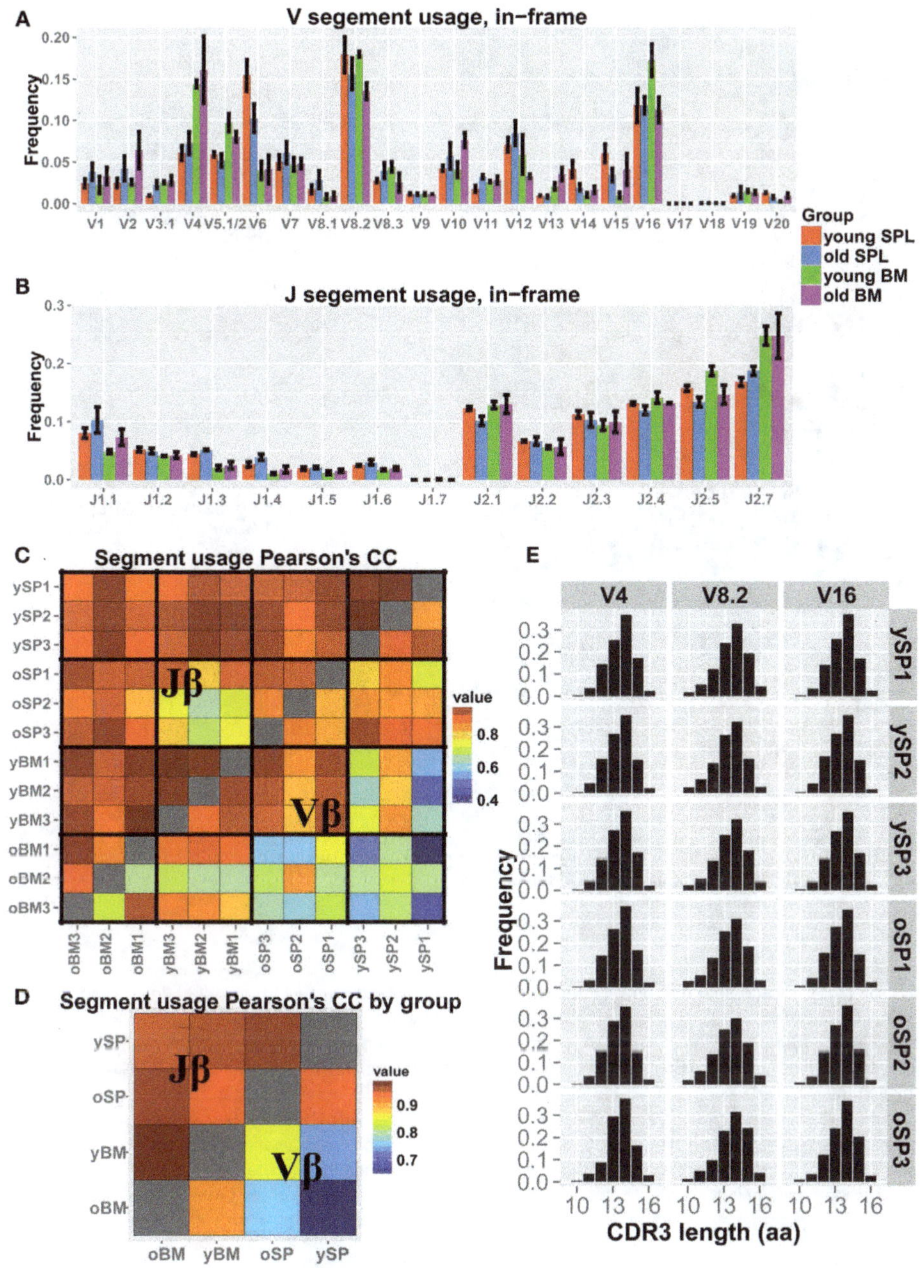

FIGURE 2 | Vβ and Jβ usage in aged mice. (A,B) Each bar represents the mean frequency of a gene segment in that group of mice. Error bars are SEM. **(C)** Pairwise correlations of Vβ and Jβ usage between all pairs of mice. We observe higher correlations between mice in Jβ usage (upper triangle) compared to Vβ usage (lower triangle). **(D)** Correlation of the gene segment usage between all pairs of mice averaged over groups. We detect a general high correlation in the data, with inter-tissue similarity across age groups. BM = bone marrow, SPL = spleen, $n = 3$ for all groups. **(E)** "Virtual" spectratypes. Each bar represents the relative frequency of a particular CDR3 length (in amino acids) for three representative Vβ segments, stated above each panel, measured across individual SPL samples. No significant changes could be detected in CDR3 length distributions across age groups.

by analysis at the level of individual TCR sequences. Hence, we assessed similarity between samples by comparing frequencies of overlapping clonotypes. This comparison is more stringent than measuring Vβ/Jβ usage, as we search for the same exact AA clonotypes and compare their observed frequency in each pair of samples. We find that, in accordance to our findings for the Vβ/Jβ usage, all BM samples, regardless of age, display a high similarity in the frequencies of shared AA clonotypes (**Figure 3A**). We also notice that the old SPL group is non-homogenous, i.e., the inter-sample similarity (between individuals) is lower when compared to that found in the young SPL group. To further illustrate this point, we calculated the mean of all pairwise correlation coefficients for each group comparison (e.g., young SPL vs. old SPL, young SPL vs. old BM, etc.). This analysis estimates the overall

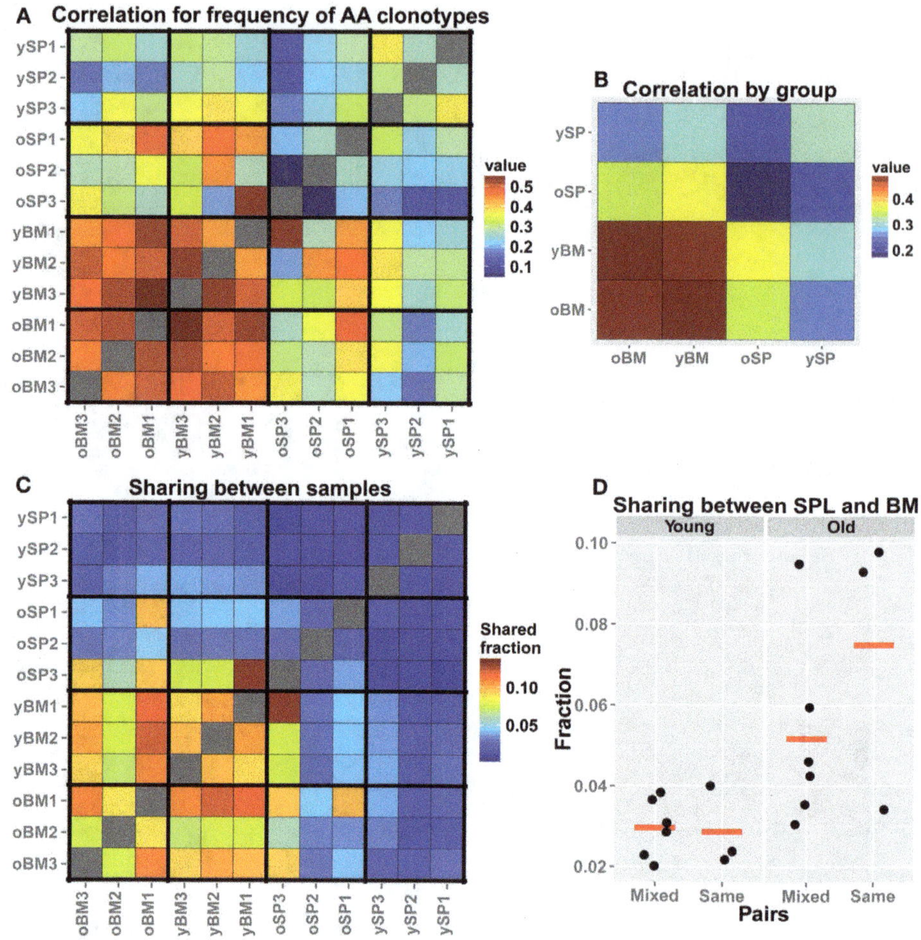

FIGURE 3 | Comparison of the TCR repertoires in different tissues and age groups at the level of AA clonotypes. **(A)** For each pair of mice, we calculated the Spearman's correlation for frequencies of clonotypes that are shared by that pair. As the frequency distribution of TCR repertoire is over-dispersed, we used the log-transformed values as input for the rank correlation test. The BM groups have high similarity between the samples, and also between age groups. **(B)** For each group of mice ($n=3$), we averaged the correlation scores of **(A)**. Scores along the diagonal indicate the intra-group similarity. Again, the homogeneity in the BM samples within groups and across age is evident. In addition, the repertoire of the old SPL group has a higher correlation with the young BM and old BM groups, and a low intra-group correlation. **(C)** Sharing of clones between samples. From each sample, we randomly chose 300 AA clones and calculated pairwise sharing. The values represent the fraction of the sample that is shared between any particular pair, averaged over 100 iterations. BM repertoires show high level of sharing between individual mice and across age groups. **(D)** A comparison of sharing between BM and SPL repertoires within the same animal or from different animals (Mixed).

similarity between groups (off-diagonal elements in the matrix of **Figure 3B**) and also between samples from the same group (diagonal elements, **Figure 3B**). We observe that the old SPL group has the lowest within-group correlation, and that it is similar to some degree to the young BM and old BM groups, but not to the young SPL group. This suggests that, in aged mice, some clones that were resident in the BM at younger age have migrated to the spleen. BM samples are similar both between and within age groups (**Figure 3B**).

As another measure for similarity, we evaluated the number of overlapping sequences between pairs of samples. In order to control for different sample sizes (**Table 1**), we randomly sampled a collection of 300 clonotypes from each sample and tested how many of these clonotypes are shared between all possible pairs of samples. We iterated this test 100 times to reduce sampling noise and calculated the mean for each pair of samples (**Figure 3C**). We found that the fraction of shared clones within the BM samples is higher than within SPL samples of both age groups. Average sharing of 10% was found between the young BM samples and 9% between the old BM samples. Sharing between SPL samples was much lower (1% for young SPL samples and 3% for old SPL samples). Moreover, 10% of clones are shared on average between young and old BM samples, whereas only 1% are shared between young and old SPL samples. This supports our previous results showing that aging of the immune system affects the composition of the SPL repertoire, but has little influence on the repertoire of BM-resident CD4^{+} T cells.

We next focused on the inter-tissue sharing of clones by comparing the overlap between SPL and BM repertoires from the same animal, to the overlap observed between SPL and BM repertoires taken from different animals (**Figure 3D**). In general, there are more clones shared across niches in old animals compared to young animals. Interestingly, we notice that in two out of three old mice, more clones are shared between SPL and BM repertoires that are derived from the same animal, compared with SPL and BM repertoires that are derived from different animals. However, we do not observe this pattern in young animals. These results suggest that with age, a private set of clones is expanded in each individual, contributing to the reduction in SPL repertoire diversity. Furthermore, as the overlap between the repertoires of the spleen and BM niches increases in old age, the repertoire of the whole animal becomes less diverse and degenerate.

CLONAL DOMINANCE IS PREVALENT IN SPLENIC CD4$^+$ T CELLS FROM OLD MICE

Following our observation that the repertoire of splenic T cells from old mice becomes less diverse, private and more similar to the BM repertoire, we next focused on analysis of properties of specific clones that contribute to these phenomena. To that end, we first pooled the top 300 AA clonotypes from each sample to a unified list of 2,108 unique AA sequences. Then, we clustered the log-transformed frequencies for all the sequences in the unified list across all samples (**Figure 4A**). We observe that young SPL samples share many of these top clonotypes, indicating a baseline similarity in the repertoire of young mice. In contrast, the old SPL samples are distinct from each other and each individual presents a unique subset of highly abundant clonotypes, which have intermediate to low frequencies in the young SPL. Furthermore, BM samples from old mice share several abundant clones with their paired SPL samples, consistent with the intra-mouse sharing we observed above (**Figure 3D**).

To reveal if the sharing of AA clonotypes in the old mice samples is also present at the nt level, we picked three representative AA clonotypes that are shared between the SPL and BM samples of old mice (**Figure 4B**). Strikingly, we found that in all three cases the same nt sequence encodes the AA clonotype that is highly frequent in both the SPL and BM. This is a strong indication that the event of clonal expansion occurred for a particular T cell clone, causing clonal dominance in aged mice, which is evident in both BM and SPL of the animal. In contrast, AA clonotypes that are highly frequent in young SPL samples typically show high convergent recombination where many nt sequences encode for the same AA clonotype (**Figure 4B**).

Following this observation, we extended this analysis and counted the number of nt clones that are shared between BM and SPL of the same animal, which are not shared by any other sample (SPL or BM) from other animals. We find that more nt sequences are shared exclusively between the BM and SPL of the same animal in old mice, but not in young mice (**Figure 4C**). This reflects again the private repertoires generated in old age, in parallel with the increased similarity between the BM and SPL repertoires.

These results suggest that expanded clonotypes in aged mice show clonal dominance, that is, the same TCR nt sequence is responsible for most observed TCRs that have the same AA sequence. To test this hypothesis, we directly calculated clonal dominance in old mice compared to young mice. For each mouse, we considered only the 300 most abundant AA clonotypes that are encoded by at least two distinct nt sequences. Then, we calculated the ratio between frequencies of the most abundant nt sequence and the least abundant nt sequence encoding each AA clonotype (**Figure 4D**). In the old SPL group, there is over a 100-fold difference on average, between the maximal frequency and the minimal frequency of nt sequences coding for the same AA sequence. This ratio, R, is significantly higher in old SPL samples ($R = 116$) than in young SPL ($R = 36$). The ratio in the BM is low for both age groups ($R = 13$ for young BM and $R = 16$ for old BM). This supports the hypothesis that expanded clonotypes in the old SPL represent events of massive clonal expansion of a particular T cell clone.

Finally, to illustrate the global changes that the repertoire undergoes with aging, we plot the number of unique nt sequences encoding for the same AA clonotype (convergent recombination level) against the frequency of that clonotype, for all AA clonotypes from all spleen samples (**Figure 4E**). We notice that the old SPL group contains a subset of clonotypes that are highly expanded and have low to moderate convergent recombination (encoded by up to 10 different nt sequences). Clonotypes with similar properties are not found in the young SPL group. This supports the hypothesis that sporadic clonal expansion is a major factor in shaping the repertoire in old mice. Also, there are very few clonotypes ($n = 3$, 0.007% of the clonotypes) with convergent recombination higher than 10 in the old SPL group, whereas in the young SPL group there are many such clonotypes ($n = 152$, 0.16%).

DISCUSSION

The immune system undergoes changes with aging, contributing to an overall increase in neurodegenerative diseases and decrease in autoimmune inflammatory diseases. In addition, susceptibility to infectious diseases inclines with age (32) due to a combination of several factors such as immune senescence (33), transcriptional changes (34), and loss of *de novo* production of naïve T cells (35). Aged individuals are particularly vulnerable to newly encountered pathogens, as TCR diversity is severely diminished in old age. Here we explored the consequences of aging on the TCR repertoire in mice, with focus on the underlying causes for loss of diversity.

We applied TCR-seq on CD4$^+$ T cells isolated from the BM and spleen of young and aged mice. First, our focus was on measuring diversity across all samples. As observed before for CD8$^+$ T cells (20), we found that the diversity of the splenic CD4$^+$ T cell compartment also declines in aged mice. Reduced diversity was revealed both by high Gini inequality coefficient and a low Simpson diversity index. However, in BM samples only a minor reduction of diversity was detected with aging, which was not statistically significant. Examining the memory phenotype of the CD4$^+$ T cells in these two niches revealed a similar pattern; while in the spleen the memory phenotype of the cells strongly shifted toward effector memory during aging, the proportions of effector and central memory T cells in the BM remained constant. This can be attributed to the nature of the BM immune niche as an immune privileged hematopoiesis site (36), allowing maintenance of only a small subset of T cell clonotypes thus less affected by clonal attrition. Clonal expansion in the BM may be inhibited due to the abundance of quiescence-inducing signals which prevent

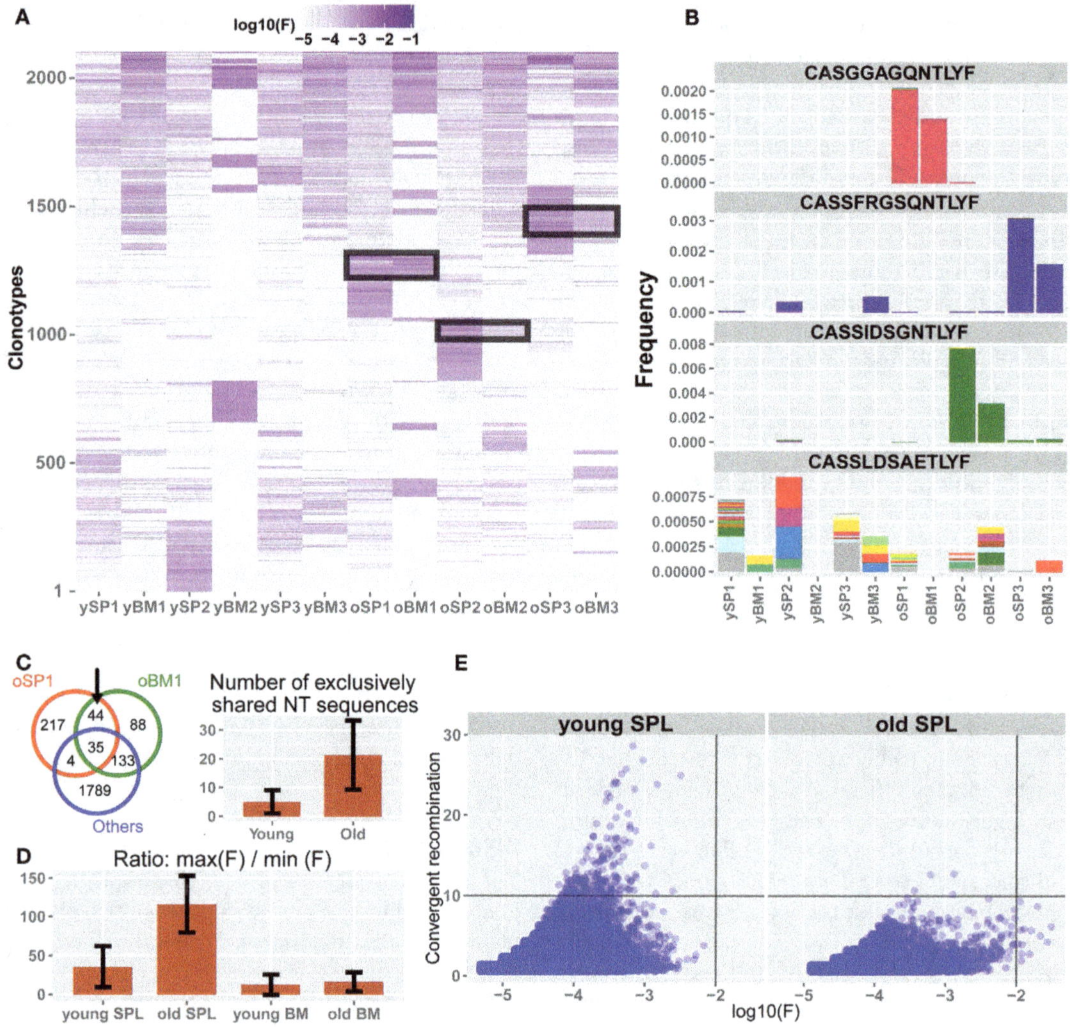

FIGURE 4 | The TCRβ repertoire of old mice is shaped by private clonal expansions. (A) Top 300 ranking AA clonotypes from all samples (total of 2,108 clonotypes) were clustered using Euclidian distance. Paired samples from the same animal are adjacent to each other. In old SPL there are subsets of enriched clones, which are unique to each mouse. Also, part of that subset is present in high frequency in the matching BM sample from the same animal (black frames). **(B)** Frequencies of four selected AA clonotypes across all samples. Stacked bars show the nt sequences, uniquely colored, that encode the AA sequence stated above the panel. Top 3 panels show representative clonotypes that are expanded and private in SPL and BM of old mice. Remarkably, these AA sequences are encoded by the same nt sequence in the spleen and BM of these animals. The bottom panel shows a typical abundant AA clonotype in young SPL samples, showing a high level of convergent recombination across most samples in which it is found. **(C)** Sharing of top 300 nt sequences between SPL and BM of the same animal. For each mouse, we calculated the number of exclusively shared nt sequences. The Venn diagram (left) shows an example in which 44 sequences are exclusively shared by BM and SPL of old mouse #1, and are not found in any other sample. Bar plot (right) shows that there are on average more exclusively shared nt sequences within SPL and BM of the same animal in old mice compared to young mice. Error bars indicate standard error. **(D)** Evaluation of clonal dominance. Bars show the average ratio between the frequency of the most frequent and the least frequent nt sequence encoding for the same AA sequence. Values were calculated for the top 300 AA clonotypes from each sample. The ratio is significantly higher in old SPL samples compared to young SPL ($p < 0.05$, Student's *t* test), suggesting clonal dominance. **(E)** Convergent recombination (# of nt sequences encoding each AA sequence) of AA clonotypes is plotted against their frequency. In old SPL the scatter shows a subset of high frequency clones that are encoded by less than 10 nt sequences (lower-right quadrant). In contrast, in young SPL many clonotypes show high convergent recombination (upper-left quadrant).

extensive proliferation of stem/progenitor cells, found in the BM as a hematopoietic niche (37).

We next evaluated the patterns of gene segment usage in our dataset. Consistent with our previous observation (23), Jβ usage is similar across samples and is not influenced significantly by tissue specificity or age. In general, the highest correlation in Vβ and Jβ usage is observed between the BM samples from both age groups, indicating a relatively stable TCR repertoire in the BM niche across age. However, analysis of distributions of gene segment usage and of CDR3 length do not show significant age-related differences that can explain the observed loss of splenic repertoire diversity. Thus, certain aspects of repertoire dynamics can be evaluated only with increased resolution, achieved by high throughput methods such as TCR-seq. This may have masked clear detection of decline in repertoire diversity with age in the $CD4^+$ compartment in previous studies that used spectratyping for evaluation of repertoire diversity (21, 38).

Gene segment usage only partially depicts the set of specificities encompassed by the TCR repertoire, thus we focused on the deepest functional level of the repertoire, the CDR3 AA sequence. Here, the similarity between the repertoires of BM niches, even between young and old mice, is emphasized. AA clonotypes in the BM are shared and their frequencies are well-correlated across the samples from different individuals, and also across age groups. This supports the notion of a relatively static composition of clonotypes in the BM niche which maintains the structure of the TCR repertoire of BM-resident $CD4^+$ T cells. In contrast, the SPL samples from aged mice display very distinct repertoires, evidenced by a low intra-group correlation for frequencies of shared AA clonotypes and a low sharing of TCR sequences between mice of this group. This suggests that the loss of diversity we detect in old mice is manifested by private immune responses during lifetime, where in each individual a particular subset of TCR specificities is amplified to dominance. This is in agreement with the pattern observed in antigen-specific response in aged mice (10) but on a more global scale. We observe tens to hundreds of clones that are private and significantly expanded in each old individual's spleen, indicating that decline in repertoire diversity is caused by expansion of a large number of clones through life. Moreover, the repertoire of the old spleen becomes more similar to that of the BM in the aged mice. Of note, in two out of three aged mice, more clonotypes are shared between BM and SPL niches of the same animal compared with sharing between different animals. This trend of exclusive sharing between BM and SPL niche of the same animal is not evident in any of the three young mice. Together with the larger similarity between repertoires of the SPL niche in aged mice to that of the BM, this suggests that specific clones from the BM niche expanded significantly in the periphery, contributing to a skewed, degenerate, and private repertoire in the old SPL. Our phenotypic analysis (**Figure 1D**) suggests that these expanded clones acquire an effector memory phenotype in the old spleen, but more specific analysis is required to validate this hypothesis. In addition, extending our dataset to include additional mice could provide further evidence for the private repertoires in the aged spleen, and for increased similarity between BM and SPL repertoires that we observe in aged mice.

Lastly, we focus on those clones that are common to SPL and BM tissues of aged mice, but exclusive to each animal. We detect clonal dominance in these expanded groups of cells, with the same nt sequence present in high frequency in both niches. The chance of this expansion to occur in two independent events of clonal expansion is highly unlikely. As we find the same exact nt sequence in the BM and SPL of the same animal, we propose that sporadic clonal expansion is the mechanism that shapes the TCR repertoire in aging. This clonal dominance can be realized in the aging immune system, as the "void" created by clonal senescence and exhaustion (39) is more easily filled with rapidly dividing T cell clones. A similar phenomenon was described in other models of similar low grade, chronic sterile innate inflammation, such as obesity, where TCR repertoire is restricted (40). The mechanisms that generate these rare expansions can be response to self-antigens (18), latent infections (32), or driven by accumulating mutations (41).

In summary, we showed that diversity of the splenic $CD4^+$ TCR repertoire declines with age, while the BM repertoire remains largely unchanged. Our results suggest that with age, the TCRβ repertoire of each individual focuses on a certain subset of few hundreds clones out of the potential repertoire, and there is large variability between the subset each individual maintains. This attrition can be explained by a reduction in thymic output of naïve cells with age along with sporadic clonal expansion, which contribute to the clonal dominance we observe in old mice. As a consequence, this phenomenon should be considered when addressing vaccination of the elderly population.

ACKNOWLEDGMENTS

This research was supported by the Minerva Foundation with funding from the Federal German Ministry for Education and Research. Nir Friedman is incumbent of the Pauline Recanati Career Development Chair of Immunology.

REFERENCES

1. Bassing CH, Swat W, Alt FW. The mechanism and regulation of chromosomal V(D)J recombination. *Cell* (2002) **109**(Suppl):S45–55. doi:10.1016/S0092-8674(02)00675-X
2. Naylor K, Li G, Vallejo AN, Lee W-W, Koetz K, Bryl E, et al. The influence of age on T cell generation and TCR diversity. *J Immunol* (2005) **174**:7446–52.
3. Nanda NK, Apple R, Sercarz E. Limitations in plasticity of the T-cell receptor repertoire. *Proc Natl Acad Sci U S A* (1991) **88**:9503–7. doi:10.1073/pnas.88.21.9503
4. Kang I, Hong MS, Nolasco H, Park SH, Dan JM, Choi J-Y, et al. Age-associated change in the frequency of memory CD4+ T cells impairs long term CD4+ T cell responses to influenza vaccine. *J Immunol* (2004) **173**:673–81.
5. Wu Y-CB, Kipling D, Dunn-Walters DK. Age-related changes in human peripheral blood IGH repertoire following vaccination. *Front Immunol* (2012) **3**:193. doi:10.3389/fimmu.2012.00193
6. Linton PJ, Dorshkind K. Age-related changes in lymphocyte development and function. *Nat Immunol* (2004) **5**:133–9. doi:10.1038/ni1033
7. Bains I, Thiébaut R, Yates AJ, Callard R. Quantifying thymic export: combining models of naive T cell proliferation and TCR excision circle dynamics gives an explicit measure of thymic output. *J Immunol* (2009) **183**:4329–36. doi:10.4049/jimmunol.0900743
8. Den Braber I, Mugwagwa T, Vrisekoop N, Westera L, Mögling R, de Boer AB, et al. Maintenance of peripheral naive T cells is sustained by thymus output in mice but not humans. *Immunity* (2012) **36**:288–97. doi:10.1016/j.immuni.2012.02.006
9. Goronzy JJ, Lee W-W, Weyand CM. Aging and T-cell diversity. *Exp Gerontol* (2007) **42**:400–6. doi:10.1016/j.exger.2006.11.016
10. Rudd BD, Venturi V, Li G, Samadder P, Ertelt JM, Way SS, et al. Nonrandom attrition of the naive CD8+ T-cell pool with aging governed by T-cell receptor:pMHC interactions. *Proc Natl Acad Sci U S A* (2011) **108**:13694–9. doi:10.1073/pnas.1107594108
11. Mosley RL, Koker MM, Miller RA. Idiosyncratic alterations of TCR size distributions affecting both CD4 and CD8 T cell subsets in aging mice. *Cell Immunol* (1998) **189**:10–8. doi:10.1006/cimm.1998.1369
12. Schwab R, Szabo P, Manavalan JS, Weksler ME, Posnett DN, Pannetier C, et al. Expanded CD4+ and CD8+ T cell clones in elderly humans. *J Immunol* (1997) **158**:4493–9.
13. Yager EJ, Ahmed M, Lanzer K, Randall TD, Woodland DL, Blackman MA. Age-associated decline in T cell repertoire diversity leads to holes in the repertoire and impaired immunity to influenza virus. *J Exp Med* (2008) **205**:711–23. doi:10.1084/jem.20071140

14. Tokoyoda K, Zehentmeier S, Hegazy AN, Albrecht I, Grün JR, Löhning M, et al. Professional memory CD4+ T lymphocytes preferentially reside and rest in the bone marrow. *Immunity* (2009) **30**:721–30. doi:10.1016/j.immuni.2009.03.015
15. Di Rosa F, Pabst R. The bone marrow: a nest for migratory memory T cells. *Trends Immunol* (2005) **26**:360–6. doi:10.1016/j.it.2005.04.011
16. Slifka MK, Whitmire JK, Ahmed R. Bone marrow contains virus-specific cytotoxic T lymphocytes. *Blood* (1997) **90**:2103–8.
17. Feuerer M, Beckhove P, Bai L, Solomayer EF, Bastert G, Diel IJ, et al. Therapy of human tumors in NOD/SCID mice with patient-derived reactivated memory T cells from bone marrow. *Nat Med* (2001) **7**:452–8. doi:10.1038/86523
18. Baruch K, Ron-Harel N, Gal H, Deczkowska A, Shifrut E, Ndifon W, et al. CNS-specific immunity at the choroid plexus shifts toward destructive Th2 inflammation in brain aging. *Proc Natl Acad Sci U S A* (2013) **110**:2264–9. doi:10.1073/pnas.1211270110
19. Ron-Harel N, Segev Y, Lewitus GM, Cardon M, Ziv Y, Netanely D, et al. Age-dependent spatial memory loss can be partially restored by immune activation. *Rejuvenation Res* (2008) **11**:903–13. doi:10.1089/rej.2008.0755
20. Ahmed M, Lanzer KG, Yager EJ, Adams PS, Johnson LL, Blackman MA. Clonal expansions and loss of receptor diversity in the naive CD8 T cell repertoire of aged mice. *J Immunol* (2009) **182**:784–92.
21. Callahan JE, Kappler JW, Marrack P. Unexpected expansions of CD8-bearing cells in old mice. *J Immunol* (1993) **151**:6657–69.
22. Quigley MF, Greenaway HY, Venturi V, Lindsay R, Quinn KM, Seder RA, et al. Convergent recombination shapes the clonotypic landscape of the naive T-cell repertoire. *Proc Natl Acad Sci U S A* (2010) **107**:19414–9. doi:10.1073/pnas.1010586107
23. Ndifon W, Gal H, Shifrut E, Aharoni R, Yissachar N, Waysbort N, et al. Chromatin conformation governs T-cell receptor Jβ gene segment usage. *Proc Natl Acad Sci U S A* (2012) **109**:15865–70. doi:10.1073/pnas.1203916109
24. Lefranc M-P, Giudicelli V, Ginestoux C, Jabado-Michaloud J, Folch G, Bellahcene F, et al. IMGT, the international ImMunoGeneTics information system. *Nucleic Acids Res* (2009) **37**:D1006–12. doi:10.1093/nar/gkn838
25. Core Team R. *R: A Language and Environment for Statistical Computing.* Vienna (2013).
26. Morgan M, Anders S, Lawrence M, Aboyoun P, Pagès H, Gentleman R. ShortRead: a Bioconductor package for input, quality assessment and exploration of high-throughput sequence data. *Bioinformatics* (2009) **25**:2607–8. doi:10.1093/bioinformatics/btp450
27. Zeileis A. *Ineq: Measuring Inequality, Concentration, and Poverty.* (2012).
28. Wickham H. *Ggplot2: Elegant Graphics for Data Analysis.* New York: Springer (2009).
29. Thomas PG, Handel A, Doherty PC, La Gruta NL. Ecological analysis of antigen-specific CTL repertoires defines the relationship between naive and immune T-cell populations. *Proc Natl Acad Sci U S A* (2013) **110**:1839–44. doi:10.1073/pnas.1222149110
30. Venturi V, Kedzierska K, Turner SJ, Doherty PC, Davenport MP. Methods for comparing the diversity of samples of the T cell receptor repertoire. *J Immunol Methods* (2007) **321**:182–95. doi:10.1016/j.jim.2007.01.019
31. Mehr R, Sternberg-Simon M, Michaeli M, Pickman Y. Models and methods for analysis of lymphocyte repertoire generation, development, selection and evolution. *Immunol Lett* (2012) **148**:11–22. doi:10.1016/j.imlet.2012.08.002
32. Nikolich-Zugich J. Ageing and life-long maintenance of T-cell subsets in the face of latent persistent infections. *Nat Rev Immunol* (2008) **8**:512–22. doi:10.1038/nri2318
33. Goronzy JJ, Weyand CM. Understanding immunosenescence to improve responses to vaccines. *Nat Immunol* (2013) **14**:428–36. doi:10.1038/ni.2588
34. Chen G, Lustig A, Weng N-P. T cell aging: a review of the transcriptional changes determined from genome-wide analysis. *Front Immunol* (2013) **4**:121. doi:10.3389/fimmu.2013.00121
35. Blackman MA, Woodland DL. The narrowing of the CD8 T cell repertoire in old age. *Curr Opin Immunol* (2011) **23**:537–42. doi:10.1016/j.coi.2011.05.005
36. Fujisaki J, Wu J, Carlson AL, Silberstein L, Putheti P, Larocca R, et al. In vivo imaging of Treg cells providing immune privilege to the haematopoietic stem-cell niche. *Nature* (2011) **474**:216–9. doi:10.1038/nature10160
37. Martinez-Agosto JA, Mikkola HKA, Hartenstein V, Banerjee U. The hematopoietic stem cell and its niche: a comparative view. *Genes Dev* (2007) **21**:3044–60. doi:10.1101/gad.1602607
38. Haynes L, Maue AC. Effects of aging on T cell function. *Curr Opin Immunol* (2009) **21**:414–7. doi:10.1016/j.coi.2009.05.009
39. Almanzar G, Schwaiger S, Jenewein B, Keller M, Herndler-Brandstetter D, Würzner R, et al. Long-term cytomegalovirus infection leads to significant changes in the composition of the CD8+ T-cell repertoire, which may be the basis for an imbalance in the cytokine production profile in elderly persons. *J Virol* (2005) **79**:3675–83. doi:10.1128/JVI.79.6.3675-3683.2005
40. Yang H, Youm Y-H, Vandanmagsar B, Ravussin A, Gimble JM, Greenway F, et al. Obesity increases the production of proinflammatory mediators from adipose tissue T cells and compromises TCR repertoire diversity: implications for systemic inflammation and insulin resistance. *J Immunol* (2010) **185**:1836–45. doi:10.4049/jimmunol.1000021
41. Johnson PLF, Yates AJ, Goronzy JJ, Antia R. Peripheral selection rather than thymic involution explains sudden contraction in naive CD4 T-cell diversity with age. *Proc Natl Acad Sci U S A* (2012) **109**:21432–7. doi:10.1073/pnas.1209283110

11

Dendritic cell subsets in type 1 diabetes: friend or foe?

Penelope A. Morel*

Department of Immunology, University of Pittsburgh, Pittsburgh, PA, USA

Edited by:
Lisa Helene Butterfield, University of Pittsburgh, USA

Reviewed by:
Bruno Laugel, Cardiff University School of Medicine, UK
Edith Janssen, Cincinnati Children's Hospital Research Foundation, USA

Correspondence:
Penelope A. Morel, Department of Immunology, University of Pittsburgh, 200 Lothrop Street, BST E1048, Pittsburgh, PA 15261, USA
e-mail: morel@pitt.edu

Type 1 diabetes (T1D) is a T cell mediated autoimmune disease characterized by immune mediated destruction of the insulin-producing β cells in the islets of Langerhans. Dendritic cells (DC) have been implicated in the pathogenesis of T1D and are also used as immunotherapeutic agents. Plasmacytoid (p)DC have been shown to have both protective and pathogenic effects and a newly described merocytic DC population has been shown to break tolerance in the mouse model of T1D, the non-obese diabetic (NOD) mouse. We have used DC populations to prevent the onset of T1D in NOD mice and clinical trials of DC therapy in T1D diabetes have been initiated. In this review we will critically examine the recent published literature on the role of DC subsets in the induction and regulation of the autoimmune response in T1D.

Keywords: dendritic cells, type 1 diabetes, T regulatory cells, autoimmunity, tolerance

INTRODUCTION

Type 1 diabetes (T1D) is an autoimmune disease characterized by immune mediated destruction of the insulin-producing β cells in the islets of Langerhans of the pancreas. The pathogenesis of T1D is multifactorial with genetic, immunological, metabolic, and environmental factors all contributing (1). It begins with a loss of self-tolerance to islet-derived self-antigens, which usually occurs early in life. This could occur as a result of a viral infection targeting the pancreas or following pancreatic remodeling. These insults lead to the death of β cells, release of self-antigens, and induction of inflammatory cytokines such as TNF-α and IL-1-β. Dendritic cells (DC) present within the pancreas take up released β-cell-derived antigens and migrate to the draining lymph nodes (LN) and activate naïve islet-specific CD4 and CD8 T cells. Depending on the signals delivered to the T cell by DCs the T cells will differentiate into either inflammatory effector cells such as T helper (Th)1 cells or anti-inflammatory Th2 or regulatory (Treg) cells. Activated islet-specific T cells then migrate to the pancreas where they infiltrate and collect around the islets. The early infiltrates appear to be dominated by Th2 and Treg cells; this is termed peri-insulitis as there is little invasion into the islet. At some point, the infiltrate becomes invasive and begins to enter and destroy the β cells, and the balance between the regulatory and inflammatory T cell populations is lost. The precise factors that trigger both loss of self-tolerance and the development of invasive insulitis are not well understood. DCs play important roles at all stages of the autoimmune response in T1D due to their pivotal role in activating naïve T cells and in maintaining self-tolerance (2). This review will explore recent developments in our understanding of the roles DC play in the pathogenesis, and prevention, of T1D (**Figure 1**) as well as the therapeutic potential of DCs for the prevention and treatment of T1D. Much of the work in this area has been focused on the non-obese diabetic (NOD) model of the disease. This mouse strain spontaneously develops diabetes and shares many of the genetic and immunological features of the human disease (3). Where possible we will highlight similarities and differences between NOD mouse studies and relevant studies in human T1D patients.

DENDRITIC CELL SUBSETS

Since their discovery by Ralph Steinman in the 1970s (4–6) DCs have been the subject of intense study. DCs are antigen presenting cells (APC) that bridge the innate and adaptive immune systems (7). They act as sentinels of the immune system through their location in peripheral tissues, where they form a dense network, and their ability to respond to pathogens through expression of pathogen recognition receptors such as Toll-like receptors (TLR). While in peripheral tissues DCs have an immature phenotype characterized by low levels of major histocompatibility complex (MHC) and co-stimulatory molecules (CD80, CD86) and a high endocytic rate; the function of tissue DCs is the detection and processing of antigen. Upon interaction with a pathogen DCs become activated, undergo maturation and migrate to the draining LN. This maturation leads to an increase in the expression of MHC, CD80, and CD86, a decrease in endocytosis and a change in the pattern of chemokine receptor expression. Mature DCs entering the T cell zone of the draining lymph node are primed to present antigen to naïve T cells. Even in the absence of pathogen there is a steady state migration of DC from the periphery to the LN and this is necessary for the maintenance of peripheral tolerance (8).

DC PHENOTYPE

There are two main classes of DC: plasmacytoid DCs (pDCs) and conventional or classical DCs (cDCs) (7). pDCs are primarily located in the blood and lymphoid organs and produce high levels of type 1 interferon (IFN) following engagement of TLRs with foreign nucleic acids (9). pDCs express a restricted set of TLRs, TLR7, and TLR9, that recognize foreign RNA and DNA respectively as well as several unique markers that distinguish them from cDCs. These include BDCA-2 and ILT7 for human pDCs and SiglecH and Bst2 for murine pDCs. In the mouse pDCs are commonly identified as $CD11c^{low}$ $B220^{+}$ $SiglecH^{+}$ $Bst2^{+}$. Human pDCs are $CD11c^{-}$ and in addition to BDCA-2 and ILT7 also express CD123 and BDCA-4 (9). There are two main populations of cDCs in mouse: $CD11c^{+}$ $CD11b^{-}$ $CD8\alpha^{+}$ $Clec9A^{+}$ and $CD11c^{+}$ $CD11b^{+}$ $CD8\alpha^{-}$ $Clec9A^{-}$ commonly referred to as CD8 DC and CD11b

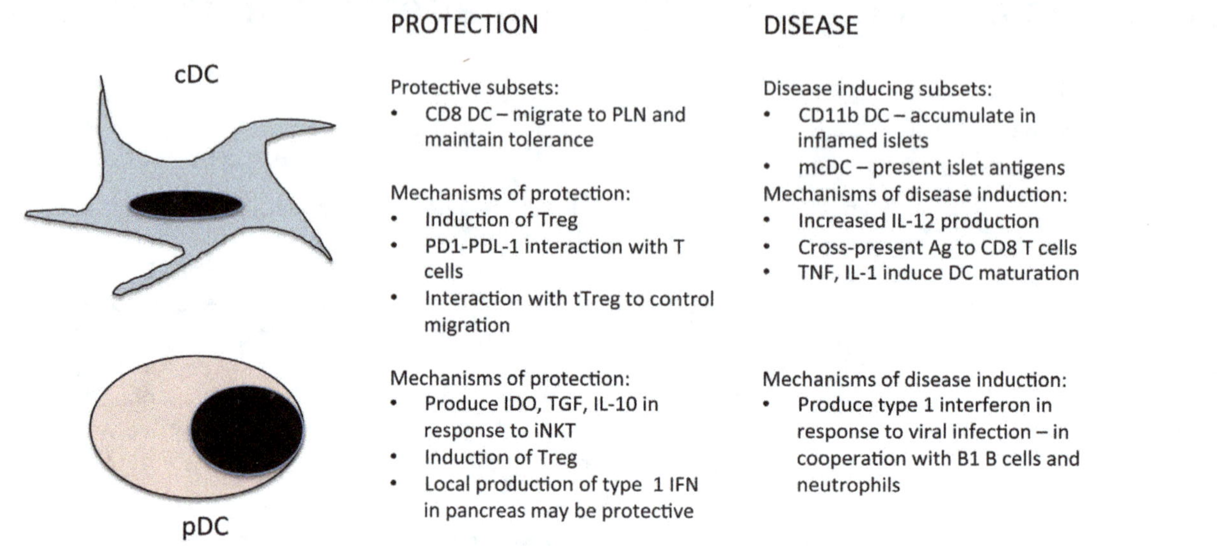

FIGURE 1 | Summary of the roles of cDC and pDC in the prevention and induction of T1D.

cDC respectively. Both CD8 and CD11b cDC arise from a common precursor characterized by expression of the C-type lectin receptor DNGR-1, but it appears that pDC arise from a distinct precursor as yet to be defined (10, 11). Recently the CD11b cDC population has been further subdivided on the basis of endothelial cell selective adhesion molecule (ESAM) expression (12). Similar populations can be identified in human such that CD11c$^+$ Clec9A$^+$ BDCA-3$^+$ DCs correspond to CD8 cDC and CD11c$^+$ CD11b$^+$ BDCA-1$^+$ DCs are analogous to CD11b cDC. These populations mainly reside in the secondary lymphoid organs and are present during steady state. Similar populations exist in peripheral tissues but they express a slightly different set of markers (7). CD11c$^+$ CD11b$^-$ CD103$^+$ DC and CD11c$^+$ CD11b$^+$ CD103$^+$ DC in the periphery are equivalent to the CD8 cDC and CD11b cDC populations respectively (13).

FUNCTIONAL DICHOTOMY IN cDC SUBSETS

The two cDC populations also have distinct functions with respect to pathogen recognition, cytokine production, and T cell activation. CD8 and CD103 cDCs express a unique pattern of TLR and other pathogen recognition receptors: they are the only subset to express TLR3 and TLR11 and also uniquely express the C-type lectin Clec9A, DEC205 (CD205), and langerin (CD207) (7, 9). CD8 and CD103 cDC are specialized in the cross-presentation of externally derived antigen on MHC class I for the activation of naïve CD8 T cells. The recent advances in the molecular mechanisms of cross-presentation are covered in a review included in this Research Topic (14). In addition, CD8 cDC appear to preferentially activate CD8 T cells due to the fact that they produce high levels of the cytokines interleukin (IL)-12 and IL-15 that are important for the differentiation and survival of CD8 T cells (15–17). CD8 and CD103 cDCs are the main producers of IL-12, an important cytokine in the differentiation of inflammatory Th1 cells (15, 16, 18). There are also reports suggesting a role for CD8 and CD103 cDCs in the maintenance of peripheral self-tolerance through the deletion of self-reactive T cells (19, 20) and the induction of Treg cells (21). While CD11b cDC are capable of cross-presentation and CD8 T cell activation they appear to be most effective in antigen presentation and activation of CD4 T cells (22) In addition the dermal and intestinal CD11b$^+$ CD103$^+$ DCs are strong inducers of Treg due to their expression of aldehyde dehydrogenase, the enzyme that converts Vitamin A to retinoic acid, necessary for Treg conversion (23, 24). Several comprehensive reviews on DC subsets and their development have recently been published and can be consulted for further details (7, 9, 13).

DC AND THE MAINTENANCE OF SELF-TOLERANCE

T and B cell tolerance to self-antigens is acquired during development through clonal deletion of self-reactive cells. DC play an important role in the process of central tolerance in the thymus as they present an array of self-antigens to developing T cells (25). If the T cells have a high affinity for self-antigen they undergo apoptosis and are deleted. Those T cells with a moderate affinity for self are induced to differentiate into forkhead transcription factor (Foxp3)$^+$ suppressor cells (26) known as thymus (t)Treg (27). In contrast, peripheral (p)Treg cells arise in the periphery upon Ag contact and several subsets of pTreg can be induced depending on the signals they encounter (28). These include IL-10 (29), TGF-β (30), retinoic acid or vitamin D3 (31, 32), low Ag dose (33), and specific DC subsets (21, 34, 35). As the study of DC biology has evolved, it has become apparent that it is possible to induce the differentiation of Treg using DCs conditioned by immunomodulatory agents (36–39). For example, the presence of TGF-β during the primary stimulation induces the production and expansion of Foxp3$^+$ Treg (35). In addition it has been possible to induce IL-10-producing T cells with DC generated using a combination of GM-CSF, TNF-α, and IL-10 (39). Studies have shown that DC producing IDO induce the generation of Treg from naïve T cells (40). Other reports have suggested that immature DC induce the development of functional suppressor cells (36) and that immature DC might, therefore, be therapeutically useful in autoimmunity (37, 38). Recent studies using both nominal and self-Ags have demonstrated that targeting Ags to CD8 cDC in the LN or spleen in the absence of an inflammatory stimulus results in the generation of Treg (41, 42). Similar results have been obtained when Ags were targeted to $CD8^-$ $DCIR2^+$ DC (21). The CD11b cDC subset has been shown to induce Treg proliferation and expansion in the presence of GM-CSF (43). A recent paper has described a feedback loop in which the number of Tregs in the periphery can be manipulated by altering the relative number of DCs suggesting that DCs play an important role in regulating pTreg numbers (44). We have recently suggested that DC in the periphery may function to maintain tolerance by presenting endogenous self-antigens to naïve T cells thereby inducing pTreg (45).

THE ROLE OF DENDRITIC CELLS IN THE PATHOGENESIS/PREVENTION OF T1D

DC DEVELOPMENT IS DEFECTIVE IN T1D

Early studies of NOD mouse revealed abnormalities in the development of myeloid cells demonstrating a reduced proliferative capacity of the bone marrow in response to GM-CSF and M-CSF (46). Several groups, including our own, have identified defects in the development of specific DC subsets in the spleen and other lymphoid organs (47–49). These defects result in a decrease in the numbers of the CD8 cDC population (50, 51), a population which has been shown to have regulatory function (52–54), with a concomitant increase in the CD11b cDC population. Recent studies have also shown that treatment of NOD with Flt 3 ligand (FL) protects mice from diabetes development and this is correlated with an enhancement in the number of CD8 cDC (55, 56). Our own studies demonstrated that treatment of NOD mice with FL increased the number of CD8 cDC and that transfer of these cells to prediabetic NOD mice could have a partial effect in preventing diabetes (50). However a recent study suggested that the timing of FL treatment was critical since disease would be exacerbated if autoimmune CD8 T cells were already present (57).

Several studies have examined the function of bone marrow-derived and isolated DC populations with respect to cytokine production and T cell differentiation and the results have not been consistent. It has been reported by some investigators that NOD DC produce higher levels of the Th1-driving cytokine IL-12 (58–60) while others failed to find such an association (49, 50, 56). Macrophages also appear to be an important source of IL-12 in NOD mice (51, 61). Adenosine plays an important role in modulating the immune response to tissue inflammation (62, 63) and a recent study found that NOD DC express higher levels of adenosine deaminase (ADA), the enzyme responsible for catabolic degradation of adenosine, and that transfer of ADA deficient DC to NOD mice protected them from diabetes (64). These studies suggest that NOD mice have imbalances in DC subsets and alterations in DC function that may contribute to pathogenesis of T1D.

DC AND THE MAINTENANCE OF TOLERANCE IN T1D

Dendritic cells are important in both central and peripheral tolerance through the deletion of self-reactive cells and the induction of Treg. NOD mice have defects in central and peripheral tolerance mechanisms (65, 66). Recent studies have shown that the number and/or function of Treg cells decrease as NOD mice age and this is associated with onset of diabetes (67). The development and maintenance of Treg in NOD mice is highly dependent on the presence of co-stimulatory molecules CD80 and CD86 (68). In addition it was recently shown that interaction between the inhibitory molecules PD-1 on T cells and PDL-1 on DC is necessary for the maintenance of tolerance in NOD mice (69). Blockade of this interaction resulted in increased DC/T cell interaction time in the islets and T cell activation leading to the generation of autoreactive effector cells (69). Another study came to the same conclusion by using different antigen constructs to increase the time of antigen presentation (70). IL-2 and signaling via IL-2R are also critical for Treg development and maintenance (71). Recent studies have identified defects in IL-2R signaling in T1D patients (72) and the diabetes susceptibility locus, Idd3, which contains IL-2 was recently shown to control Treg function through an effect on APC (73–75). Several early reports demonstrated that the inflammatory cytokine TNF-α plays an important role in the initiation of T1D (76) and more recently this has been attributed to effects of TNF-α on DC subsets (77). In this study administration of TNF-α to NOD mice was shown to decrease the number of CD8 DC, increase the CD11b DC population, and the DC had a more mature phenotype and activated islet-specific T cells (77) A recent study describing the depletion of Treg in NOD mice showed that the increase in diabetes in these animals was associated with aggressive infiltration of pancreatic islets by DC rather than CD4 T cells (78). These results suggest that tTreg in this context may prevent autoimmunity by controlling the migration of cDC into the islet.

DC CONTRIBUTE TO THE DEVELOPMENT OF T1D

Analysis of the phenotype and function of BM-derived DC in NOD mice have suggested that these cells produce higher levels of IL-12p70, and that this related to increased expression of NFκB (58). Our own studies suggest that BM-derived DC from NOD can produce higher or lower levels of IL-12p70 depending on the culture conditions and activation stimuli used (49, 79, 80). Recent studies using DTR transgenic mice that allow the targeted depletion of macrophages or DC have demonstrated that the CD11b cDC population is responsible for presenting antigen to autoreactive T cells (81). Ablation of these cells protected NOD mice from diabetes development. The interaction of iNKT cells with cDC was shown to lead to either protection via induction of Treg or exacerbation of disease if the interaction occurred at the same time as TLR4 ligation (82).

The role of pDC in diabetes pathogenesis is somewhat more controversial and there are conflicting reports in the literature. Depletion of pDC using the CD11c-DTR system caused accelerated disease (81), suggesting a protective role for pDC. The protection induced by pDC was correlated with increased local production of IDO and increased numbers of NKT cells in the pancreas. In a model of virus infection it was shown that activation of iNKT cells stimulated TGF-β production from pDC, which led to the induction of Treg and protection from diabetes (83). In contrast, another study found that IFN-α could be detected in the pancreas of NOD mice at early ages and that blocking the ability of mice to respond to IFN-α prevented diabetes (84). Furthermore these investigators showed that depletion of pDC using a depleting antibody reduced the incidence of diabetes (85). Another study revealed a crosstalk between B-1a B cells, neutrophils and pDC that contributed to the induction of diabetes via type 1 IFN production (86). This study suggests that DNA from dying β cells together with antibodies from B-1a B cells form complexes that are potentiated by neutrophils and lead to the induction of type 1 IFN by pDC (86). The authors show that this is seen only in NOD mice and speculate that this is related to the defects in the ability of NOD macrophages to clear debris (87). Several studies have examined the role of pDC, type 1 IFN and viral infection in the induction of T1D; reviewed in Swiecki et al. (88). The situation is complex with some studies showing exacerbation of diabetes (89, 90) with viral infection and others showing protection (91, 92). It has been suggested that whether viral infection leads to diabetes induction is related to the tropism of the virus and the local environment in which type 1 IFN is produced (88). Thus a virus infecting the pancreas may induce local type 1 IFN, which protects islets from infection and damage, whereas in other situations the type 1 IFN, produced by pDC following viral infection, could result in activation of autoreactive T cells and diabetes exacerbation (88). It has been reported that pDC also accumulate in the islets of NOD mice (93) at a later time point, around 10 weeks of age. The infiltrating pDC were shown to express IDO, which is characteristic of a more tolerogenic phenotype of DC (94) leading to the speculation that these cells may be attempting to control ongoing T cell activation. Studies in the next few years will hopefully clarify these contrasting results on the role that pDC play in diabetes pathogenesis.

A novel population of cDC, termed merocytic (mc)DC, have recently been identified and shown to be responsible for cross-presentation of islet antigens to CD8 T cells and direct presentation to CD4 T cells (95, 96). The mcDC express CD11c but are negative for both CD11b and CD8, they accumulate in the spleen as NOD mice age and were shown to secrete large amounts of type 1 IFN (95, 96). In addition transfer of mcDC pulsed with irradiated islets to non-diabetic NOD mice accelerated the onset of diabetes (95, 96). The number of mcDC was recently mapped to the *Idd13* congenic interval suggesting that the relative number of these cells is genetically determined (97). Further studies are required to determine the significance of this DC population, and whether a counterpart of these cells exists in human.

Dendritic cells are constitutively present within islets of normal mice and have been shown to express peptide-MHC (pMHC) complexes containing peptides derived from islet antigens (98). Two major DC subsets can be found within islets; the CD11b cDC and CD103 cDC (99, 100). CD103 DC depend on FL for their homeostasis whereas islet CD11b DC appear to arise from monocytes and are unaffected by the absence of FL (101). The number of DCs in the islets remains relatively stable but these numbers increase following T cell infiltration and inflammation (98, 99, 102). In addition the phenotype of the DC becomes more inflammatory with increases in the expression of co-stimulatory molecules and MHC (2). The evidence suggests that the initiation of the autoimmune response occurs within the draining pancreatic lymph node (PLN) since removal of the PLN prevents diabetes (103) and several studies have shown that the initial proliferation of islet-specific CD4 and CD8 T cells takes place in the PLN (104, 105). Islet CD103 DC migrate to the PLN where they present islet antigens to specific CD4 and CD8 T cells (2, 101), and when T cells infiltrate the islet they localize to DC-rich areas (2). The movement of DC and T cells within the islet can now be visualized using a novel two-photon imaging technique (106). In addition pancreatic CD103 DC from NOD mice have been shown to express less IL-10 than similar populations from non-diabetic strains suggesting that these have lost their ability to induce tolerance (107). Islet CD11b DC are relatively poor at presenting antigen under steady state conditions but they accumulate as inflammation increases and become more mature. Since CD11b DC do not appear to migrate to PLN their role appears to be in the modulating the local tissue response (101).

DC IN HUMAN T1D

Several studies have examined the blood of newly diagnosed T1D patients for the presence of DC subsets. pDCs have been shown to be increased (108) or decreased (109) at the time of diagnosis. A recent detailed longitudinal analysis of immune parameters in newly diagnosed T1D children has revealed that reduced numbers of cDC1s and NKT cells at the time of diagnosis are correlated with reduced residual β cell function 1 year later (110). Another study found decreased numbers of cDCs and pDCs in newly diagnosed pediatric T1D patients and also observed a decrease in the expression of CCR2 on these cells (111). Other studies have found correlations with vitamin D levels and immune cells in T1D patients (112). A study of pancreatic biopsies on a small number of new onset T1D patients revealed the presence of infiltrating macrophages and DC that produce TNF-α (113). A recent description of three cases of fulminant T1D secondary to enterovirus infection revealed marked islet infiltration of activated DC and macrophages and the presence of inflammatory cytokines (114). Thus it is likely that DCs will be shown to contribute to the onset of human T1D.

DENDRITIC CELLS AS THERAPY FOR T1D

The fact that DCs play an important role in the induction and maintenance of self-tolerance has made them attractive targets for therapeutic interventions. Three main strategies have been employed and these include the adoptive transfer of specific DC subsets, the *in vitro* expansion of Tregs with specific DCs and the *in vivo* targeting of DC subsets (115). As discussed above the complexity of DC subsets and the plasticity of their function have made this a challenging objective, since there is a fine balance between the immunostimulatory and immunoregulatory functions of DC (45, 116, 117). DCs with a so called semi-mature phenotype, which consists of increased MHC and co-stimulatory molecule expression but low inflammatory cytokine production are thought to be most effective in inducing tolerance in the context of autoimmunity (118, 119). This maturation state can be induced by exposing DC to the cytokine TNF-α and DCs treated in this way have been shown to prevent experimental allergic encephalomyelitis (EAE) (118). In general the function of these DCs is to induce the expansion of Treg or other regulatory mechanisms such as Th2 cells. The attraction for using DCs as therapeutic agents is that since they present specific antigen to T cells it is possible to envision the generation of antigen-specific tolerance (120).

ADOPTIVE TRANSFER OF THERAPEUTIC DC

Dendritic cells were first used as therapeutic agents to prevent diabetes in NOD mice over 20 years ago by Clare-Salzler et al. (121). In this study DCs isolated from the PLN of NOD mice and transferred to prediabetic NOD mice were able to prevent disease onset whereas DCs from other LN or spleen were not effective. Later studies by the same group have suggested that DC in the PLN are more mature and that this is important for their therapeutic effect (122). We have previously shown that the injection of semi-mature bone marrow-derived DC prior to the onset of destructive insulitis prevents the subsequent development of diabetes (123, 124). The therapeutic DC populations expressed high levels of co-stimulatory molecules (CD80, CD86, and CD40) and produced low levels of IL-12p70 following CD40 ligation (49). Further investigation revealed that the therapeutic DC population changed the cytokine milieu in treated NOD mice. Whereas NOD mice generally exhibit a strong bias toward type 1 cytokine production, injection of DC induced the production of type 2 cytokines (125). In addition we (124) and others (126, 127) showed that injection of DC transduced with the IL-4 gene could effectively prevent diabetes in NOD mice when given at later time points, past the onset of invasive insulitis. We also confirmed, using *in vitro* studies, that therapeutic DC could drive the differentiation of Th2 cells (79), whereas non-therapeutic DC did not. The therapeutic DCs were not treated with any tolerogenic agents and did not require the addition of islet-derived peptides but the cultures were performed in FBS, which was subsequently shown to induce a Th2 environment that may have been non-specifically contributing to the therapeutic effect (128). In more recent experiments we have shown that the therapeutic DC population induces the expansion of Treg in the presence of low dose antigen (129) and DCs cultured in the absence of FBS are equally able to induce Treg expansion (unpublished observations). In addition it has been shown that DC grown in autologous serum were able to prevent diabetes but only when pulsed with insulin-derived peptides (130).

In order to ensure that DCs maintain a tolerogenic phenotype and drive tolerance rather than immunity several approaches aimed at conditioning the DC have been explored. These have included treating DC with cytokines such as IL-10 (130, 131), IL-10/TGF-β (132), and TSLP (IL-25) (133), pharmacological agents such as dexamethasone and vitamin D_3 (134), carbon monoxide (CO) (135), anti-CTLA-4 antibody (136), secretory IgA (137) among others. In general, the treatment of DCs with these agents induces a semi-mature phenotype in the DC characterized by reduced expression of co-stimulatory molecules, reduced inflammatory cytokine production and resistance to further maturation stimuli. The infusion of these modified DC into NOD mice results in the deletion of autoreactive CD4 T cells and the generation of islet-specific Treg (130, 131, 133, 136, 137). One exception to this was the treatment of NOD mice with CO-treated DC, which reduced β1-integrin expression by CD8 T cells and thus inhibited their migration into the islet (135). Another approach has been the use of anti-sense oligonucleotides to down-regulate the expression of the co-stimulatory molecules, CD40, CD80, and CD86 on DC (138). This approach prevented diabetes in NOD mice through the induction of Treg and a phase 1 clinical trial using this approach was initiated (139).

DC USED TO EXPAND REGULATORY T CELLS *IN VITRO*

Dendritic cells have also been used *in vitro* in order to expand Treg cells, and these Treg can be adoptively transferred into individuals with autoimmunity with the hope of curbing or arresting the inflammatory response. An early study expanded Treg, isolated from an islet-specific TCR transgenic NOD mice (BDC2.5), with peptide pulsed DC and IL-2 and showed that these cells could prevent diabetes in prediabetic NOD mice (34). Further studies from this group indicated that DC expressing higher levels of the co-stimulatory molecule, CD86 were the most efficient at inducing Treg expansion (140). The CD11b cDC subset has been shown to induce Treg proliferation and expansion in the presence of GM-CSF (43). A recent study examining the mechanism by which GM-CSF treatment prevents diabetes has further suggested that the expression of OX40L and the Notch3 ligand Jagged1 on DC was necessary for Treg expansion *in vitro*, although this study did not determine whether these polyclonal expanded Treg were effective in preventing diabetes (141). Some of the approaches to generate tolerogenic DC are being developed for clinical trial in the context of transplantation (142) but these are not yet being fully developed for use in autoimmune disease. A recent study compared the ability of several DC conditioning regimens to induce suppressive Treg in the human system (143). This study found that DC pretreated with IL-10 induced the most suppressive Treg, while TGF-β, rapamycin, and dexamethasone were less effective (143).

IN VIVO TARGETING OF DC

In general these types of therapies have involved the use of reagents that deliberately target specific DC subsets but these can also include approaches that, while not directly targeting DC, act by changing the local DC environment. Recent studies using both nominal and self-antigens have demonstrated that targeting antigens to CD8 cDC in the LN or spleen using anti-CD205 antibodies coupled to specific antigens in the absence of an inflammatory stimulus results in the generation of Treg (41, 42). Similar results have been obtained when antigens were targeted to CD11b cDC (21). A recent study used anti-CD205 antibodies coupled to the peptide mimetope for the CD4 BDC2.5 T cell to target DC in NOD mice (144). This resulted in the generation of long-lived and stable BDC2.5 Treg but this had no impact on the development of diabetes. However when the anti-CD205 was coupled to the proinsulin protein diabetes was prevented (144). Similar studies using an anti-CD205 coupled to HA and given to INS-HA/TCR-HA mice also demonstrated efficacy in the prevention of diabetes (145). In this mouse model the foreign antigen HA is expressed in the pancreas under the control of the rat insulin promoter and the T cells are all transgenic for an HA-specific TCR (145). These results suggest that the choice of antigen for targeting will be critical if this approach is to move forward. A similar approach has been used to induce tolerance in islet-specific CD8 T cells. These studies reported initial activation of adoptively transferred islet-specific CD8 cells followed by deletion of these cells, but the impact of these on diabetes development was not reported (146).

It has been known for some time that varying the dose of the stimulating antigen has a profound effect on T cell differentiation (147–149). Interest in this area has been renewed by the observation that the induction of Treg is optimal in situations of low

TCR signal strength (33, 129, 150). The induction of Treg by low dose antigen occurs optimally when DC are presenting the antigen (129), and while the addition of TGF-β is not necessary a recent study showed that TGF-β production by T cells is required (151). Interestingly the most effective induction of Treg *in vivo* occurs when low doses of a high affinity peptide are used, rather than higher doses of low affinity peptides (152). Furthermore it was recently shown that the affinity of the peptide affects the duration of DC/T cell contacts *in vivo* providing an explanation for why low dose of more potent pMHC complexes are most effective at driving Treg expansion *in vivo* (153). Several approaches have been attempted to deliver low dose antigen *in vivo* including the continuous delivery of low dose antigen via osmotic pump (154) and the direct targeting of DC subsets as discussed above (21, 41, 42). In the context of T1D a recent study demonstrated that low doses of a high affinity insulin peptide mimetope was more effective at preventing diabetes than the native peptide (155). These results suggest that long-lasting peripheral tolerance could be achieved by delivering the appropriate dose of antigen to steady state DC in the periphery. The challenge will be translating this to the human situation although a recent paper showed that human insulin-specific Treg could be induced by low dose stimulation (156).

Another way to target DC *in vivo* is to use microparticles (157). A recent study used microspheres loaded with anti-sense oligonucleotides specific for CD40, CD80, and CD86 and showed prevention of diabetes along with an increase in Treg in treated NOD mice (158). These investigators further showed that repeated treatment with these microspheres could reverse diabetes in newly diagnosed NOD mice. The microspheres were taken up by resident DC in the spleen and these DC showed reduced expression of the co-stimulatory molecules (158).

In a study of combined therapy with oral anti-CD3 and intravenous anti-CD20 antibodies the prevention of diabetes seen in these animals was correlated with an increase in Treg and IL-10-producing T cells. Furthermore a population of IL-27 producing DCs was found to be responsible for the induction of IL-10-producing T cells in this system (159). As discussed above FL treatment of NOD mice in some circumstances prevents T1D (55, 56) but the timing of FL administration has to be before the onset of autoimmunity otherwise disease is exacerbated (57). Treatment of NOD mice with soluble CTLA-4 has been shown to restore the tolerance inducing properties of DC through the IFN-γ dependent activation of IDO. In this model CTLA-A binds to B7 molecules on DC and this stimulates the release of IFN-γ, which activates the immunosuppressive mechanism of tryptophan catabolism (160). A novel approach has been to induce accumulation of thymic DC populations which results in an increase in suppressive Tregs. A recent study identified the delta-like ligand 4 (Dll4)-Notch signaling pathway as important in controlling the number of thymic DCs (161). These investigators found that blockade of the Dll4-Notch pathway resulted in an increase in thymic DC numbers and thymic Treg. Treatment of NOD mice with these blockers not only prevented the establishment of disease in prediabetic animals but also was able to reverse disease in newly diagnosed diabetic animals (161). This protection was dependent on the presence of Treg since treatment of non-diabetic animals with a Treg-depleting antibody reversed the protection (161). Several studies have reported the use of α-GalCer, an agonist for iNKT cells, as a means to prevent disease in NOD mice (162–164). Recent studies have suggested that α-GalCer treatment induces tolerogenic DC populations that induce non-inflammatory islet-specific T cells (165), and novel derivatives of α-GalCer have been developed that have the same effect without some of the profound suppressive effects on iNKT function (166).

CLINICAL TRIALS IN T1D INVOLVING DC

As discussed above a phase I clinical trial utilizing autologous monocyte-derived DC treated with anti-sense oligonucleotides to down-modulate co-stimulatory molecules has been conducted. In this trial of 10 patients with established T1D, 7 were given the immunosuppressive DC and 3 were given unmanipulated DC. In this trial no adverse events were observed and there were few changes noted in terms of insulin requirements, immune cell phenotype, and cytokine production (139). Interestingly, further analysis of this clinical trial revealed an increase in certain B cell populations and subsequent *in vitro* studies revealed that human DC treated with these anti-sense oligonucleotides could induce the proliferation of immunosuppressive B cells (167). A second trial using this same approach is now ongoing but results are not yet available. The field of DC-based vaccines is much more advanced in the setting of cancer and many clinical trials have been conducted; reviewed in the current Research Topic (Butterfileld, under review). Many features of cancer DC vaccines have been studied and it has become apparent that characteristics such as the form of the antigen used to pulse the DC, the conditioning regimen of the DC, and the route of administration all play critical roles in determining the outcome of the DC-based immunization. These features will need to be taken into consideration as more DC-based therapies are proposed for the treatment of T1D. There have been numerous clinical trials in T1D with the aim of inducing antigen-specific tolerance (168). These trials utilize islet-derived antigens, such as insulin GAD65 or hsp 70, and various routes of administration have been tested including oral, nasal, and intradermal. So far these trials have failed to have a significant impact on disease although in some cases evidence for immune tolerance was observed (168). It is to be expected that the success of such trials will depend on the APC, most likely a DC, targeted by these antigen formulations. At the present time not much attention is being paid to the nature of the DC presenting the antigen in these trials but, in view of our increasing understanding of the complexity of DC phenotype and function this is likely to change.

FUTURE PERSPECTIVES

As discussed at the beginning of this review many of the studies that examine the therapeutic potential of DC in the treatment/prevention of T1D have been performed in the NOD mouse. This has been a very useful model for identifying susceptibility genes and understanding the progression to disease but therapeutic approaches that have successful in this mouse model have not translated well to the clinic (169). DCs play a pivotal role in setting the tone of the immune response. On the one hand they contribute to the development and maintenance of self-tolerance and on the other they contribute to the breaking of that tolerance and the initiation of disease. A deeper understanding of how DC can influence the development of autoimmune diabetes will aid in the development of novel therapeutic strategies. A great deal of progress has been achieved in the last several years and we have a better understanding of how DC can both maintain and break self-tolerance. The challenge in the future will be to use this knowledge to achieve the ultimate goal of inducing antigen-specific tolerance to prevent autoimmunity without causing widespread immune suppression.

REFERENCES

1. Atkinson MA, Bluestone JA, Eisenbarth GS, Hebrok M, Herold KC, Accili D, et al. How does type 1 diabetes develop? The notion of homicide or beta-cell suicide revisited. *Diabetes* (2011) **60**(5):1370–9. doi:10.2337/db10-1797
2. Calderon B, Unanue ER. Antigen presentation events in autoimmune diabetes. *Curr Opin Immunol* (2012) **24**(1):119–28. doi:10.1016/j.coi.2011.11.005
3. Leiter EH, Prochazka M, Coleman DL. Animal model of human disease, the nonobese diabetic (NOD) mouse. *Am J Pathol* (1987) **128**:380–3.
4. Steinman RM, Cohn ZA. Identification of a novel cell type in peripheral lymphoid organs of mice. I. Morphology, quantitation, tissue distribution. *J Exp Med* (1973) **137**(5):1142–62. doi:10.1084/jem.137.5.1142
5. Steinman RM, Lustig DS, Cohn ZA. Identification of a novel cell type in peripheral lymphoid organs of mice. 3. Functional properties in vivo. *J Exp Med* (1974) **139**(6):1431–45. doi:10.1084/jem.139.6.1431
6. Steinman RM, Cohn ZA. Identification of a novel cell type in peripheral lymphoid organs of mice. II. Functional properties in vitro. *J Exp Med* (1974) **139**(2):380–97. doi:10.1084/jem.139.6.1431
7. Merad M, Sathe P, Helft J, Miller J, Mortha A. The dendritic cell lineage: ontogeny and function of dendritic cells and their subsets in the steady state and the inflamed setting. *Annu Rev Immunol* (2013) **31**(1):563–604. doi:10.1146/annurev-immunol-020711-074950
8. Steinman RM, Nussenzweig MC. Avoiding horror autotoxicus: the importance of dendritic cells in peripheral T cell tolerance. *Proc Natl Acad Sci U S A* (2002) **99**(1):351–8. doi:10.1073/pnas.231606698
9. Reizis B, Bunin A, Ghosh HS, Lewis KL, Sisirak V. Plasmacytoid dendritic cells: recent progress and open questions. *Annu Rev Immunol* (2011) **29**(1):163–83. doi:10.1146/annurev-immunol-031210-101345
10. Onai N, Kurabayashi K, Hosoi-Amaike M, Toyama-Sorimachi N, Matsushima K, Inaba K, et al. A clonogenic progenitor with prominent plasmacytoid dendritic cell developmental potential. *Immunity* (2013) **38**(5):943–57. doi:10.1016/j.immuni.2013.04.006
11. Schraml Barbara U, van Blijswijk J, Zelenay S, Whitney Paul G, Filby A, Acton Sophie E, et al. Genetic tracing via DNGR-1 expression history defines dendritic cells as a hematopoietic lineage. *Cell* (2013) **154**(4):843–58. doi:10.1016/j.cell.2013.07.014
12. Lewis Kanako L, Caton Michele L, Bogunovic M, Greter M, Grajkowska Lucja T, Ng D, et al. Notch2 receptor signaling controls functional differentiation of dendritic cells in the spleen and intestine. *Immunity* (2011) **35**(5):780–91. doi:10.1016/j.immuni.2011.08.013
13. Ganguly D, Haak S, Sisirak V, Reizis B. The role of dendritic cells in autoimmunity. *Nat Rev Immunol* (2013) **13**(8):566–77. doi:10.1038/nri3477
14. Nair-Gupta P, Blander JM. An updated view of the intracelluair mechanisms regulating cross-presentation. *Front Immunol* (2013) **4**:401. doi:10.3389/fimmu.2013.00401
15. Hochrein H, Shortman K, Vremec D, Scott B, Hertzog P, O'Keeffe M. Differential production of IL-12, IFN-alpha, and IFN-gamma by mouse dendritic cell subsets. *J Immunol* (2001) **166**(9):5448–55.
16. Farrand KJ, Dickgreber N, Stoitzner P, Ronchese F, Petersen TR, Hermans IF. Langerin+ CD8alpha+ dendritic cells are critical for cross-priming and IL-12 production in response to systemic antigens. *J Immunol* (2009) **183**(12):7732–42. doi:10.4049/jimmunol.0902707
17. Mattei F, Schiavoni G, Belardelli F, Tough DF. IL-15 is expressed by dendritic cells in response to type I IFN, double-stranded RNA, or lipopolysaccharide and promotes dendritic cell activation. *J Immunol* (2001) **167**(3):1179–87.
18. Pulendran B, Lingappa J, Kennedy MK, Smith J, Teepe M, Rudensky A, et al. Developmental pathways of dendritic cells in vivo: distinct function, phenotype, and localization of dendritic cell subsets in FLT3 ligand-treated mice. *J Immunol* (1997) **159**(5):2222–31.
19. Ohnmacht C, Pullner A, King SB, Drexler I, Meier S, Brocker T, et al. Constitutive ablation of dendritic cells breaks self-tolerance of CD4 T cells and results in spontaneous fatal autoimmunity. *J Exp Med* (2009) **206**(3):549–59. doi:10.1084/jem.20082394
20. Liu K, Iyoda T, Saternus M, Kimura Y, Inaba K, Steinman RM. Immune tolerance after delivery of dying cells to dendritic cells in situ. *J Exp Med* (2002) **196**(8):1091–7. doi:10.1084/jem.20021215
21. Yamazaki S, Dudziak D, Heidkamp GF, Fiorese C, Bonito AJ, Inaba K, et al. CD8+CD205+ splenic dendritic cells are specialized to induce Foxp3+ regulatory t cells. *J Immunol* (2008) **181**(10):6923–33.
22. Dudziak D, Kamphorst AO, Heidkamp GF, Buchholz VR, Trumpfheller C, Yamazaki S, et al. Differential antigen processing by dendritic cell subsets in vivo. *Science* (2007) **315**(5808):107–11. doi:10.1126/science.1136080
23. Sun CM, Hall JA, Blank RB, Bouladoux N, Oukka M, Mora JR, et al. Small intestine lamina propria dendritic cells promote de novo generation of Foxp3 T reg cells via retinoic acid. *J Exp Med* (2007) **204**(8):1775–85. doi:10.1084/jem.20070602
24. Coombes JL, Siddiqui KR, Arancibia-Carcamo CV, Hall J, Sun CM, Belkaid Y, et al. A functionally specialized population of mucosal CD103+ DCs induces Foxp3+ regulatory T cells via a TGF-beta and retinoic acid-dependent mechanism. *J Exp Med* (2007) **204**(8):1757–64. doi:10.1084/jem.20070590
25. Proietto AI, van Dommelen S, Zhou P, Rizzitelli A, D'Amico A, Steptoe RJ, et al. Dendritic cells in the thymus contribute to T-regulatory cell induction. *Proc Natl Acad Sci U S A* (2008) **105**(50):19869–74. doi:10.1073/pnas.0810268105
26. Hori S, Nomura T, Sakaguchi S. Control of regulatory T cell development by the transcription factor Foxp3. *Science* (2003) **299**(5609):1057–61. doi:10.1126/science.1079490
27. Abbas AK, Benoist C, Bluestone JA, Campbell DJ, Ghosh S, Hori S, et al. Regulatory T cells: recommendations to simplify the nomenclature. *Nat Immunol* (2013) **14**(4):307–8. doi:10.1038/ni.2554
28. Wing K, Fehérvári Z, Sakaguchi S. Emerging possibilities in the development and function of regulatory T cells. *Int Immunol* (2006) **18**(7):991–1000. doi:10.1093/intimm/dxl044
29. Bergmann C, Strauss L, Zeidler R, Lang S, Whiteside TL. Expansion and characteristics of human T regulatory type 1 cells in co-cultures simulating tumor microenvironment. *Cancer Immunol Immunother* (2007) **56**(9):1429–42. doi:10.1007/s00262-007-0280-9
30. Fantini MC, Becker C, Monteleone G, Pallone F, Galle PR, Neurath MF. Cutting edge: TGF-beta induces a regulatory phenotype in $CD4^{+}CD25^{-}$ T cells through Foxp3 induction and down-regulation of Smad7. *J Immunol* (2004) **172**(9):5149–53.
31. Chambers ES, Hawrylowicz CM. The impact of vitamin D on regulatory T cells. *Curr Allergy Asthma Rep* (2011) **11**(1):29–36. doi:10.1007/s11882-010-0161-8
32. Mucida D, Park Y, Kim G, Turovskaya O, Scott I, Kronenberg M, et al. Reciprocal TH17 and regulatory T cell differentiation mediated by retinoic acid. *Science* (2007) **317**(5835):256–60. doi:10.1126/science.1145697
33. Kretschmer K, Apostolou I, Hawiger D, Khazaie K, Nussenzweig MC, von Boehmer H. Inducing and expanding regulatory T cell populations by foreign antigen. *Nat Immunol* (2005) **6**(12):1219–27. doi:10.1038/ni1265
34. Tarbell KV, Yamazaki S, Olson K, Toy P, Steinman RM. CD25+ CD4+ T cells, expanded with dendritic cells presenting a single autoantigenic peptide, suppress autoimmune diabetes. *J Exp Med* (2004) **199**(11):1467–77. doi:10.1084/jem.20040180
35. Yamazaki S, Bonito AJ, Spisek R, Dhodapkar M, Inaba K, Steinman RM. Dendritic cells are specialized accessory cells along with TGF^{-} for the differentiation of $Foxp3^{+}$ $CD4^{+}$ regulatory T cells from peripheral Foxp3 precursors. *Blood* (2007) **110**(13):4293–302. doi:10.1182/blood-2007-05-088831
36. Jonuleit H, Schmitt E, Schuler G, Knop J, Enk AH. Induction of interleukin 10-producing, nonproliferating CD4(+) T cells with regulatory properties by repetitive stimulation with allogeneic immature human dendritic cells. *J Exp Med* (2000) **192**(9):1213–22. doi:10.1084/jem.192.9.1213
37. Jonuleit H, Schmitt E, Steinbrink K, Enk AH. Dendritic cells as a tool to induce anergic and regulatory T cells. *Trends Immunol* (2001) **22**(7):394–400. doi:10.1016/S1471-4906(01)01952-4
38. Roncarolo MG, Levings MK, Traversari C. Differentiation of T regulatory cells by immature dendritic cells. *J Exp Med* (2001) **193**(2):F5–9. doi:10.1084/jem.193.2.F5
39. Wakkach A, Fournier N, Brun V, Breittmayer JP, Cottrez F, Groux H. Characterization of dendritic cells that induce tolerance and T regulatory 1 cell

differentiation in vivo. *Immunity* (2003) **18**(5):605–17. doi:10.1016/S1074-7613(03)00113-4

40. Fallarino F, Grohmann U, You S, McGrath BC, Cavener DR, Vacca C, et al. The combined effects of tryptophan starvation and tryptophan catabolites down-regulate T cell receptor {zeta}-chain and induce a regulatory phenotype in naive T cells. *J Immunol* (2006) **176**(11):6752–61.
41. Bonifaz L, Bonnyay D, Mahnke K, Rivera M, Nussenzweig MC, Steinman RM. Efficient targeting of protein antigen to the dendritic cell receptor DEC-205 in the steady state leads to antigen presentation on major histocompatibility complex class I products and peripheral CD8+ T cell tolerance. *J Exp Med* (2002) **196**(12):1627–38. doi:10.1084/jem.20021598
42. Kretschmer K, Heng TS, von Boehmer H. De novo production of antigen-specific suppressor cells in vivo. *Nat Protoc* (2006) **1**(2):653–61. doi:10.1038/nprot.2006.105
43. Zou T, Caton AJ, Koretzky GA, Kambayashi T. Dendritic cells induce regulatory T cell proliferation through antigen-dependent and -independent interactions. *J Immunol* (2010) **185**(5):2790–9. doi:10.4049/jimmunol.0903740
44. Darrasse-Jeze G, Deroubaix S, Mouquet H, Victora GD, Eisenreich T, Yao KH, et al. Feedback control of regulatory T cell homeostasis by dendritic cells in vivo. *J Exp Med* (2009) **206**(9):1853–62. doi:10.1084/jem.20090746
45. Morel PA, Turner MS. Dendritic cells and the maintenance of self-tolerance. *Immunol Res* (2011) **50**(2–3):124–9. doi:10.1007/s12026-011-8217-y
46. Serreze DV, Gaskins HR, Leiter EH. Defects in the differentiation and function of antigen presenting cells in NOD/Lt mice. *J Immunol* (1993) **150**(6):2534–43.
47. Prasad SJ, Goodnow CC. Cell-intrinsic effects of non-MHC NOD genes on dendritic cell generation in vivo. *Int Immunol* (2002) **14**(6):677–84. doi:10.1093/intimm/dxf034
48. Steptoe RJ, Ritchie JM, Harrison LC. Increased generation of dendritic cells from myeloid progenitors in autoimmune-prone nonobese diabetic mice. *J Immunol* (2002) **168**:5032–41.
49. Feili-Hariri M, Morel PA. Phenotypic and functional characteristics of BM-derived DC from NOD and non diabetes-prone strains. *Clin Immunol* (2001) **98**:133–42. doi:10.1006/clim.2000.4959
50. Vasquez AC, Feili-Hariri M, Tan RJ, Morel PA. Qualitative and quantitative abnormalities in splenic dendritic cell populations in NOD mice. *Clin Exp Immunol* (2004) **135**(2):209–18. doi:10.1111/j.1365-2249.2003.02359.x
51. Marleau AM, Summers KL, Singh B. Differential contributions of APC subsets to T cell activation in nonobese diabetic mice. *J Immunol* (2008) **180**(8):5235–49.
52. den Haan JM, Lehar SM, Bevan MJ. CD8(+) but not CD8(−) dendritic cells cross-prime cytotoxic T cells in vivo. *J Exp Med* (2000) **192**(12):1685–96. doi:10.1084/jem.192.12.1685
53. Pettersson A, Wu XC, Ciumas C, Lian H, Chirsky V, Huang YM, et al. CD8alpha dendritic cells and immune protection from experimental allergic encephalomyelitis. *Clin Exp Immunol* (2004) **137**(3):486–95. doi:10.1111/j.1365-2249.2004.02556.x
54. Hawiger D, Inaba K, Dorsett Y, Guo M, Mahnke K, Rivera M, et al. Dendritic cells induce peripheral T cell unresponsiveness under steady state conditions in vivo. *J Exp Med* (2001) **194**(6):769–80. doi:10.1084/jem.194.6.769
55. Chilton PM, Rezzoug F, Fugier-Vivier I, Weeter LA, Xu H, Huang Y, et al. Flt3-ligand treatment prevents diabetes in NOD mice. *Diabetes* (2004) **53**(8):1995–2002. doi:10.2337/diabetes.53.8.1995
56. O'Keeffe M, Brodnicki TC, Fancke B, Vremec D, Morahan G, Maraskovsky E, et al. Fms-like tyrosine kinase 3 ligand administration overcomes a genetically determined dendritic cell deficiency in NOD mice and protects against diabetes development. *Int Immunol* (2005) **17**(3):307–14. doi:10.1093/intimm/dxh210
57. Van Belle TL, Juntti T, Liao J, von Herrath MG. Pre-existing autoimmunity determines type 1 diabetes outcome after Flt3-ligand treatment. *J Autoimmun* (2010) **34**(4):445–52. doi:10.1016/j.jaut.2009.11.010
58. Poligone B, Weaver DJJ, Sen P, Baldwin ASJ, Tisch R. Elevated NF-kappaB activation in nonobese diabetic mouse dendritic cells results in enhanced APC function. *J Immunol* (2002) **168**:188–96.
59. Weaver DJJ, Poligone B, Bui T, Abdel-Motal UM, Baldwin ASJ, Tisch R. Dendritic cells from nonobese diabetic mice exhibit a defect in NF-kappa B regulation due to a hyperactive I kappa B kinase. *J Immunol* (2001) **167**:1461–8.
60. Marleau AM, Singh B. Myeloid dendritic cells in non-obese diabetic mice have elevated costimulatory and T helper-1-inducing abilities. *J Autoimmun* (2002) **19**(1–2):23–35. doi:10.1006/jaut.2002.0597
61. Liu J, Beller D. Aberrant production of IL-12 by macrophages from several autoimmune-prone mouse strains is characterized by intrinsic and unique patterns of NF-kappa B expression and binding to the IL-12 p40 promoter. *J Immunol* (2002) **169**(1):581–6.
62. Deaglio S, Dwyer KM, Gao W, Friedman D, Usheva A, Erat A, et al. Adenosine generation catalyzed by CD39 and CD73 expressed on regulatory T cells mediates immune suppression. *J Exp Med* (2007) **204**(6):1257–65. doi:10.1084/jem.20062512
63. Mandapathil M, Hilldorfer B, Szczepanski MJ, Czystowska M, Szajnik M, Ren J, et al. Generation and accumulation of immunosuppressive adenosine by human CD4+CD25highFOXP3+ regulatory T cells. *J Biol Chem* (2010) **285**(10):7176–86. doi:10.1074/jbc.M109.047423
64. Ghaemi Oskouie F, Shameli A, Yang A, Desrosiers MD, Mucsi AD, Blackburn MR, et al. High levels of adenosine deaminase on dendritic cells promote autoreactive T cell activation and diabetes in nonobese diabetic mice. *J Immunol* (2011) **186**(12):6798–806. doi:10.4049/jimmunol.1004222
65. Liston A, Lesage S, Gray DH, O'Reilly LA, Strasser A, Fahrer AM, et al. Generalized resistance to thymic deletion in the NOD mouse; a polygenic trait characterized by defective induction of Bim. *Immunity* (2004) **21**(6):817–30. doi:10.1016/j.immuni.2004.10.014
66. Kreuwel HT, Biggs JA, Pilip IM, Pamer EG, Lo D, Sherman LA. Defective CD8+ T cell peripheral tolerance in nonobese diabetic mice. *J Immunol* (2001) **167**(2):1112–7.
67. Tritt M, Sgouroudis E, d'Hennezel E, Albanese A, Piccirillo CA. Functional waning of naturally occurring CD4+ regulatory T-cells contributes to the onset of autoimmune diabetes. *Diabetes* (2008) **57**(1):113–23. doi:10.2337/db06-1700
68. Salomon B, Lenschow DJ, Rhee L, Ashourian N, Singh B, Sharpe A, et al. B7/CD28 costimulation is essential for the homeostasis of the CD4+CD25+ immunoregulatory T cells that control autoimmune diabetes. *Immunity* (2000) **12**(4):431–40. doi:10.1016/S1074-7613(00)80195-8
69. Fife BT, Pauken KE, Eagar TN, Obu T, Wu J, Tang Q, et al. Interactions between PD-1 and PD-L1 promote tolerance by blocking the TCR-induced stop signal. *Nat Immunol* (2009) **10**(11):1185–92. doi:10.1038/ni.1790
70. Obst R, van Santen HM, Melamed R, Kamphorst AO, Benoist C, Mathis D. Sustained antigen presentation can promote an immunogenic T cell response, like dendritic cell activation. *Proc Natl Acad Sci U S A* (2007) **104**(39):15460–5. doi:10.1073/pnas.0707331104
71. Malek TR, Castro I. Interleukin-2 receptor signaling: at the interface between tolerance and immunity. *Immunity* (2010) **33**(2):153–65. doi:10.1016/j.immuni.2010.08.004
72. Long SA, Cerosaletti K, Bollyky PL, Tatum M, Shilling H, Zhang S, et al. Defects in IL-2R signaling contribute to diminished maintenance of FOXP3 expression in CD4(+)CD25(+) regulatory T-cells of type 1 diabetic subjects. *Diabetes* (2010) **59**(2):407–15. doi:10.2337/db09-0694
73. Anderson AC, Chandwaskar R, Lee DH, Kuchroo VK. Cutting edge: the Idd3 genetic interval determines regulatory T cell function through CD11b+CD11c-APC. *J Immunol* (2008) **181**(11):7449–52.
74. Hamilton-Williams EE, Martinez X, Clark J, Howlett S, Hunter KM, Rainbow DB, et al. Expression of diabetes-associated genes by dendritic cells and CD4 T cells drives the loss of tolerance in nonobese diabetic mice. *J Immunol* (2009) **183**(3):1533–41. doi:10.4049/jimmunol.0900428
75. Sgouroudis E, Kornete M, Piccirillo CA. IL-2 production by dendritic cells promotes Foxp3(+) regulatory T-cell expansion in autoimmune-resistant NOD congenic mice. *Autoimmunity* (2011) **44**(5):406–14. doi:10.3109/08916934.2010.536795
76. Yang XD, Tisch R, Singer SM, Cao ZA, Liblau RS, Schreiber RD, et al. Effect of tumor necrosis factor alpha on insulin-dependent diabetes mellitus in NOD mice. I. The early development of autoimmunity and the diabetogenic process. *J Exp Med* (1994) **180**(3):995–1004. doi:10.1084/jem.180.3.995
77. Lee LF, Xu B, Michie SA, Beilhack GF, Warganich T, Turley S, et al. The role of TNF-alpha in the pathogenesis of type 1 diabetes in the nonobese diabetic mouse: analysis of dendritic cell maturation. *Proc Natl Acad Sci U S A* (2005) **102**(44):15995–6000. doi:10.1073/pnas.0508122102
78. Lee MH, Lee WH, Todorov I, Liu CP. CD4+ CD25+ regulatory T cells prevent type 1 diabetes preceded by dendritic cell-dominant invasive insulitis by affecting chemotaxis and local invasiveness of dendritic cells. *J Immunol* (2010) **185**(4):2493–501. doi:10.4049/jimmunol.1001036

79. Feili-Hariri M, Falkner DH, Morel PA. Polarization of naive T cells into Th1 or Th2 by distinct cytokine-driven murine dendritic cell populations: implications for immunotherapy. *J Leukoc Biol* (2005) **78**:656–64. doi:10.1189/jlb.1104631
80. Feili-Hariri M, Flores RR, Vasquez AC, Morel PA. Dendritic cell immunotherapy for autoimmune diabetes. *Immunol Res* (2006) **36**(1–3):167–73. doi:10.1385/IR:36:1:167
81. Saxena V, Ondr JK, Magnusen AF, Munn DH, Katz JD. The countervailing actions of myeloid and plasmacytoid dendritic cells control autoimmune diabetes in the nonobese diabetic mouse. *J Immunol* (2007) **179**(8):5041–53.
82. Caielli S, Conforti-Andreoni C, Di Pietro C, Usuelli V, Badami E, Malosio ML, et al. On/off TLR signaling decides proinflammatory or tolerogenic dendritic cell maturation upon CD1d-mediated interaction with invariant NKT cells. *J Immunol* (2010) **185**(12):7317–29. doi:10.4049/jimmunol.1000400
83. Diana J, Brezar V, Beaudoin L, Dalod M, Mellor A, Tafuri A, et al. Viral infection prevents diabetes by inducing regulatory T cells through NKT cell-plasmacytoid dendritic cell interplay. *J Exp Med* (2011) **208**(4):729–45. doi:10.1084/jem.20101692
84. Li Q, Xu B, Michie SA, Rubins KH, Schreriber RD, McDevitt HO. Interferon-alpha initiates type 1 diabetes in nonobese diabetic mice. *Proc Natl Acad Sci U S A* (2008) **105**(34):12439–44. doi:10.1073/pnas.0806439105
85. Li Q, McDevitt HO. The role of interferon alpha in initiation of type I diabetes in the NOD mouse. *Clin Immunol* (2011) **140**(1):3–7. doi:10.1016/j.clim.2011.04.010
86. Diana J, Simoni Y, Furio L, Beaudoin L, Agerberth B, Barrat F, et al. Crosstalk between neutrophils, B-1a cells and plasmacytoid dendritic cells initiates autoimmune diabetes. *Nat Med* (2013) **19**(1):65–73. doi:10.1038/nm.3042
87. Creusot RJ. Initiating type I diabetes: new suspects in the lineup. *Nat Med* (2013) **19**(1):18–20. doi:10.1038/nm.3044
88. Swiecki M, McCartney SA, Wang Y, Colonna M. TLR7/9 versus TLR3/MDA5 signaling during virus infections and diabetes. *J Leukoc Biol* (2011) **90**(4):691–701. doi:10.1189/jlb.0311166
89. Alba A, Planas R, Clemente X, Carrillo J, Ampudia R, Puertas MC, et al. Natural killer cells are required for accelerated type 1 diabetes driven by interferon-beta. *Clin Exp Immunol* (2008) **151**(3):467–75. doi:10.1111/j.1365-2249.2007.03580.x
90. Dotta F, Censini S, van Halteren AG, Marselli L, Masini M, Dionisi S, et al. Coxsackie B4 virus infection of beta cells and natural killer cell insulitis in recent-onset type 1 diabetic patients. *Proc Natl Acad Sci U S A* (2007) **104**(12):5115–20. doi:10.1073/pnas.0700442104
91. von Herrath M. Diabetes: a virus-gene collaboration. *Nature* (2009) **459**(7246):518–9. doi:10.1038/459518a
92. Filippi CM, Estes EA, Oldham JE, von Herrath MG. Immunoregulatory mechanisms triggered by viral infections protect from type 1 diabetes in mice. *J Clin Invest* (2009) **119**(6):1515–23. doi:10.1172/JCI38503
93. Welzen-Coppens JM, van Helden-Meeuwsen CG, Leenen PJ, Drexhage HA, Versnel MA. The kinetics of plasmacytoid dendritic cell accumulation in the pancreas of the NOD mouse during the early phases of insulitis. *PLoS One* (2013) **8**(1):e55071. doi:10.1371/journal.pone.0055071
94. Grohmann U, Fallarino F, Puccetti P. Tolerance, DCs and tryptophan: much ado about IDO. *Trends Immunol* (2003) **24**(5):242–8. doi:10.1016/S1471-4906(03)00072-3
95. Katz JD, Janssen EM. Breaking T cell tolerance to beta cell antigens by merocytic dendritic cells. *Cell Mol Life Sci* (2011) **68**(17):2873–83. doi:10.1007/s00018-011-0730-6
96. Katz JD, Ondr JK, Opoka RJ, Garcia Z, Janssen EM. Cutting edge: merocytic dendritic cells break T cell tolerance to beta cell antigens in nonobese diabetic mouse diabetes. *J Immunol* (2010) **185**(4):1999–2003. doi:10.4049/jimmunol.1001398
97. Pelletier AN, Lesage S. The Idd13 congenic interval defines the number of merocytic dendritic cells, a novel trait associated with autoimmune diabetes susceptibility. *J Autoimmun* (2013) **43**:70–7. doi:10.1016/j.jaut.2013.04.004
98. Calderon B, Suri A, Miller MJ, Unanue ER. Dendritic cells in islets of Langerhans constitutively present beta cell-derived peptides bound to their class II MHC molecules. *Proc Natl Acad Sci U S A* (2008) **105**(16):6121–6. doi:10.1073/pnas.0801973105
99. Melli K, Friedman RS, Martin AE, Finger EB, Miao G, Szot GL, et al. Amplification of autoimmune response through induction of dendritic cell maturation in inflamed tissues. *J Immunol* (2009) **182**(5):2590–600. doi:10.4049/jimmunol.0803543
100. Ginhoux F, Liu K, Helft J, Bogunovic M, Greter M, Hashimoto D, et al. The origin and development of nonlymphoid tissue CD103+ DCs. *J Exp Med* (2009) **206**(13):3115–30. doi:10.1084/jem.20091756
101. Yin N, Xu J, Ginhoux F, Randolph GJ, Merad M, Ding Y, et al. Functional specialization of islet dendritic cell subsets. *J Immunol* (2012) **188**(10):4921–30. doi:10.4049/jimmunol.1103725
102. Calderon B, Carrero JA, Miller MJ, Unanue ER. Cellular and molecular events in the localization of diabetogenic T cells to islets of Langerhans. *Proc Natl Acad Sci U S A* (2011) **108**(4):1561–6. doi:10.1073/pnas.1018973108
103. Gagnerault MC, Luan JJ, Lotton C, Lepault F. Pancreatic lymph nodes are required for priming of beta cell reactive T cells in NOD mice. *J Exp Med* (2002) **196**(3):369–77. doi:10.1084/jem.20011353
104. Hoglund P, Mintern J, Waltzinger C, Heath W, Benoist C, Mathis D. Initiation of autoimmune diabetes by developmentally regulated presentation of islet cell antigens in the pancreatic lymph nodes. *J Exp Med* (1999) **189**(2):331–9. doi:10.1084/jem.189.2.331
105. Zhang Y, O'Brien B, Trudeau J, Tan R, Santamaria P, Dutz JP. In situ beta cell death promotes priming of diabetogenic CD8 T lymphocytes. *J Immunol* (2002) **168**(3):1466–72.
106. Coppieters K, Martinic MM, Kiosses WB, Amirian N, von Herrath M. A novel technique for the in vivo imaging of autoimmune diabetes development in the pancreas by two-photon microscopy. *PLoS One* (2010) **5**(12):e15732. doi:10.1371/journal.pone.0015732
107. Welzen-Coppens JM, van Helden-Meeuwsen CG, Leenen PJ, Drexhage HA, Versnel MA. Reduced numbers of dendritic cells with a tolerogenic phenotype in the prediabetic pancreas of NOD mice. *J Leukoc Biol* (2012) **92**(6):1207–13. doi:10.1189/jlb.0312168
108. Allen JS, Pang K, Skowera A, Ellis R, Rackham C, Lozanoska-Ochser B, et al. Plasmacytoid dendritic cells are proportionally expanded at diagnosis of type 1 diabetes and enhance islet autoantigen presentation to T-cells through immune complex capture. *Diabetes* (2009) **58**(1):138–45. doi:10.2337/db08-0964
109. Vuckovic S, Withers G, Harris M, Khalil D, Gardiner D, Flesch I, et al. Decreased blood dendritic cell counts in type 1 diabetic children. *Clin Immunol* (2007) **123**(3):281–8. doi:10.1016/j.clim.2007.03.002
110. Galgani M, Nugnes R, Bruzzese D, Perna F, De Rosa V, Procaccini C, et al. Meta-immunological profiling of children with type 1 diabetes identifies new biomarkers to monitor disease progression. *Diabetes* (2013) **62**(7):2481–91. doi:10.2337/db12-1273
111. Nieminen JK, Vakkila J, Salo HM, Ekstrom N, Harkonen T, Ilonen J, et al. Altered phenotype of peripheral blood dendritic cells in pediatric type 1 diabetes. *Diabetes Care* (2012) **35**(11):2303–10. doi:10.2337/dc11-2460
112. Rose K, Penna-Martinez M, Klahold E, Karger D, Shoghi F, Kahles H, et al. Influence of the vitamin D plasma level and vitamin D-related genetic polymorphisms on the immune status of patients with type 1 diabetes: a pilot study. *Clin Exp Immunol* (2013) **171**(2):171–85. doi:10.1111/cei.12013
113. Uno S, Imagawa A, Okita K, Sayama K, Moriwaki M, Iwahashi H, et al. Macrophages and dendritic cells infiltrating islets with or without beta cells produce tumour necrosis factor-alpha in patients with recent-onset type 1 diabetes. *Diabetologia* (2007) **50**(3):596–601. doi:10.1007/s00125-006-0569-9
114. Aida K, Nishida Y, Tanaka S, Maruyama T, Shimada A, Awata T, et al. RIG-I- and MDA5-initiated innate immunity linked with adaptive immunity accelerates beta-cell death in fulminant type 1 diabetes. *Diabetes* (2011) **60**(3):884–9. doi:10.2337/db10-0795
115. Mukherjee G, Dilorenzo TP. The immunotherapeutic potential of dendritic cells in type 1 diabetes. *Clin Exp Immunol* (2010) **161**(2):197–207. doi:10.1111/j.1365-2249.2010.04157.x
116. Morel PA, Feili-Hariri M, Coates PT, Thomson AW. Dendritic cells, T cell tolerance and therapy of adverse immune reactions. *Clin Exp Immunol* (2003) **133**(1):1–10. doi:10.1046/j.1365-2249.2003.02161.x
117. Morelli AE, Thomson AW. Tolerogenic dendritic cells and the quest for transplant tolerance. *Nat Rev Immunol* (2007) **7**(8):610–21. doi:10.1038/nri2132
118. Menges M, Rossner S, Voigtlander C, Schindler H, Kukutsch NA, Bogdan C, et al. Repetitive injections of dendritic cells matured with tumor necrosis factor alpha induce antigen-specific protection of mice from autoimmunity. *J Exp Med* (2002) **195**(1):15–21. doi:10.1084/jem.20011341

119. Lutz MB, Schuler G. Immature, semi-mature and fully mature dendritic cells: which signals induce tolerance or immunity? *Trends Immunol* (2002) **23**(9):445–9. doi:10.1016/S1471-4906(02)02281-0
120. Clemente-Casares X, Tsai S, Huang C, Santamaria P. Antigen-specific therapeutic approaches in Type 1 diabetes. *Cold Spring Harbor Perspect Med* (2012) **2**(2):a007773. doi:10.1101/cshperspect.a007773
121. Clare-Salzler MJ, Brooks J, Chai A, Van Herle K, Anderson C. Prevention of diabetes in nonobese diabetic mice by dendritic cell transfer. *J Clin Invest* (1992) **90**(3):741–8. doi:10.1172/JCI115946
122. Naumov YN, Bahjat KS, Gausling R, Abraham R, Exley MA, Koezuka Y, et al. Activation of CD1d-restricted T cells protects NOD mice from developing diabetes by regulating dendritic cell subsets. *Proc Natl Acad Sci U S A* (2001) **98**(24):13838–43. doi:10.1073/pnas.251531798
123. Feili-Hariri M, Dong X, Alber SM, Watkins SC, Salter RD, Morel PA. Immunotherapy of NOD mice with bone marrow-derived dendritic cells. *Diabetes* (1999) **48**:2300–8. doi:10.2337/diabetes.48.12.2300
124. Feili-Hariri M, Falkner DH, Gambotto A, Papworth GD, Watkins SC, Robbins PD, et al. Dendritic cells transduced to express IL-4 prevent diabetes in nonobese diabetic mice with established insulitis. *Human Gene Ther* (2003) **14**:13–23. doi:10.1089/10430340360464679
125. Feili-Hariri M, Falkner DH, Morel PA. Regulatory Th2 response induced following adoptive transfer of dendritic cells in prediabetic NOD mice. *Eur J Immunol* (2002) **32**:2021–30. doi:10.1002/1521-4141(200207)32:7<2021::AID-IMMU2021>3.0.CO;2-J
126. Creusot RJ, Chang P, Healey DG, Tcherepanova IY, Nicolette CA, Fathman CG. A short pulse of IL-4 delivered by DCs electroporated with modified mRNA can both prevent and treat autoimmune diabetes in NOD mice. *Mol Ther* (2010) **18**(12):2112–20. doi:10.1038/mt.2010.146
127. Ruffner MA, Robbins PD. Dendritic cells transduced to express interleukin 4 reduce diabetes onset in both normoglycemic and prediabetic nonobese diabetic mice. *PLoS One* (2010) **5**(7):e11848. doi:10.1371/journal.pone.0011848
128. Haase C, Ejrnaes M, Juedes AE, Wolfe T, Markholst H, von Herrath MG. Immunomodulatory dendritic cells require autologous serum to circumvent nonspecific immunosuppressive activity in vivo. *Blood* (2005) **106**(13):4225–33. doi:10.1182/blood-2005-03-0975
129. Turner MS, Kane LP, Morel PA. Dominant role of antigen dose in CD4+Foxp3+ regulatory T cell induction and expansion. *J Immunol* (2009) **183**(8):4895–903. doi:10.4049/jimmunol.0901459
130. Haase C, Yu L, Eisenbarth G, Markholst H. Antigen-dependent immunotherapy of non-obese diabetic mice with immature dendritic cells. *Clin Exp Immunol* (2010) **160**(3):331–9. doi:10.1111/j.1365-2249.2010.04104.x
131. Tai N, Yasuda H, Xiang Y, Zhang L, Rodriguez-Pinto D, Yokono K, et al. IL-10-conditioned dendritic cells prevent autoimmune diabetes in NOD and humanized HLA-DQ8/RIP-B7.1 mice. *Clin Immunol* (2011) **139**(3):336–49. doi:10.1016/j.clim.2011.03.003
132. Torres-Aguilar H, Sanchez-Torres C, Jara LJ, Blank M, Shoenfeld Y. IL-10/TGF-beta-treated dendritic cells, pulsed with insulin, specifically reduce the response to insulin of CD4+ effector/memory T cells from type 1 diabetic individuals. *J Clin Immunol* (2010) **30**(5):659–68. doi:10.1007/s10875-010-9430-5
133. Besin G, Gaudreau S, Menard M, Guindi C, Dupuis G, Amrani A. Thymic stromal lymphopoietin and thymic stromal lymphopoietin-conditioned dendritic cells induce regulatory T-cell differentiation and protection of NOD mice against diabetes. *Diabetes* (2008) **57**(8):2107–17. doi:10.2337/db08-0171
134. Kleijwegt FS, Jansen DT, Teeler J, Joosten AM, Laban S, Nikolic T, et al. Tolerogenic dendritic cells impede priming of naive CD8(+) T cells and deplete memory CD8(+) T cells. *Eur J Immunol* (2013) **43**(1):85–92. doi:10.1002/eji.201242879
135. Simon T, Pogu S, Tardif V, Rigaud K, Remy S, Piaggio E, et al. Carbon monoxide-treated dendritic cells decrease beta1-integrin induction on CD8(+) T cells and protect from type 1 diabetes. *Eur J Immunol* (2013) **43**(1):209–18. doi:10.1002/eji.201242684
136. Karumuthil-Melethil S, Perez N, Li R, Prabhakar BS, Holterman MJ, Vasu C. Dendritic cell-directed CTLA-4 engagement during pancreatic beta cell antigen presentation delays type 1 diabetes. *J Immunol* (2010) **184**(12):6695–708. doi:10.4049/jimmunol.0903130
137. Diana J, Moura IC, Vaugier C, Gestin A, Tissandie E, Beaudoin L, et al. Secretory IgA induces tolerogenic dendritic cells through SIGNR1 dampening autoimmunity in mice. *J Immunol* (2013) **191**(5):2335–43. doi:10.4049/jimmunol.1300864
138. Machen J, Harnaha J, Lakomy R, Styche A, Trucco M, Giannoukakis N. Antisense oligonucleotides down-regulating costimulation confer diabetes-preventive properties to nonobese diabetic mouse dendritic cells. *J Immunol* (2004) **173**(7):4331–41.
139. Giannoukakis N, Phillips B, Finegold D, Harnaha J, Trucco M. Phase I (safety) study of autologous tolerogenic dendritic cells in type 1 diabetic patients. *Diabetes Care* (2011) **34**(9):2026–32. doi:10.2337/dc11-0472
140. Tarbell KV, Yamazaki S, Steinman RM. The interactions of dendritic cells with antigen-specific, regulatory T cells that suppress autoimmunity. *Semin Immunol* (2006) **18**(2):93–102. doi:10.1016/j.smim.2006.01.009
141. Gopisetty A, Bhattacharya P, Haddad C, Bruno JC Jr, Vasu C, Miele L, et al. OX40L/Jagged1 cosignaling by GM-CSF-induced bone marrow-derived dendritic cells is required for the expansion of functional regulatory T cells. *J Immunol* (2013) **190**(11):5516–25. doi:10.4049/jimmunol.1202298
142. Moreau A, Varey E, Bouchet-Delbos L, Cuturi MC. Cell therapy using tolerogenic dendritic cells in transplantation. *Transplant Res* (2012) **1**(1):13. doi:10.1186/2047-1440-1-13
143. Boks MA, Kager-Groenland JR, Haasjes MSP, Zwaginga JJ, van Ham SM, ten Brinke A. IL-10-generated tolerogenic dendritic cells are optimal for functional regulatory T cell induction – a comparative study of human clinical-applicable DC. *Clin Immunol* (2012) **142**(3):332–42. doi:10.1016/j.clim.2011.11.011
144. Petzold C, Riewaldt J, Koenig T, Schallenberg S, Kretschmer K. Dendritic cell-targeted pancreatic beta-cell antigen leads to conversion of self-reactive CD4(+) T cells into regulatory T cells and promotes immunotolerance in NOD mice. *Rev Diabet Stud* (2010) **7**(1):47–61. doi:10.1900/RDS.2010.7.47
145. Bruder D, Westendorf AM, Hansen W, Prettin S, Gruber AD, Qian Y, et al. On the edge of autoimmunity: T-cell stimulation by steady-state dendritic cells prevents autoimmune diabetes. *Diabetes* (2005) **54**(12):3395–401. doi:10.2337/diabetes.54.12.3395
146. Mukhopadhaya A, Hanafusa T, Jarchum I, Chen YG, Iwai Y, Serreze DV, et al. Selective delivery of beta cell antigen to dendritic cells in vivo leads to deletion and tolerance of autoreactive CD8+ T cells in NOD mice. *Proc Natl Acad Sci U S A* (2008) **105**(17):6374–9. doi:10.1073/pnas.0802644105
147. Constant S, Pfeiffer C, Woodard A, Pasqualini T, Bottomly K. Extent of T cell receptor ligation can determine the functional differentiation of naive CD4+ T cells. *J Exp Med* (1995) **182**(5):1591–6. doi:10.1084/jem.182.5.1591
148. Constant SL, Bottomly K. Induction of Th1 and Th2 CD4+ T cell responses: the alternative approaches. *Annu Rev Immunol* (1997) **15**:297–322. doi:10.1146/annurev.immunol.15.1.297
149. Hosken NA, Shibuya K, Heath AW, Murphy KM, O'Garra A. The effect of antigen dose on CD4+ T helper cell phenotype development in a T cell receptor-alpha beta-transgenic model. *J Exp Med* (1995) **182**(5):1579–84. doi:10.1084/jem.182.5.1579
150. Sauer S, Bruno L, Hertweck A, Finlay D, Leleu M, Spivakov M, et al. T cell receptor signaling controls Foxp3 expression via PI3K, Akt, and mTOR. *Proc Natl Acad Sci U S A* (2008) **105**(22):7797–802. doi:10.1073/pnas.0800928105
151. Gabryšová L, Christensen JR, Wu X, Kissenpfennig A, Malissen B, O'Garra A. Integrated T-cell receptor and costimulatory signals determine TGF-β-dependent differentiation and maintenance of Foxp3+ regulatory T cells. *Eur J Immunol* (2011) **41**(5):1242–8. doi:10.1002/eji.201041073
152. Gottschalk RA, Corse E, Allison JP. TCR ligand density and affinity determine peripheral induction of Foxp3 in vivo. *J Exp Med* (2010) **207**(8):1701–11. doi:10.1084/jem.20091999
153. Gottschalk RA, Hathorn MM, Beuneu H, Corse E, Dustin ML, Altan-Bonnet G, et al. Distinct influences of peptide-MHC quality and quantity on in vivo T-cell responses. *Proc Natl Acad Sci U S A* (2012) **109**(3):881–6. doi:10.1073/pnas.1119763109
154. von Boehmer H. Peptide-based instruction of suppressor commitment in naive T cells and dynamics of immunosuppression in vivo. *Scand J Immunol* (2005) **62**(Suppl 1):49–54. doi:10.1111/j.1365-3083.2005.01609.x
155. Daniel C, Weigmann B, Bronson R, von Boehmer H. Prevention of type 1 diabetes in mice by tolerogenic vaccination with a strong agonist insulin mimetope. *J Exp Med* (2011) **208**(7):1501–10. doi:10.1084/jem.20110574
156. Long SA, Rieck M, Tatum M, Bollyky PL, Wu RP, Muller I, et al. Low-dose antigen promotes induction of FOXP3 in human CD4+ T cells. *J Immunol* (2011) **187**(7):3511–20. doi:10.4049/jimmunol.1003880

157. Keselowsky BG, Xia CQ, Clare-Salzler M. Multifunctional dendritic cell-targeting polymeric microparticles: engineering new vaccines for type 1 diabetes. *Hum Vaccin* (2011) **7**(1):37–44. doi:10.4161/hv.7.1.12916
158. Phillips B, Nylander K, Harnaha J, Machen J, Lakomy R, Styche A, et al. A microsphere-based vaccine prevents and reverses new-onset autoimmune diabetes. *Diabetes* (2008) **57**(6):1544–55. doi:10.2337/db07-0507
159. Hu C, Ding H, Zhang X, Wong FS, Wen L. Combination treatment with anti-CD20 and oral anti-CD3 prevents and reverses autoimmune diabetes. *Diabetes* (2013) **62**(8):2849–58. doi:10.2337/db12-1175
160. Fallarino F, Bianchi R, Orabona C, Vacca C, Belladonna ML, Fioretti MC, et al. CTLA-4-Ig activates forkhead transcription factors and protects dendritic cells from oxidative stress in nonobese diabetic mice. *J Exp Med* (2004) **200**(8):1051–62. doi:10.1084/jem.20040942
161. Billiard F, Lobry C, Darrasse-Jeze G, Waite J, Liu X, Mouquet H, et al. Dll4-Notch signaling in Flt3-independent dendritic cell development and autoimmunity in mice. *J Exp Med* (2012) **209**(5):1011–28. doi:10.1084/jem.20111615
162. Hong S, Wilson MT, Serizawa I, Wu L, Singh N, Naidenko OV, et al. The natural killer T-cell ligand alpha-galactosylceramide prevents autoimmune diabetes in non-obese diabetic mice. *Nat Med* (2001) **7**(9):1052–6. doi:10.1038/nm0901-1052
163. Sharif S, Arreaza GA, Zucker P, Mi QS, Sondhi J, Naidenko OV, et al. Activation of natural killer T cells by alpha-galactosylceramide treatment prevents the onset and recurrence of autoimmune Type 1 diabetes. *Nat Med* (2001) **7**(9):1057–62. doi:10.1038/nm0901-1057
164. Wang B, Geng YB, Wang CR. CD1-restricted NK T cells protect nonobese diabetic mice from developing diabetes. *J Exp Med* (2001) **194**(3):313–20. doi:10.1084/jem.194.3.313
165. Wang J, Cho S, Ueno A, Cheng L, Xu BY, Desrosiers MD, et al. Ligand-dependent induction of noninflammatory dendritic cells by anergic invariant NKT cells minimizes autoimmune inflammation. *J Immunol* (2008) **181**(4):2438–45.
166. Tohn R, Blumenfeld H, Haeryfar SM, Veerapen N, Besra GS, Porcelli SA, et al. Stimulation of a shorter duration in the state of anergy by an invariant natural killer T cell agonist enhances its efficiency of protection from type 1 diabetes. *Clin Exp Immunol* (2011) **164**(1):26–41. doi:10.1111/j.1365-2249.2011.04323.x
167. Di Caro V, Phillips B, Engman C, Harnaha J, Trucco M, Giannoukakis N. Retinoic acid-producing, ex vivo-generated human tolerogenic dendritic cells induce the proliferation of immunosuppressive B-lymphocytes. *Clin Exp Immunol* (2013) **174**(2):302–17. doi:10.1111/cei.12177
168. Coppieters KT, Harrison LC, von Herrath MG. Trials in type 1 diabetes: antigen-specific therapies. *Clin Immunol* (2013) **149**(3):345–55. doi:10.1016/j.clim.2013.02.002
169. Shoda LK, Young DL, Ramanujan S, Whiting CC, Atkinson MA, Bluestone JA, et al. A comprehensive review of interventions in the NOD mouse and implications for translation. *Immunity* (2005) **23**(2):115–26. doi:10.1016/j.immuni.2005.08.002

12

An interaction library for the FcεRI signaling network

Lily A. Chylek[1,2], David A. Holowka[1], Barbara A. Baird[1]* and William S. Hlavacek[2]*

[1] Department of Chemistry and Chemical Biology, Cornell University, Ithaca, NY, USA
[2] Los Alamos National Laboratory, Theoretical Division, Center for Non-linear Studies, Los Alamos, NM, USA

Edited by:
Rob J. De Boer, Utrecht University, Netherlands

Reviewed by:
Christopher E. Rudd, University of Cambridge, UK
Grégoire Altan-Bonnet, Memorial Sloan-Kettering Cancer Center, USA

***Correspondence:**
Barbara A. Baird, Department of Chemistry and Chemical Biology, Cornell University, Ithaca, NY 14853, USA
e-mail: bab13@cornell.edu;
William S. Hlavacek, Los Alamos National Laboratory, Theoretical Division, Center for Nonlinear Studies, Los Alamos, NM 87545, USA
e-mail: wish@lanl.gov

Antigen receptors play a central role in adaptive immune responses. Although the molecular networks associated with these receptors have been extensively studied, we currently lack a systems-level understanding of how combinations of non-covalent interactions and post-translational modifications are regulated during signaling to impact cellular decision-making. To fill this knowledge gap, it will be necessary to formalize and piece together information about individual molecular mechanisms to form large-scale computational models of signaling networks. To this end, we have developed an interaction library for signaling by the high-affinity IgE receptor, FcεRI. The library consists of executable rules for protein–protein and protein–lipid interactions. This library extends earlier models for FcεRI signaling and introduces new interactions that have not previously been considered in a model. Thus, this interaction library is a toolkit with which existing models can be expanded and from which new models can be built. As an example, we present models of branching pathways from the adaptor protein Lat, which influence production of the phospholipid PIP_3 at the plasma membrane and the soluble second messenger IP_3. We find that inclusion of a positive feedback loop gives rise to a bistable switch, which may ensure robust responses to stimulation above a threshold level. In addition, the library is visualized to facilitate understanding of network circuitry and identification of network motifs.

Keywords: immunoreceptor signaling, IgE receptors (FcεRI), mast cells, knowledge engineering, computational modeling, network motifs, feed-forward loops, visualization

INTRODUCTION

Cell signaling plays a key part in regulation of the immune system. Adaptive immune responses are controlled by multichain immune recognition receptors, or immunoreceptors, which include the T cell receptor (TCR) (1), the B cell antigen receptor (BCR) (2), and the high-affinity receptor for IgE, which is also known as FcεRI (3). Each of these receptors is the gatekeeper of complex signaling machineries that translate extracellular stimuli into cellular responses. Individual interactions in immunoreceptor signaling systems have been studied extensively, and there is now a need to form a cohesive picture of how these interactions combine to mediate information processing. This need is driven in part by emerging data that reveal complex dynamical behaviors that arise from molecular interactions (4, 5), as well as by a growing appreciation of network features, such as crosstalk (6), which may only be apparent when one considers the interplay of multiple interactions.

Knowledge about signaling can be combined and synthesized into multiple forms, of which we employ two that are versatile and extensible: a visual map drawn in accordance with recommended standard conventions, and a rule-based model. The value of a standardized map, as opposed to an *ad hoc* cartoon, in depicting molecular interactions has been well appreciated: such maps can be used to organize information concisely, can be interpreted with minimal ambiguity, and can aid in logical analysis (7–11). After creation of a map, construction of a computational model can be viewed as the next level of information formalization (12). Through modeling, assumptions about molecular interactions (e.g., whether or not two interactions are competitive) are made more concrete and can thus be better assessed. In addition, modeling can extend our predictive capabilities when quantitative factors are important, enabling us to develop more sophisticated hypotheses. Modeling has become an increasingly important part of studies of immunoreceptor signaling (13).

Of the modeling frameworks that have been used to investigate biochemical systems, the framework of chemical kinetics is useful for studying dynamical behaviors that evolve on >1 ms time scales and that can be characterized using measurable parameters, such as protein copy numbers and binding rate constants. Among the modeling techniques of chemical kinetics is rule-based modeling (14), which provides a means to represent individual biomolecular sites, which is essential when, for example, different phosphorylation sites can recruit different binding partners (15). Rule-based modeling also enables simulation of the behavior of a large number of distinct chemical species. Myriad multicomponent protein complexes and protein phosphoforms, for example, can potentially arise in cell signaling systems and this complexity poses a challenge for other modeling techniques (16, 17). Rule-based models are built from executable rules. Rules in a model have a certain degree of interdependence, but tend to be more modular than the component parts used in other modeling techniques, such as ordinary differential equations (17). Thus, it is not only possible to formulate rules for a specific model, but to construct general rule libraries from which different models may be built.

To further our systems-level understanding of immunoreceptor signaling, we have developed a map and a rule library for early signaling mediated by FcεRI, which shares features with other related immunoreceptors. The FcεRI signaling system has a special feature of experimental tractability because the receptor can be stimulated using structurally defined antigens (18–20), making it a valuable model system for understanding how signaling is initiated. Furthermore, FcεRI has been the subject of several past modeling studies that have elucidated early events following receptor crosslinking (21, 22), the flow of information during signaling (23), aggregation of adaptor proteins (24, 25), and the impact of ligand dose and binding kinetics on kinase activation (26, 27). Aspects of the models used in these studies form a foundation for the rule library presented here. The library extends previous work by adding rules for interactions not previously included in models for FcεRI signaling. Thus, the library serves as a bridge between past studies of relatively small scope, and potential future studies that integrate information about more network elements to, for example, analyze multiplexed signaling data (28). As a first example of library use, we present simulations of recruitment of signaling proteins to the adaptor Lat, which is phosphorylated in response to FcεRI stimulation (29).

METHODS

We developed a library of rules based on known protein–protein and protein–lipid interactions, which were identified through a survey of the FcεRI literature. The rules can be assembled into different sets to form different models that capture the chemical kinetics of FcεRI signaling with site-specific resolution (14, 16, 30). Here, the term "site" is used to refer to a generic functional site in a biomolecule, which in the case of a protein may be a domain, linear motif, or amino acid residue subject to post-translational modification. In a rule-based model, rules capture knowledge about biomolecular interactions of interest. The rules in a model specify what interactions can occur in a system and under what conditions these interactions occur. A rule provides necessary and sufficient conditions for testing its applicability, a definition of the consequences of an interaction, and a rate law. A detailed example of a rule is illustrated graphically in Figure S1 in Supplementary Material. Rules, in combination with parameters and initial conditions, can be processed to simulate the time-dependent behavior of a signaling system, including the time-dependent formation of protein complexes and post-translational modifications of proteins at specific sites. A benefit of a rule-based approach is that it enables concise specification and efficient simulation of models that include multivalent interactions and multi-site phosphorylation, which are two inherent characteristics of immunoreceptor signaling systems that are otherwise difficult or impossible to fully capture in a physicochemical model. We specified our library using a domain-specific language for rule-based modeling, the BioNetGen language (BNGL) (30), which is compatible with several software tools for simulation and analysis.

Our simulations are based on the law of mass action and an assumption of well-mixed reaction compartments. In the example model, the following compartments are considered implicitly: the cytosol, the plasma membrane, and the extracellular fluid surrounding a single-cell. Simulations were performed using CVODE (31), the built-in deterministic simulator of BioNetGen, which takes as input the ODEs derived from a rule-specified reaction network. Our illustrations of rules are based on published guidelines for model visualization (10) and were drawn with the help of a template available online (http://bionetgen.org/index.php/Extended_Contact_Maps).

In our bifurcation analyses, we found stable steady states through simulations that were started from arbitrary initial conditions or nearby steady states. The bifurcation parameter was an input signal taken in the model of interest to control the rate of activation of Syk and Fyn, which were each deactivated through a first-order process. Thus, as the input signal increases, so too do the steady-state levels of active Syk and Fyn. In simulations performed to find stable steady states, the bifurcation parameter was systematically varied from a low to high value, and vice versa.

To characterize signaling dynamics for specific observables (i.e., model outputs), we calculated rise time as the time required for the observable to reach 95% of its final steady-state value. For comparison between two models, a ratio of rise times was calculated.

RESULTS AND DISCUSSION

LIBRARY

In this section, we present a collection of rules, which can be viewed as a single model or as an assemblage of multiple models. Our main purpose is not to simulate the full set of interactions represented by these rules, but to formalize available knowledge about the FcεRI system to facilitate future modeling studies aimed at addressing specific questions. Rules in the library are provided in File S1 in Supplementary Material.

Rule-based models are compositional, meaning that rules can be specified somewhat independently of each other, enabling construction of new models from components of existing models. We have taken advantage of this feature to build on three previously reported models: one for ligand–receptor interactions and two for intracellular signaling. Below, we briefly review these models and the processes that they capture. A visual overview of the intracellular processes captured in the library is provided in **Figure 1**.

Initiation of signaling by FcεRI requires aggregation of receptors, which can be induced by reagents such as haptenated proteins and polymers, as well as by anti-receptor antibodies (32). Several models have been developed to investigate the interactions that lead to receptor aggregation. The model that we consider here is that of Xu et al. (33) for interactions of IgE-FcεRI with DNP–BSA, a multivalent antigen (haptenated protein). We chose this model because DNP–BSA is commonly used for stimulation of mast cells sensitized with anti-DNP IgE, and receptor aggregation induced by this antigen has been studied in detail (34). In this model, the effective valence of the ligand was taken to be two. The model includes transient hapten exposure, initial binding of a ligand to a receptor, crosslinking of neighboring receptors, and dissociation of ligand–receptor bonds. In this model, it was assumed that receptor sites (antigen-combining sites in cell-surface IgE) are equivalent and that the single-site dissociation rate constant is the same for both ligand sites, regardless of whether the second site is bound or free. Cyclic aggregates are not considered. For use in this study, the model was translated from its original form to rules, which was also done in another recent study (35). The model of Xu et al. is illustrated in **Figure 2**.

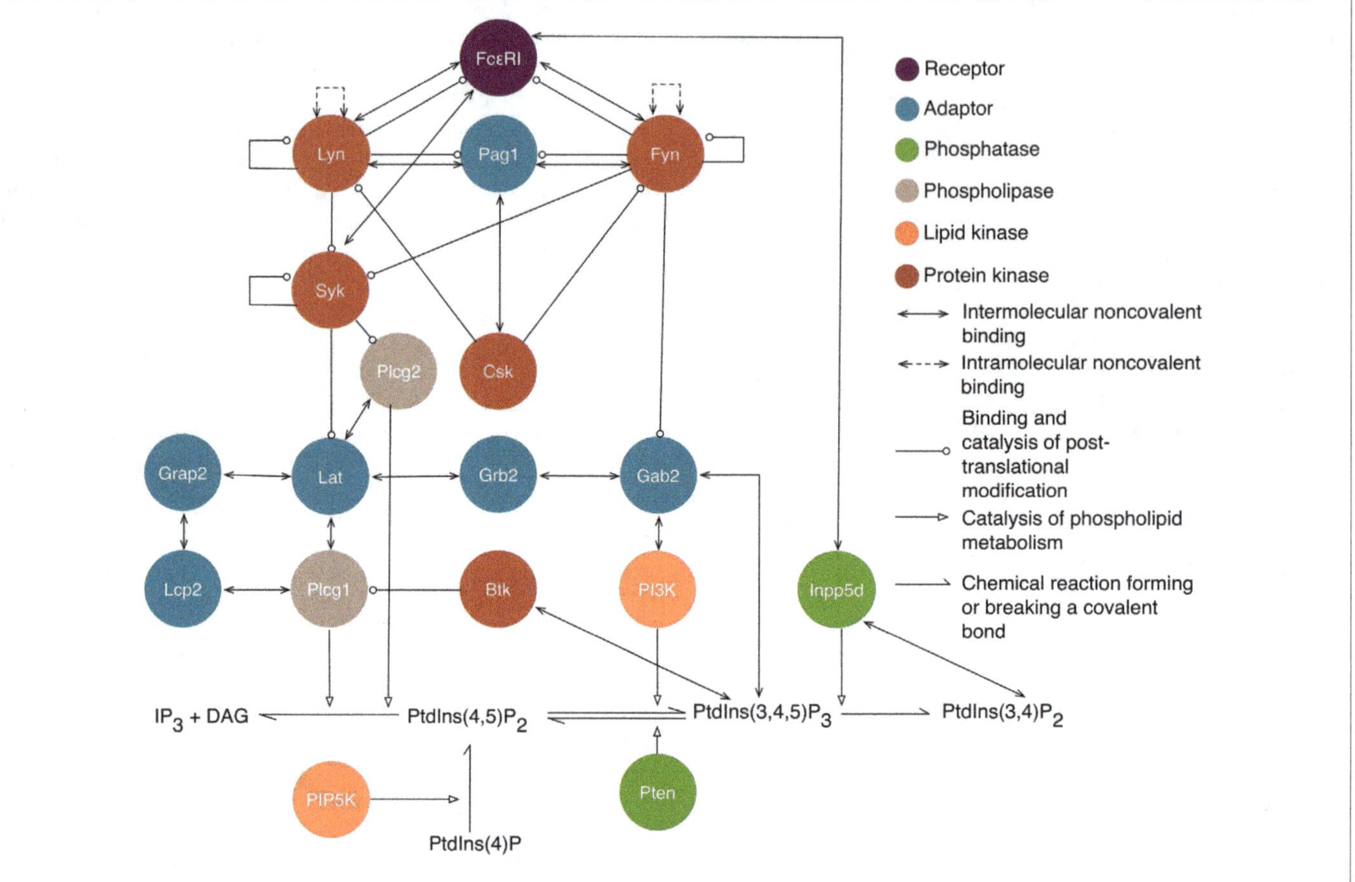

FIGURE 1 | An overview of intracellular signaling interactions included in the model/library for FcεRI signaling. Rules are included in the library for the interactions depicted here. Proteins are represented as circles that are color-coded according to their function, as indicated in the legend. Standard UniProt names are used, and we note that Grap2 is commonly known as Gads, Lcp2 is commonly known as Slp76, and Inpp5d is commonly known as Ship1. The legend also indicates the arrows that are used to represent different types of interactions and influences. Reactions of lipid species are illustrated at the bottom. Arrows from proteins that point to lipid reactions indicate that the reaction is catalyzed by that protein. Arrows from protein to lipid species indicate that the protein binds that lipid. Not shown are implicit phosphatase reactions that cause dephosphorylation of all sites that can be phosphorylated. Ligand–receptor interactions are shown in **Figure 2**. A subset of interactions is illustrated with site-specific detail in **Figure 3**.

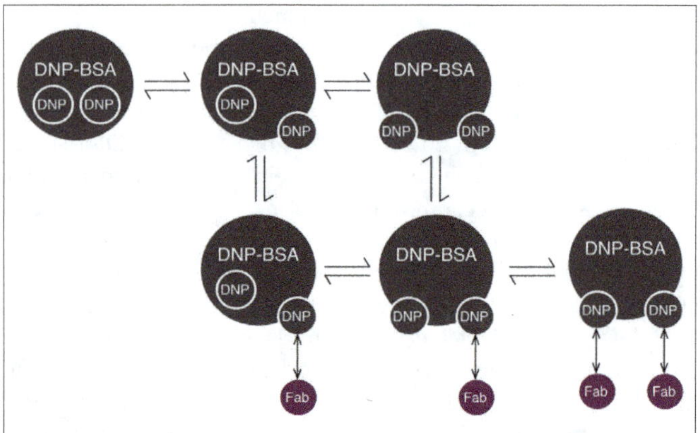

FIGURE 2 | Reaction scheme for DNP–BSA interactions with cell-surface IgE. BSA (bovine serum albumin) is haptenated with multiple DNP groups, which are assumed to transition between two states: inaccessible (represented as being inside the molecule) and accessible (represented as being on the edge of the molecule). Accessible DNP can bind Fab arms of IgE. Each IgE antibody has two Fab arms, and is thus bivalent.

Receptor aggregation initiates signaling by bringing receptors into proximity with the Src-family kinase (SFK) Lyn. Lyn's association with receptors may be facilitated by several complementary mechanisms, including regulation by the membrane lipid environment (36) and constitutive direct binding to FcεRI via Lyn's unique N-terminal domain (37). For simplicity, we explicitly model the latter mechanism because it allows the plasma membrane to be treated as well-mixed and has been formalized in past modeling studies (21, 22). Lyn mediates phosphorylation of other receptors in an aggregate, thereby generating binding sites for the SH2 domain of Lyn. In this model, FcεRI constitutively associates with the unique N-terminal domain of Lyn. Crosslinking of receptors enables Lyn to *trans* phosphorylate a second receptor at sites in the receptor's cytoplasmic subunits. These subunits, a β chain (Ms4a2) and a homodimer of two γ chains (Fcer1g), each contain an immunoreceptor tyrosine-based activation motif (ITAM). Each ITAM contains two (canonical) tyrosine residues that can be phosphorylated. The β chain contains an additional, non-canonical tyrosine in the middle of the ITAM sequence. In the original model, the tyrosines in the β chain were treated as a single-site, as were tyrosines in the γ chains. Here, we consider the β chain's N-terminal (canonical) and middle (non-canonical) tyrosines separately because they are capable of recruiting distinct binding partners. The phosphorylated N-terminal tyrosine recruits Lyn to aggregated receptors via SH2 domain binding, and enhances Lyn's catalytic activity by disruption of an inhibitory intramolecular bond, forming a positive feedback loop. The non-canonical phosphotyrosine binds the lipid phosphatase Inpp5d (Ship1), which we will discuss below. The dually phosphorylated γ ITAM binds the tandem SH2 domains of the kinase Syk. Tyrosine residues in the linker region of Syk are phosphorylated by Lyn. Syk *trans* phosphorylates the activation loop in a second Syk molecule that is co-localized by being bound to cross-linked receptor, which constitutes positive feedback.

Rules for additional interactions among signaling proteins, which include mediators of negative regulation, were adapted from a model for BCR signaling (38). Lyn and a second SFK, Fyn, bind the transmembrane adaptor protein Pag1. Pag1 can then be phosphorylated by these kinases, generating additional binding sites for Lyn and Fyn, as well as for the kinase Csk. When co-localized on Pag1, Csk can phosphorylate Lyn and Fyn at an inhibitory C-terminal tyrosine. In this model, it was assumed that phosphorylation occurs in *cis*, meaning that Csk mediates phosphorylation of an SFK only when both are bound to the same Pag1 molecule. The C-terminal phosphotyrosine of an SFK forms an intramolecular bond with the SFK's SH2 domain, resulting in autoinhibition of the SFK's kinase domain.

The new rules of our library join the proximal signaling events described above to downstream processes that have not previously been considered in mechanistic models of FcεRI signaling. New rules are discussed in the sections that follow and are illustrated in **Figure 3**. The nomenclature and residue numbers used are consistent with UniProt conventions for rat proteins (39), because rat cells are commonly used in experimental studies of FcεRI signaling. If we view the rules of our library as constituting a single model, then the terminal output of the model is production of IP_3, which is a second messenger. Binding of IP_3 to its receptor on the endoplasmic reticulum leads to release of Ca^{2+} ions from intracellular stores, which is a key step for several processes in mast cell function, including degranulation and chemotaxis (40). Finally, we note that the interactions included in this library are not all unique to FcεRI signaling and are shared by pathways operative in TCR and BCR signaling. Thus, to facilitate identification of rules applicable to multiple pathways/cell types, in Table S1

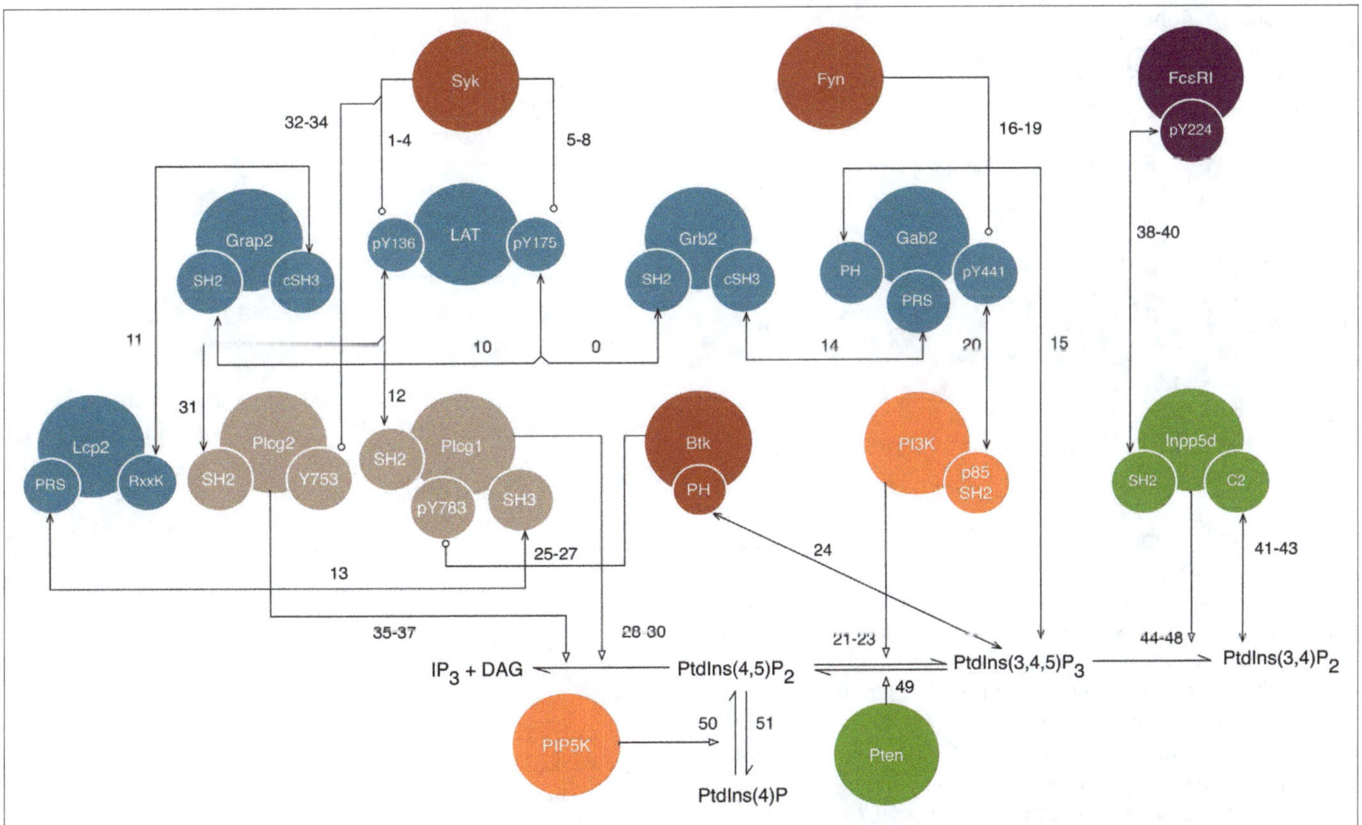

FIGURE 3 | A detailed illustration of new interactions included in the model for FcεRI signaling. This diagram shows a subset of the interactions shown in **Figure 1**, but with illustration of additional details, namely the sites responsible for interactions. Conventions for color-coding and arrow symbols are the same as in **Figure 1**. Large circles represent proteins. Small circles, overlapping the edges of large circles, represent protein sites/components, such as domains, motifs, and amino acid residues. Standard UniProt names are used, and we note that Grap2 is commonly known as Gads, Lcp2 is commonly known as Slp76, and Inpp5d is commonly known as Ship1. Arrows represent interactions and are numbered to correspond to the numbering of rules given in the text. Phosphatase activity is considered implicitly as dephosphorylation reactions that apply to all sites, and is not illustrated in this figure.

in Supplementary Material, we list protein–protein interactions included in the FcεRI library and whether each interaction is part of TCR and BCR signaling according to the NetPath database (41).

PHOSPHORYLATION OF LAT

Lat is a transmembrane, palmitoylated adaptor protein (42) that is involved in many signaling processes in both T cells and mast cells (43, 44). Syk phosphorylates Lat at multiple tyrosine residues (43), of which we focus on two: Y136 and Y175, which are better known as Y132 and Y191 in human Lat. Recent imaging studies suggest that Lat and the receptor become co-clustered after antigen-mediated receptor aggregation (45, 46). However, it is not clear if Syk-mediated phosphorylation of Lat takes place within the context of a signaling complex that co-localizes Syk and Lat, or if instead, Syk-mediated phosphorylation of Lat takes place through random collisions between Syk's kinase domain and tyrosine substrates in Lat that generate short-lived enzyme–substrate complexes, as in a Michaelis–Menten mechanism. It has previously been assumed that the latter mechanism holds (47) and we follow this approach, using rules capturing enzyme–substrate binding, dissociation, and catalysis. For example, the rules listed below, which are written using the conventions of BNGL (30), represent Syk-catalyzed phosphorylation of Y136 in Lat. Mass action kinetics are assumed. Bond indices are prefixed with the "!" symbol and internal state labels are prefixed with the "~" symbol. Here, internal state labels indicate whether a tyrosine residue is phosphorylated ("P") or unphosphorylated ("0").

```
(1) Syk(tSH2!+,PTK) + Lat(Y136~0) ->
    Syk(tSH2!+,PTK!1).Lat(Y136~0!1)
    kfSykLat
(2) Syk(PTK!1).Lat(Y136~0!1) -> Syk(PTK) +
    Lat(Y136~0) krSykLat
(3) Syk(PTK!1,Y519_Y520~P).Lat(Y136~0!1) ->
    Syk(PTK,Y519_Y520~P) + Lat(Y136~P)
    kpSykLat136_1
(4) Syk(PTK!1,Y519_Y520~0).Lat(Y136~0!1) ->
    Syk(PTK,Y519_Y520~0) + Lat(Y136~P)
    kpSykLat136_2
```

The first rule represents binding of Syk to Lat. In general, for rules in our library, protein components' names are consistent with terminology used in the biological literature. Here, the PTK component of Syk represents the protein tyrosine kinase domain of the protein. We assume that the interaction represented by Rule 1 only occurs when Syk is recruited to the plasma membrane, through binding of its tandem SH2 domains (tSH2) to phosphorylated FcεRI. Thus, the rule specifies that the tSH2 component must be bound for the reaction to occur (indicated by "!+"). The second rule represents the reverse reaction, which occurs independently of the binding state of Syk. Thus, the tSH2 component of Syk is not included in this rule. Rules 3 and 4 represent phosphorylation of Lat Y136 by Syk. These two rules differ in whether Syk is phosphorylated at its activation loop tyrosine residues Y519 and Y520, which are treated as a single site for simplicity. Phosphorylation of the activation loop enhances the catalytic activity of Syk (48). Rate constants consistent with this regulatory mechanism are given after each rule, and are assigned values in the "parameters" block of the model specification (File S1 in Supplementary Material). A similar set of rules are used to capture phosphorylation of Y175 in Lat.

```
(5) Syk(tSH2!+,PTK) + Lat(Y175~0) ->
    Syk(tSH2!+,PTK!1).Lat(Y175~0!1)
    kfSykLat
(6) Syk(PTK!1).Lat(Y175~0!1) -> Syk(PTK) +
    Lat(Y175~0) krSykLat
(7) Syk(PTK!1,Y519_Y520~P).Lat(Y175~0!1) ->
    Syk(PTK,Y519_Y520~P) + Lat(Y175~P)
    kpSykLat175_2
(8) Syk(PTK!1,Y519_Y520~0).Lat(Y175~0!1) ->
    Syk(PTK,Y519_Y520~0) + Lat(Y175~P)
    kpSykLat175_1
```

INTERACTIONS AMONG LAT AND ITS BINDING PARTNERS

Phosphorylated Y136 and Y175 have preferences for distinct binding partners, although crosstalk occurs between the pathways that branch from each site. Phosphorylated Y175 binds Grb2 and Grap2 (commonly known as Gads) (49), which are two related cytosolic adaptor proteins that each contain an SH2 domain flanked by two SH3 domains (50). These adaptors are also able to bind other sites in Lat, with Grb2 being more promiscuous (51), but for simplicity we focus on Y175. The interactions of Lat pY175 with Grb2 and Grap2, which are taken to be mutually exclusive, are modeled as follows:

```
(9)  Lat(Y175~P) + Grb2(SH2) <->
     Lat(Y175~P!1).Grb2(SH2!1) kfLatGrb2,
     krLatGrb2
(10) Lat(Y175~P) + Grap2(SH2) <->
     Lat(Y175~P!1).Grap2(SH2!1) kfLatGrap2,
     krLatGrap2
```

These rules are nearly as general as possible, in that minimal molecular context is included on the left-hand side of either of these rules (i.e., the only requirements for a bond to form is availability of the cognate binding sites in each molecule). For this reason, a large number of distinct reactions are implicitly defined by each rule. This feature is a generic aspect of rules and what allows for concise model specification.

Grap2 binds Lcp2, which is also known as Slp76. This high-affinity interaction occurs through the SH3 domain of Grap2 and an unconventional RxxK motif in Lcp2 (52).

```
(11) Grap2(SH3) + Lcp2(RxxK) <->
     Grap2(SH3!1).Lcp2(RxxK!1) kfGrap2Lcp,
     krGrap2Lcp
```

Phosphorylated Y136 in Lat binds phospholipase Cγ1 (Plcg1) with high specificity (49), and the interaction is modeled with the following rule:

```
(12) Lat(Y136~P) + Plcg1(SH2) <->
     Lat(Y136~P!1).Plcg1(SH2!1) kfLatPlcg,
     krLatPlcg
```

Both of the tandem SH2 domains of Plcg1 contribute to co-localization of this enzyme with FcεRI upon stimulation (53), and there is evidence both SH2 domains are capable of binding Lat (54). However, for simplicity, we only consider a single SH2 domain in this model.

Plcg1 also interacts with Lcp2, via the SH3 domain of Plcg1 (55).

```
(13) Lcp2(PRS) + Plcg1(SH3) <-> Lcp2(PRS!1).
     Plcg1(SH3!1) kfLcp2Plcg1,krLcp2Plcg1
```

The final adaptor protein that we consider is Gab2. A linear motif in Gab2 can bind to the C-terminal SH3 domain of Grb2. We designate this motif as a proline-rich sequence (PRS), although its sequence differs from conventional SH3 binding motifs (56).

```
(14) Grb2(cSH3) + Gab2(PRS) <-> Grb2(cSH3!1).
     Gab2(PRS!1) kfGrb2Gab2,krGrb2Gab2
```

In addition, Gab2 can be recruited by binding of its PH domain to phosphatidylinositol 3,4,5-trisphosphate [PtdIns(3,4,5)P_3], also abbreviated as PIP_3, in the plasma membrane (57).

```
(15) PI345P3(headgroup) + Gab2(PH) <->
     PI345P3(headgroup!1).Gab2(PH!1)
     kfGab2Pip3,krGab2Pip3
```

The "headgroup" component in these rules represents the head-group of the lipid, which is responsible for interactions with proteins.

RECRUITMENT OF PI3K TO Gab2

PI3K association with Gab2 is dependent on Gab2 phosphorylation. Gab2 is phosphorylated by Fyn (58), which we assume catalyzes phosphorylation through a Michaelis–Menten mechanism.

```
(16) Fyn(U!+,SH2,PTK) + Lat(Y175~P!1).
     Grb2(SH2!1,cSH3!2).Gab2(PRS!2,Y441~0) ->
     Fyn(U!+,SH2,PTK!3).Lat(Y175~P!1).
     Grb2(SH2!1,cSH3!2).Gab2(PRS!2,Y441~0!3)
     kfFynGab2
(17) Rec(b_Y210~P!4).Fyn(U,SH2!4,PTK) +
     Lat(Y175~P!1).Grb2(SH2!1,cSH3!2).
     Gab2(PRS!2,Y441~0) -> Rec(b_Y210~P!4).
     Fyn(U,SH2!4,PTK!3).Lat(Y175~P!1).
     Grb2(SH2!1,cSH3!2).Gab2(PRS!2,Y441~0!3)
     kfFynGab2
(18) Fyn(PTK!1).Gab2(Y441~0!1) ->
     Fyn(PTK) + Gab2(Y441~0) krFynGab2
(19) Fyn(PTK!1).Gab2(Y441~0!1) ->
     Fyn(PTK) + Gab2(Y441~P) kpFynGab2
```

The first two rules differ with respect to the mechanism by which Fyn is bound to a receptor. In the first rule, Fyn is taken to be bound by its unique domain (U). In the second rule, Fyn is taken to be bound by its SH2 domain.

Phosphorylated Gab2 binds the SH2 domain in the p85 subunit of PI3K (p85_SH2). Y441 of Gab2 lies in a consensus sequence for p85 binding (59).

```
(20) Gab2(Y441~P) + Pi3k(p85_SH2) <->
     Gab2(Y441~P!1).Pi3k(p85_SH2!1)
     kfGab2Pi3k,krGab2Pi3k
```

PI3K ACTIVITY

Once recruited, PI3K phosphorylates the 3rd position in the inositol ring of phosphatidylinositol 4,5-bisphosphate [PtdIns(4,5)P_2], also abbreviated as PIP_2, generating PIP_3.

```
(21) Lat(Y175~P!1).Grb2(SH2!1,cSH3!2).
     Gab2(PRS!2,Y441~P!3).Pi3k(p85_SH2!3,
     PI3Kc) + PI45P2(headgroup) ->
     Lat(Y175~P!1).Grb2(SH2!1,cSH3!2).
     Gab2(PRS!2,Y441~P!3).Pi3k(p85_SH2!3,
     PI3Kc!4).PI45P2(headgroup!4) kfPi3kPip2
(22) Pi3k(PI3Kc!1).PI45P2(headgroup!1) ->
     Pi3k(PI3Kc) + PI45P2(headgroup)
     krPi3kPip2
(23) Pi3k(PI3Kc!1).PI45P2(headgroup!1) ->
     Pi3k(PI3Kc) + PI345P3(headgroup)
     kpPi3k DeleteMolecules
```

In these rules, lipid phosphorylation is treated as consumption and production of different lipid species. For this reason, the BNGL keyword "DeleteMolecules" is used to indicate removal of reactant molecules (30).

Btk-MEDIATED ACTIVATION OF Plcg1

PtdIns(3,4,5)P_3 is a binding partner for multiple proteins, including the Tec-family kinase Btk, which is involved in activating Plcg1. The PH domain of Btk mediates this interaction.

```
(24) Btk(PH) + PI345P3(headgroup) <->
     Btk(PH!1).PI345P3(headgroup!1)
     kfBtkPip3,krBtkPip3
```

Recruited Btk can phosphorylate Plcg1 at sites that are associated with enhancement of phospholipase activity (60). In this way, pathways that branch from the two Lat phosphosites, Y136 and Y175, converge in contributing to IP_3 production.

```
(25) Btk(PH!+,PTK) + Plcg1(SH2!+,Y783~0) ->
     Btk(PH!+,PTK!1).Plcg1(SH2!+,Y783~0!1)
     kfBtkPlcg
(26) Btk(PTK!1).Plcg1(Y783~0!1) -> Btk(PTK) +
     Plcg1(Y783~0) krBtkPlcg
(27) Btk(PTK!1).Plcg1(Y783~0!1) -> Btk(PTK) +
     Plcg1(Y783~P) kpBtkPlcg
```

Plcg1 ACTIVITY

Plcg1 cleaves PtdIns(4,5)P_2 to generate the second messengers diacyl glycerol (DAG) and inositol 1,4,5-trisphosphate (IP_3) (61). The cleavage reaction is taken to occur through a Michaelis–Menten mechanism:

```
(28) Plcg1(SH2!+,PLC)+PI45P2(headgroup) ->
     Plcg1(SH2!+,PLC!1).PI45P2(headgroup!1)
     kfPlcgPip2
(29) Plcg1(PLC!1).PI45P2(headgroup!1) ->
     Plcg1(PLC)+PI45P2(headgroup) krPlcgPip2
(30) Plcg1(PLC!1,Y783~P).PI45P2(headgroup!1)
     -> Plcg1(PLC,Y783~P)+IP3()+DAG()
     kcPlcg DeleteMolecules
```

RECRUITMENT AND ACTIVITY OF Plcg2

In addition to Plcg1, we also include Plcg2 in the library because isoform-specific differences between these two proteins have been found in FcεRI signaling. It has been observed that phosphorylation and activation of Plcg2 is less sensitive to PI3K inhibition than Plcg1 (62). Thus, we include a mechanism by which Plcg2 is activated by Syk rather than by Btk. However, we note that other studies have found phosphorylation of Plcg2 to be reduced in the absence of Btk (63), suggesting that Btk may act on Plcg2.

```
(31) Lat(Y136~P)+Plcg2(SH2) <->
     Lat(Y136~P!1).Plcg2(SH2!1) kfLatPlcg,
     krLatPlcg
(32) Syk(tSH2!+,PTK)+Plcg2(SH2!+,Y753~0)
     -> Syk(tSH2!+,PTK!1).Plcg2(SH2!+,
     Y753~0!1) kfSykPlcg
(33) Syk(PTK!1).Plcg2(Y753~0!1) -> Syk(PTK)+
     Plcg2(Y753~0) krSykPlcg
(34) Syk(PTK!1).Plcg2(Y753~0!1) -> Syk(PTK)+
     Plcg2(Y753~P) kpSykPlcg
(35) Plcg2(SH2!+,PLC)+PI45P2(headgroup) ->
     Plcg2(SH2!+,PLC!1).PI45P2(headgroup!1)
     kfPlcgPip2
(36) Plcg2(PLC!1).PI45P2(headgroup!1) ->
     Plcg2(PLC)+PI45P2(headgroup) krPlcgPip2
(37) Plcg2(PLC!1,Y753~P).PI45P2(headgroup!1)
     -> Plcg2(PLC,Y753~P)+IP3()+DAG()
     kcPlcg DeleteMolecules
```

Rule 31 represents binding to Lat. Rules 32–34 represent phosphorylation of Plcg2 through a Michaelis–Menten mechanism. Rule 35–37 represent catalyzed hydrolysis of PIP_2.

ACTIVATION OF Inpp5d

The final regulator of lipid signaling explicitly considered in our model is Inpp5d, also known as Ship1, a phosphatase that can be recruited to FcεRI by binding a non-canonical ITAM tyrosine in the β subunit of the receptor (64, 65). Although Inpp5d and Lyn both bind the β subunit, they have preferences for different phosphotyrosines and thus we treat these interactions as non-competitive. Inpp5d dephosphorylates the 5th position of the inositol ring of PtdIns(3,4,5)P_3 to form PtdIns(3,4)P_2. This product of Inpp5d activity can in turn bind the Inpp5d C2 domain (66), forming a positive feedback loop that has an overall negative impact on FcεRI-mediated degranulation. The following rules are used to model binding of Inpp5d to the receptor:

```
(38) Inpp5d(SH2,C2)+Rec(b_Y224~P) ->
     Inpp5d(SH2!1,C2).Rec(b_Y224~P!1)
     kfShipRec
(39) Inpp5d(IPP,C2!+)+Rec(b_Y224~P) ->
     Inpp5d(IPP!1,C2!+).Rec(b_Y224~P!1)
     100*kfShipRec
(40) Inpp5d(SH2!1).Rec(b_Y224~P!1) ->
     Inpp5d(SH2)+Rec(b_Y224~P) krShipRec
```

In the first rule, Inpp5d is cytosolic, because its SH2 and C2 domains are both free and, in the model, these are the only domains that mediate membrane recruitment. In the second rule, Inpp5d is already membrane associated through binding of its C2 domain to PtdIns(3,4)P_2. For this reason, receptor binding occurs more quickly (we assume a 100-fold enhancement). The third rule represents dissociation of Inpp5d from the receptor.

Binding of Inpp5d to PtdIns(3,4)P_2 is modeled similarly, with different rules for membrane-recruited and cytosolic Inpp5d:

```
(41) Inpp5d(SH2,C2)+PI34P2(headgroup) ->
     Inpp5d(SH2,C2!1).PI34P2(headgroup!1)
     kfShipPip2
(42) Inpp5d(SH2!+,C2)+PI34P2(headgroup) ->
     Inpp5d(SH2!+,C2!1).PI34P2(headgroup!1)
     100*kfShipPip2
(43) Inpp5d(C2!1).PI34P2(headgroup!1) ->
     Inpp5d(C2)+PI34P2(headgroup) krShipPip2
```

In the first rule, Inpp5d is cytosolic, whereas in the second rule, it is localized to the membrane through binding of its SH2 domain to the receptor. As above, a 100-fold enhancement is assumed. The third rule represents dissociation.

Inpp5d ACTIVITY

The following rules capture the catalytic activity of Inpp5d:

```
(44) Inpp5d(SH2!+,C2,IPP)+PI345P3
     (headgroup) -> Inpp5d(SH2!+,C2,IPP!1).
     PI345P3(headgroup!1) kfShipPip3
(45) Inpp5d(SH2,C2!+,IPP)+PI345P3
     (headgroup) -> Inpp5d(SH2,C2!+,IPP!1).
     PI345P3(headgroup!1) kfShipPip3
(46) Inpp5d(SH2!+,C2!+,IPP)+PI345P3
     (headgroup) -> Inpp5d(SH2!+,C2!+,
     IPP!1).PI345P3(headgroup!1) kfShipPip3
(47) Inpp5d(IPP!1).PI345P3(headgroup!1) ->
     Inpp5d(IPP)+PI345P3(headgroup)
     krShipPip3
(48) Inpp5d(IPP!1).PI345P3(headgroup!1) ->
     Inpp5d(IPP)+PI34P2(headgroup)
     kdpShipPip3 DeleteMolecules
```

In the rules above, "IPP" represents the catalytic domain of Inpp5d.

ADDITIONAL LIPID REACTIONS

Conversion of PtdIns(3,4,5)P_3 to PtdIns(4,5)P_2 by Pten is considered implicitly as a first-order reaction. Conversions between PtdIns(4,5)P_2 and PtdIns(4)P are modeled similarly.

```
(49) PI345P3(headgroup) -> PI45P2(headgroup)
     kPten DeleteMolecules
(50) PI4P(headgroup) -> PI45P2(headgroup)
     kfP5 DeleteMolecules
(51) PI45P2(headgroup) -> PI4P(headgroup)
     krP5 DeleteMolecules
```

IDENTIFICATION OF NETWORK MOTIFS

It has been hypothesized that relatively simple network motifs with specialized functions play important roles in cellular regulatory systems and that understanding the design principles of these motifs can help us better understand the complex systems in which they are embedded (67, 68). Network motifs, such as feedback loops, have the potential to generate and/or regulate non-linear dynamical behavior (69), which may, for example, enable precise encoding of information about a stimulus (70). We assessed the FcεRI signaling network for the presence of network motifs, and identified motifs from four classes: positive feedback loops, negative feedback loops, incoherent feed-forward loops, and coherent feed-forward loops. Several of the positive and negative feedbacks contribute to regulation of the SFKs Lyn and Fyn, as well as Syk. One positive feedback loop arises because SFKs phosphorylate tyrosine residues in FcεRI, which serve as binding sites that recruit additional Lyn and Fyn molecules. Furthermore, Lyn and Fyn can each *trans* phosphorylate their own activation loop, which enhances catalytic activity. A similar mechanism also activates the kinase Syk. Negative feedback arises because Lyn and Fyn can phosphorylate the adaptor Pag1, which recruits Csk to negatively regulate SFK activity. This set of interactions has been predicted to lead to oscillations in BCR signaling (38).

Other positive feedback loops are involved in regulating lipid metabolism. PI3K generates PIP_3, which recruits Gab2. Gab2 can in turn recruit additional PI3K. An additional positive feedback loop regulates Inpp5d, because it is capable of binding its own product. Inpp5d is also involved in an incoherent feed-forward loop, meaning a process in which two parallel mechanisms have opposite influences on an output. Here, the output is PIP_3. Inpp5d is recruited to FcεRI and dephosphorylates PIP_3. Incoherence arises because FcεRI contributes to activation of PI3K, which generates PIP_3. In this way, opposing influences are exerted on the abundance of PIP_3 upon stimulation of FcεRI signaling. Such circuitry has been hypothesized to be involved in adaptation, the capacity of a system to respond to an input and then reset itself to a pre-stimulated state (71). Thus, PIP_3 level may be raised and then lowered after a period of FcεRI stimulation, with Inpp5d-mediated positive feedback reinforcing negative regulation over time.

Finally, we identified a pair of coherent feed-forward loops stemming from the adaptor Lat. In a coherent feed-forward loop, two processes exert the same influence (either positive or negative) on an output. In each of the feed-forward loops of interest here, both processes in the network motif have a positive influence on Plcg1 activity. In the first feed-forward loop, Lat recruits Plcg1 via one of its phosphotyrosines. Other Lat phosphotyrosines are involved in assembly of a signaling complex that ultimately recruits PI3K. The product of PI3K, PIP_3, binds the kinase Btk, which phosphorylates Plcg1 at an activating site. In the second feed-forward loop, Lat contributes to Plcg1 recruitment through direct binding as well as through recruitment of another adaptor, Lcp2. What function could be achieved by these (overlapping) feed-forward loops? In transcriptional regulatory networks, it has been found that feed-forward loops can act as sign-sensitive delay elements, meaning that they enable rapid responses to changes in an input in one direction, and slow responses to changes in the input in the opposite direction (72, 73). Thus, the feed-forward loops initiated by Lat may influence the timing of Plcg1 activation and deactivation after increases or decreases in, for example, upstream receptor phosphorylation.

It is worth noting that Plcg1 and PI3K act on the same substrate, PIP_2. Thus, although PI3K can positively influence Plcg1, these two enzymes also compete with one another and could together deplete available PIP_2, assuming both access the same lipid pool. In this way, the feed-forward loop may be self-limiting. For example, if Plcg1 causes rapid conversion of PIP_2 to IP_3, less PIP_2 would be available to PI3K and as a result, less PIP_3 would be generated and the impact of the feed-forward loop would be reduced. The strength of the feed-forward loop would also be influenced by the rate of production of PIP_2 by specific lipid kinases and phosphatases. A caveat is that Plcg1 and PI3K may act on spatially distinct lipid pools, which PIP_2 has been found to exist in (74). These factors are not immediately evident from examination of isolated circuitry. This example highlights the importance of considering broader context and physical parameters (e.g., concentrations and binding affinities) in assessment of network motif functionality.

SENSITIVITY OF PHOSPHOLIPID METABOLISM TO PROTEIN TYROSINE KINASE ACTIVATION

We next used our rule library to develop models for investigation of signaling dynamics. We focused on the adaptor protein Lat, which is known for its role as a signaling hub in both T cells and mast cells (44). This role arises in large part from its capacity to recruit multiple adaptors and enzymes that regulate lipid metabolism and production of second messengers. Most of Lat's interactions depend on prior Lat phosphorylation, which is catalyzed primarily by Syk. However, studies of FcεRI signaling induced by structurally defined antigens have revealed that not all "downstream" events are equally dependent on Lat phosphorylation. Specifically, a panel of rigid antigens, composed of haptenated DNA sequences and differing in the distance between DNP hapten groups, was evaluated for the ability to induce phosphorylation of signaling proteins, Ca^{2+} mobilization, and degranulation. It was found that phosphorylation of FcεRI and Lat, as well as store-operated Ca^{2+} entry and degranulation, were strongly dependent on hapten spacing, with the shortest spacing examined associated with the strongest responses. In contrast, it was also found that release of Ca^{2+} from intracellular stores did not show as strong a dependence on the distance between hapten sites (19). Given that Ca^{2+} release is thought to occur as a result of activities of proteins

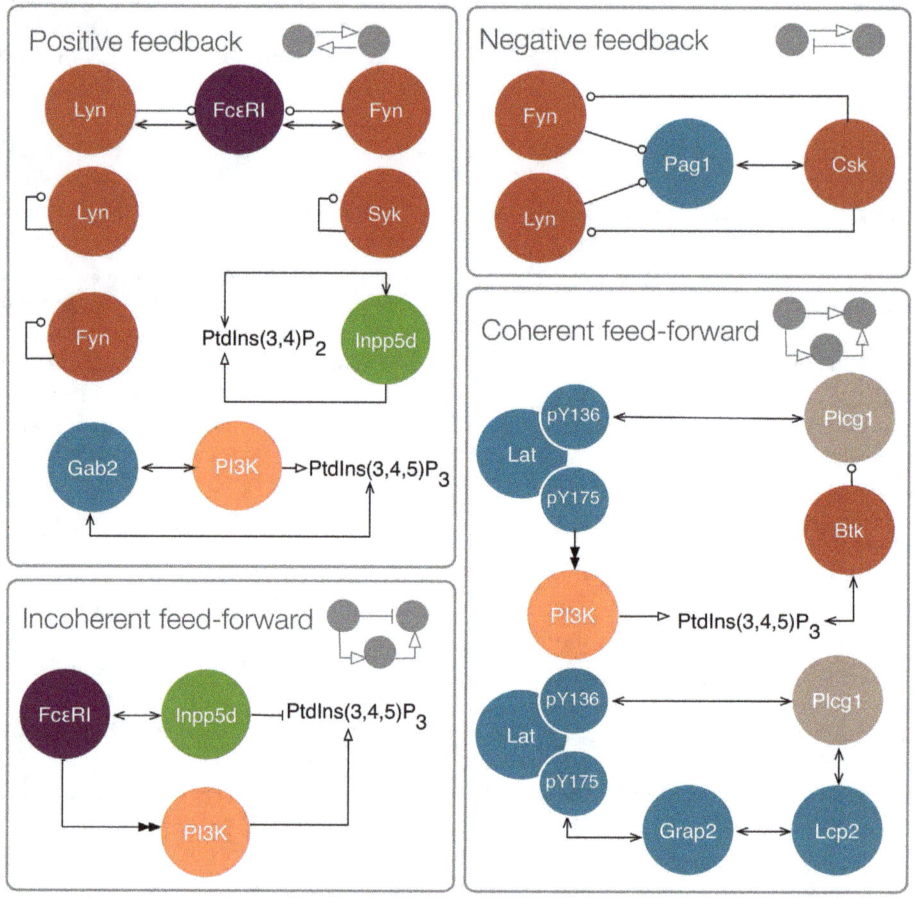

FIGURE 4 | Motifs in the FcεRI signaling network. Positive feedbacks include interactions between FcεRI and Lyn and Fyn, because Lyn and Fyn catalyze phosphorylation of additional binding sites for these kinases. Lyn, Fyn, and Syk are subject to *trans* autophosphorylation at activating sites. Inpp5d binds its own product. Gab2 recruits PI3K, which generates PIP_3, which can recruit additional Gab2. Negative feedback includes inhibition of Lyn and Fyn by Csk. Incoherent feed-forward includes FcεRI stimulation leading to activation of both PI3K and Inpp5d, which exert opposing influences on PIP_3 level. Coherent feed-forwards include recruitment and activation of Plcg1, and recruitment of Plcg1 through two pathways.

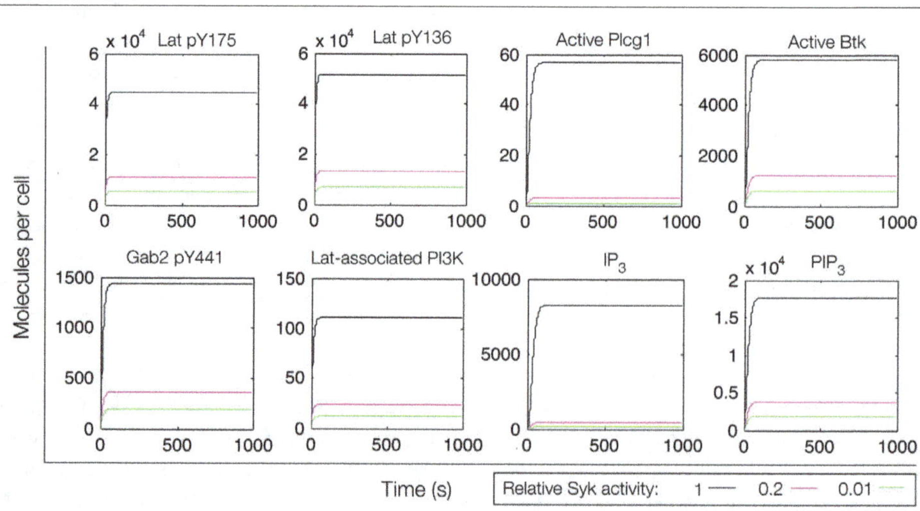

FIGURE 5 | Simulation of a model of the feed-forward loop connecting Lat to IP_3 production. Different color lines indicate different relative levels of Syk activity. In these simulations, Syk activity was set at the indicated level and held constant.

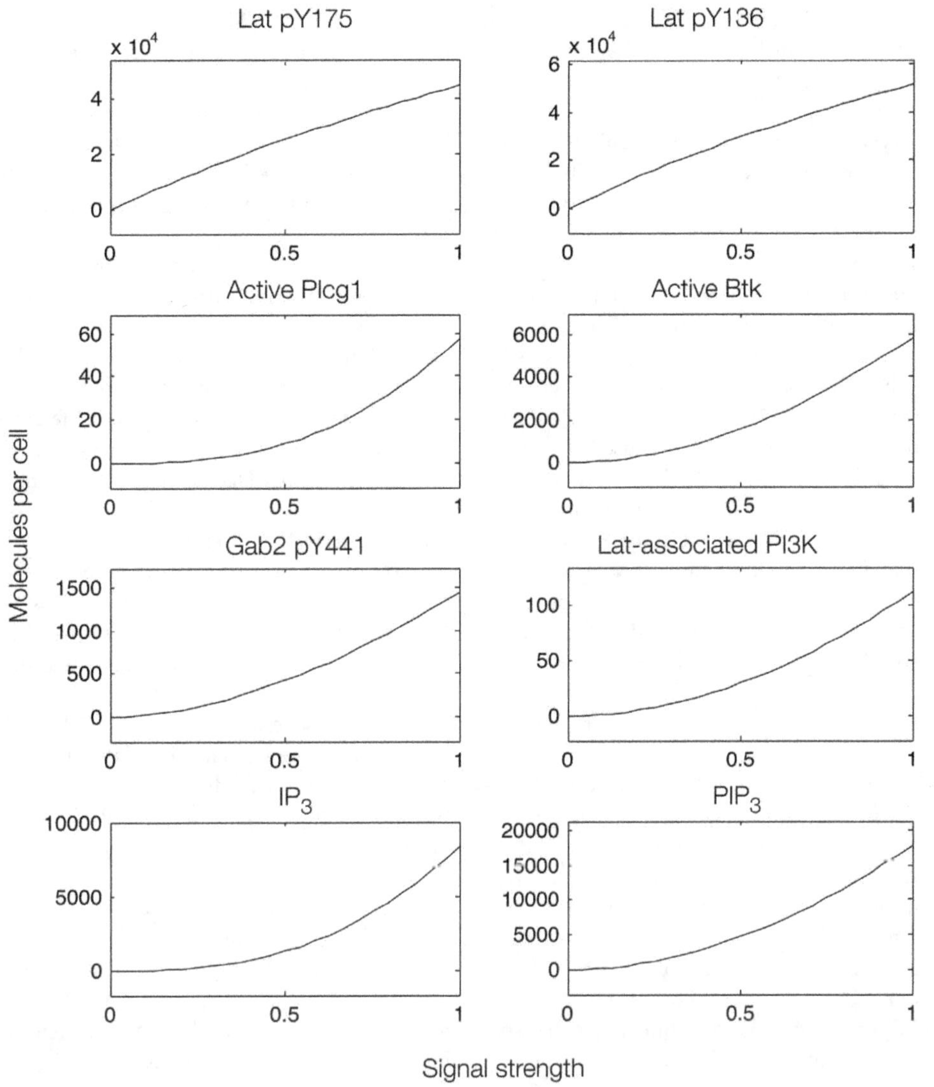

FIGURE 6 | Steady-state dose–response curves, which were found by simulation of the feed-forward loop connecting Lat to IP_3 production. The differences in phosphorylation level between the two phosphorylation sites in Lat (top panels) results from different affinities of the binding partners that interact with each site. Active Plcg1 is taken to be Plcg1 that is both recruited to Lat and phosphorylated, and active Btk is taken to be Btk recruited to PIP_3.

that depend on Lat, how can this apparent uncoupling between Lat phosphorylation and Ca^{2+} mobilization be explained?

We hypothesize that compensatory mechanisms mediated by Fyn and Gab2 (58) are involved in this phenomenon. Gab2 can be phosphorylated by Fyn, and can then recruit PI3K. As discussed above, production of PIP_3 by PI3K contributes to activation of Plcg1. A product of Plcg1 is IP_3, which induces release of Ca^{2+} from intracellular stores. Thus, if Gab2 recruitment and activation is robust to differences in Lat phosphorylation level, then Gab2 may open an avenue by which Ca^{2+} mobilization could escape control of Lat. We used our rule library to build models to determine if Gab2 could potentially enable Ca^{2+} mobilization when Lat phosphorylation is diminished.

We first considered a model in which Syk and Fyn were independent inputs. Our initial model (File S2 in Supplementary Material) essentially consists of the first coherent feed-forward loop shown in **Figure 4**: lat recruits Plcg1, as well as PI3K through Gab2 and Grb2. Btk is recruited to PIP_3 and activates Plcg1 through phosphorylation. Fyn participates by phosphorylating Gab2. To model the differences between antigens observed to induce the most and least Lat phosphorylation, we considered different levels of active Syk consistent with the approximately fourfold difference in Lat phosphorylation observed experimentally (19). The level of active Fyn was kept constant. Simulations of this model revealed that differences in Lat phosphorylation level were maintained or amplified in downstream events. According to the model, a decrease in Lat phosphorylation (arising from lowered Syk activity) causes at least proportionate decreases in the levels of activated Plcg1, activated Btk, Lat-associated PI3K, PIP_3, and IP_3 (**Figure 5**). We also considered a scenario in which activity of Syk and Fyn are both controlled by the magnitude of an input signal, which may be a more realistic scenario because both kinases are recruited to phosphorylated receptors. We varied the strength of this signal and evaluated the resulting steady-state levels of outputs (**Figure 6**). Consistent with results from the first scenario, decreased signal strength led to decreased Lat phosphorylation, and was accompanied by even steeper decreases in activation of other signaling molecules. Thus, the interactions included in this model are insufficient to explain the experimental observation of Ca^{2+} mobilization in the absence of strong Lat phosphorylation.

In an extension of the initial model (File S3 in Supplementary Material), we incorporated additional interactions from the rule library, those responsible for the positive feedback involving Gab2 interaction with PIP_3 (see **Figure 4**). We reasoned that, with the addition of these interactions, once PIP_3 production is initiated, PIP_3 production may become self-sustaining, because PIP_3 is able to recruit Gab2 to the plasma membrane, which in turn is able to recruit PI3K. Simulated time courses with the same level of active Fyn and different levels of active Syk, as in **Figure 5**, are shown in **Figure 7**. These results indicate that certain signaling readouts downstream of Lat are buffered against reduced Lat phosphorylation. For example, there is less than a fourfold difference in peak IP_3 levels between the conditions of high (black line) and intermediate (magenta line) Lat phosphorylation. In contrast, the model without Gab2-mediated positive feedback predicted a greater than 100-fold difference.

To further investigate the role of positive feedback, we modulated an input signal controlling both Fyn and Syk activity, as in **Figure 6**. Steady-state simulation results from this model are shown in **Figure 8**, which differ from those obtained with the first model. First, the total numbers of signaling molecules in activated forms are greater than for the case without feedback, as long as the signal strength is above a certain level. Second, within certain input ranges, the model shows bistability, i.e., existence of two stable steady states, as indicated by signal strength values that correspond to more than one steady-state output value. Bistability has also been characterized in TCR signaling (75, 76) and BCR signaling (38, 77). Third, we found that certain signaling readouts downstream of Lat are now buffered against reduced Lat phosphorylation (**Figure 7**), decreasing less sharply when signal is reduced. Together, these results suggest that Gab2-mediated positive feedback may enable committed, all-or-none decisions that lead to high levels of IP_3 as long as Lat phosphorylation is above a threshold. When input level falls below this threshold, positive feedback is unable to enhance IP_3 production (**Figure 7**). Thus, some amount of PIP_3 must be generated through Lat-dependent mechanisms before the Fyn/Gab2 pathway can contribute to production of IP_3.

We also considered how positive feedback affects the dynamics of signaling. We calculated the rise time for IP_3 at different input levels as predicted by the models with and without positive feedback. We found that positive feedback caused IP_3 level to reach its steady state more slowly (**Figure 9A**). Rise time for the model with positive feedback peaked in the bistable region, where the system transitions from a low steady state to a higher steady state (**Figure 9B**). The slower rise in IP_3 level qualitatively mimics the experimentally observed dynamics of Ca^{2+} release from stores caused by antigens that induce low levels of Lat phosphorylation (19). These same antigens induce minimal store-operated calcium entry (SOCE) and minimal degranulation, which suggests that SOCE may be sensitive to the kinetics of IP_3 production.

There are several experimental tests that could be pursued to evaluate the role of Gab2-mediated positive feedback. One predicted effect of the feedback loop is bistability of several signaling readouts (**Figure 8**), including PIP_3. Testing for bistability usually benefits from single-cell measurements, because cell-to-cell variability may result in different cells having different bifurcation points. At the single-cell level, PIP_3 production can be monitored using PH domain constructs (78). When the strength of an input signal, such as ligand-induced receptor aggregation, crosses a threshold level, the quantity of PIP_3 is expected to increase dramatically in a switch-like manner. Another characteristic arising from bistability is hysteresis, meaning history dependence. As

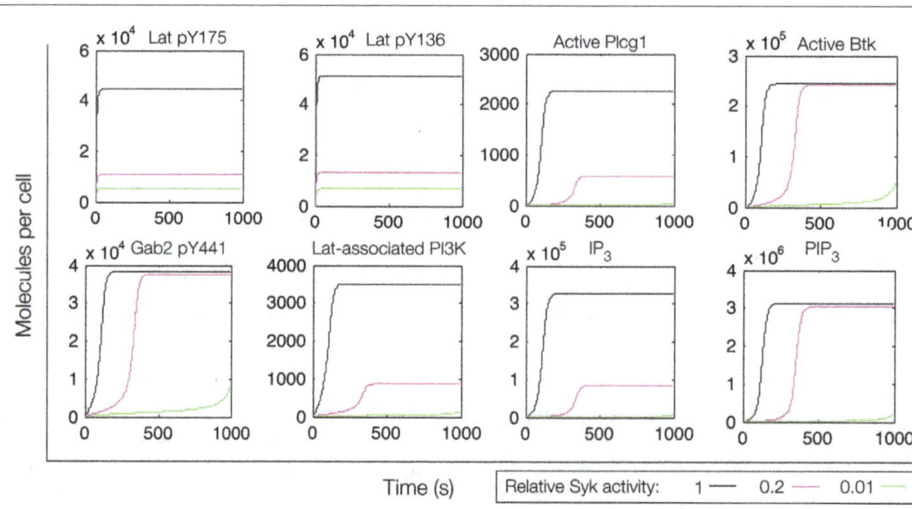

FIGURE 7 | Simulation of a model of the feed-forward loop connecting Lat to IP_3 production with consideration of a Gab2-mediated positive feedback loop. Different color lines indicate different relative levels of Syk activity.

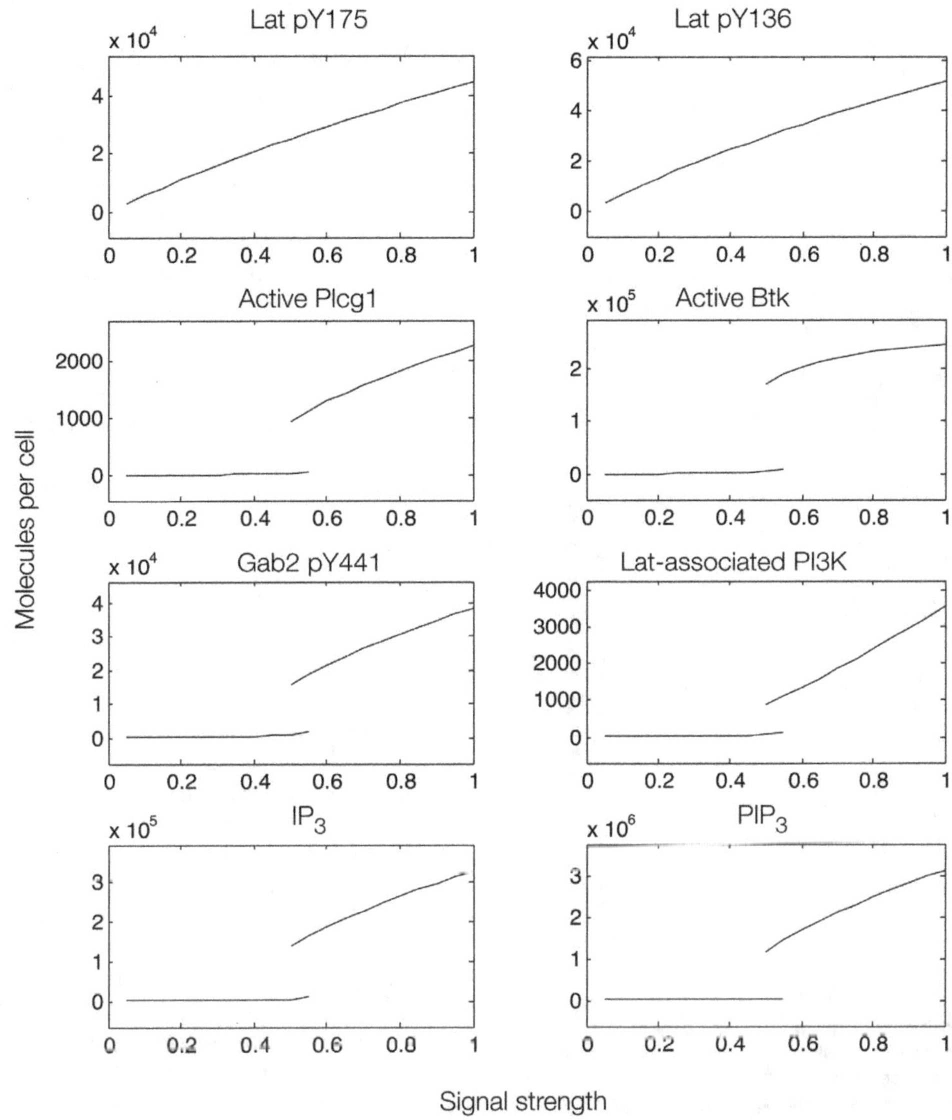

FIGURE 8 | Steady-state dose–response curves, which were found by simulation of the feed-forward loop connecting Lat to IP_3 production when Gab2-mediated positive feedback is considered. Each plot is a bifurcation diagram; the bifurcation parameter is signal strength, which governs the rate of production of active Syk and Fyn. Only stable steady states are shown. As can be seen, the model predicts the possibility of bistability.

signal strength is reduced from a high level [e.g., by breaking up receptor aggregates with a monovalent hapten (34)], PIP_3 level is expected to switch back to a low state. However, this switch is predicted to occur at a lower input level than that required to induce a transition from low signaling to high signaling. Controlling input level would require an understanding of how ligand dose relates to receptor aggregation, which can be obtained with a model for ligand–receptor interactions (79).

A second approach would involve disruption of the Gab2 feedback loop, which would be expected to increase sensitivity to Lat phosphorylation. Mutation of the Gab2 PH domain, which binds PIP_3 and is therefore a key component of the feedback, would be expected to inhibit Ca^{2+} mobilization. However, such manipulation of endogenous Gab2 would be technically challenging, making this strategy potentially difficult to implement. An alternative approach would be to knock down either Gab2 or Fyn, which would be predicted to similarly inhibit Ca^{2+} mobilization.

CONCLUSION

As a step toward systems-level understanding of FcεRI signaling, we have synthesized information about a relatively large number of interactions and proteins into a formalized interaction library. This library consists of executable rules that can be used to extend existing models and to build new models. The rules are annotated with information from the primary literature, thereby facilitating reuse of information. The rules are also visualized to illustrate the scope and detail of the library's contents. Analysis of the library reveals multiple feedback and

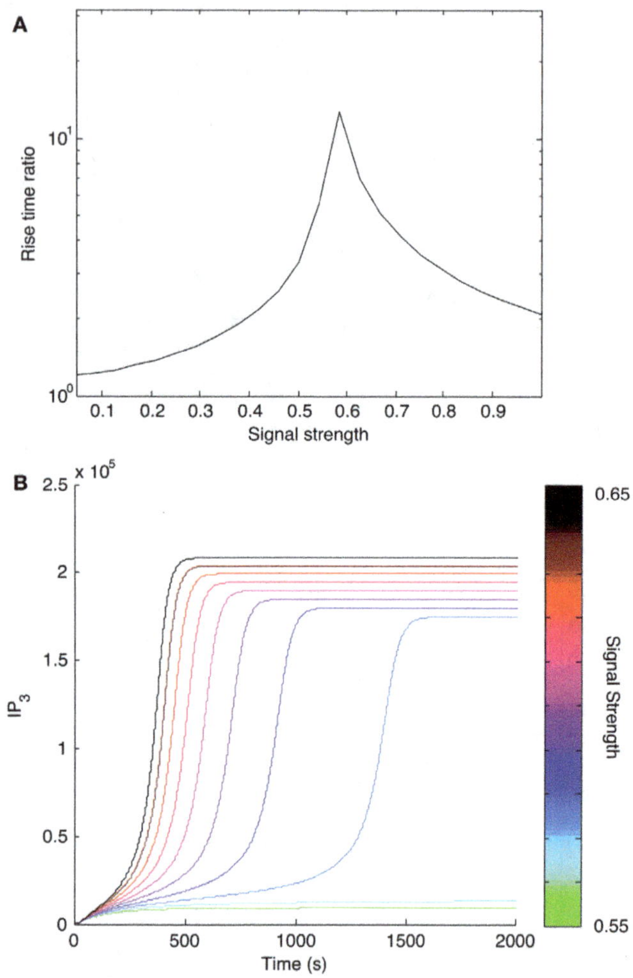

FIGURE 9 | Effect of positive feedback on signaling dynamics. **(A)** Rise time for IP_3 synthesis was calculated as the time needed to reach 95% of the final steady-state level. Rise times were calculated for different levels of input, or signal strength. Rise times for the model with positive feedback were divided by rise times for the model without positive feedback and plotted against corresponding input level. All indicated rise time ratios are greater than one, meaning that the model with positive feedback takes more time to reach its final steady state. **(B)** Time courses for IP_3 production in a narrow range of input levels surrounding the peak shown in **(A)**. The input level corresponding to each curve is indicated with the color bar at the right.

feed-forward loops in FcεRI signaling, the behavior of which can be investigated quantitatively through simulation and complementary quantitative experiments. We used the library to model events involved in phosphoinositide metabolism at different levels of Syk activity, and found that a Gab2-mediated positive feedback can compensate for reduced Lat phosphorylation, which provides a potential explanation for how antigens that induce dramatically different levels of Lat phosphorylation can induce similar Ca^{2+} fluxes (19).

We anticipate that the approach presented here will have several potential applications in linking computational and experimental investigations of cellular information processing. First, a library of rules could be used to build a model of broad scope and site-specific detail for use in analysis of multiplexed, high-resolution data, such as proteomic measurements of site-specific post-translational modifications (80). Currently, such data are often analyzed using clustering, enrichment analysis, and other techniques that reveal trends in dynamics and functions of detected proteins (81), but that do not necessarily provide a concrete picture of the mechanisms at work. Modeling will enable us to better leverage information about mechanisms and physical parameters, complementing current analysis techniques. A combination of modeling and quantitative high-throughput experimentation could, for example, be used to characterize the distribution of signaling complexes that can be nucleated by Lat. Binding partners of Lat have shared binding sites and a range of affinities (49). To understand how binding of these proteins is balanced, it would be necessary to measure binding affinities of SH2 domains to each phosphosite (82) and to quantify protein copy numbers (83). A model could then be used to integrate such data and determine the expected distribution of signaling complexes.

Second, rule libraries could facilitate the extension of models by increments. The benefit of such an approach is that a model of an idealized network motif (71, 84) could be extended piece by piece to form a more complete representation of the motif's context. Studies of such models could reveal how well the predicted behavior of an isolated motif is maintained when additional interactions are considered, and what complicating factors may need to be taken into account in experimental assessments of motif function or in synthetic biology efforts aimed at engineering regulatory systems on the basis of network motif design principles.

Finally, rule libraries may help address problems in knowledge engineering, i.e., the task of gathering, organizing, and interpreting large quantities of information. Rule-based models have already been annotated using interactive wikis (85, 86), which could open the door to community-based model development and curation, making it easier to assemble and assess data for model building. Furthermore, a widely used approach in knowledge engineering is natural language processing (NLP), the automated derivation of information from text. A major bioinformatics goal of NLP is to extract networks and quantitative models from the primary biomedical literature (87). A limiting factor in this task is the availability of "gold standard" networks against which to compare an automatically constructed network or model, which is necessary to assess the performance of network/model construction algorithms. For many biological systems, reliable network representations and models are non-existent. Furthermore, even when a reliable network is available, it may be in a format (e.g., ordinary differential equations) that does not map to underlying interactions in a clear manner. This problem is addressed by a rule library, because rules not only serve as the basis for simulations but also provide precise, human- and machine-readable representations of biomolecular interactions. NLP could aid in library construction through automatic extraction of rules from the literature. As information about cell signaling systems continues to expand, we anticipate that formalization and synthesis of knowledge will become increasingly important for informing hypotheses, making quantitative predictions, and elucidating systems-level properties of cellular regulatory systems.

ACKNOWLEDGMENTS

This work was supported by NIH grants R01 AI018306 and P50GM085273 and by US Department of Energy Contract DE-AC52-06NA25396 through the Los Alamos Center for Non-linear Studies (CNLS) and the Laboratory-Directed Research and Development (LDRD) Program. We thank Leonard A. Harris for technical advice.

REFERENCES

1. Smith-Garvin JE, Koretzky GA, Jordan MS. T cell activation. *Annu Rev Immunol* (2009) **27**:591–619. doi:10.1146/annurev.immunol.021908.132706
2. Packard TM, Cambier JC. B lymphocyte antigen receptor signaling: initiation, amplification, and regulation. *F1000Prime Rep* (2013) **5**:40. doi:10.12703/P5-40
3. Kraft S, Kinet JP. New developments in FcεRI regulation, function and inhibition. *Nat Rev Immunol* (2007) **7**:365–78. doi:10.1038/nri2072
4. Wollman R, Meyer T. Coordinated oscillations in cortical actin and Ca^{2+} correlate with cycles of vesicle secretion. *Nat Cell Biol* (2012) **14**:1261–9. doi:10.1038/ncb2614
5. Wu M, Wu X, De Camilli P. Calcium oscillations-coupled conversion of actin travelling waves to standing oscillations. *Proc Natl Acad Sci U S A* (2013) **110**:1339–44. doi:10.1073/pnas.1221538110
6. Fraser I, Germain R. Navigating the network: signaling cross-talk in hematopoietic cells. *Nat Immunol* (2009) **10**:327–31. doi:10.1038/ni.1711
7. Kohn K, Aladjem M, Weinstein J, Pommier Y. Network architecture of signaling from uncoupled helicase-polymerase to cell cycle checkpoints and trans-lesion DNA synthesis. *Cell Cycle* (2009) **8**:2281–99. doi:10.4161/cc.8.14.9102
8. Le Novère N, Hucka M, Mi H, Moodie S, Schreiber F, Sorokin A, et al. The systems biology graphical notation. *Nat Biotechnol* (2009) **27**:735–41. doi:10.1038/nbt.1558
9. Caron E, Ghosh S, Matsuoka Y, Ashton-Beaucage D, Therrien M, Lemieux S, et al. A comprehensive map of the mTOR signaling network. *Mol Syst Biol* (2010) **6**:453. doi:10.1038/msb.2010.108
10. Chylek LA, Hu B, Blinov ML, Emonet T, Faeder JR, Goldstein B, et al. Guidelines for visualizing and annotating rule-based models. *Mol Biosyst* (2011) **7**:2779–95. doi:10.1039/c1mb05077j
11. Tiger C, Krause F, Cedersund G, Palmér R, Klipp E, Hohmann S, et al. A framework for mapping, visualisation and automatic model creation of signal-transduction networks. *Mol Syst Biol* (2012) **8**:578. doi:10.1038/msb.2012.12
12. Kirouac D, Saez-Rodriguez J, Swantek J, Burke JM, Lauffenburger D, Sorger P. Creating and analyzing pathway and protein interaction compendia for modelling signal transduction networks. *BMC Syst Biol* (2012) **6**:29. doi:10.1186/1752-0509-6-29
13. Germain RN, Meier-Schellersheim M, Nita-Lazar A, Fraser ID. Systems biology in immunology: a computational modeling perspective. *Annu Rev Immunol* (2011) **29**:527–85. doi:10.1146/annurev-immunol-030409-101317
14. Chylek LA, Harris LA, Tung C-S, Faeder JR, Lopez CF, Hlavacek WS. Rule-based modeling: a computational approach for studying biomolecular site dynamics in cell signaling systems. *Wiley Interdiscip Rev Syst Biol Med* (2014) **6**:13–36. doi:10.1002/wsbm.1245
15. Chylek LA. Decoding the language of phosphorylation site dynamics. *Sci Signal* (2013) **6**:jc2. doi:10.1126/scisignal.2004061
16. Hlavacek WS, Faeder JR, Blinov ML, Posner RG, Hucka M, Fontana W. Rules for modeling signal-transduction systems. *Sci STKE* (2006) **2006**:re6. doi:10.1126/stke.3442006re6
17. Chylek LA, Stites EC, Posner RG, Hlavacek WS. Innovations of the rule-based modeling approach. In: Prokop A, Csukás B, editors. *Systems Biology: Integrative Biology and Simulation Tools* (Vol. 1). Dordrecht: Springer (2013). p. 273–300.
18. Paar J, Harris N, Holowka D, Baird B. Bivalent ligands with rigid double-stranded DNA spacers reveal structural constraints on signaling by FcεRI. *J Immunol* (2002) **169**:856–64.
19. Sil D, Lee J, Luo D, Holowka D, Baird B. Trivalent ligands with rigid DNA spacers reveal structural requirements for IgE receptor signaling in RBL mast cells. *ACS Chem Biol* (2007) **2**:674–84. doi:10.1021/cb7001472
20. Posner R, Geng D, Haymore S, Bogert J, Pecht I, Licht A, et al. Trivalent antigens for degranulation of mast cells. *Org Lett* (2007) **9**:3551–4. doi:10.1021/ol071175h
21. Goldstein B, Faeder JR, Hlavacek WS, Blinov ML, Redondo A, Wofsy C. Modeling the early signaling events mediated by FcεRI. *Mol Immunol* (2002) **38**:1213–9. doi:10.1016/S0161-5890(02)00066-4
22. Faeder JR, Hlavacek WS, Reischl I, Blinov ML, Metzger H, Redondo A, et al. Investigation of early events in FcεRI-mediated signaling using a detailed mathematical model. *J Immunol* (2003) **170**:3769–81.
23. Faeder JR, Blinov ML, Goldstein B, Hlavacek WS. Combinatorial complexity and dynamical restriction of network flows in signal transduction. *Syst Biol (Stevenage)* (2005) **2**:5–15. doi:10.1049/sb:20045031
24. Nag A, Monine MI, Faeder JR, Goldstein B. Aggregation of membrane proteins by cytosolic cross-linkers: theory and simulation of the LAT-Grb2-SOS1 system. *Biophys J* (2009) **96**:2604–23. doi:10.1016/j.bpj.2009.01.019
25. Nag A, Monine M, Perelson A, Goldstein B. Modeling and simulation of aggregation of membrane protein LAT with molecular variability in the number of binding sites for cytosolic Grb2-SOS1-Grb2. *PLoS One* (2012) **7**:e28758. doi:10.1371/journal.pone.0028758
26. Nag A, Faeder JR, Goldstein B. Shaping the response: the role of FcεRI and Syk expression levels in mast cell signaling. *IET Syst Biol* (2010) **33**(4–47):334–47. doi:10.1049/iet-syb.2010.0006
27. Nag A, Monine MI, Blinov ML, Goldstein B. A detailed mathematical model predicts that serial engagement of IgE-Fc epsilon RI complexes can enhance Syk activation in mast cells. *J Immunol* (2010) **185**:3268–76. doi:10.4049/jimmunol.1000326
28. Cao L, Yu K, Banh C, Nguyen V, Ritz A, Raphael B, et al. Quantitative time-resolved phosphoproteomic analysis of mast cell signaling. *J Immunol* (2007) **179**:5864–76.
29. Gilfillan A, Tkaczyk C. Integrated signalling pathways for mast-cell activation. *Nat Rev Immunol* (2006) **16**:218–30. doi:10.1038/nri1782
30. Faeder JR, Blinov ML, Hlavacek WS. Rule-based modeling of biochemical systems with BioNetGen. *Methods Mol Biol* (2009) **500**:113–67. doi:10.1007/978-1-59745-525-1_5
31. Hindmarsh AC, Brown PN, Grant KE, Lee SL, Serban R, Shumaker DE, et al. Sundials: suite of nonlinear and differential/algebraic equation solvers. *ACM Trans Math Softw* (2005) **31**:363–96. doi:10.1145/1089014.1089020
32. Holowka D, Sil D, Torigoe C, Baird B. Insights into immunoglobulin E receptor signaling from structurally defined ligands. *Immunol Rev* (2007) **217**:269–79. doi:10.1111/j.1600-065X.2007.00517.x
33. Xu K, Goldstein B, Holowka D, Baird B. Kinetics of multivalent antigen DNP-BSA binding to IgE-Fc epsilon RI in relationship to the stimulated tyrosine phosphorylation of Fc epsilon RI. *J Immunol* (1998) **160**:3225–35.
34. Shelby SA, Holowka D, Baird B, Veatch SL. Distinct stages of stimulated FcεRI receptor clustering and immobilization are identified through superresolution imaging. *Biophys J* (2013) **105**:2343–54. doi:10.1016/j.bpj.2013.09.049
35. Liu Y, Barua D, Liu P, Wilson BS, Oliver JM, Hlavacek WS, et al. Single-cell measurements of IgE-mediated FcεRI signaling using an integrated microfluidic platform. *PLoS One* (2013) **8**:e60159. doi:10.1371/journal.pone.0060159
36. Young RM, Holowka D, Baird B. A lipid raft environment enhances Lyn kinase activity by protecting the active site tyrosine from dephosphorylation. *J Biol Chem* (2003) **278**:20746–52. doi:10.1074/jbc.M211402200
37. Jouvin MH, Adamczewski M, Numerof R, Letourneur O, Vallé A, Kinet JP. Differential control of the tyrosine kinases Lyn and Syk by the two signaling chains of the high affinity immunoglobulin E receptor. *J Biol Chem* (1994) **269**:5918–25.
38. Barua D, Hlavacek WS, Lipniacki T. A computational model for early events in B cell antigen receptor signaling: analysis of the roles of Lyn and Fyn. *J Immunol* (2012) **189**:646–58. doi:10.4049/jimmunol.1102003

39. Consortium TU. Activities at the Universal Protein Resource (UniProt). *Nucleic Acids Res* (2014) **42**:D191–8. doi:10.1093/nar/gkt1140
40. Holowka D, Calloway N, Cohen R, Gadi D, Lee J, Smith NL, et al. Roles for Ca^{2+} mobilization and its regulation in mast cell functions. *Front Immunol* (2012) **3**:104. doi:10.3389/fimmu.2012.00104
41. Kandasamy K, Mohan SS, Raju R, Keerthikumar S, Kumar GS, Venugopal AK, et al. NetPath: a public resource of curated signal transduction pathways. *Genome Biol* (2010) **11**:R3. doi:10.1186/gb-2010-11-1-r3
42. Zhang W, Trible RP, Samelson LE. LAT palmitoylation: its essential role in membrane microdomain targeting and tyrosine phosphorylation during T cell activation. *Immunity* (1998) **9**:239–46. doi:10.1016/S1074-7613(00)80606-8
43. Zhang W, Sloan-Lancaster J, Kitchen J, Trible RP, Samelson LE. LAT: the ZAP-70 tyrosine kinase substrate that links T cell receptor to cellular activation. *Cell* (1998) **92**:83–92. doi:10.1016/S0092-8674(00)80901-0
44. Saitoh S, Arudchandran R, Manetz T, Zhang W, Sommers C, Love P, et al. Lat is essential for FcεRI-mediated mast cell activation. *Immunity* (2000) **12**:525–35. doi:10.1016/S1074-7613(00)80204-6
45. Das R, Hammond S, Holowka D, Baird B. Real-time cross-correlation image analysis of early events in IgE receptor signaling. *Biophys J* (2008) **94**:4996–5008. doi:10.1529/biophysj.107.105502
46. Veatch SL, Chiang EN, Sengupta P, Holowka DA, Baird BA. Quantitative nanoscale analysis of IgE-FcεRI clustering and coupling to early signaling proteins. *J Phys Chem B* (2012) **116**:6923–35. doi:10.1021/jp300197p
47. Barua D, Goldstein B. A mechanistic model of early FcεRI signaling: lipid rafts and the question of protection from dephosphorylation. *PLoS One* (2012) **7**:e51669. doi:10.1371/journal.pone.0051669
48. Zhang J, Billingsley ML, Kincaid RL, Siraganian RP. Phosphorylation of Syk activation loop tyrosines is essential for Syk function. An in vivo study using a specific anti-Syk activation loop phosphotyrosine antibody. *J Biol Chem* (2000) **275**:35442–7. doi:10.1074/jbc.M004549200
49. Houtman JC, Higashimoto Y, Dimasi N, Cho S, Yamaguchi H, Bowden B, et al. Binding specificity of multiprotein signaling complexes is determined by both cooperative interactions and affinity preferences. *Biochemistry* (2004) **43**:4170–8. doi:10.1021/bi0357311
50. Jang IK, Zhang J, Gu H. Grb2, a simple adapter with complex roles in lymphocyte development, function, and signaling. *Immunol Rev* (2009) **232**:150–9. doi:10.1111/j.1600-065X.2009.00842.x
51. Cho S, Velikovsky C, Swaminathan CP, Houtman JC, Samelson LE, Mariuzza RA. Structural basis for differential recognition of tyrosine-phosphorylated sites in the linker for activation of T cells (LAT) by the adaptor gads. *EMBO J* (2004) **23**:1441–51. doi:10.1038/sj.emboj.7600168
52. Seet BT, Berry DM, Maltzman JS, Shabason J, Raina M, Koretzky GA, et al. Efficient T-cell receptor signaling requires a high-affinity interaction between the Gads C-SH3 domain and the SLP-76 RxxK motif. *EMBO J* (2007) **26**:678–89. doi:10.1038/sj.emboj.7601535
53. Stauffer TP, Meyer T. Compartmentalized IgE receptor-mediated signal transduction in living cells. *J Cell Biol* (1997) **139**:1447–54. doi:10.1083/jcb.139.6.1447
54. Samelson LE. Signal transduction mediated by the T cell antigen receptor: the role of adapter proteins. *Annu Rev Immunol* (2002) **20**:371–94. doi:10.1146/annurev.immunol.20.092601.111357
55. Yablonski D, Kadlecek T, Weiss A. Identification of a phospholipase C-gamma1 (PLC-gamma1) SH3 domain-binding site in SLP-76 required for T-cell receptor-mediated activation of PLC-gamma1 and NFAT. *Mol Cell Biol* (2001) **21**:4208–18. doi:10.1128/MCB.21.13.4208-4218.2001
56. Lewitzky M, Kardinal C, Gehring NH, Schmidt EK, Konkol B, Eulitz M, et al. The C-terminal SH3 domain of the adapter protein Grb2 binds with high affinity to sequences in Gab1 and SLP-76 which lack the SH3-typical P-x-x-P core motif. *Oncogene* (2001) **20**:1052–62. doi:10.1038/sj.onc.1204202
57. Edmead CE, Fox BC, Stace C, Ktistakis N, Welham MJ. The pleckstrin homology domain of Gab-2 is required for optimal interleukin-3 signalsome-mediated responses. *Cell Signal* (2006) **18**:1147–55. doi:10.1016/j.cellsig.2005.09.002
58. Parravicini V, Gadina M, Kovarova M, Odom S, Gonzalez-Espinosa C, Furumoto Y, et al. Fyn kinase initiates complementary signals required for IgE-dependent mast cell degranulation. *Nat Immunol* (2002) **3**:741–8. doi:10.1038/ni817
59. Gu H, Maeda H, Moon JJ, Lord JD, Yoakim M, Nelson BH, et al. New role for Shc in activation of the phosphatidylinositol 3-kinase/Akt pathway. *Mol Cell Biol* (2000) **20**:7109–20. doi:10.1128/MCB.20.19.7109-7120.2000
60. Qiu Y, Kung HJ. Signaling network of the Btk family kinases. *Oncogene* (2000) **19**:5651–61. doi:10.1038/sj.onc.1203958
61. Oh-hora M, Rao A. Calcium signaling in lymphocytes. *Curr Opin Immunol* (2008) **20**:250–8. doi:10.1016/j.coi.2008.04.004
62. Barker S, Caldwell K, Pfeiffer J, Wilson B. Wortmannin-sensitive phosphorylation, translocation, and activation of PLCγ1, but not PLCγ2, in antigen-stimulated RBL-2H3 mast cells. *Mol Biol Cell* (1998) **9**:483–96. doi:10.1091/mbc.9.2.483
63. Kawakami Y, Kitaura J, Satterthwaite AB, Kato RM, Asai K, Hartman SE, et al. Redundant and opposing functions of two tyrosine kinases, Btk and Lyn, in mast cell activation. *J Immunol* (2000) **165**:1210–9.
64. Kimura T, Sakamoto H, Appella E, Siraganian RP. The negative signaling molecule SH2 domain-containing inositol-polyphosphate 5-phosphatase (SHIP) binds to the tyrosine-phosphorylated beta subunit of the high affinity IgE receptor. *J Biol Chem* (1997) **272**:13991–6. doi:10.1074/jbc.272.21.13991
65. On M, Billingsley JM, Jouvin MH, Kinet JP. Molecular dissection of the FcRβ signaling amplifier. *J Biol Chem* (2004) **279**:45782–90. doi:10.1074/jbc.M404890200
66. Condé C, Gloire G, Piette J. Enzymatic and non-enzymatic activities of SHIP-1 in signal transduction and cancer. *Biochem Pharmacol* (2011) **82**:1320–34. doi:10.1016/j.bcp.2011.05.031
67. Milo R, Shen-Orr S, Itzkovitz S, Kashtan N, Chklovskii D, Alon U. Network motifs: simple building blocks of complex networks. *Science* (2002) **298**:842–7. doi:10.1126/science.298.5594.824
68. Lim WA, Lee C, Tang C. Design principles of regulatory networks: searching for the molecular algorithms of the cell. *Mol Cell* (2013) **49**:202–12. doi:10.1016/j.molcel.2012.12.020
69. Tyson J, Novak B. Functional motifs in biochemical reaction networks. *Annu Rev Phys Chem* (2010) **61**:219–40. doi:10.1146/annurev.physchem.012809.103457
70. Dolmetsch R, Xu K, Lewis R. Calcium oscillations increase the efficiency and specificity of gene expression. *Nature* (1998) **392**:933–6. doi:10.1038/31960
71. Ma W, Trusina A, El-Samad H, Lim W, Tang C. Defining network topologies that can achieve biochemical adaptation. *Cell* (2009) **138**:760–73. doi:10.1016/j.cell.2009.06.013
72. Mangan S, Alon U. Structure and function of the feed-forward loop network motif. *Proc Natl Acad Sci U S A* (2003) **100**:11980–5. doi:10.1073/pnas.2133841100
73. Mangan S, Zaslaver A, Alon U. The coherent feedforward loop serves as a sign-sensitive delay element in transcription networks. *J Mol Biol* (2003) **334**:197–204. doi:10.1016/j.jmb.2003.09.049
74. Calloway N, Owens T, Corwith K, Rodgers W, Holowka D, Baird B. Stimulated association of STIM1 and Orai1 is regulated by the balance of Ptdins(4,5)P_2 between distinct membrane pools. *J Cell Sci* (2011) **124**:2602–10. doi:10.1242/jcs.084178
75. Lipniacki T, Hat B, Faeder JR, Hlavacek WS. Stochastic effects and bistability in T cell receptor signaling. *J Theor Biol* (2008) **254**:110–22. doi:10.1016/j.jtbi.2008.05.001
76. Das J, Ho M, Zikherman J, Govern C, Yang M, Weiss A, et al. Digital signaling and hysteresis characterize ras activation in lymphoid cells. *Cell* (2009) **136**:337–51. doi:10.1016/j.cell.2008.11.051
77. Mukherjee S, Zhu J, Zikherman J, Parameswaran R, Kadlecek TA, Wang Q, et al. Monovalent and multivalent ligation of the B cell receptor exhibit differential dependence upon Syk and Src family kinases. *Sci Signal* (2013) **6**:ra1. doi:10.1126/scisignal.2003220
78. Halet G. Imaging phosphoinositide dynamics using GFP-tagged protein domains. *Biol Cell* (2005) **97**:501–18. doi:10.1042/BC20040080
79. Monine MI, Posner RG, Savage PB, Faeder JR, Hlavacek WS. Modeling multivalent ligand-receptor interactions with steric constraints on configurations of cell-surface receptor aggregates. *Biophys J* (2010) **98**:48–56. doi:10.1016/j.bpj.2009.09.043
80. Rigbolt K, Blagoev B. Quantitative phosphoproteomics to characterize signaling networks. *Semin Cell Dev Biol* (2012) **23**:863–71. doi:10.1016/j.semcdb.2012.05.006
81. Kumar C, Mann M. Bioinformatics analysis of mass spectrometry-based proteomics data sets. *FEBS Lett* (2009) **583**:1703–12. doi:10.1016/j.febslet.2009.03.035
82. Hause RJJ, Leung KK, Barkinge JL, Ciaccio M, Chuu C, Jones RB. Comprehensive binary interaction mapping of SH2 domains via fluorescence polarization

reveals novel functional diversification of ErbB receptors. *PLoS One* (2012) **7**:e44471. doi:10.1371/journal.pone.0044471

83. Nagaraj N, Wisniewski JR, Geiger T, Cox J, Kircher M, Kelso J, et al. Deep proteome and transcriptome mapping of a human cancer cell line. *Mol Syst Biol* (2011) **7**:578. doi:10.1038/msb.2011.81
84. Rowland M, Fontana W, Deeds E. Crosstalk and competition in signaling networks. *Biophys J* (2012) **3**:2389–98. doi:10.1016/j.bpj.2012.10.006
85. Thomson TM, Benjamin KR, Bush A, Love T, Pincus D, Resnekov O, et al. Scaffold number in yeast signaling system sets tradeoff between system output and dynamic range. *Proc Natl Acad Sci U S A* (2011) **108**:20265–70. doi:10.1073/pnas.1004042108
86. Barua D, Hlavacek WS. Modeling the effect of APC truncation on destruction complex function in colorectal cancer cells. *PLoS Comput Biol* (2013) **9**:e1003217. doi:10.1371/journal.pcbi.1003217
87. Li C, Liakata M, Rebholz-Schuhmann D. Biological network extraction from scientific literature: state of the art and challenges. *Brief Bioinform* (2013). doi:10.1093/bib/bbt006

13

Mathematical modeling of oncogenesis control in mature T-cell populations

Sebastian Gerdes[1], Sebastian Newrzela[2], Ingmar Glauche[1], Dorothee von Laer[3], Martin-Leo Hansmann[2] and Ingo Roeder[1]*

[1] Institute for Medical Informatics and Biometry, Medical Faculty Carl Gustav Carus, Dresden, Germany
[2] Senckenberg Institute of Pathology, Goethe-University Hospital Frankfurt, Frankfurt, Germany
[3] Department of Hygiene, Medical University Innsbruck, Innsbruck, Austria

Edited by:
Carmen Molina-Paris, University of Leeds, UK

Reviewed by:
Antonio A. Freitas, Institut Pasteur, France
Tomasz Zal, University of Texas MD Anderson Cancer Center, USA

***Correspondence:**
Ingo Roeder, Institute for Medical Informatics and Biometry, Medical Faculty Carl Gustav Carus, TU Dresden, Fetscherstr. 74, 01307 Dresden, Germany
e-mail: ingo.roeder@tu-dresden.de

T-cell receptor (TCR) polyclonal mature T cells are surprisingly resistant to oncogenic transformation after retroviral insertion of T-cell oncogenes. In a mouse model, it has been shown that mature T-cell lymphoma/leukemia (MTCLL) is not induced upon transplantation of mature, TCR polyclonal wild-type (WT) T cells, transduced with gammaretroviral vectors encoding potent T-cell oncogenes, into RAG1-deficient recipients. However, further studies demonstrated that quasi-monoclonal T cells treated with the same protocol readily induced MTCLL in the recipient mice. It has been hypothesized that in the TCR polyclonal situation, outgrowth of preleukemic cells and subsequent conversion to overt malignancy is suppressed through regulation of clonal abundances on a per-clone basis due to interactions between TCRs and self-peptide-MHC-complexes (spMHCs), while these mechanisms fail in the quasi-monoclonal situation. To quantitatively study this hypothesis, we applied a mathematical modeling approach. In particular, we developed a novel ordinary differential equation model of T-cell homeostasis, in which T-cell fate depends on spMHC-TCR-interaction-triggered stimulatory signals from antigen-presenting cells (APCs). Based on our mathematical modeling approach, we identified parameter configurations of our model, which consistently explain the observed phenomena. Our results suggest that the preleukemic cells are less competent than healthy competitor cells in acquiring survival stimuli from APCs, but that proliferation of these preleukemic cells is less dependent on survival stimuli from APCs. These predictions now call for experimental validation.

Keywords: T-cell homeostasis, T-cell niche, gene therapy, mature T-cell lymphoma, MTCL

1. INTRODUCTION

Mature T cells are an essential component of the adaptive immune system. They carry the so-called *T-cell receptor* (TCR) on their surface. This receptor enables them to recognize peptides that are presented to them via major histocompatibility complex (MHC) molecules on antigen-presenting cells (APCs). A vast number of different TCRs is expressed in T cells in healthy individuals, estimated to be in the order of 10^6 in mice (1) and 10^7 in humans (2). An individual T cell expresses a single TCR variant, and passes this variant on to its daughter cells. The set of all T cells expressing the same TCR is called a *T-cell clone* (or simply referred to as *clone*). The enormous TCR diversity is created during T-cell maturation in the thymus through genomic rearrangement of the TCR gene locus (3). A series of selection processes ensures that mature T cells can bind with low to moderate affinity to self-peptide-MHC complexes (spMHCs) on APCs (4–6). After maturation, T cells enter the peripheral T-cell pool.

The peripheral T-cell pool is remarkably stable in terms of cell numbers and clonal diversity throughout the lifetime of mice and humans. In order to explain this stability, concepts have emerged that are based on competition between T cells for limiting trophic resources needed for survival and proliferation (7). The limiting trophic resources can be divided in public and TCR-specific resources (8). In principle, public trophic resources are equally accessible to all T cells, and include stimulatory cytokines (e.g. interleukin 7), nutrients, costimulatory molecules, or physical space. In contrast, access to TCR-specific resources depends on the particular TCR that is expressed on a T cell. TCR-specific resources are represented mainly by stimulatory interactions with APCs due to binding of the TCR to spMHCs (9–11).

Different spMHCs may vary substantially in their suitability to mediate a stimulatory interaction for particular T-cell clones. Consequently, a *T-cell niche* concept has been proposed, in which different spMHCs represent distinct T-cell niches (12). The niches provide vital resources that different T-cell clones compete for. A particular clone may not receive resources from all niches equally well. This concept implies that the TCR diversity is stabilized by the diversity of the available spMHCs (13).

When the regulation of cellular proliferation in the T-cell system is corrupted, mature T-cell lymphoma/leukemia (MTCLL) formation may occur. However, oncogenesis is comparatively rare in mature T cells. For example, the incidence of B-cell lymphoid neoplasms is substantially higher than the incidence of T-cell/natural killer cell lymphoid neoplasms, as shown in a study from the United States ($26.13/10^5$/year vs. $1.79/10^5$/year (14)). Furthermore, several studies from the field of retroviral gene therapy confirm the relative resistance of mature T cells to oncogenesis. Despite long follow-up times, retroviral vector-induced oncogenesis has never been observed in clinical gene therapy trials involving gene-modified mature T cells (15–17). In contrast, genotoxicity was observed in several studies involving retroviral gene transfer into hematopoietic stem and progenitor cells (HSPCs) (18, 19).

Motivated by these observations, we here focus on the analysis of oncogenesis control in mature T-cell populations.

In order to explicitly investigate the relative resistance of mature T cells to malignant transformation in a gene therapeutic context, HSPCS, and mature T cells were exposed to an identical transformation assay in a defined experimental setting (20). In this assay, HSPCs and mature T cells were isolated from wild-type mice and were each transduced independently with high copy numbers of gammaretroviral vectors encoding potent T-cell oncogenes. Subsequently, the cells were transplanted into immunoincompetent RAG1-deficient mice. HSPC-transplanted animals consistently developed MTCLL. In contrast, MTCLL has not been observed in any of the recipients that were transplanted with mature T cells. This finding corroborated the relative resistance of mature T cells to malignant transformation.

In a subsequent study, the impact of TCR diversity on T-cell resistance to malignant transformation has been further assessed (21). In this study, T-cell populations were isolated from OT1- or P14-mice, i.e. mice expressing a transgenic TCR. T-cell populations from these mouse models are quasi-monoclonal, i.e. they express predominantly one specific TCR. By applying a similar, yet refined, transformation assay as in the previous study MTCLL readily developed in the recipient RAG1-deficient mice (see **Figure 1**). Moreover, addition of untransduced TCR polyclonal T cells to quasi-monoclonal, transduced cell populations prevented malignancy development, demonstrating that TCR polyclonality plays a pivotal role in malignancy control in mature T cells.

Building on these observations, we hypothesize that in the TCR polyclonal situation, prohomeostatic signals, due to interactions between TCRs and spMHCs, suppress the outgrowth of preleukemic T cells (i.e. in this context, T cells that have been transformed by retroviral insertion of an oncogene), while these mechanisms fail in the TCR quasi-monoclonal situation, and vigorous cell expansion occurs. In this paper, we aim to quantitatively assess the implications of this hypothesis using a mathematical modeling approach. Specifically, we develop a mathematical model of a niche-dependent mature T-cell regulation [similar to previous published models, e.g. Ref. (22)], which will be applied to model the physiological situation and MTCLL formation. Using this model of T-cell homeostasis, we present an *in silico* simulation scenario that is suited to mimic the experimental procedures performed by Newrzela et al. (20, 21). In an extensive parameter screen, we evaluate if, and under which parameter constellations the experimental observations can be explained.

2. MATERIALS AND METHODS

2.1. MODEL DESCRIPTION

The two major entities in our model are *T-cell species* (also called simply *species*) and *T-cell niches* (also called simply *niches*). With the term *species*, we refer to a set of T cells that is homogeneous in terms of our model parameters. In the physiological situation, a T-cell clone can be represented as a particular species. However, in order to model the aforementioned experimental situation (20, 21), we will represent each T-cell clone by two species, namely a species representing healthy cells within a clone and a preleukemic species representing cells that potentially give rise to MTCLL.

Our model is constructed to describe the temporal dynamics of species abundances, i.e. the number of cells belonging to a particular T-cell species at any point of time. The number of species in the system is denoted by the symbol m. The species abundances at time t are represented by the vector $\mathbf{c}(t) = (c_i(t))$ with $i = 1, 2, \ldots, m$. The initial species abundances $\mathbf{c}(0)$ are defined by an m-dimensional vector denoted $\mathbf{c}^0 = \left(c_i^0\right)$.

In the model, T-cell species compete for resources needed for survival and proliferation that are supplied by T-cell niches. The number of niches in the system is denoted by the symbol n. It is assumed that the niches supply resources at constant rates, represented by the n-dimensional vector $\mathbf{p} = (p_j)$, where $j = 1, 2, \ldots, n$.

The competition for niche resources between species is defined by the $m \times n$ matrix $\mathbf{A} = [a_{ij}]$, called *niche affinity matrix*, in which a_{ij} is a measure of the capability of species i to acquire resources from niche j.

At any time point t, species receive resources from niches according to instantaneous rates. These rates, which are termed *resource acquisition rates*, are stored in an $m \times n$ matrix $\mathbf{R}(t) = [r_{ij}(t)]$. $r_{ij}(t)$ denotes the rate at which the i-th species receives resources from the j-th niche at time t, and is the affinity- and abundance-weighted proportion of the total rate p_j at which

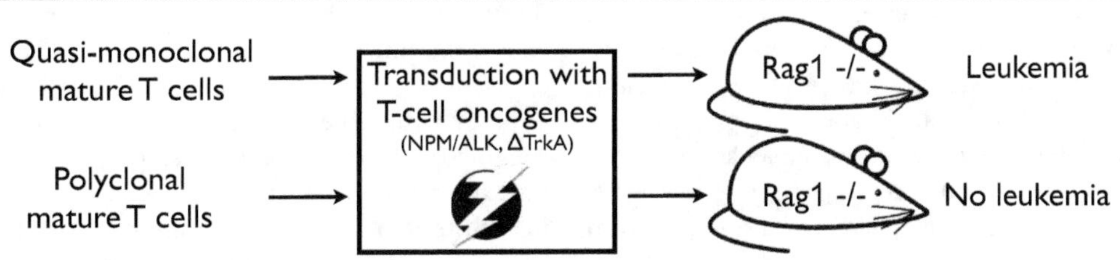

FIGURE 1 | Experimental strategy as described in Newrzela et al. (21). TCR quasi-monoclonal T-cell populations transduced with potent T-cell oncogenes developed mature T-cell lymphoma/leukemia in RAG1-deficient recipient mice, while TCR polyclonal T-cell populations that have been subjected to the same transformation assay did not.

niche j provides resources. Thus, $r_{ij}(t)$ is calculated as follows:

$$r_{ij}(t) = \begin{cases} \frac{a_{ij}c_i(t)}{\sum_{k=1}^{m} a_{kj}c_k(t)} p_j & \text{if } \sum_{k=1}^{m} a_{kj}c_k(t) > 0 \\ 0 & \text{otherwise} \end{cases}$$

The sum of the resource acquisition rates over all niches yields the net resource acquisition rate for a particular species.

Different T-cell species may differ in the amount of resources needed to sustain an individual cell. Therefore, we introduce the m-dimensional vector $\mathbf{v} = (v_i)$, which we term *resource utilization efficiency*. This parameter determines for each species, how many T cells can be sustained by one resource unit per unit of time. The product of the resource acquisition rates and the resource utilization efficiencies yields the time-dependent carrying capacities of the individual species, stored in the vector $\mathbf{k}(t) = (k_i(t))$:

$$k_i(t) = v_i \sum_{j=1}^{n} r_{ij}(t)$$

The carrying capacities indicate how many cells of a given species can be sustained by the system, given the current resource distribution among the species. The carrying capacities may change dynamically in time, as the species abundances vary. The relation between the actual size of a species and the carrying capacity determines whether the species abundance decreases or increases. Due to lack of biological data determining a particular growth model for T-cell clones, we chose a rather general logistic growth dynamics, where τ denotes the minimum cell cycle time:

$$\frac{dc_i(t)}{dt} = \begin{cases} \frac{c_i(t)}{\tau}\left(1 - \frac{c_i(t)}{k_i(t)}\right) & \text{if } k_i(t) > 0 \\ 0 & \text{if } k_i(t) = 0 \end{cases}$$

We require c_i^0, a_{ij}, p_j, and v_i to be greater than or equal to zero, and τ to be greater than zero.

2.2. PARAMETER CHOICE

In its general form, the model presented in the previous subsection has $nm + 2m + n + 1$ scalar parameters. In the following, we sketch our numerical approach and reparameterize the model in order to reduce the effective number of parameters.

In our approach, the number of TCR-defined clones is denoted by q. Each clone is represented by two species (thus $m = 2q$). Without loss of generality, species 1 to q represent the presumably healthy cells within the q clones (referred to as *healthy species*) and species $q+1$ to $2q$ represent the cells that potentially give rise to leukemia/lymphoma (referred to as *preleukemic species*). The specific case of the monoclonal situation is represented by setting all but the first healthy and the first preleukemic initial species abundances to zero ($c_i = 0$ except $c_1 > 0$, $c_{q+1} > 0$). We assume that each species may in principle receive a stimulus from each niche due to unspecific affinity. The magnitude of the unspecific affinity is denoted $u^{(h)}$ for the healthy species and $u^{(p)}$ for the preleukemic species. In addition, we assume that each species has a preferred niche, to which it has an additional affinity [*specific affinity*, denoted $s^{(h)}$ for the healthy species and $s^{(p)}$ for the preleukemic species]. Biologically, the specific affinity could be interpreted as affinity to cognate self-peptide, and the unspecific affinity as affinity to the MHC itself.

The scalar parameters describing the specific and the unspecific affinities are used to define the niche affinity matrix $\mathbf{A}$. Formally, we construct the matrices $\mathbf{A}^{(h)} = \left[a_{ij}^{(h)}\right]$ describing the niche affinities of the healthy species and $\mathbf{A}^{(p)} = \left[a_{ij}^{(p)}\right]$ describing the niche affinities of the preleukemic species as follows,

$$a_{ij}^{(h)} = \begin{cases} s^{(h)} + u^{(h)} & \text{if } i = j \\ u^{(h)} & \text{if } i \neq j \end{cases}$$

$$a_{ij}^{(p)} = \begin{cases} s^{(p)} + u^{(p)} & \text{if } i = j \\ u^{(p)} & \text{if } i \neq j \end{cases}$$

$$i \in \{1, 2, \ldots, q\}, \qquad j \in \{1, 2, \ldots, n\}$$

and use these matrices in order to construct the actual niche affinity matrix $\mathbf{A}$ by vertical concatenation of $\mathbf{A}^{(h)}$ and $\mathbf{A}^{(p)}$:

$$\mathbf{A} = \begin{bmatrix} \mathbf{A}^{(h)} \\ \mathbf{A}^{(p)} \end{bmatrix}$$

Furthermore, we introduce the symbols $v^{(h)}$ and $v^{(p)}$ to describe the resource utilization efficiencies of the healthy and preleukemic species, respectively. $v^{(h)}$ and $v^{(p)}$ are used to construct the actual resource utilization efficiencies (superscript T denoting the transpose of a vector):

$$\mathbf{v} = (\underbrace{v^{(h)}, \ldots, v^{(h)}}_{q \text{ times}}, \underbrace{v^{(p)}, \ldots, v^{(p)}}_{q \text{ times}})^T$$

Note that no interspecies heterogeneity with respect to the magnitudes of the specific and unspecific affinities of the healthy species ($s^{(h)}$, $u^{(h)}$) and their resource utilization efficiency $v^{(h)}$ is considered. The same applies to the preleukemic species, with parameters $s^{(p)}$, $u^{(p)}$, and $v^{(p)}$.

In order to make numerical simulations feasible, while still preserving the niche-based regulation, we are using a system with 100 niches ($n = 100$) and 100 clones ($q = 100$), i.e. 200 species ($m = 200$) for the numerical simulations.

As mentioned above, the real number of T-cell clones in mice is estimated in the order of 10^6, while the total number of T cells in a mouse is estimated to be in the order of 10^8 (23). Assuming that in the physiological situation the number of niches in mice equals the number of T-cell clones, a niche nourishes 100 cells on average. Therefore, we consider the niche sizes $p_j = 100$ for all $j = 1, \ldots, 100$. The minimum cell cycle time τ is set to 8 h as a rough estimate of vigorous T-cell proliferation (24). Since an initial exploratory screen did not reveal a qualitative effect of changes in niche size $\mathbf{p}$ and the minimum cell cycle time τ on the model behavior, we keep $\mathbf{p}$ and τ fixed to the above described values.

Additionally, and without loss of generality, we can fix one of the four niche affinity parameters $s^{(h)}$, $s^{(p)}$, $u^{(h)}$, and $u^{(p)}$ as the distribution of resources depends on relative affinities only. We chose to fix the unspecific affinity of the healthy cells $u^{(h)} = 1/n = 0.01$

(n being the number of niches) as our reference. The specific affinity of the healthy species $s^{(h)}$ is set to 1 [except for the results shown in **Figure 6**, in which we are also considering the values $s^{(h)} = 0.2$ and $s^{(h)} = 5$]. Furthermore, we set the resource utilization efficiency of the healthy cells $v^{(h)}$ to 1, thus interpreting the corresponding value of the preleukemic cells $v^{(p)}$ as a relative measure compared to the healthy situation.

Hence, at this point the scalar parameters $s^{(p)}$ (specific affinity of the preleukemic species), $u^{(p)}$ (unspecific affinity of the preleukemic species), $v^{(p)}$ (resource utilization efficiency of the preleukemic species), and the vector-valued initial condition $\mathbf{c}^0$ are not yet fixed. How they are varied in the parameter screen is described in the following subsection.

2.3. SIMULATION PROCEDURE

2.3.1. Physiological situation

In order to study the behavior of the system, we *in silico* transplant 500 cells into an empty system. TCR diversities $q = 1$ and $q = 100$ are considered. In the TCR polyclonal situation, the initial species abundances $\mathbf{c}^0$ are obtained by distributing the 500 cells according to a uniform distribution over the healthy species. $s^{(h)}$ is set to 1. The parameters $s^{(p)}$, $u^{(p)}$, and $v^{(p)}$, which describe the properties of the preleukemic species, do not influence the model behavior here, since no preleukemic cells are transplanted into the system. All other model parameters are fixed to the above described values. We let the system evolve for 400 time-steps. To demonstrate the system response to perturbations, we simulate a significant cell loss by removing 99% of the cells at time $t = 200$. The simulation results are presented in subsection 1.

2.3.2. Oncogenic situation

In order to systematically evaluate the effect of the parameters describing the properties of the preleukemic cells [i.e. their specific affinity $s^{(p)}$, their unspecific affinity $u^{(p)}$, their resource utilization efficiency $v^{(p)}$] and the initial abundances $\mathbf{c}^0$, we perform an extensive parameter screen. $s^{(p)}$, $u^{(p)}$, and $v^{(p)}$ are varied in multiples of their healthy counterparts, ranging from ~1/40 to ~40. The relative distances between two neighboring values is 20%, so that 41 different fold-changes are considered per parameter.

The fraction of transplanted cells that have been transformed into preleukemic cells is currently not known for the used experimental protocol. Therefore, we consider three scenarios, denoted P1, P10, and P100, which consider 1, 10, and 100 initial preleukemic cells, respectively. All three scenarios are evaluated for each combination of the specific affinity of the preleukemic species $s^{(p)}$, their unspecific affinity $u^{(p)}$, and their resource utilization efficiency $v^{(p)}$. All cases are initiated by 500 cells that are *in silico-transplanted* into an empty system.

This corresponds to 5 cells per clone in the polyclonal situation on average, in accordance with the experimental situation (5×10^6 transplanted cells, TCR diversity estimated in the order of 10^6). In scenario P1, one T cell (0.2%) is assigned to the preleukemic cell compartment, in scenario P10, 10 T cells (2%), belonging to 10 different species in the TCR polyclonal situation, are assigned to the preleukemic cell compartment, and in scenario P100, 100 T cells (20%), belonging to 100 different species in the polyclonal situation. In all three scenarios, the remaining cells are distributed randomly according to a uniform probability distribution over the healthy species in the polyclonal situation. In addition to the polyclonal settings we construct a corresponding monoclonal situation, in which the fraction of 0.2% (P1), 2% (P10), or 20% (P100) preleukemic cells is assigned to only a single clone.

The number of parameter sets evaluated in each of the three scenarios is 41^3 (since 41 different fold-changes are considered for $s^{(p)}$, $u^{(p)}$, and $v^{(p)}$). Hence, in total $3 \times 41^3 \approx 2 \times 10^5$ parameter sets are evaluated for both the polyclonal and the monoclonal situation.

As we are not primarily interested in transient phenomena but in the long-term behavior of the system, our aim is the identification and characterization of stable steady states, namely whether the preleukemic cells are able to dominate the system or not. Therefore, simulations are run until the relative change of all species abundances between two successive time steps are below 10^{-6}. For this situation we assume that the system is sufficiently close to a steady state. If this criterion is not fulfilled after 10^8 simulation steps, the current simulation is stopped, and the stability of the system will be assessed manually.

For each individual parameter set, we evaluate if the corresponding simulations for the mono- and polyclonal situation are consistent with the experimental phenomena, i.e. if we observe a stable and considerably enlarged population of preleukemic cells in the monoclonal situation, and control of the preleukemic cells in the polyclonal situation (i.e. the contribution of the preleukemic cell population remains below a certain threshold). The specific criteria used for the classification are listed in **Table 1**. If a parameter set fulfills all criteria, we consider it consistent with the observed phenomena as described in (20, 21).

The simulation results of the parameter screen are presented in subsection 2.

3. RESULTS

3.1. PHYSIOLOGICAL SITUATION

First, we investigate the behavior of the described system in the absence of preleukemic cells. As can be seen in **Figure 2**, the system quickly converges to a steady state, both in the mono- and the

Table 1 | Criteria used for classification.

	Total cell count	Contribution of preleukemic cells
TCR monoclonal situation	At least 300% of physiological cell count	At least 80% of total cell count
TCR polyclonal situation	At most 120% of physiological cell count	At most 50% of total cell count

A particular tested parameter set is classified as consistent with the experimental phenomena, if the total cell count and the contribution of the preleukemic cells fulfill the criteria specified in the table, i.e. a leukemia-like situation in the TCR monoclonal situation, and a state of non-dominance of the preleukemic species in the TCR polyclonal situation. The total cell count at the steady state is compared to the physiological cell count, which is established based on the simulations shown in subsection 1. The contribution of the preleukemic cells is the ratio between the number of preleukemic cells and the total cell count at the steady state.

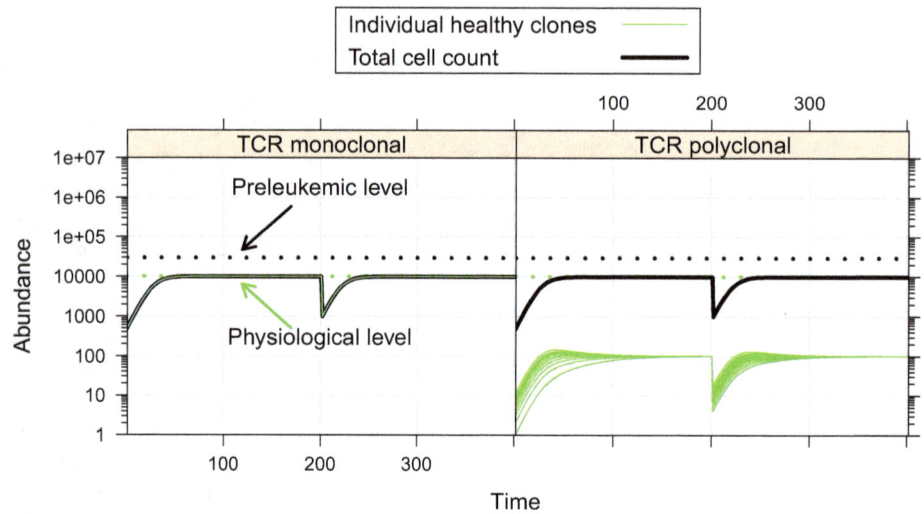

FIGURE 2 | Simulation results of physiological situation. The left panel documents the dynamic system behavior in the monoclonal situation. In the right panel, the individual green lines represent the abundance of different clones. The system quickly converges to a steady state. The total cell count in the steady state of the physiological situation is indicated by the horizontal dashed green line at 10^4. The horizontal red line at 3×10^4 represents the total cell count that is required as a minimum in order to qualify a situation as premalignant. At $t = 200$, 99% of the cells are removed from the system. Both in the mono- and the polyclonal situation the system quickly reestablishes the previous steady state.

polyclonal situation. In the polyclonal situation, all clones have an abundance of 100 cells at the steady state due to the parameter symmetry among the healthy species (i.e. all species have the same specific affinity $s^{(h)} = 1$ to their preferred niche, and the same unspecific affinity $u^{(h)} = 1/n$ to all niches). The total cell count at the steady state amounts to $v^{(h)} \cdot \sum_{j=1}^{n} p_j = 10^4$ both in the monoclonal and the polyclonal situation. After a perturbation, e.g. due to cell kill, the system quickly reestablishes its previous state, unless individual species are completely eliminated within the cell kill simulation.

The steady state with equal-sized clones is reached regardless of the initial abundances of the healthy cells, given that the abundances of all healthy species are >0 (data not shown). Transient changes of the niche sizes or transient addition of niches (e.g. to model infections) can entail the transient expansion of one more species/clones (data not shown).

3.2. ONCOGENIC SITUATION

For the oncogenic situation, we evaluate whether a certain proportion of preleukemic cells (represented by the three scenarios P1, P10, and P100) can develop into a (pre)leukemic situation in the monoclonal case, while being controlled by healthy competitor cells in the polyclonal case. The evaluation is carried out based on prespecified formal criteria (see **Table 1**). In all tested parameter settings, the steady state (i.e. convergence) criterion is reached both in the mono- and the polyclonal situation. **Figure 3** shows representative simulation results to provide some intuition about the spectrum of possible simulation outcomes for the three scenarios P1, P10, and P100.

Out of the $\approx 2 \times 10^5$ tested parameter configurations, 1050 parameter sets are consistent with the experimental phenomena according to the defined criteria (c.f. **Table 1**). Further, it should be emphasized that the consistent parameter sets are identifiable as a confined region in the parameter space in all three scenarios (see **Figure 4**) and that the regions in scenarios P1, P10, and P100 overlap considerably. In all three scenarios, we identify a region that is characterized by lowered specific and unspecific affinities as well as an increased resources utilization of preleukemic compared to normal T cells. Technically, this refers to triangular prisms in the $u^{(p)}_{low} s^{(p)}_{low} v^{(p)}_{high}$ octant of the parameter cube (**Figure 4**). In scenario P1, the region of consistent parameter sets additionally extends to the $u^{(p)}_{low} s^{(p)}_{high} v^{(p)}_{high}$ octant. Our results indicate that the overall systems behavior displays only a minor dependency on the initial number of preleukemic cells with respect to the phenomena in focus.

Assessing the set of consistent parameter constellations in more detail, we find that the resource utilization efficiency parameter for the preleukemic species $v^{(p)}$ had to be chosen at least three-fold higher than the resource utilization efficiency for healthy cells, in order to be consistent with the experimental observations. This is more clearly seen in **Figure 5**, which further characterizes the parameter sets that are consistent with the predefined criteria. The fact that a three-fold increase of $v^{(p)}$ is required, directly reflects criterion from **Table 1**, stating that the cell counts have to be increased at least three-fold in the monoclonal situation.

Concerning the niche affinities of the preleukemic cells, a clear pattern can be observed, likewise apparent in **Figure 5**. In scenarios P10 and P100, the specific affinity of the preleukemic cells $s^{(p)}$ is decreased (i.e. $s^{(p)} < s^{(h)}$) in all consistent parameter sets. In scenario P1, however, the specific affinity can be considerably increased without rendering a tested parameter set inconsistent. This is due to the fact that in scenario P1, only a single cell is preleukemic initially. Therefore, the fitness of the preleukemic cell

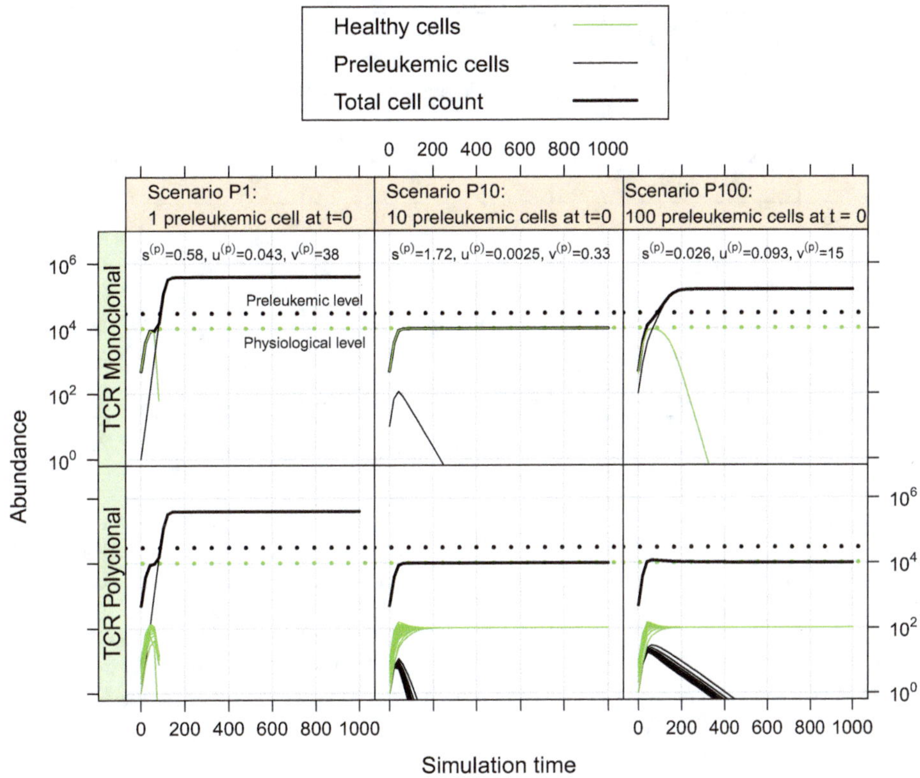

FIGURE 3 | Simulation results of three representative parameter sets. For each scenario, we show the simulation results of one possible parameter set. The parameter set picked for scenario P1 is not consistent with the experimental observations as specified in **Table 1**. The preleukemic cells expand more than threefold both in the mono- and polyclonal situation. The parameter set chosen for P10 is also not consistent with the specified criteria. Using this parameter set, the preleukemic cells are less fit than the healthy cells, and die out both in the mono- and the polyclonal situation. The parameter set chosen for scenario P100 is consistent with the specified criteria.

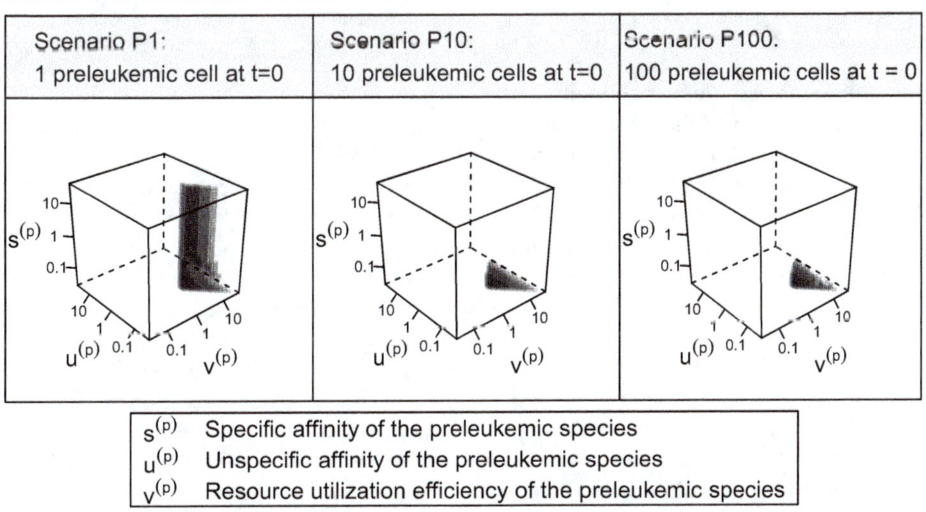

FIGURE 4 | 3D scatter plot of consistent parameter sets. Each tested parameter set can be represented by a point in one of the three presented cubes, the coordinates representing the fold-changes of $s^{(p)}$, $t^{(p)}$, and $v^{(p)}$ in comparison with their healthy counterparts $s^{(h)}$, $u^{(h)}$, and $v^{(h)}$. In the center of each cube, the parameters $s^{(p)}$, $u^{(p)}$, and $v^{(p)}$ are equal to their counterparts describing the healthy cells. Only the parameter sets that are consistent with the experimental observations (criteria in **Table 1**) are plotted. Transparency is used in order to give an impression of the shape of the consistent parameter region.

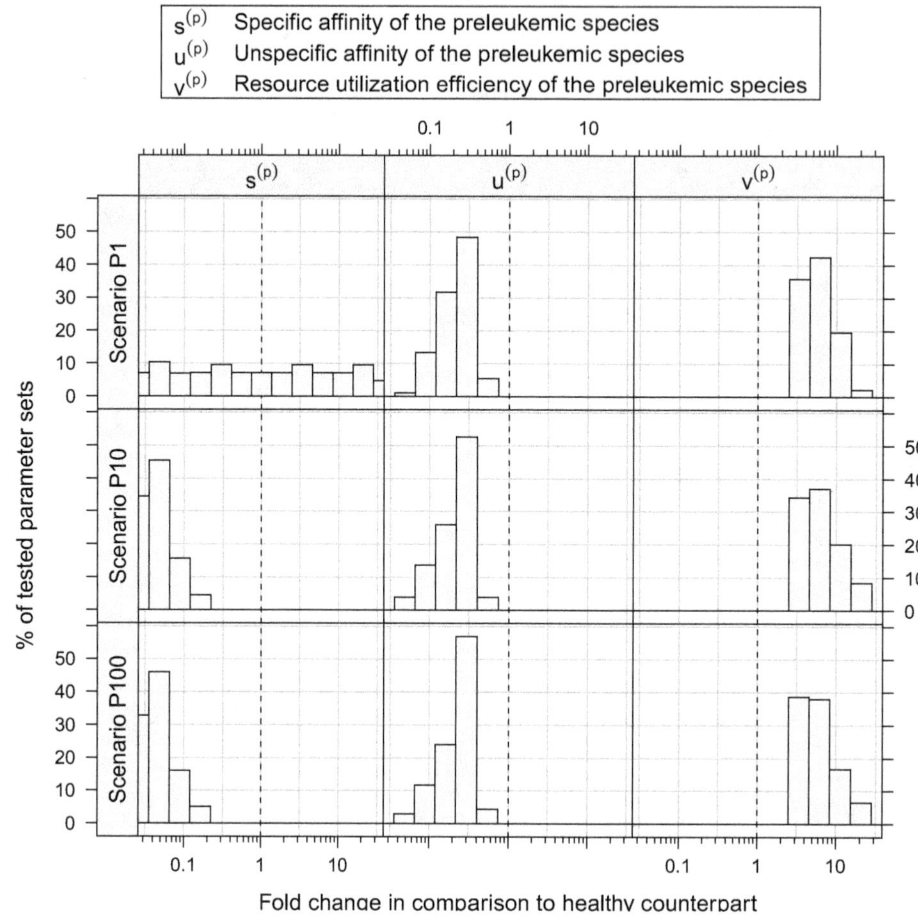

FIGURE 5 | Histograms of consistent parameter values. These histograms show the distribution of the specific affinity of the preleukemic species $s^{(p)}$, their unspecific affinity $u^{(p)}$, and their resource utilization efficiency $v^{(p)}$ of the consistent parameter sets. $s^{(p)}$ is decreased in all consistent parameter sets of scenario P10 and P100, while it is indifferent in scenario P1. $u^{(p)}$ is decreased and $v^{(p)}$ is increased in all consistent parameter sets.

pool (i.e. proliferative potential) increases only marginally in the polyclonal situation if the specific affinity of the preleukemic cells $s^{(p)}$ is increased. In contrast, in scenario P10 and P100, the fitness of the preleukemic cell population in the polyclonal situation responds more sensitively to an increase of the specific affinity of the preleukemic cells due the greater TCR diversity within the preleukemic cell population. Because of that, the preleukemic cells cannot be controlled by healthy competitor cells in the polyclonal situation, even if the specific affinity is only mildly increased, rendering such parameter sets inconsistent.

The unspecific affinity of the preleukemic cells is decreased in all consistent parameter sets (i.e. $u^{(p)} < u^{(h)}$). This reduction generates a disadvantage of preleukemic species for accessing resources from non-preferred niches, thus prohibiting a dominating expansion. Nonetheless, the preleukemic species must have at least some residual unspecific affinity in order to generate results that are consistent with the experimental situation. Specifically, the residual unspecific affinity allows them to access resources from the unprotected niches in the monoclonal situation. Without this ability, these cells cannot outgrow the healthy species in this situation. When comparing the decrease of the specific and the unspecific affinity of the preleukemic cells ($u^{(p)}$), it stands out that in scenarios P10 and P100, the specific affinity of the preleukemic cells ($s^{(p)}$) is decreased to a greater degree than the unspecific affinity ($u^{(p)}$) in all consistent parameter sets. In contrast, the decrease of the specific affinity of preleukemic cells ($s^{(p)}$) is greater than their decrease in unspecific affinity ($u^{(p)}$) in only ≈30% of the consistent parameter sets in scenario P1. Hence, if only a single preleukemic cell is present initially, the ability to receive a stimulus due to interaction with cognate self-peptide may be preserved or even increased, while in the situation of many initially present preleukemic cells the simulation results are not consistent with the experimental phenomena.

Furthermore, our simulations demonstrate that there is a rather strict functional relation between the unspecific affinity of the preleukemic cells ($u^{(p)}$) and their resource utilization efficiency ($v^{(p)}$) for all consistent parameters (see **Figure 6**). In other words, a certain acquired growth advantage, which is mediated by an increase in resource utilization ($v^{(p)}$), requires a corresponding decrease in the unspecific affinity ($u^{(p)}$) to guarantee consistency. Interestingly, the stringency of this relation depends crucially on the specific affinity of the healthy cells ($s^{(h)}$). To illustrate this

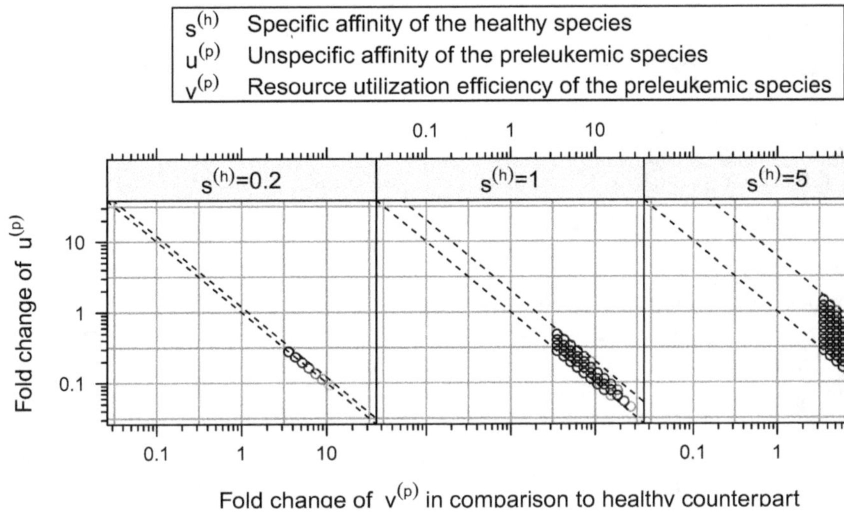

FIGURE 6 | Relation between resource utilization efficiency $v^{(p)}$ and unspecific affinity $u^{(p)}$ in the consistent parameter sets. Here, the fold-changes of the unspecific affinities of the preleukemic cells $u^{(p)}$ in the consistent parameter sets is plotted against their resource utilization efficiencies $v^{(p)}$. The relation between these quantities is relatively strict. All points are contained between two parallel lines. In this plot, we show additional simulation results, in which also the specific affinity of the healthy cells $s^{(h)}$ is varied.

relationship, we tested the system behavior also for $s^{(h)} = 0.2$ and $s^{(h)} = 5$ in addition to the value $s^{(h)} = 1$ used so far. Although varying values of $s^{(h)}$ do not qualitatively change the system behavior, the size of the consistent parameter region, i.e. the number of consistent parameter sets, is affected considerably by the particular choice of $s^{(h)}$: it is larger for $s^{(h)} = 5$ and smaller for $s^{(h)} = 0.2$. This can be seen in **Figure 6**, which illustrates the relationship for different values of $s^{(h)}$.

Interpreting the specific affinity as affinity to cognate self-peptide, and the unspecific affinity as affinity to the MHC itself, the ratio of the specific and the unspecific affinity of the healthy cells (i.e. $s^{(h)}/u^{(h)}$) determines how strict the regulation exerted by the self-peptide defined niches is. If the ratio is large, the niche regulation is strict, i.e. T cells can hardly access resources from niches other than their preferred niche. If the ratio is small, T cells can acquire more resources from niches other than their preferred niche. Our simulation results indicate that the stronger the niche regulation (i.e. a larger $s^{(h)}$), the larger is the consistent parameter region, and hence the more robust are the modeling results and the biological behavior of the system.

4. DISCUSSION

Oncogenesis in mature T cells and especially the resistance to malignant transformation of these cells even in potent oncogenic transformation assays have raised substantial interest in these cell populations. In a series of experiments, it has been shown that the resistance of mature T cells depends on the diversity of the TCR repertoire. Specifically, MTCLLs could readily be induced in T-cell populations that are quasi-monoclonal with respect to their TCR, while oncogenesis occurred only in rare cases in the TCR polyclonal situation, despite identical experimental conditions (20, 21). This observation led to the hypothesis that in the polyclonal situation, regulation based on competition for survival stimuli mediated by interaction between TCRs and spMHCs on APCs can prevent the expansion of preleukemic cells. Furthermore, the hypothesis implies that this regulation fails in the quasi-monoclonal situation, and the preleukemic cells expand, and eventually give rise to overt malignancy.

We have developed and applied a mathematical model of T-cell homeostasis to qualitatively and quantitatively challenge this concept. In the model, mature T cells compete for resources that are provided by T-cell niches. Biologically, the resources correspond to survival stimuli from APCs due to interactions between spMHCs and the TCR. The different T-cell niches are defined by the different spMHCs found on APCs. Due to differential affinities of different TCRs to spMHCs, T cells may differ in their capability to acquire resources from a particular niche.

Within this modeling framework we systematically evaluated the effect of the model parameters. For each specific parameter set, we tested if it is consistent with the observed phenomena according to the criteria in **Table 1**.

In order to achieve consistency with the criteria, the niche affinities of the preleukemic cells had to be decreased (i.e. $s^{(p)} < s^{(h)}$ and $u^{(p)} < u^{(h)}$, while their resource utilization efficiency had to be increased (i.e. $v^{(p)} > v^{(h)}$). Biologically, this suggests that the preleukemic cells are less dependent on niche resources (decreased affinities). In particular, our results predict a stronger decrease of the specific affinity of the preleukemic cells ($s^{(p)}$) compared to the unspecific affinity ($u^{(p)}$).

This implies that in the presence of healthy competitor cells with preference for the same niche, the preleukemic cells can be outcompeted. In the polyclonal situation this preventive effect acts on almost all niches, thus keeping the preleukemic cells at a minimum or even making them disappear.

In contrast, in the monoclonal situation the vast majority of niches is unguarded by healthy cells, and their resources can, therefore, be accessed by the preleukemic cells due to their albeit small, but non-zero unspecific affinity ($u^{(p)}$). In this situation, the decrease in the affinities can be compensated by the increase of the resource utilization efficiency of the preleukemic cells ($v^{(p)}$). Metaphorically speaking, the polyclonal healthy competitor cells protect the niche resources against the aggressive preleukemic cells in the polyclonal situation. If the polyclonal guards in the form of healthy competitor cells are not present, the preleukemic cells are able to claim all or most of the niche resources and promote MTCLL occurrence.

Transferring our findings back into a mechanistic context, we speculate that the decreased model affinities correspond to a down-regulation of TCR-mediated regulations and/or impairment of intracellular TCR signaling, i.e. a reduced T-cell avidity (25). A more efficient utilization of these signals (i.e. an increase in $v^{(p)}$) can be interpreted as a partial independence of preleukemic cells from environment-mediated growth signals, or as failure to respond adequately to inhibitory signals. On an intracellular level this independence might be achieved by a constitutive up-regulation of growth-promoting pathways.

In order to describe the T-cell system, and in particular the experiments performed by Newrzela et al. in mathematical terms we made a number of simplifying assumptions. It is a long-standing notion that oncogenesis often develops in a multi-step process (26). Also, in the context of gene therapy, it has been described that oncogenesis may occur directly (*single hit induction*), or may require additional lesions (*cooperating hit induction*) (27, 28). In our simulation scenario, however, we consider the effect of a first but fully effective hit only, i.e. we assume a virtually instantaneous effect of the oncogene affecting all preleukemic cells after transduction. In principle, it would be possible to incorporate cooperating hits into our model that are subsequently acquired after transplantation. We refrained from doing so, since only preliminary experimental data on tumor evolution in the context of the phenomena in focus are available to date.

Similarly, we did not account for heterogeneity concerning the effect of the oncogene, i.e. all cells belonging to the preleukemic cell compartment are assigned the same functional alteration in the model. Also, it is not clear, if our model adequately describes the emergence of preleukemic cells on an individual clone level. Hopefully, such individual clone data will be available in the future, so that we will be able to validate our model in this regard.

In order to make numeric simulations feasible, we considered a system with only 100 niches and 100 T-cell clones in the polyclonal situation. This is several orders of magnitude below the estimated TCR diversity in mice, and the estimated number of self-peptides that can be presented per allele [$\sim 10^5$ Ref. (13)]. However, there is significant cross-reactivity (i.e. presence of TCRs that may recognize more than one spMHC) in the T-cell system (29), so that the number of functionally relevant, distinct niches may be considerably lower. Being well aware of these simplifications, we consider the proposed system dimensions as sufficient in order to capture the general niche-based structure of the mature T-cell system.

Although we successfully demonstrated that suppression of preleukemic T cells due to TCR-related regulation in the polyclonal situation can consistently explain the experimental observations, we are aware that alternative explanations could also account for the observed phenomena. Definitive proof or disproof of the niche regulation hypothesis will require further experimental work.

Therefore, our conceptual understanding of T-cell oncogenesis will be challenged in further experiments. Specifically, we suggest to compare the phenotype of the leukemic/preleukemic cells with the phenotype of the healthy competitors regarding, e.g. their gene expression profile, their activation of relevant signaling pathways and their functional properties (30). This will allow assessing whether our assertions about the properties of the preleukemic cells (i.e. down-regulation of the TCR/TCR signaling and up-regulation of growth-promoting pathways) are correct. Our modeling results predict that there is a minimum clonal diversity that is needed in order to control preleukemic T cells as produced in the previous experiments. Further transplantation experiments are planned to determine the minimum TCR diversity in clonality titration experiments.

All simulations presented in this publication start with a hypocellular condition. However, additional simulations (data not shown) demonstrated that the model results are generally not dependent on the initial abundance of a species, as long as it is present at all. Therefore, our results apply also to leukemogenesis with physiological onset conditions as it occurs in clinical settings. The situation in which the malignancy develops from a single mutated cell (as can be expected for the majority of patients) corresponds to the presented scenario P1.

Central to this work is our assumption that the abundances of individual TCR-defined clones are regulated on a per-clone basis due to interactions with spMHCs. However, many aspects of the insinuated regulation are elusive to date. This is at least partially due to the fact that in the *in vivo* situation, accurate and precise time-dependent quantification of individual TCR-defined clones with abundances in the physiological range is technologically challenging, if not impossible, to date. Nonetheless, such a concept is intellectually appealing, and seems plausible on a mechanistic level. We hypothesize that this regulation is (at least in part) responsible for the relatively low incidence of mature T-cell malignancies relative to mature B-cell malignancies. This hypothesis would imply less effective control mechanisms in the mature B-cell system, which might be caused by the fact that clonal homeostasis in the mature B-cell system is presumably more complex than in the T-cell system, due to affinity maturation of the B-cell receptor, and ongoing influx of newly generated mature B-cell clones from the bone marrow. These complicating factors may undermine the effectiveness of the leukemia control mechanisms proposed for the mature T-cell system in the mature B-cell system.

So far in this publication, the unspecific affinities $u^{(h)}$ and $u^{(p)}$ are interpreted in terms of TCR affinity for the MHC molecule itself. However, these unspecific affinities could also represent the reliance of T-cell survival on survival cytokines, e.g. interleukin 7. Further studies could aim to disentangle these two potential components of the unspecific affinity. To do so, the use of mouse models with a restricted MHC repertoire might be useful.

As exemplified in this paper, mathematical modeling approaches allow for the quantitative assessment of functional principles of T-cell interactions, their integration into a consistent conceptual framework and the derivation of testable hypotheses. Our results add a new puzzle piece to the complex picture of mature T-cell homeostasis. The hypothesis that regulation based on TCR-defined clonal membership suppresses MTCLL emergence may serve as a novel starting point to delve deeper into the mechanisms governing the homeostatic behavior of mature T cells.

Our modeling results prompt further experimental research to clarify the nature of the differential transformability of mature T cells. Moreover, our work demonstrates the general ability of theoretical approaches to formalize and conceptually validate the results of experimental research and promotes the idea of an iterative, interdisciplinary approach to research in immunology.

5. AUTHORS CONTRIBUTION

Sebastian Gerdes performed mathematical modeling and wrote the paper, Sebastian Newrzela provided conceptual input and wrote the paper, Ingmar Glauche performed mathematical modeling and wrote the paper, Martin-Leo Hansmann provided conceptual input, Dorothee von Laer provided conceptual input, Ingo Roeder wrote the paper, provided conceptual input, and guided research.

ACKNOWLEDGMENTS

Ingo Roeder, Sebastian Newrzela, and Martin-Leo Hansmann are funded by the German Research Foundation (DFG) under RO3500/4-1, NE1438/4-1, and HA1284/8-1 as part of the collaborative research group on mature T-cell lymphomas, "CONTROL-T." Furthermore, Sebastian Gerdes and Ingo Roeder were funded by the DFG grant RO3500/1-2.

REFERENCES

1. Casrouge A, Beaudoing E, Dalle S, Pannetier C, Kanellopoulos J, Kourilsky P. Size estimate of the αßTCR repertoire of naive mouse splenocytes. *J Immunol* (2000) **164**(11):5782–7.
2. Naylor K, Li G, Vallejo AN, Lee W-W, Koetz K, Bryl E, et al. The influence of age on T cell generation and TCR diversity. *J Immunol* (2005) **174**(11):7446–52.
3. Jung D, Alt FW. Unraveling V(D)J recombination: insights into gene regulation. *Cell* (2004) **116**(2):299–311. doi:10.1016/S0092-8674(04)00039-X
4. Huesmann M, Scott B, Kisielow P, von Boehmer H. Kinetics and efficacy of positive selection in the thymus of normal and T cell receptor transgenic mice. *Cell* (1991) **66**(3):533–40. doi:10.1016/0092-8674(81)90016-7
5. Minter LM, Osborne BA. Cell death in the thymus – it' s all a matter of contacts. *Semin Immunol* (2003) **15**(3):135–44. doi:10.1016/S1044-5323(03)00029-0
6. Zal T, Volkmann A, Stockinger B. Mechanisms of tolerance induction in major histocompatibility complex class II-restricted T cells specific for a blood-borne self-antigen. *J Exp Med* (1994) **180**(6):2089–99. doi:10.1084/jem.180.6.2089
7. Freitas AA, Rocha B. Population biology of lymphocytes: the flight for survival. *Annu Rev Immunol* (2000) **18**(1):83–111. doi:10.1146/annurev.immunol.18.1.83
8. Singh NJ, Bando JK, Schwartz RH. Subsets of nonclonal neighboring CD4+ T cells specifically regulate the frequency of individual antigen-reactive T cells. *Immunity* (2012) **37**(4):735–46. doi:10.1016/j.immuni.2012.08.008
9. Brocker T. Survival of mature CD4 T lymphocytes is dependent on major histocompatibility complex class II-expressing dendritic cells. *J Exp Med* (1997) **186**(8):1223–32. doi:10.1084/jem.186.8.1223
10. Kirberg J, Berns A, von Boehmer H. Peripheral T cell survival requires continual ligation of the T cell receptor to major histocompatibility complex-encoded molecules. *J Exp Med* (1997) **186**(8):1269–75. doi:10.1084/jem.186.8.1269
11. Martin B, Bécourt C, Bienvenu B, Lucas B. Self-recognition is crucial for maintaining the peripheral CD4+ T-cell pool in a nonlymphopenic environment. *Blood* (2006) **108**(1):270–7. doi:10.1182/blood-2006-01-0017
12. Hataye J, Moon JJ, Khoruts A, Reilly C, Jenkins MK. Naive and memory CD4+ T cell survival controlled by clonal abundance. *Science* (2006) **312**(5770):114–6. doi:10.1126/science.1124228
13. Mahajan VS, Leskov IB, Chen JZ. Homeostasis of T cell diversity. *Cell Mol Immunol* (2005) **2**(1):1–10.
14. Morton LM, Wang SS, Devesa SS, Hartge P, Weisenburger DD, Linet MS. Lymphoma incidence patterns by WHO subtype in the United States, 1992-2001. *Blood* (2006) **107**(1):265–76. doi:10.1182/blood-2005-06-2508
15. Deeks S, Wagner B, Anton P, Mitsuyasu R, Scadden D, Haung C, et al. A phase II randomized study of HIV-specific T-cell gene therapy in subjects with undetectable plasma viremia on combination antiretroviral therapy. *Mol Ther* (2002) **5**(6):788–97. doi:10.1006/mthe.2002.0611
16. Recchia A, Bonini C, Magnani Z, Urbinati F, Sartori D, Muraro S, et al. Retroviral vector integration deregulates gene expression but has no consequence on the biology and function of transplanted T cells. *Proc Natl Acad Sci U S A* (2006) **103**(5):1457–62. doi:10.1073/pnas.0507496103
17. Scholler J, Brady TL, Binder-Scholl G, Hwang W-T, Plesa G, Hege KM, et al. Decade-long safety and function of retroviral-modified chimeric antigen receptor T cells. *Sci Transl Med* (2012) **4**(132):ra53–132. doi:10.1126/scitranslmed.3003761
18. Hacein-Bey-Abina S, Von Kalle C, Schmidt M, McCormack M, Wulffraat N, Leboulch P, et al. LMO2-associated clonal T cell proliferation in two patients after gene therapy for SCID-X1. *Science* (2003) **302**(5644):415–9. doi:10.1126/science.1088547
19. Ott M, Schmidt M, Schwarzwaelder K, Stein S, Siler U, Koehl U, et al. Correction of X-linked chronic granulomatous disease by gene therapy, augmented by insertional activation of MDS1-EVI1, PRDM16 or SETBP1. *Nat Med* (2006) **12**(4):401–9. doi:10.1038/nm1393
20. Newrzela S, Cornils K, Li Z, Baum C, Brugman MH, Hartmann M, et al. Resistance of mature T cells to oncogene transformation. *Blood* (2008) **112**(6):2278–86. doi:10.1182/blood-2007-12-128751
21. Newrzela S, Al-Ghaili N, Heinrich T, Petkova M, Hartmann S, Rengstl B, et al. T-cell receptor diversity prevents T-cell lymphoma development. *Leukemia* (2012) **26**(12):2499–507. doi:10.1038/leu.2012.142
22. De Boer RJ, Perelson AS. T cell repertoires and competitive exclusion. *J Theor Biol* (1994) **169**(4):375–90. doi:10.1006/jtbi.1994.1160
23. Doherty P, Riberdy J, Belz G. Quantitative analysis of the CD8+ T-cell response to readily eliminated and persistent viruses. *Philos Trans R Soc Lond B Biol Sci* (2000) **355**(1400):1093–101. doi:10.1098/rstb.2000.0647
24. De Boer RJ, Perelson AS, Ribeiro RM. Modelling deuterium labelling of lymphocytes with temporal and/or kinetic heterogeneity. *J R Soc Interface* (2012) **9**(74):2191–200. doi:10.1098/rsif.2012.0149
25. McKee MD, Roszkowski JJ, Nishimura MI. T cell avidity and tumor recognition: implications and therapeutic strategies. *J Transl Med* (2005) **3**(1):35. doi:10.1186/1479-5876-3-35
26. Rous P, Beard J. The progression to carcinoma of virus-induced rabbit papillomas (shope). *J Exp Med* (1935) **62**(4):523–48. doi:10.1084/jem.62.4.523
27. Baum C, von Kalle C, Staal FJ, Li Z, Fehse B, Schmidt M, et al. Chance or necessity? Insertional mutagenesis in gene therapy and its consequences. *Mol Ther* (2004) **9**(1):5–13. doi:10.1016/j.ymthe.2003.10.013
28. Fehse B, Roeder I. Insertional mutagenesis and clonal dominance: biological and statistical considerations. *Gene Ther* (2007) **15**(2):143–53. doi:10.1038/sj.gt.3303052
29. Yin Y, Mariuzza RA. The multiple mechanisms of T cell receptor cross-reactivity. *Immunity* (2009) **31**(6):849–51. doi:10.1016/j.immuni.2009.12.002
30. Wu S, Jin L, Vence L, Radvanyi LG. Development and application of phosphoflow as a tool for immunomonitoring. *Expert Rev Vaccines* (2010) **9**(6):631–43. doi:10.1586/erv.10.59

14

Autoimmunity as a double agent in tumor killing and cancer promotion

Kevin H. Toomer[1] and Zhibin Chen[1,2]*

[1] Department of Microbiology and Immunology, University of Miami Miller School of Medicine, Miami, FL, USA
[2] Sylvester Comprehensive Cancer Center, University of Miami Miller School of Medicine, Miami, FL, USA

Edited by:
Fang-Ping Huang, Imperial College London, UK

Reviewed by:
Amedeo Amedei, University of Florence, Italy
Carlos Alfaro, Clínica Universidad de Navarra, Spain

***Correspondence:**
Zhibin Chen, Department of Microbiology and Immunology, University of Miami Miller School of Medicine, RMSB 3035, 1600 NW 10th Avenue, Miami, FL 33136, USA
e-mail: zchen@med.miami.edu

Cancer immunotherapy through manipulation of the immune system holds great potential for the treatment of human cancers. However, recent trials targeting the negative immune regulators cytotoxic T-lymphocyte antigen 4, programed death 1 (PD-1), and PD-1 receptor ligand (PD-L1) demonstrated that clinically significant antitumor responses were often associated with the induction of autoimmune toxicity. This finding suggests that the same immune mechanisms that elicit autoimmunity may also contribute to the destruction of tumors. Given the fact that the immunological identity of tumors might be largely an immunoprivileged self, autoimmunity may not represent a wholly undesirable outcome in the context of cancer immunotherapy. Rather, targeted killing of cancer cells and autoimmune damage to healthy tissues may be intricately linked through molecular mechanisms, in particular inflammatory cytokine signaling. On the other hand, since chronic inflammation is a well-recognized condition that promotes tumor development, it appears that autoimmunity can be a "double agent" in mediating either pro-tumor or antitumor effects. This review surveys the tumor-promoting and tumoricidal activities of several prominent cytokines: IFN-γ, TNF-α, TGF-β, IL-17, IL-23, IL-4, and IL-13, produced by three major subsets of T helper cells that interact with innate immune cells. Many of these cytokines exert divergent and seemingly contradictory effects on cancer development in different human and animal models, suggesting a high degree of context dependence in their functions. We hypothesize that these inflammatory cytokines could mediate a feedback loop of autoimmunity, antitumor immunity, and tumorigenesis. Understanding the diverse and paradoxical roles of cytokines from autoimmune responses in the setting of cancer will advance the long-term goal of improving cancer immunotherapy, while minimizing the hazards of immune-mediated tissue damage and the possibility of *de novo* tumorigenesis, through proper monitoring and preventive measures.

Keywords: autoimmunity, antitumor, tumorigenesis, inflammation, cytokine

INTRODUCTION: PARADOXICAL RELATIONSHIPS BETWEEN AUTOIMMUNITY AND TUMOR

The process of inducing the immune system to selectively destroy tumor tissues *in vivo* faces numerous conceptual as well as practical hurdles. Foremost among these is the self-derived immunological identity of tumors (1, 2). The prevalence of self-antigen expression on cancer cells implies that many tumors will be protected from cytotoxic immune responses via intrinsic host mechanisms of self-tolerance. It is therefore evident that any biologic therapy capable of provoking a therapeutically useful antitumor immune response will carry some risk of off-target autoimmune toxicity. The resulting destruction of normal host tissues, besides contributing to morbidity and mortality in its own right, can potentially lead to *de novo* tumorigenesis by initiating chronic inflammation, which is a feature of premalignant states in numerous organs including breast, bladder, prostate, cervix, ovary, stomach, and lungs (3). The molecular sequence that links chronic inflammation to cancer development involves intricate and context-dependent interactions among differentiated tissue cells, immune cells, organ-specific stem cells, and other cell types present at the incipient tumor site (4). In light of these disparate outcomes, autoimmunity may be regarded as a "double agent" implicated in both immune-mediated tumor elimination and the cellular, genetic, and epigenetic changes that underlie carcinogenesis. Given the complexity and interconnections of the associated signaling networks, navigating this new therapeutic realm demands a formidable balancing act: any cancer treatment that seeks to modify immune system function must induce a degree of self-reactivity that leads to immune-mediated tumor killing while containing the destructive and cancer-promoting aspects of that self-reactivity within tolerable limits.

After decades of hard struggle in cancer immunotherapy, exciting opportunities have emerged, especially in monoclonal-antibody-based therapies designed to elicit antitumor immunity either through inhibition of negative immune system regulators or activation of costimulatory receptors (5). Remarkable benefits in patient survival have been demonstrated in clinical trials of novel monoclonal antibodies blocking immune checkpoints,

Table 1 | Anti- and pro-tumor activities of selected cytokines.

Cytokine	Antitumor activities	Pro-tumor activities
IFN-γ	Required for Th1 differentiation, effective cytotoxic antitumor immune responses, and transplanted tumor rejection induced by bacterial endotoxin (10); mediates immune surveillance against spontaneous tumor development (11); enhances tumor antigenicity by upregulating expression of antigen presentation machinery (12); has immunosuppressive functions that can restrain chronic inflammation in certain contexts (13, 14)	Mediates chronic inflammation in gastric epithelium (15, 16); protects tumor cells from CTL lysis by altering their surface MHC expression (17, 18)
TNF-α	Mediates transplanted tumor rejection induced by bacterial endotoxin (19); local administration damages tumor vasculature, and has been used in isolated limb perfusion to treat melanomas and soft tissue sarcomas (20)	Mediates chronic inflammation, oxidative stress, and genomic damage, promoting malignant transformation in various organs (21–23); activates growth and survival-promoting pathways that drive angiogenesis, proliferation, invasion, and metastasis in established tumors (24, 25)
TGF-β	Regulates the cell cycle and inhibits proliferation in stromal and epithelial tissues (26, 27); restrains chronic inflammation by opposing Th1 differentiation and downregulating IFN-γ production by NK cells and DCs (28–30)	Induces tolerant, cancer-promoting phenotypes in tumor-associated macrophages (M2) and neutrophils (31); promotes differentiation and recruitment of immunosuppressive Treg cells in the tumor microenvironment (32, 33); promotes angiogenesis, invasion, and metastasis of cancer cells (34); may suppress antitumor immunity by inhibiting Th1 signaling (35)
IL-17/IL-23	May promote IFN-γ secretion and Th1 differentiation (36, 37); possible mediator of innate and adaptive antitumor immunity through interactions with the Th1 signaling axis (38–41), or direct cytotoxicity of Th17 cells (42)	Mediates chronic inflammation in the liver (43–46); drives differentiation and expansion of Th17 cells in the tumor microenvironment, which has been shown to favor disease progression and suppress antitumor immunity (47, 48); activates proliferative and survival-promoting pathways in cancer cells (49–51)
IL-4/IL-13	Poorly characterized	Drives differentiation of tolerogenic CD4+ Th2 cells in the tumor microenvironment (52); induces cancer-promoting phenotypes in tumor-associated macrophages (M2) and DCs (31, 53); IL-4 mediates survival and proliferation of cancer stem cells (54–56); IL-13Rα2 signaling promotes tumor invasion and metastasis (57–59)

including cytotoxic T-lymphocyte antigen 4 (CTLA4) (6), programed death 1 (PD-1) (7), and PD-1 receptor ligand (PD-L1) (8). In practice, however, many biologic therapies have fallen short of expectations in clinical trials, failing to deliver enhancements in disease-free or overall patient survival (9). A partial explanation for this disappointment is the context-dependent nature of immune signaling pathways themselves. In many cases, a given signal can exert diverse, and often opposing, effects on the progression of cancer depending on a variety of factors including the tissues involved, expression level of the signal molecule(s), tumor stage and antigenic profile, and host genetic background. Thus, there is a remarkable degree of overlap between the signaling mechanisms that mediate the desired outcome of tumor destruction, and those which fuel the detrimental processes of cancer development, tumor progression, and autoimmunity. Many cytokines with therapeutic potential have demonstrated these paradoxical effects, revealing both tumoricidal and tumor-promoting activities under different experimental conditions. The task of eliciting potent cytotoxic immune responses, while managing the concomitant dangers of autoimmunity, therefore requires detailed mechanistic knowledge of immune system signaling. This review will summarize the current understanding of the pro- and antitumor activities of several major cytokines (**Table 1**): interferon-gamma (IFN-γ); tumor necrosis factor-alpha (TNF-α); transforming growth factor-beta (TGF-β); the Th17 cytokines IL-17 and IL-23; and the Th2 cytokines IL-4 and IL-13. Concluding remarks will address a hypothetical loop of autoimmunity-mediated antitumor immunity, leading to further induction of autoimmune responses, inflammatory cytokine signaling, and tumor promotion, including potential *de novo* tumorigenesis in solid organs such as the gastrointestinal tract with demonstrated susceptibility to inflammatory carcinogenesis.

ANTI- AND PRO-TUMOR ROLES OF AUTOIMMUNITY COULD BE MEDIATED THROUGH INFLAMMATORY CYTOKINES OF Th CELLS

The pathological correlation between inflammation and cancer has been known to clinical science for 150 years (60). However, it is only in recent times that our understanding of the immune system has become sophisticated enough to yield practical applications in the realm of cancer biology. For example, ample evidence has been gathered for the roles of inflammatory signals derived from innate immune response in promoting tumor growth and progression [for recent reviews, please see Ref. (4, 61, 62)]. There is emerging evidence for a tumor-promoting role by inflammatory effectors from the adaptive immune system, for example, in the TRAMP model of prostate cancer initiated with transgenic expression of an oncogene (the SV40 large T antigen) (63, 64), or implanted model of melanoma (65). Given the long-lasting nature of memory responses that is characteristic of adaptive immunity and the potency of autoimmune memory T cells [for review see Ref. (66)], one might speculate that inflammatory signals originated from the adaptive immune system, compared to their innate-derived counterparts, might sustain a longer effect, regardless of their pro- or antitumor nature. However, we should also emphasize that in a complex *in vivo* setting of immune responses, it is likely that the intimate interaction between innate and adaptive immune cells determines an immunological outcome (67–69). Nevertheless, definitive evidence remains to be gathered to show whether an inflammatory signal(s), at a physiologically relevant setting, can initiate *de novo* tumorigenesis.

Numerous parameters of immune system function have been correlated with clinical outcomes in cancer patients, including the cellular composition of tumor inflammatory infiltrate (70), expression of pro- and anti-apoptotic genes in circulating PBMCs (71), and cytokine profiles measured in peripheral blood (72). It has long been recognized that the same inflammatory cytokine may play a prominent role in either tumor killing or cancer promotion. Although the original stimuli of inflammatory cytokine production are unknown in most cancer settings, given the largely "self" constituents of tumors, we reasoned that autoimmune T cells, especially the three main T helper subsets, Th1, Th2, and Th17, could be a major source of these cytokines, or play a major role in driving other immune cells to produce them.

Early experimental models offered hope that the induction of selective antitumor immune responses, even those mediated by CTL recognition of self-antigens, was possible without clinically significant autoimmunity. One study reported the eradication of established p53-overexpressing tumor cells in mice, achieved through adoptive transfer of a clone of cytotoxic T cells, which recognized wild-type p53. No autoimmune damage was observed in normal tissues, despite the p53+/+ genotype of the treated mice (73). *In vitro* assays also suggested that epitope-specific CTL clones had the capacity to initiate cytotoxic immune responses against non-mutated, tumor-associated p53, while simultaneously avoiding reactivity with the same antigen when endogenously expressed (74). Other experiments used transgenic models to search for evidence of autoimmune pathology in an organ-specific fashion. In one study, transgenic mice were engineered to express low levels of Friend murine leukemia virus envelope protein (FMuLV) from an immunoglobulin promoter; adoptive transfer of FMuLV-specific T cells mediated complete destruction of leukemia tumor cells, without concurrent autoimmunity. Lymphoid tissues in the treated mice were unharmed, despite the fact that they expressed the targeted cancer-associated antigen in a "self" context (75). Another study employed transgenic mice with tissue-specific expression of influenza virus hemagglutinin (HA) in pancreatic islet β cells. Administration of an anti-HA vaccine to these animals produced CTL-mediated rejection of renal carcinoma cells, which had also been genetically engineered to express HA. Prior to vaccination, the immune systems of the transgenic mice exhibited HA self-tolerance, and supported growth of implanted tumors expressing this antigen. Remarkably, in addition to tumor rejection, immunohistologic analysis of treated mice showed intact structure and function in the pancreatic islets (76).

Despite these favorable preclinical results, most types of cancer immunotherapy tested in human patients have revealed serious and persistent risks of treatment-associated autoimmunity. Reported manifestations include vitiligo, uveitis, psoriasis, and colitis, with potential consequences ranging from cosmetic complaints to permanent disability and death (77). However, it has been suggested that autoimmunity, in addition to mediating these adverse events, makes an essential contribution to antitumor immunity. Indeed, it may be the case that effective cancer immunotherapy requires a significant degree of self-reactivity, since antitumor immune responses must surmount both the preexisting tolerance to self-derived tumor antigens and immunosuppressive signals from the tumor microenvironment (1, 77). For some cancer immunotherapies, such as blockade of the inhibitory T cell signaling molecule CTLA4, autoimmune toxicity shows a positive correlation with therapeutic response (78). Meanwhile, antitumor vaccines, probably the category of cancer immunotherapy least associated with severe autoimmunity in human studies (77), have generally failed to show therapeutic efficacy in large-scale Phase 3 trials (79). Thus, it appears that the future of cancer immunotherapy will not feature the elimination of autoimmunity, which is unlikely to be feasible or wholly desirable. Rather, the cytokines that mediate autoinflammation can be harnessed as effective agents in tumor destruction, if their toxic and tumor-promoting potentials are understood and judiciously managed.

IFN-γ

Interferons (IFNs) are a family of cytokines that bind to cell-surface receptors and mediate numerous functions related to pathogen defenses, immune function, cell survival and differentiation, and angiogenesis (12, 80). Type I interferons are broadly expressed (80), while IFN-γ, the sole member of the Type II interferon family, is produced mainly by T lymphocytes, NKT cells, and natural killer (NK) cells as a crucial component of the inflammatory response (10). IFN-γ is integral to the development of Th1 adaptive immunity, by maintaining IL-12 signaling in $CD4^+$ T lymphocytes while simultaneously suppressing Th2 differentiation (10). Murine models support a range of anti-carcinogenic properties for IFN-γ (11). Antibody-mediated suppression of IFN-γ signaling has revealed that this cytokine is required for LPS-stimulated rejection of transplantable tumors in mice. IFN-γ receptor knockout mice (IFN-$\gamma R1^{-/-}$) exhibit susceptibility to both spontaneous and chemically induced tumors, in addition to poor resistance to a variety of pathogens (10, 11). IFN-γ is a powerful inducer of Class I and Class II antigen presentation machinery, suggesting its primary importance in the production of specific antitumor immune responses (12). *In vitro* assays have also revealed pro-apoptotic, antiangiogenic, and antiproliferative effects (10–12, 81). Indeed, reduced IFN-γ production has been observed in a variety of human malignancies, including melanoma, gastric cancer, lung cancer, glioblastoma, nasopharyngeal carcinoma, colorectal cancer, and head and neck cancer (72).

Certain human cancers, notably melanoma, are known to develop resistance to IFN-γ through various mutations in downstream molecules in the IFN signal transduction pathway, such as JAK and STAT1 (12, 81).

Despite this promising body of experimental evidence, anticancer therapy with exogenous IFN-γ has generated mixed results. A 2003 clinical trial in malignant melanoma patients showed no positive responses to intratumoral injections of IFN-γ (82). A Phase 3 trial for ovarian cancer and peritoneal carcinoma was prematurely ended in 2006, due to decreased survival and more frequent adverse events in patients treated with subcutaneous IFN-γ, as compared to conventional platinum-based chemotherapy (82). To understand why this cytokine has not demonstrated the broad therapeutic efficacy that prior data would suggest, it is necessary to examine the dual nature of the inflammatory process. While inflammation can promote the cell-mediated destruction of tumor cells, its chronic forms may lead to pathological changes that promote cancer development in a variety of tissues. These changes include accumulation of reactive oxygen species, epithelial hyperplasia, extracellular matrix generation, and angiogenesis (3, 83, 84). Besides mediating anticancer immunity, IFN-γ is a major player in chronic inflammation, as illustrated by its contributions to Th1-driven autoimmune disease. In clinical trials, anti-IFN-γ antibodies have been useful in treating a variety of inflammatory disorders, including rheumatoid arthritis, Crohn's disease, corneal transplant rejection, and skin diseases such as vitiligo and alopecia areata (82, 85, 86).

The interplay between IFN-γ signaling, aberrant chronic inflammation, and neoplastic disease has been explored in the pathogenesis of gastric cancer, one of the classic models of human malignancy precipitated by chronic inflammation (87–90). With regard to gastric carcinogenesis, the role of Th subsets would also perhaps be best surveyed while keeping in mind the robust evidence of innate immunity in gastric cancer development (91–93). In the natural course of this disease, infection with the bacterium *Helicobacter pylori* during childhood precipitates a chronic inflammatory response which, in a small portion of patients (<5%), progresses to malignancy decades in the future (84, 94). Studies of mice infected with the related pathogen *Helicobacter felis* showed that a Th1-biased inflammatory response is involved in gastric cancer development (94). Knockout of the transcription factor T-bet, which controls commitment to the Th1 lineage (95), curtailed gastric tumorigenesis induced in mice infected with *H. felis* (15). A recent experiment employed a murine model that directly implicates IFN-γ in this course of preneoplastic change. The transgenic mice, which were engineered to overexpress IFN-γ from a stomach-specific, H/K ATPase β promoter, exhibited a prominent inflammatory infiltrate along with accelerated histological changes characteristic of a premalignant phenotype: metaplasia, loss of parietal and chief cells, gastric gland atrophy, and dysplasia beginning as early as 3 months of age (16).

IFN-γ can thus be seen as an essential mediator of both immune-mediated tumor rejection and the destructive chronic inflammation that precedes malignant transformation. There is, however, another vital dimension to this cytokine's effects, that of a master regulator which restrains inflammation in a variety of contexts. In two key murine model systems of Th1-driven autoimmunity, collagen-induced arthritis (CIA) and experimental autoimmune encephalitis (EAE), it has been established that abrogation of IFN-γ signaling through monoclonal antibody therapy or genetic knockout produces a seemingly paradoxical increase in disease susceptibility and severity (13, 14). The mechanisms for this apparent downregulation of the inflammatory response are not yet clear, but suppression of pro-inflammatory Th17 cytokines, induction of T cell apoptosis, and enhanced Treg cell differentiation appear to play prominent roles (13, 14, 96). Another mechanism of IFN-γ mediated immunosuppression is suggested by its ability to alter tumor cell MHC presentation in a manner that *decreases* tumor antigenicity and protects tumor cells from CTL killing. One *in vitro* experiment demonstrated that IFN-γ could protect ovarian carcinoma cell lines from CTL-mediated lysis by upregulating HLA-E on cancer cells, which engaged the inhibitory CD94/NKG2A receptor on $CD8^+$ effector T cells (18). A similar cancer-promoting role for IFN-γ was revealed in a mouse model of melanoma, where tumor protection from CTL killing was associated with IFN-γ-stimulated upregulation of non-cognate MHC-I molecules (17).

Given the evidence above, IFN-γ-mediated downregulation of the inflammatory response can be regarded as an obstacle to effective cancer immunotherapy. However, it remains an important physiological mechanism for preserving tolerance to self-antigens and protecting tissues from the damaging effects of autoimmunity (80, 97). In keeping with this fact, experimental data also suggest that IFN-γ mediated suppression of inflammation may be protective in certain contexts. One recent experiment employed a transgenic mouse line engineered to overexpress IFN-γ in a stomach-specific manner, using the same H/K ATPase β promoter as Syu et al. (16). In this case, however, no spontaneous gastritis or metaplasia occurred (98). Moreover, IFN-γ was reported to be protective against gastric dysplasia produced by either *H. felis* infection or stomach-specific overexpression of the cytokine IL-1β (a well established mediator of gastric carcinogenesis). IFN-γ was also shown to inhibit proliferation of gastric epithelial cells, enhance autophagy in a manner recognized as protective against tumor development (99), and diminish expression of pro-inflammatory Th1 and Th17 cytokines (98). As noted by Syu et al. (16), the seemingly contradictory results of these two studies can most likely be explained by differing degrees of overexpression. These findings underscore the challenges of discerning which aspect of IFN-γ will prevail in a particular patient, tumor type, and stage of malignancy. Attempts to broaden the therapeutic use of this cytokine must take into account these intricate and context-dependent multidirectional effects.

TNF-α

Activated macrophages and T lymphocytes produce TNF-α in response to pro-inflammatory stimuli. This cytokine stimulates inflammation through multiple mechanisms, including recruitment of neutrophils and monocytes and induction of cell adhesion molecule expression on the endothelial surface (72, 100). TNF-α is involved in the classical pathway of macrophage activation (M1), which plays a central role in immune defenses against tumors and intracellular parasites (31). Although usually undetectable in the tissues and circulation of healthy people, TNF-α exerts important effects on immune homeostasis during states of disease. It is known, for instance, that systemic TNF-α mediates the wasting observed in humans and animals afflicted with chronic illness (24, 100, 101). As with IFN-γ, aberrant TNF-α signaling is associated with a variety of autoimmune disorders. Five TNF inhibitors have been approved for clinical use in the United States for the treatment of inflammatory illnesses such as Crohn's disease, ankylosing spondylitis, and rheumatoid arthritis (100, 102).

The observation that the human body's response to infection is capable of producing regression of tumors has been recorded by clinicians since at least the eighteenth century (103). It was not until 1975, however, that TNF-α was identified as one of the principal mediators of this anticancer immune response. The name "tumor necrosis factor" reflects early experiments, which demonstrated this cytokine's capacity to induce hemorrhagic necrosis of subcutaneously transplanted sarcomas, leukemias, and mastocytomas in mice whose immune systems were primed by exposure to bacterial endotoxin (19). However, 38 years of data subsequent to this discovery have not fulfilled the early promise of TNF-α as a safe, potent, or selective tumoricidal agent. Unlike mice with abrogated IFN-γ signaling, TNF-α-knockout animals do not develop spontaneous tumors, and peritoneal tumors transplanted into them do not show accelerated growth (104). These knockout animals have also shown an unexpected resistance to chemically induced skin tumors (105). Indeed, there seem to be numerous contexts in which TNF-α signaling helps to initiate carcinogenesis and sustain tumor growth. In obese patients, TNF-α is suggested to be a key mediator of cancer-promoting inflammation in various organs, including the pancreas (22), colon (21), and liver (23). Picogram amounts of TNF-α are constitutively secreted by many tumor types, and appear to stimulate cancer growth, although the underlying signaling mechanisms are not completely understood (24, 106). The pro-carcinogenic functions of TNF-α appear to be mediated predominantly through downstream activation of the proliferative and survival-promoting pathways NF-κB and AP-1 (20, 21, 100, 104). Elevated serum concentrations of TNF-α have been described as a clinical feature of eight independent cancer types (72). A direct link between the pro-inflammatory effects of TNF-α and carcinogenesis can be seen by returning to the example of gastric cancer. The presence of a specific, inflammation-associated single nucleotide polymorphism in the *TNF-A* gene has been found to increase the odds ratio of non-cardia gastric cancer (83). The importance of this association has been further established by examining the genome of the initiating pathogen: *H. pylori* harbors the Tipα gene family, whose members are known to induce high levels of TNF-α expression in the gastric epithelium (24, 106). Experimental transfection of a transformed BALB/3T3 cell line with *H. pylori* genes revealed that tumor progression was dependent on Tipα-induced production of TNF-α (106).

TNF-α has also been implicated as a disease promoter in hepatocellular carcinoma (HCC), from chronic inflammation to tumor progression including invasion, metastasis, and angiogenesis in established HCC tumors (107). *In vitro* studies of numerous cell types, including murine hepatocytes, have demonstrated that TNF-α-mediated inflammation leads to an increase in markers of oxidative stress, which in turn can lead to genomic damage (108–111). Moreover, the development of obesity-induced hepatosteatosis and steatohepatitis in mice is dependent on signaling by TNF-α, along with IL-6 (21). In the Mdr2-knockout mouse, an experimental model of inflammation-induced HCC, the spontaneous development of hepatic malignancy is dependent on TNF signaling, and can be attenuated through downstream inhibition of NF-κB (23). Overall, experiments on HCC and many other tumor types have established that TNF-α is intimately involved in all aspects of cancer development, including transformation, proliferation, angiogenesis, invasion, and metastasis (25).

Owing to a high frequency of inflammation-related adverse events, the therapeutic applications of exogenous TNF-α in cancer have been quite limited (24). Localized TNF-α infusion has demonstrated antitumor efficacy against melanomas and soft tissue sarcomas in human patients. In this context, high concentrations of TNF-α were shown to induce hyperpermeability and structural disruption in tumor vasculature, thus promoting tumor necrosis and enhancing the efficacy of traditional cytostatic drugs. However, this intervention was aimed at limb sparing and had no impact on patient survival (20). Given the broad range of cancer-promoting activities of TNF-α, blockade of its signaling remains a tempting therapeutic approach. Unfortunately, the fundamental role of TNF-α in pathogen defense represents a formidable obstacle to implementation (24). The feasibility of modifying TNF-α signaling without triggering destructive autoimmunity on one hand, or vulnerability to opportunistic infections on the other, remains to be seen.

TGF-β

Transforming growth factor-beta mediates a vast array of functions related to wound healing, immune responses, cell proliferation and differentiation, and carcinogenesis, via receptors expressed on nearly all human cells. It plays a crucial role in T cell tolerance (112). Its classical signal transducers are transcription factors known as Smads, which combine with each other as well as additional cofactors to form a variety of DNA-binding complexes. These intricate assemblies of transcriptional regulators allow TGF-β to implement a versatile, yet precisely controlled, range of downstream effects. Additional "Smad-independent" signaling pathways are known to further augment this functional repertoire (27, 29, 34, 35). This cytokine has been extensively characterized as a negative regulator of immune responses, with anti-inflammatory, antiproliferative, and immunosuppressive activities (27, 29, 34, 35). Thus, TGF-β helps restrain the destructive effects of uncontrolled inflammation and proliferation that might otherwise occur in the context of infection or tissue damage. Mouse models reveal that knockout of TGF-β or its receptor produces a phenotype characterized by lethal autoimmune disease (113, 114). One recent study featured a murine model with the TGF-β receptor gene deleted in stromal fibroblasts. The transgenic animals experienced an excessive, aberrant inflammatory response in adjacent epithelial tissue, characterized by molecular markers of DNA damage, oxidative stress, cell cycle dysregulation, and death from invasive squamous cell carcinoma by the age of 7 weeks (26). Other models have examined the specific effects of TGF-β silencing in the innate immune and T cell compartments. One experiment blockaded TGF-β signaling in mouse NK cells through transgenic expression of a dominant negative receptor. NK cells were more numerous in lymphatic tissues of the transgenic mice, and showed enhanced secretion of IFN-γ. Consistent with the Th1-promoting effects of IFN-γ signaling, transgenic mice also demonstrated an enhanced Th1 inflammatory response, which protected against infection with cutaneous Leishmaniasis (28). These effects suggest the importance of TGF-β in maintaining NK cell homeostasis, as well as downregulating Th1 differentiation. Another study reported a dendritic cell-specific deletion of the TGF-β receptor gene, which resulted in multiorgan autoimmunity, a pro-inflammatory DC phenotype characterized by IFN-γ overproduction, and reduced Foxp3 expression in Treg cells (30). Accumulating evidence suggests that TGF-β is directly involved in many aspects of T cell homeostasis, including differentiation of Treg cells and $CD8^+$ effectors, maintenance of peripheral tolerance, and preservation of naïve T cell populations (112). The precise molecular mechanisms behind these effects are largely unresolved, and represent an area of active investigation.

In the early stages of carcinogenesis, TGF-β is known to suppress tumor growth through induction of cell cycle inhibitors and promotion of apoptosis. However, in many advanced cancers, paracrine and autocrine TGF-β signaling drives tumor progression and metastasis. TGF-β is produced in large quantities by a variety of human cancers, to the extent that it is arguably the most ubiquitous immunosuppressive mediator in cancer progression (34). Elevated systemic levels of TGF-β have been reported in breast cancer, lung cancer, pancreatic cancer, glioblastoma multiforme, colorectal carcinoma, HCC, renal cell carcinoma, and gastric carcinoma (72). TGF-β is a crucial inducer of pro-tumor phenotypes in both tumor-associated macrophages (TAMs) and tumor-associated neutrophils (TANs), leading to cancer cell proliferation and the curtailing of antitumor immune responses (31). The capacity of TGF-β to promote the differentiation of Treg cells appears to be highly deleterious in this context, since Treg cells are key inducers of immune tolerance in the tumor microenvironment. The association between TGF-β signaling and Treg cell recruitment has been experimentally demonstrated in a lung cancer cell line (115), as well as in animal models of pancreatic cancer (32) and HCC (33). One key observation from these studies is that a tolerogenic immune microenvironment is not exclusively the result of tumor-secreted cytokines. Rather, it requires elaboration of TGF-β and other anti-inflammatory signals from immune cell populations such as dendritic cells and TAMs.

Several other mechanisms are believed to underlie the procarcinogenic role of TGF-β, including enhanced extracellular matrix formation, cytoskeletal rearrangements to facilitate epithelial-to-mesenchymal transition (EMT), angiogenesis, and cell cycle dysregulation (27, 29, 34, 35). In a clinical context, TGF-β serves as a marker of metastasis and poor prognosis for many malignancies (35, 72). The transition of TGF-β from a protective role early in tumor development to a tumor-promoting one in more advanced disease appears to be a watershed moment in many cancers, reflecting global derangement of signal transduction through genetic and epigenetic mechanisms. Indeed, *in vitro* experiments have linked specific forms of oncogenic transformation to alterations in TGF-β responsiveness. One study found that engineered overexpression of HER2 in mesenchymal human breast cancer cells caused a loss of sensitivity to the antiproliferative effects of TGF-β (116). Another reported that loss of TGF-β growth inhibition correlated with the loss of c-myc downregulation in ovarian carcinoma cells (117).

The prevalence of TGF-β overexpression across a broad range of human malignancies has made this cytokine a tantalizing therapeutic target. Four classes of TGF-β inhibiting molecules have already been tested in clinical trials, with responses that generally fell short of hopes (118). At least one class of TGF-β inhibitor has also shown the capacity to elicit biochemical resistance in mouse models (119). This observation, coupled with the integral roles of TGF-β in wound healing and tissue homeostasis, suggests that long-term inhibition of TGF-β signaling may be a dangerous prospect. Rather, it has been suggested that TGF-β inhibition will find its first clinical applications as part of a combined drug regimen, administered to cancer patients over relatively brief spans of time to minimize resistance and adverse events (118).

IL-17 AND IL-23

The Th17 subset of $CD4^+$ T cells has added a new dimension of complexity to the Th1/Th2 paradigm since its initial discovery in 2005. Extensive studies in murine models have implicated this T cell population in a number of pro-inflammatory functions, including the pathogenesis of autoimmune diseases of the brain (EAE) and joints (CIA), mediated by the characteristic cytokine IL-17 (36, 120–122). Knockout mice have also revealed an important role for IL-17 signaling in the defense of mucosal surfaces against a variety of bacterial and fungal pathogens, including *Staphylococcus aureus*, *Klebsiella pneumoniae*, *Citrobacter rodentium*, and *Candida albicans* (36, 120). Th17 cells also engage in physiologically important interactions with key cytokines of the Th1 immune system. One attribute, noted in the initial characterization of this helper T cell subset, is the inhibitory effect of IFN-γ on Th17 differentiation and production of IL-17 (123, 124). Meanwhile, IL-23, a cytokine that is essential to sustain the survival and proliferation of Th17 populations, appears to participate in divergent regulatory pathways with the Th1-associated cytokine IL-12, whose release is promoted by IFN-γ (125–127). The dichotomous signaling of IL-12/IL-23 is especially intriguing, as these two cytokines share a common subunit: IL-12 is formed through the covalent linkage of p40 and p35 subunits, whereas IL-23 is a combination of p40 and p19 (128). TGF-β signaling also appears to make a major contribution to Th17 differentiation, although the precise nature and mechanism of this association remains a subject of intense controversy (122, 129).

Th17 signaling through the canonical IL-23/IL-17 pathway has been shown to contribute to cancer development in a variety of experimental contexts. During the preneoplastic stage, excessive Th17-mediated signaling is a probable contributor to the chronic inflammation that can precipitate cancer in a variety of tissues. In the case of Hepatitis B-induced inflammation, evidence from human and animal experiments suggests that Th17, not Th1, signaling is the primary mechanism underlying liver immunopathology and eventual malignant transformation to HCC (43–46). Th17 cells have been discovered in human tumors in many different organs, and a growing body of evidence suggests that their presence, like that of immunosuppressive Treg cells, may be a general feature of the tumor microenvironment (37, 121). One comprehensive examination of gene expression profiles in human cancers revealed overexpression of IL-23 in the vast majority of human carcinomas, when compared to expression profiles of adjacent, non-cancerous tissue (130). A recent quantitative PCR analysis revealed statistically significant IL-23 upregulation across a panel of non-small cell lung carcinoma (NSCLC) patient samples, in comparison to matched normal tissue controls (49). In mouse models, knockout of IL-23 conferred resistance to both chemically induced and transplanted epithelial tumors, whereas knockout of IL-12 produced the opposite effects (130). Moreover, there is mounting evidence that tumor cells produce chemokines in order to selectively recruit Th17 lymphocytes (121). In the 4T1 mouse model of breast cancer, Qian et al. reported that signaling via mammary tumor-derived prostaglandin E_2 (PGE_2) caused overexpression of IL-23 (but not IL-12) in the tumor microenvironment (48). This overexpression, in turn, was associated with expansion of Th17 cell populations in the tumor tissue, spleens, and peripheral blood of experimental animals (48). This discovery is likely to have significant implications in a variety of human cancers, since PGE_2 is the most abundant prostanoid in epithelial cell tumors (127). In the same study, exposure of murine dendritic cells to tumor-conditioned medium enhanced their expression of the IL-23 subunit p19, and also reduced expression of p40 and the IL-12 subunit p35, in a dose-dependent manner (48). These changes collectively indicate a shift from Th1 to Th17 immune phenotype, which seems to be favorable for cancer persistence. As in the case of experimental models of TGF-β signaling, cells of the innate immune system were key participants in the generation of an immune microenvironment promoting carcinogenesis.

The pathways through which Th17 signaling exerts its tumor-promoting effects are not yet clear, but a variety of relevant observations have emerged. One probable mechanism is the stimulation of angiogenesis and cell proliferation: the p19 subunit of IL-23 is transcriptionally upregulated by growth-promoting signals from NF-κB and AP-1 (48). Administration of recombinant IL-23 has been shown to enhance proliferation in an IL-23 receptor-positive lung adenocarcinoma cell line (49, 51). One study reported IL-23-mediated enhancement of cancer growth and proliferation in cultures of human oral squamous cell carcinoma; in this case, IL-23 exposure was accompanied by enhanced nuclear translocation of NF-κB (50). Mouse models have also furnished valuable mechanistic clues. In one experiment, IL-17 knockout mice showed reduced growth of transplanted B16 melanoma and MB49 bladder carcinoma, whereas acceleration of tumor growth occurred with knockout of IFN-γ. In mice with both knockouts, tumor growth was reduced relative to WT controls (65). In the IFN-γ knockout mice, elevated concentrations of IL-17 were measured in tumor tissue compared to tumors in wild-type controls. Moreover, IL-17 was found to enhance signaling by the pro-survival, pro-angiogenic transcription factor Stat3 in both tumor and stromal cells (65). Another study reported similar results using receptor knockouts: IL-17 receptor-deficient mice showed diminished tumor growth of transplanted melanoma and lymphoma cell lines, while IFN-γ receptor knockout led to growth enhancement. The double-knockout genotype was also protective in comparison to WT controls (47). In addition, IL-17 receptor deficiency was correlated with increased tumor infiltration of $CD8^+$ effector T cells, and decreased numbers of myeloid-derived suppressor cells (MDSCs), both favorable indications for the generation of antitumor immunity (47). Interestingly, these pro- and antitumor effects were successfully reproduced in wild-type mice through administration of either recombinant IL-17 (which accelerated tumor growth) or antibody-mediated IL-17 blockade (which suppressed it), hinting at the viability of anticancer therapies targeting this pathway (47). It is also notable that elimination of IL-17 signaling in both studies produced an antitumor effect that was potent enough to compensate for the concurrent loss of IFN-γ signaling, despite the role of IFN-γ as a potent mediator of Th1-driven antitumor immunity.

The complex and heterogeneous functions of the Th17 signaling axis, and their relationships to cancer progression, are only beginning to be elucidated. Despite the results mentioned above, numerous studies support the existence of antitumor Th17 effects, including those which may be mediated through signals other than IL-17 and IL-23 (121). For instance, subsets of Th17 cells are capable of producing IFN-γ, indicating possible cross-talk with the Th1 pathway of differentiation, as well as the ability to stimulate cytotoxic and tumoricidal immune responses (36, 37). In human pancreatic ductal adenocarcinomas, one recent study found correlation of protective benefit with activity of Th17 cells specific to α-enolase, a pancreatic tumor-associated antigen (42). Another recent study reported that a mouse model deficient in RORγt (a transcription factor required for Th17 differentiation) exhibited accelerated growth of transplanted melanoma tumors, along with a diminished percentage of Th1 $CD4^+$ cells at the tumor site; this phenotype was rescued by adoptive transfer of Th17 cells, a portion of which began to produce measurable quantities of IFN-γ (41). One study of IL-17 knockout mice demonstrated increased susceptibility to lung melanoma. Subsequent treatment by Th17 adoptive transfer served to prevent tumor development by inducing a specific $CD8^+$ antitumor response (40). It has also been found that systemic administration of high-dose IL-23 led to reduced tumor growth and prolonged survival in a mouse fibrosarcoma, due to Th1-mediated activation of cytotoxic T cells, helper T cells, and NK cells (38). Increased growth and lung metastasis of murine colon carcinoma has also been reported in IL-17 deficient animals, with corresponding reductions in IFN-γ^+ NK cells and IFN-γ^+ tumor-specific T cells (39).

Although characterized less than a decade ago, the Th17 lymphocyte population has already become the focus of a vast and diverse body of scientific literature. However, this expanded knowledge contains apparent contradictions, which will challenge the field of cancer immunology for years to come. As with the pathways and cytokines previously discussed, the tumor-related effects of IL-17 and IL-23 exhibit a high degree of context dependence. Some of these discordant results may therefore be attributable to the source of tumor cells, the tissue involved, the stage of cancer growth, the genetic background of the organism, and other features of the experimental model employed in a particular study. Meanwhile, our understanding of Th17 interactions with other elements of the immune system, including NK cells, antigen-presenting cells and other helper T cell subsets, remains incomplete. Experiments designed to address the cross-talk between Th17 cytokines and other branches of the immune system should help resolve some of the inconsistencies in their reported effects. While a variety of IL-17/IL-23 antagonists are currently being developed for the treatment of autoimmune diseases (131), safe and effective modification of Th17 signaling in cancer therapy will require a more thorough understanding of the forces which underlie Th17 differentiation, recruitment, and interaction with malignant cells.

IL-4 AND IL-13

The Th2 subset of $CD4^+$ T cells plays an important physiological role in implementing immune defenses against helminths and other extracellular parasites. Th2-mediated responses include generation of high-affinity IgE antibodies, mucus overproduction, and heightened smooth muscle contractility, all of which function in the clearance of invasive multicellular organisms. However, aberrant and excessive Th2 activation also provides the foundations for allergic disease (132). The major cytokine responsible for differentiation of naïve $CD4^+$ T cells into the Th2 phenotype is IL-4, while Th2 effector functions are mediated through a combination of IL-4, IL-13, and IL-5 (133). All three of these cytokines exert varied effects on cancer development, which remain an area of ongoing investigation. Th2 cytokines appear to be involved in shifting the immune response to forms favorable to tumor growth, particularly in the context of innate immunity. IL-4, IL-13, and IL-5 promote the differentiation of macrophages into an "M2" or alternatively activated form, which displays poor antigen-presenting capacity and local anti-inflammatory effects (31, 83, 134). M2 macrophages play a variety of physiological roles in tissue homeostasis, including wound healing, extracellular matrix remodeling, and scavenging of debris (132, 134). This M2 phenotype contrasts with the classically activated (M1) macrophage, which is specialized for the production of pro-inflammatory cytokines (e.g., IFN-γ), cytotoxic immune responses, and efficient destruction of phagocytosed microbes (132, 134). In the context of cancer, M2 polarization of TAMs is associated with suppression of antitumor immune responses, disease progression, and poor prognosis (31, 83). Moreover, it has been established that tumors are capable of producing Th2 cytokines in order to bias innate and adaptive immune responses toward this more favorable phenotype (134). A study of pancreatic cancer patients demonstrated that tumor-produced cytokines (TNF and IL-1β) triggered activation of a Th2 phenotype in cancer-associated fibroblasts, dendritic cells, and naïve $CD4^+$ T cells. Moreover, the ratio of Th2:Th1 $CD4^+$ T lymphocytes present at the tumor site was negatively correlated with patient survival (52). In a humanized mouse model implanted with human breast carcinoma, Th2 cytokine expression was detected in both cancer cells and tumor-promoting $CD4^+$ T cells within the tumor microenvironment. Dendritic cells isolated from these tumors also potently induced Th2 cytokine secretion from naïve $CD4^+$ T cells *in vitro*, suggesting that tumor growth is facilitated by a complex network of Th2 paracrine signals (53).

The Th2 cytokine IL-4 is capable of signaling through two distinct cell-surface receptor complexes. The Type I receptor, found on cells of hematopoietic stem cell origin, is composed of IL-4Rα and the common gamma chain γc. The Type II receptor, expressed on cells of non-hematopoietic origin, contains IL-4Rα and IL-13Rα1, and also binds the cytokine IL-13 (135). IL-13Rα2 is a second type of IL-13 binding receptor, whose physiological role remains uncertain. The receptor bears structural similarities to IL-13Rα1, but is expressed in two forms: as soluble IL-13Rα2, and as a transmembrane protein, which interacts with a number of signal transduction pathways (54). IL-4 and IL-13 exert both overlapping and distinct physiological effects by binding these receptors, whose structure and function have been extensively studied as potential therapeutic targets in asthma and other allergic diseases (135, 136). Emerging evidence indicates that these receptors can influence cancer development through pathways other than macrophage polarization, although the molecular details of this process are only starting to become clear.

The Type II IL-4/IL-13 receptor has been found to be overexpressed in a variety of epithelial tumors, and treatment of cancer cell lines with IL-4 is associated with pro-proliferative and anti-apoptotic effects (54, 137). The effects of IL-4 signaling have been studied extensively in the development of colon cancer: one study found pro-proliferative effects of IL-4Rα signaling in mouse colon tumors, as well as human and mouse colon adenocarcinoma cell lines examined *in vitro* (55). Of particular interest is the relationship between intestinal malignancies and multipotent stem cells, which have been identified in recent experiments as an integral driving force in the growth of both premalignant adenomas and established tumors (138, 139). It now appears that IL-4 signaling is vital to the functioning of at least some of these tumorigenic stem cells. Research on colon cancer has identified a subset of tumor cells with a $CD133^+$ stem-like phenotype, which was found to be necessary and sufficient for the establishment of transplanted human colon tumors in immunodeficient mice (56). In keeping with the cancer stem cell (CSC) hypothesis (4), these cells possess self-renewing capacity, an especially high resistance to death-promoting signals, and the ability to effect regeneration of the overall tumor mass (56, 140). One study revealed that resistance to drug-induced apoptosis in $CD133^+$ colon cancer cells was mediated through increased production of IL-4 (56). Preliminary experiments suggest that this IL-4-mediated, pro-survival pathway may be a promising therapeutic target. In the same study, blockade with either IL-4 neutralizing antibody or a mutant, inhibitory form of IL-4 (IL-4DM) reduced the viability of $CD133^+$ and $CD133^-$ tumor cell cultures, while increasing the efficacy of cytotoxic treatment with standard chemotherapeutic agents: oxaliplatin, 5-fluorouracil, and the death receptor ligand TRAIL. IL-4 antagonism also enhanced the effectiveness and duration of chemotherapy response in mice bearing transplanted tumors, suggesting a role for combined therapy in the treatment of human disease (56). Both the *in vitro* and *in vivo* effects of IL-4 blockade were mediated by decreases in the anti-apoptotic molecules cFlip, Bcl-xL, and Ped (56, 140).

Another remarkable finding has been the role of IL-13Rα2 in models of cancer development, indicating signaling functions far beyond the previously suggested role of a decoy receptor (141). This receptor is known to be overexpressed in several human cancers. An immunohistochemical analysis of human tissues found IL-13Rα2 overexpression in 71% of pancreatic ductal adenocarcinoma samples in comparison to normal pancreas controls (142). Indeed, experiments in an orthotopic mouse model of pancreatic cancer suggest that IL-13Rα2 is an important mediator of the pro-tumor effects of IL-13, including activation of AP-1 growth signals, production of immunomodulatory cytokines such as TGF-β, and promotion of metastasis (58, 142). Similar IL-13Rα2-dependent effects have been demonstrated in other cancer models, including ovarian carcinoma (59), colorectal cancer (57), head and neck squamous cell carcinoma (143), and malignant glioma (144). As with IL-4, IL-13 signaling has been suggested as a possible target of anticancer therapy. To this end, recombinant cytotoxic proteins have been developed, which consisted of IL-4 or IL-13 joined to a mutant form of *Pseudomonas* exotoxin. These agents have been found to restrain tumor growth in numerous animal models (142–144). However, in a Phase 3 clinical trial, IL-13 *Pseudomonas* exotoxin failed to improve median survival time in patients with glioblastoma multiforme when compared to conventional chemotherapy (145). While this agent may still find use as an adjuvant therapy (146), the outcome suggests that the development of Th2-targeted treatments with robust antitumor efficacy will require further exploration.

Despite considerable progress in the field, many Th2-mediated influences on tumor development remain poorly characterized. For instance, populations of eosinophils and mast cells, crucial mediators of Th2-driven allergic responses, also contribute to the inflammatory infiltrate in numerous human tumors. However, experimental data exploring their effects are lacking, and conflicting results have been published regarding their impact on clinical prognosis (83). This ambiguity underscores the fearsomely complex, and incompletely understood, nature of signaling among discrete immune system components in the context of cancer development. Owing to these knowledge gaps, the possibility that an anti-Th2 intervention could impede antitumor immune responses *in vivo* cannot be prematurely dismissed. Systemic therapies to antagonize Type I or Type II receptors will also confront a high risk of adverse events, owing to the global effects of Th2 cytokines on immune homeostasis and other physiological functions. Nevertheless, a fascinating body of experimental and clinical data suggests that the pro-carcinogenic effects of IL-4 and IL-13 will remain a source of therapeutic interest for years to come.

POTENTIAL FEEDBACK BETWEEN AUTOINFLAMMATION AND TUMOR: IMPLICATIONS FOR CANCER IMMUNOTHERAPY

Virtually all of the immune signaling pathways relevant to tumor biology play major physiological roles in the maintenance of self-tolerance and tissue homeostasis. Moreover, most well-characterized tumor-associated antigens are self-antigens, meaning that they are also expressed by normal cells in the course of growth and differentiation. Conversely, antigenic proteins expressed exclusively in cancerous tissue, such as viral products or mutated oncogenes, have been characterized in only a small number of tumor types. Overall, it seems that tumors, despite their aberrant characteristics, may remain antigenically "self" entities first and foremost (1, 2). In the clinical context, this suggests that useful antitumor immune responses elicited in patients may be functionally inseparable from those directed against healthy tissues. The seemingly inextricable association between off-target autoimmune damage to healthy tissues and antitumor immunity induced by effective cancer immunotherapy during recent clinical trials can be seen as supporting this hypothesis. Evidence from molecular studies in this regard and a large body of research on inflammation and cancer suggest a feedback loop of autoimmunity, antitumor immunity, inflammation, and *de novo* tumorigenesis that reinforces the remarkable entanglement between autoimmunity and cancer (**Figure 1**). In particular, the persistence of antigens in most autoimmune conditions likely leads to the formation of a type of autoimmune memory cells called effector memory T (T_{EM}) cells [for review see Ref. (66)], which could further perpetuate this feedback loop. Advances in not only experimental and clinical research, but also in computational biology tools for large datasets, will be needed to understand the complexity of molecular and cellular interactions in such chronic human disease settings (66, 147).

Along this line, one may argue that a combination of immunomodulation with conventional cancer therapies such as chemotherapy could be used to augment tumor-specific immune responses. Despite the severe immunosuppression produced by many standard chemotherapeutic agents, current data suggest that patients with chemotherapy-induced leukopenia retain a functional T cell compartment that is capable of mediating clinically significant antitumor immunity (148). Within solid tumors, it has been demonstrated that chemotherapy can deplete immune suppressor cells (MDSCs and Treg cells) in the tumor microenvironment, increase tumor antigenicity, and upregulate the expression of costimulatory molecules for CTL activation (79). All of these mechanisms point toward possible synergistic effects that could enhance the clinical efficacy of existing cancer immunotherapies, including agents that have shown meager benefits when administered alone. Indeed, synergy between cancer vaccines and chemotherapy has already been demonstrated in studies of advanced small-cell lung cancer and follicular B-cell lymphoma (149).

Immunological research continues to produce crucial mechanistic insights into the tumor-related effects of major cytokines. For instance, a recent murine experimental model has demonstrated that IFN-γ and TNF-α produced by Th1 cells are capable of inducing prolonged senescence in pancreatic tumors, by inducing expression of the transcription factors JUNB and INK4A (150). The identification of specific signaling pathways for tumor cell growth inhibition and apoptosis heralds a new and improved generation of cytokine-based therapies. More broadly, this knowledge may eventually enable a combinatorial approach to cancer immunotherapy, in which multiple treatments can be jointly administered to yield superior therapeutic outcomes. The current field of cancer immunotherapy is divided between treatments that encourage global activation of cytotoxic immune responses, such as exogenous cytokines and antibodies targeting T cell-inhibitory signals (e.g., anti-PD-1, anti-PD-L1, anti-CTLA4), and treatments based on tumor antigens, which aim to stimulate destruction of cancerous tissues by engaging a specific population of tumor-reactive CTLs (e.g., cancer vaccines and autologous T cell transfers). With further advancement in the clinical and investigative realms, it may become possible for these two approaches to complement each other within the same patient. A cancer vaccine that produces a meager antitumor response *in vivo* could have enhanced efficacy when administered alongside a treatment that

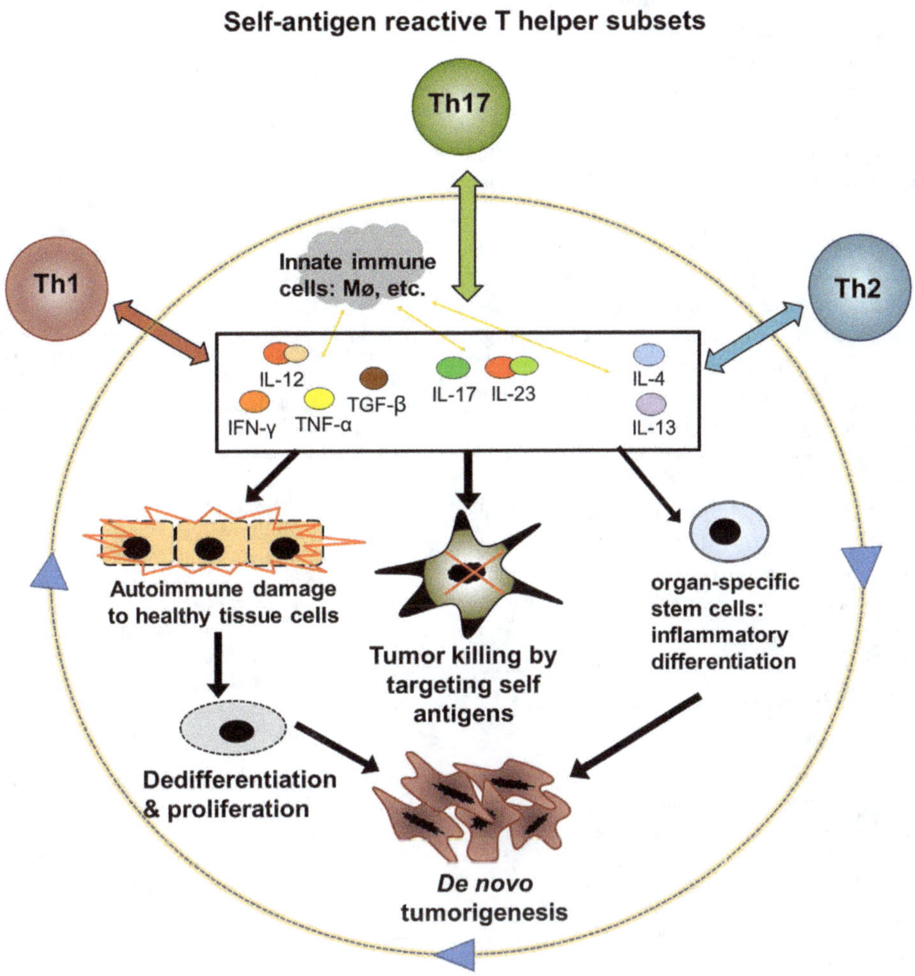

FIGURE 1 | A hypothetic feedback loop between autoimmunity, antitumor immunity, and inflammatory tumorigenesis. Three major subsets of autoantigen reactive T helper cells, Th1, Th2, and Th17, could mediate both antitumor and pro-tumor effects through interaction with innate immune cells and CD8 T cell effectors. (1) Th1, Th2, and Th17 cells release cytokines after encountering autoantigens. These cytokines may exert direct and indirect effects on cell cycle regulation, apoptosis, and differentiation in both tumors and healthy tissues. (2) Cytokines can promote tumor killing by various mechanisms including stimulation of CD8 effectors, innate immune cell activation, and direct toxicity. (3) Inflammation in healthy tissues, particularly when chronic, could contribute to loss of antiproliferative signals and aberrant differentiation in normal cells, leading to a premalignant phenotype. Continued proliferation of these abnormal cells, with accumulation of DNA damage, leads to the emergence of cancer. (4) Chronic cytokine signaling may induce abnormal differentiation of organ-specific stem cells or other precursor cells and drive a cascade of cancer development. The feedback between autoinflammation and cancer may particularly affect solid organs such as the gastrointestinal tract that are demonstrated to be susceptible to inflammatory carcinogenesis.

elicits global T cell activation, such as CTLA4 blockade. Moreover, the systemic autoimmune toxicity produced by these broad-acting treatments might be mitigated if a lower dose was combined with a cancer vaccine or other antigen-focused immune stimulus. Adding to the possibilities, multiple immunomodulatory agents from either treatment category could theoretically be combined (e.g., anti-PD-1 in combination with one or more exogenous cytokines) to provide unprecedented control over the targeting, intensity, and duration of the induced immune response. The potential advantages of a combined regimen are already supported by data from numerous preclinical models (5). The true capabilities of cancer immunotherapy may only be realized once multiple treatments can be synthesized into a therapeutic strategy tailored to the pathological and molecular characteristics of every patient's disease. Although the harmful clinical sequelae of autoimmunity may never be banished entirely, this integrative approach has the potential to harness its tumoricidal functions better than any single agent administered in isolation.

In summary, clinical data suggest that both the anticipated benefits of cancer immunotherapy and its associated adverse events share autoimmunity as a common originating process. Thus autoimmunity, regarded until recently as a "side effect" of cancer immunotherapy, may be more properly considered a correlate of antitumor immunity, or even more appropriately as an antitumor effector in its own right. Despite the lopsided benefit versus risk ratio in cancer immunotherapies that succeed in providing substantial survival benefit, it should be noted that autoimmune damage to healthy tissues is a justifiably dreaded cause of morbidity and mortality in patients receiving these treatments. This hazard may be even more dire if one considers that an immunosuppressive microenvironment effectively designates tumors as an immunoprivileged self, which is more resistant to immune targeting than its healthy counterpart (1, 2). Furthermore, the calculation of benefit versus risk must account for the possibility that inflammatory signals arising from therapeutically induced autoimmunity may ultimately contribute to *de novo* tumorigenesis in the clinical setting. Therefore, achieving optimal benefit of cancer immunotherapies awaits advances in tumor-specific targeting, either by site or by unique antigens, coupled with proper monitoring and prevention of potentially catastrophic autoimmune damage or long-term risks of *de novo* tumorigenesis.

ACKNOWLEDGMENTS

This work was supported in part by grants from the National Institute of Cancer (1R21CA178675-01 to Zhibin Chen) and the Bankhead-Coley Research Program of Florida Department of Health (09BN-05 to Zhibin Chen). We sincerely apologize to all colleagues whose studies have contributed importantly to the understanding of the topics surveyed in this article, but not cited due to the limit of the length of the article as well as the scope of our knowledge.

REFERENCES

1. Miska J, Bas E, Devarajan P, Chen Z. Autoimmunity-mediated antitumor immunity: tumor as an immunoprivileged self. *Eur J Immunol* (2012) **42**:2584–2596. doi:10.1002/eji.201242590
2. Miska J, Devarajan P, Chen Z. The immunological identity of tumor: self implications. *Oncoimmunology* (2013) **2**:e23794. doi:10.4161/onci.23794
3. Balkwill F, Mantovani A. Inflammation and cancer: back to Virchow? *Lancet* (2001) **357**:539–45. doi:10.1016/S0140-6736(00)04046-0
4. Hanahan D, Weinberg RA. Hallmarks of cancer: the next generation. *Cell* (2011) **144**:646–74. doi:10.1016/j.cell.2011.02.013
5. Melero I, Hervas-Stubbs S, Glennie M, Pardoll DM, Chen L. Immunostimulatory monoclonal antibodies for cancer therapy. *Nat Rev Cancer* (2007) **7**:95–106. doi:10.1038/nrc2051
6. Hodi FS, O'Day SJ, McDermott DF, Weber RW, Sosman JA, Haanen JB, et al. Improved survival with ipilimumab in patients with metastatic melanoma. *N Engl J Med* (2010) **363**:711–23. doi:10.1056/NEJMoa1003466
7. Topalian SL, Hodi FS, Brahmer JR, Gettinger SN, Smith DC, McDermott DF, et al. Safety, activity, and immune correlates of anti-PD-1 antibody in cancer. *N Engl J Med* (2012) **366**:2443–54. doi:10.1056/NEJMoa1200690
8. Brahmer JR, Tykodi SS, Chow LQ, Hwu WJ, Topalian SL, Hwu P, et al. Safety and activity of anti-PD-L1 antibody in patients with advanced cancer. *N Engl J Med* (2012) **366**:2455–65. doi:10.1056/NEJMoa1200694
9. Whiteside TL. Inhibiting the inhibitors: evaluating agents targeting cancer immunosuppression. *Expert Opin Biol Ther* (2010) **10**:1019–35. doi:10.1517/14712598.2010.482207
10. Schroder K, Hertzog PJ, Ravasi T, Hume DA. Interferon-gamma: an overview of signals, mechanisms and functions. *J Leukoc Biol* (2004) **75**:163–89. doi:10.1189/jlb.0603252
11. Ikeda H, Old LJ, Schreiber RD. The roles of IFN gamma in protection against tumor development and cancer immunoediting. *Cytokine Growth Factor Rev* (2002) **13**:95–109. doi:10.1016/S1359-6101(01)00038-7
12. Seliger B, Ruiz-Cabello F, Garrido F. IFN inducibility of major histocompatibility antigens in tumors. *Adv Cancer Res* (2008) **101**:249–76. doi:10.1016/S0065-230X(08)00407-7
13. Kelchtermans H, Billiau A, Matthys P. How interferon-gamma keeps autoimmune diseases in check. *Trends Immunol* (2008) **29**:479–86. doi:10.1016/j.it.2008.07.002
14. Zhang J. Yin and yang interplay of IFN-gamma in inflammation and autoimmune disease. *J Clin Invest* (2007) **117**:871–3. doi:10.1172/JCI31860
15. Stoicov C, Fan X, Liu JH, Bowen G, Whary M, Kurt-Jones E, et al. T-bet knockout prevents *Helicobacter felis*-induced gastric cancer. *J Immunol* (2009) **183**:642–9. doi:10.4049/jimmunol.0900511
16. Syu LJ, El-Zaatari M, Eaton KA, Liu Z, Tetarbe M, Keeley TM, et al. Transgenic expression of interferon-gamma in mouse stomach leads to inflammation, metaplasia, and dysplasia. *Am J Pathol* (2012) **181**:2114–25. doi:10.1016/j.ajpath.2012.08.017
17. Cho HI, Lee YR, Celis E. Interferon gamma limits the effectiveness of melanoma peptide vaccines. *Blood* (2011) **117**:135–44. doi:10.1182/blood-2010-08-298117
18. Malmberg KJ, Levitsky V, Norell H, de Matos CT, Carlsten M, Schedvins K, et al. IFN-gamma protects short-term ovarian carcinoma cell lines from CTL lysis via a CD94/NKG2A-dependent mechanism. *J Clin Invest* (2002) **110**:1515–23. doi:10.1172/JCI200215564
19. Carswell EA, Old LJ, Kassel RL, Green S, Fiore N, Williamson B. An endotoxin-induced serum factor that causes necrosis of tumors. *Proc Natl Acad Sci U S A* (1975) **72**:3666–70. doi:10.1073/pnas.72.9.3666
20. van Horssen R, Ten Hagen TL, Eggermont AM. TNF-alpha in cancer treatment: molecular insights, antitumor effects, and clinical utility. *Oncologist* (2006) **11**:397–408. doi:10.1634/theoncologist.11-4-397
21. Grivennikov SI, Karin M. Inflammatory cytokines in cancer: tumour necrosis factor and interleukin 6 take the stage. *Ann Rheum Dis* (2011) **70**(Suppl 1):i104–8. doi:10.1136/ard.2010.140145
22. Gukovsky I, Li N, Todoric J, Gukovskaya A, Karin M. Inflammation, autophagy, and obesity: common features in the pathogenesis of pancreatitis and pancreatic cancer. *Gastroenterology* (2013) **144**:1199.e–209.e. doi:10.1053/j.gastro.2013.02.007
23. Park EJ, Lee JH, Yu GY, He G, Ali SR, Holzer RG, et al. Dietary and genetic obesity promote liver inflammation and tumorigenesis by enhancing IL-6 and TNF expression. *Cell* (2010) **140**:197–208. doi:10.1016/j.cell.2009.12.052
24. Balkwill F. Tumour necrosis factor and cancer. *Nat Rev Cancer* (2009) **9**:361–71. doi:10.1038/nrc2628
25. Wu Y, Zhou BP. TNF-alpha/NF-kappaB/Snail pathway in cancer cell migration and invasion. *Br J Cancer* (2010) **102**:639–44. doi:10.1038/sj.bjc.6605530
26. Achyut BR, Bader DA, Robles AI, Wangsa D, Harris CC, Ried T, et al. Inflammation-mediated genetic and epigenetic alterations drive cancer development in the neighboring epithelium upon stromal abrogation of TGF-beta signaling. *PLoS Genet* (2013) **9**:e1003251. doi:10.1371/journal.pgen.1003251
27. Chaudhury A, Howe PH. The tale of transforming growth factor-beta (TGF-beta) signaling: a soigne enigma. *IUBMB Life* (2009) **61**:929–39. doi:10.1002/iub.239
28. Laouar Y, Sutterwala FS, Gorelik L, Flavell RA. Transforming growth factor-beta controls T helper type 1 cell development through regulation of natural killer cell interferon-gamma. *Nat Immunol* (2005) **6**:600–7. doi:10.1038/ni1197
29. Prud'homme GJ. Pathobiology of transforming growth factor beta in cancer, fibrosis and immunologic disease, and therapeutic considerations. *Lab Invest* (2007) **87**:1077–91. doi:10.1038/labinvest.3700669
30. Ramalingam R, Larmonier CB, Thurston RD, Midura-Kiela MT, Zheng SG, Ghishan FK, et al. Dendritic cell-specific disruption of TGF-beta receptor II leads to altered regulatory T cell phenotype and spontaneous multiorgan autoimmunity. *J Immunol* (2012) **189**:3878–93. doi:10.4049/jimmunol.1201029
31. Galdiero MR, Garlanda C, Jaillon S, Marone G, Mantovani A. Tumor associated macrophages and neutrophils in tumor progression. *J Cell Physiol* (2013) **228**:1404–12. doi:10.1002/jcp.24260
32. Moo-Young TA, Larson JW, Belt BA, Tan MC, Hawkins WG, Eberlein TJ, et al. Tumor-derived TGF-beta mediates conversion of CD4+Foxp3+ regulatory T cells in a murine model of pancreas cancer. *J Immunother* (2009) **32**:12–21. doi:10.1097/CJI.0b013e318189f13c
33. Yang P, Li QJ, Feng Y, Zhang Y, Markowitz GJ, Ning S, et al. TGF-beta-miR-34a-CCL22 signaling-induced Treg cell recruitment promotes venous metastases of HBV-positive hepatocellular carcinoma. *Cancer Cell* (2012) **22**:291–303. doi:10.1016/j.ccr.2012.07.023
34. Yang L. TGFbeta and cancer metastasis: an inflammation link. *Cancer Metastasis Rev* (2010) **29**:263–71. doi:10.1007/s10555-010-9226-3

35. Massague J. TGFbeta in cancer. *Cell* (2008) **134**:215–30. doi:10.1016/j.cell.2008.07.001
36. Kurebayashi Y, Nagai S, Ikejiri A, Koyasu S. Recent advances in understanding the molecular mechanisms of the development and function of Th17 cells. *Genes Cells* (2013) **18**:247–65. doi:10.1111/gtc.12039
37. Zou W, Restifo NP. T(H)17 cells in tumour immunity and immunotherapy. *Nat Rev Immunol* (2010) **10**:248–56. doi:10.1038/nri2742
38. Kaiga T, Sato M, Kaneda H, Iwakura Y, Takayama T, Tahara H. Systemic administration of IL-23 induces potent antitumor immunity primarily mediated through Th1-type response in association with the endogenously expressed IL-12. *J Immunol* (2007) **178**:7571–80.
39. Kryczek I, Wei S, Szeliga W, Vatan L, Zou W. Endogenous IL-17 contributes to reduced tumor growth and metastasis. *Blood* (2009) **114**:357–9. doi:10.1182/blood-2008-09-177360
40. Martin-Orozco N, Muranski P, Chung Y, Yang XO, Yamazaki T, Lu S, et al. T helper 17 cells promote cytotoxic T cell activation in tumor immunity. *Immunity* (2009) **31**:787–98. doi:10.1016/j.immuni.2009.09.014
41. Nuñez S, Saez JJ, Fernandez D, Flores-Santibanez F, Alvarez K, Tejon G, et al. T helper type 17 cells contribute to anti-tumour immunity and promote the recruitment of T helper type 1 cells to the tumour. *Immunology* (2013) **139**:61–71. doi:10.1111/imm.12055
42. Amedei A, Niccolai E, Benagiano M, Della Bella C, Cianchi F, Bechi P, et al. Ex vivo analysis of pancreatic cancer-infiltrating T lymphocytes reveals that ENO-specific Tregs accumulate in tumor tissue and inhibit Th1/Th17 effector cell functions. *Cancer Immunol Immunother* (2013) **62**:1249–60. doi:10.1007/s00262-013-1429-3
43. Huang Z, van Velkinburgh JC, Ni B, Wu Y. Pivotal roles of the interleukin-23/T helper 17 cell axis in hepatitis B. *Liver Int* (2012) **32**:894–901. doi:10.1111/j.1478-3231.2012.02764.x
44. Wu W, Li J, Chen F, Zhu H, Peng G, Chen Z. Circulating Th17 cells frequency is associated with the disease progression in HBV infected patients. *J Gastroenterol Hepatol* (2010) **25**:750–7. doi:10.1111/j.1440-1746.2009.06154.x
45. Yang W, Ding X, Deng J, Lu Y, Matsuda Z, Thiel A, et al. Interferon-gamma negatively regulates Th17-mediated immunopathology during mouse hepatitis virus infection. *J Mol Med (Berl)* (2011) **89**:399–409. doi:10.1007/s00109-010-0711-5
46. Ye Y, Xie X, Yu J, Zhou L, Xie H, Jiang G, et al. Involvement of Th17 and Th1 effector responses in patients with Hepatitis B. *J Clin Immunol* (2010) **30**:546–55. doi:10.1007/s10875-010-9416-3
47. He D, Li H, Yusuf N, Elmets CA, Li J, Mountz JD, et al. IL-17 promotes tumor development through the induction of tumor promoting microenvironments at tumor sites and myeloid-derived suppressor cells. *J Immunol* (2010) **184**:2281–8. doi:10.4049/jimmunol.0902574
48. Qian X, Gu L, Ning H, Zhang Y, Hsueh EC, Fu M, et al. Increased Th17 cells in the tumor microenvironment is mediated by IL-23 via tumor-secreted prostaglandin E2. *J Immunol* (2013) **190**:5894–902. doi:10.4049/jimmunol.1203141
49. Baird AM, Leonard J, Naicker KM, Kilmartin L, O'Byrne KJ, Gray SG. IL-23 is pro-proliferative, epigenetically regulated and modulated by chemotherapy in non-small cell lung cancer. *Lung Cancer* (2013) **79**:83–90. doi:10.1016/j.lungcan.2012.10.003
50. Fukuda M, Ehara M, Suzuki S, Ohmori Y, Sakashita H. IL-23 promotes growth and proliferation in human squamous cell carcinoma of the oral cavity. *Int J Oncol* (2010) **36**:1355–65. doi:10.3892/ijo_00000620
51. Li J, Zhang L, Zhang J, Wei Y, Li K, Huang L, et al. Interleukin 23 regulates proliferation of lung cancer cells in a concentration-dependent way in association with the interleukin-23 receptor. *Carcinogenesis* (2013) **34**:658–66. doi:10.1093/carcin/bgs384
52. De Monte L, Reni M, Tassi E, Clavenna D, Papa I, Recalde H, et al. Intratumor T helper type 2 cell infiltrate correlates with cancer-associated fibroblast thymic stromal lymphopoietin production and reduced survival in pancreatic cancer. *J Exp Med* (2011) **208**:469–78. doi:10.1084/jem.20101876
53. Aspord C, Pedroza-Gonzalez A, Gallegos M, Tindle S, Burton EC, Su D, et al. Breast cancer instructs dendritic cells to prime interleukin 13-secreting CD4+ T cells that facilitate tumor development. *J Exp Med* (2007) **204**:1037–47. doi:10.1084/jem.20061120
54. Hallett MA, Venmar KT, Fingleton B. Cytokine stimulation of epithelial cancer cells: the similar and divergent functions of IL-4 and IL-13. *Cancer Res* (2012) **72**:6338–43. doi:10.1158/0008-5472.CAN-12-3544
55. Koller FL, Hwang DG, Dozier EA, Fingleton B. Epithelial interleukin-4 receptor expression promotes colon tumor growth. *Carcinogenesis* (2010) **31**:1010–7. doi:10.1093/carcin/bgq044
56. Todaro M, Alea MP, Di Stefano AB, Cammareri P, Vermeulen L, Iovino F, et al. Colon cancer stem cells dictate tumor growth and resist cell death by production of interleukin-4. *Cell Stem Cell* (2007) **1**:389–402. doi:10.1016/j.stem.2007.08.001
57. Barderas R, Bartolome RA, Fernandez-Acenero MJ, Torres S, Casal JI. High expression of IL-13 receptor alpha2 in colorectal cancer is associated with invasion, liver metastasis, and poor prognosis. *Cancer Res* (2012) **72**:2780–90. doi:10.1158/0008-5472.CAN-11-4090
58. Fujisawa T, Joshi B, Nakajima A, Puri RK. A novel role of interleukin-13 receptor alpha2 in pancreatic cancer invasion and metastasis. *Cancer Res* (2009) **69**:8678–85. doi:10.1158/0008-5472.CAN-09-2100
59. Fujisawa T, Joshi BH, Puri RK. IL-13 regulates cancer invasion and metastasis through IL-13Ralpha2 via ERK/AP-1 pathway in mouse model of human ovarian cancer. *Int J Cancer* (2012) **131**:344–56. doi:10.1002/ijc.26366
60. Virchow RLK. *Cellular Pathology as based upon Physiological and Pathological Histology*. Philadelphia: J. B. Lippincott (1863).
61. Gabrilovich DI, Nagaraj S. Myeloid-derived suppressor cells as regulators of the immune system. *Nat Rev Immunol* (2009) **9**:162–74. doi:10.1038/nri2506
62. Qian BZ, Pollard JW. Macrophage diversity enhances tumor progression and metastasis. *Cell* (2010) **141**:39–51. doi:10.1016/j.cell.2010.03.014
63. Ammirante M, Luo JL, Grivennikov S, Nedospasov S, Karin M. B-cell-derived lymphotoxin promotes castration-resistant prostate cancer. *Nature* (2010) **464**:302–5. doi:10.1038/nature08782
64. He Y, Zha J, Wang Y, Liu W, Yang X, Yu P. Tissue damage-associated "danger signals" influence T-cell responses that promote the progression of preneoplasia to cancer. *Cancer Res* (2013) **73**:629–39. doi:10.1158/0008-5472.CAN-12-2704
65. Wang L, Yi T, Kortylewski M, Pardoll DM, Zeng D, Yu H. IL-17 can promote tumor growth through an IL-6-Stat3 signaling pathway. *J Exp Med* (2009) **206**:1457–64. doi:10.1084/jem.20090207
66. Devarajan P, Chen Z. Autoimmune effector memory T cells: the bad and the good. *Immunol Res* (2013) **57**:12–22. doi:10.1007/s12026-013-8448-1
67. Germain RN, Robey EA, Cahalan MD. A decade of imaging cellular motility and interaction dynamics in the immune system. *Science* (2012) **336**:1676–81. doi:10.1126/science.1221063
68. Miska J, Abdulreda MH, Devarajan P, Lui JB, Suzuki J, Pileggi A, et al. Real-time immune cell interactions in target tissue during autoimmune-induced damage and graft tolerance. *J Exp Med* (2014) **211**:441–56. doi:10.1084/jem.20130785
69. Suzuki J, Ricordi C, Chen Z. Immune tolerance induction by integrating innate and adaptive immune regulators. *Cell Transplant* (2010) **19**:253–68. doi:10.3727/096368909X480314
70. Tomsova M, Melichar B, Sedlakova I, Steiner I. Prognostic significance of CD3+ tumor-infiltrating lymphocytes in ovarian carcinoma. *Gynecol Oncol* (2008) **108**:415–20. doi:10.1016/j.ygyno.2007.10.016
71. Tano T, Okamoto M, Kan S, Nakashiro K, Shimodaira S, Koido S, et al. Prognostic impact of expression of Bcl-2 and Bax genes in circulating immune cells derived from patients with head and neck carcinoma. *Neoplasia* (2013) **15**:305–14. doi:10.1593/neo.121528
72. Lippitz BE. Cytokine patterns in patients with cancer: a systematic review. *Lancet Oncol* (2013) **14**:e218–28. doi:10.1016/S1470-2045(12)70582-X
73. Vierboom MP, Nijman HW, Offringa R, van der Voort EI, van Hall T, van den Broek L, et al. Tumor eradication by wild-type p53-specific cytotoxic T lymphocytes. *J Exp Med* (1997) **186**:695–704. doi:10.1084/jem.186.5.695
74. Hilburger Ryan M, Abrams SI. Characterization of CD8+ cytotoxic T lymphocyte/tumor cell interactions reflecting recognition of an endogenously expressed murine wild-type p53 determinant. *Cancer Immunol Immunother* (2001) **49**:603–12. doi:10.1007/s002620000156
75. Hu J, Kindsvogel W, Busby S, Bailey MC, Shi YY, Greenberg PD. An evaluation of the potential to use tumor-associated antigens as targets for antitumor T cell therapy using transgenic mice expressing a retroviral tumor antigen in normal lymphoid tissues. *J Exp Med* (1993) **177**:1681–90. doi:10.1084/jem.177.6.1681
76. Morgan DJ, Kreuwel HT, Fleck S, Levitsky HI, Pardoll DM, Sherman LA. Activation of low avidity CTL specific for a self epitope results in tumor rejection but not autoimmunity. *J Immunol* (1998) **160**:643–51.
77. Caspi RR. Immunotherapy of autoimmunity and cancer: the penalty for success. *Nat Rev Immunol* (2008) **8**:970–6. doi:10.1038/nri2438

78. Attia P, Phan GQ, Maker AV, Robinson MR, Quezado MM, Yang JC, et al. Autoimmunity correlates with tumor regression in patients with metastatic melanoma treated with anti-cytotoxic T-lymphocyte antigen-4. *J Clin Oncol* (2005) **23**:6043–53. doi:10.1200/JCO.2005.06.205
79. Andersen MH, Junker N, Ellebaek E, Svane IM, Thor Straten P. Therapeutic cancer vaccines in combination with conventional therapy. *J Biomed Biotechnol* (2010) **2010**:237623. doi:10.1155/2010/237623
80. Zaidi MR, Merlino G. The two faces of interferon-gamma in cancer. *Clin Cancer Res* (2011) **17**:6118–24. doi:10.1158/1078-0432.CCR-11-0482
81. Fojtova M, Boudny V, Kovarik A, Lauerova L, Adamkova L, Souckova K, et al. Development of IFN-gamma resistance is associated with attenuation of SOCS genes induction and constitutive expression of SOCS 3 in melanoma cells. *Br J Cancer* (2007) **97**:231–7. doi:10.1038/sj.bjc.6603849
82. Miller CH, Maher SG, Young HA. Clinical use of interferon-gamma. *Ann N Y Acad Sci* (2009) **1182**:69–79. doi:10.1111/j.1749-6632.2009.05069.x
83. Demaria S, Pikarsky E, Karin M, Coussens LM, Chen YC, El-Omar EM, et al. Cancer and inflammation: promise for biologic therapy. *J Immunother* (2010) **33**:335–51. doi:10.1097/CJI.0b013e3181d32e74
84. Moss SF, Blaser MJ. Mechanisms of disease: Inflammation and the origins of cancer. *Nat Clin Pract Oncol* (2005) **2**:90–7. doi:10.1038/ncponc0081 quiz 91 p following 113,
85. Skurkovich B, Skurkovich S. Anti-interferon-gamma antibodies in the treatment of autoimmune diseases. *Curr Opin Mol Ther* (2003) **5**:52–7.
86. Skurkovich S, Skurkovich B, Kelly J. Anticytokine therapy, particularly anti-IFN-gamma, in Th1-mediated autoimmune diseases. *Expert Rev Clin Immunol* (2005) **1**:11–25. doi:10.1586/1744666X.1.1.11
87. Fox JG, Wang TC. Inflammation, atrophy, and gastric cancer. *J Clin Invest* (2007) **117**:60–9. doi:10.1172/JCI30111
88. Merchant JL. What lurks beneath: IL-11, via Stat3, promotes inflammation-associated gastric tumorigenesis. *J Clin Invest* (2008) **118**:1628–31. doi:10.1172/JCI35344
89. Polk DB, Peek RM Jr. *Helicobacter pylori*: gastric cancer and beyond. *Nat Rev Cancer* (2010) **10**:403–14. doi:10.1038/nrc2857
90. Toh BH, van Driel IR, Gleeson PA. Pernicious anemia. *N Engl J Med* (1997) **337**:1441–8. doi:10.1056/NEJM199711133372007
91. El-Omar EM, Rabkin CS, Gammon MD, Vaughan TL, Risch HA, Schoenberg JB, et al. Increased risk of noncardia gastric cancer associated with proinflammatory cytokine gene polymorphisms. *Gastroenterology* (2003) **124**:1193–201. doi:10.1016/S0016-5085(03)00157-4
92. Judd LM, Alderman BM, Howlett M, Shulkes A, Dow C, Moverley J, et al. Gastric cancer development in mice lacking the SHP2 binding site on the IL-6 family co-receptor gp130. *Gastroenterology* (2004) **126**:196–207. doi:10.1053/j.gastro.2003.10.066
93. Tu S, Bhagat G, Cui G, Takaishi S, Kurt-Jones EA, Rickman B, et al. Overexpression of interleukin-1beta induces gastric inflammation and cancer and mobilizes myeloid-derived suppressor cells in mice. *Cancer Cell* (2008) **14**:408–19. doi:10.1016/j.ccr.2008.10.011
94. Weis VG, Goldenring JR. Current understanding of SPEM and its standing in the preneoplastic process. *Gastric Cancer* (2009) **12**:189–97. doi:10.1007/s10120-009-0527-6
95. Szabo SJ, Kim ST, Costa GL, Zhang X, Fathman CG, Glimcher LH. A novel transcription factor, T-bet, directs Th1 lineage commitment. *Cell* (2000) **100**:655–69. doi:10.1016/S0092-8674(00)80702-3
96. Li X, McKinstry KK, Swain SL, Dalton DK. IFN-gamma acts directly on activated CD4+ T cells during mycobacterial infection to promote apoptosis by inducing components of the intracellular apoptosis machinery and by inducing extracellular proapoptotic signals. *J Immunol* (2007) **179**:939–49.
97. Mellor AL, Munn DH. Creating immune privilege: active local suppression that benefits friends, but protects foes. *Nat Rev Immunol* (2008) **8**:74–80. doi:10.1038/nri2233
98. Tu SP, Quante M, Bhagat G, Takaishi S, Cui G, Yang XD, et al. IFN-gamma inhibits gastric carcinogenesis by inducing epithelial cell autophagy and T-cell apoptosis. *Cancer Res* (2011) **71**:4247–59. doi:10.1158/0008-5472.CAN-10-4009
99. White E, DiPaola RS. The double-edged sword of autophagy modulation in cancer. *Clin Cancer Res* (2009) **15**:5308–16. doi:10.1158/1078-0432.CCR-07-5023
100. Bradley JR. TNF-mediated inflammatory disease. *J Pathol* (2008) **214**:149–60. doi:10.1002/path.2287
101. Palladino MA, Bahjat FR, Theodorakis EA, Moldawer LL. Anti-TNF-alpha therapies: the next generation. *Nat Rev Drug Discov* (2003) **2**:736–46. doi:10.1038/nrd1175
102. Murdaca G, Colombo BM, Cagnati P, Gulli R, Spano F, Puppo F. Update upon efficacy and safety of TNF-alpha inhibitors. *Expert Opin Drug Saf* (2012) **11**:1–5. doi:10.1517/14740338.2012.630388
103. Hobohm U. Fever and cancer in perspective. *Cancer Immunol Immunother* (2001) **50**:391–6.
104. Kruglov AA, Kuchmiy A, Grivennikov SI, Tumanov AV, Kuprash DV, Nedospasov SA. Physiological functions of tumor necrosis factor and the consequences of its pathologic overexpression or blockade: mouse models. *Cytokine Growth Factor Rev* (2008) **19**:231–44. doi:10.1016/j.cytogfr.2008.04.010
105. Moore RJ, Owens DM, Stamp G, Arnott C, Burke F, East N, et al. Mice deficient in tumor necrosis factor-alpha are resistant to skin carcinogenesis. *Nat Med* (1999) **5**:828–31. doi:10.1038/10552
106. Fujiki H, Sueoka E, Suganuma M. Tumor promoters: from chemicals to inflammatory proteins. *J Cancer Res Clin Oncol* (2013) **139**:1603–14. doi:10.1007/s00432-013-1455-8
107. Capece D, Fischietti M, Verzella D, Gaggiano A, Cicciarelli G, Tessitore A, et al. The inflammatory microenvironment in hepatocellular carcinoma: a pivotal role for tumor-associated macrophages. *Biomed Res Int* (2013) **2013**:187204. doi:10.1155/2013/187204
108. Natarajan M, Gibbons CF, Mohan S, Moore S, Kadhim MA. Oxidative stress signalling: a potential mediator of tumour necrosis factor alpha-induced genomic instability in primary vascular endothelial cells. *Br J Radiol* (2007) **80**(1):S13–22. doi:10.1259/bjr/15316848
109. Pierce RH, Campbell JS, Stephenson AB, Franklin CC, Chaisson M, Poot M, et al. Disruption of redox homeostasis in tumor necrosis factor-induced apoptosis in a murine hepatocyte cell line. *Am J Pathol* (2000) **157**:221–36. doi:10.1016/S0002-9440(10)64533-6
110. Suematsu N, Tsutsui H, Wen J, Kang D, Ikeuchi M, Ide T, et al. Oxidative stress mediates tumor necrosis factor-alpha-induced mitochondrial DNA damage and dysfunction in cardiac myocytes. *Circulation* (2003) **107**:1418–23. doi:10.1161/01.CIR.0000055318.09997.1F
111. Wheelhouse NM, Chan YS, Gillies SE, Caldwell H, Ross JA, Harrison DJ, et al. TNF-alpha induced DNA damage in primary murine hepatocytes. *Int J Mol Med* (2003) **12**:889–94. doi:10.3892/ijmm.12.6.889
112. Li MO, Flavell RA. TGF-beta: a master of all T cell trades. *Cell* (2008) **134**:392–404. doi:10.1016/j.cell.2008.07.025
113. Kulkarni AB, Huh CG, Becker D, Geiser A, Lyght M, Flanders KC, et al. Transforming growth factor beta 1 null mutation in mice causes excessive inflammatory response and early death. *Proc Natl Acad Sci U S A* (1993) **90**:770–4. doi:10.1073/pnas.90.2.770
114. Leveen P, Larsson J, Ehinger M, Cilio CM, Sundler M, Sjostrand LJ, et al. Induced disruption of the transforming growth factor beta type II receptor gene in mice causes a lethal inflammatory disorder that is transplantable. *Blood* (2002) **100**:560–8. doi:10.1182/blood.V100.2.560
115. Ni XY, Sui HX, Liu Y, Ke SZ, Wang YN, Gao FG. TGF-beta of lung cancer microenvironment upregulates B7H1 and GITRL expression in dendritic cells and is associated with regulatory T cell generation. *Oncol Rep* (2012) **28**:615–21. doi:10.3892/or.2012.1822
116. Wilson CA, Cajulis EE, Green JL, Olsen TM, Chung YA, Damore MA, et al. HER-2 overexpression differentially alters transforming growth factor-beta responses in luminal versus mesenchymal human breast cancer cells. *Breast Cancer Res* (2005) **7**:R1058–79. doi:10.1186/bcr1343
117. Baldwin RL, Tran H, Karlan BY. Loss of c-myc repression coincides with ovarian cancer resistance to transforming growth factor beta growth arrest independent of transforming growth factor beta/Smad signaling. *Cancer Res* (2003) **63**:1413–9.
118. Connolly EC, Freimuth J, Akhurst RJ. Complexities of TGF-beta targeted cancer therapy. *Int J Biol Sci* (2012) **8**:964–78. doi:10.7150/ijbs.4564
119. Connolly EC, Saunier EF, Quigley D, Luu MT, De Sapio A, Hann B, et al. Outgrowth of drug-resistant carcinomas expressing markers of tumor aggression after long-term TbetaRI/II kinase inhibition with LY2109761. *Cancer Res* (2011) **71**:2339–49. doi:10.1158/0008-5472.CAN-10-2941

120. Ishigame H, Kakuta S, Nagai T, Kadoki M, Nambu A, Komiyama Y, et al. Differential roles of interleukin-17A and -17F in host defense against mucoepithelial bacterial infection and allergic responses. *Immunity* (2009) **30**:108–19. doi:10.1016/j.immuni.2008.11.009
121. Ye J, Livergood RS, Peng G. The role and regulation of human Th17 cells in tumor immunity. *Am J Pathol* (2013) **182**:10–20. doi:10.1016/j.ajpath.2012.08.041
122. Yosef N, Shalek AK, Gaublomme JT, Jin H, Lee Y, Awasthi A, et al. Dynamic regulatory network controlling TH17 cell differentiation. *Nature* (2013) **496**:461–8. doi:10.1038/nature11981
123. Harrington LE, Hatton RD, Mangan PR, Turner H, Murphy TL, Murphy KM, et al. Interleukin 17-producing CD4+ effector T cells develop via a lineage distinct from the T helper type 1 and 2 lineages. *Nat Immunol* (2005) **6**:1123–32. doi:10.1038/ni1254
124. Park H, Li Z, Yang XO, Chang SH, Nurieva R, Wang YH, et al. A distinct lineage of CD4 T cells regulates tissue inflammation by producing interleukin 17. *Nat Immunol* (2005) **6**:1133–41. doi:10.1038/ni1261
125. Langowski JL, Kastelein RA, Oft M. Swords into plowshares: IL-23 repurposes tumor immune surveillance. *Trends Immunol* (2007) **28**:207–12. doi:10.1016/j.it.2007.03.006
126. McKenzie BS, Kastelein RA, Cua DJ. Understanding the IL-23-IL-17 immune pathway. *Trends Immunol* (2006) **27**:17–23. doi:10.1016/j.it.2005.10.003
127. Murugaiyan G, Saha B. Protumor vs antitumor functions of IL-17. *J Immunol* (2009) **183**:4169–75. doi:10.4049/jimmunol.0901017
128. Oppmann B, Lesley R, Blom B, Timans JC, Xu Y, Hunte B, et al. Novel p19 protein engages IL-12p40 to form a cytokine, IL-23, with biological activities similar as well as distinct from IL-12. *Immunity* (2000) **13**:715–25. doi:10.1016/S1074-7613(00)00070-4
129. Hatton RD. TGF-beta in Th17 cell development: the truth is out there. *Immunity* (2011) **34**:288–90. doi:10.1016/j.immuni.2011.03.009
130. Langowski JL, Zhang X, Wu L, Mattson JD, Chen T, Smith K, et al. IL-23 promotes tumour incidence and growth. *Nature* (2006) **442**:461–5. doi:10.1038/nature04808
131. Toussirot E. The IL23/Th17 pathway as a therapeutic target in chronic inflammatory diseases. *Inflamm Allergy Drug Targets* (2012) **11**:159–68. doi:10.2174/187152812800392805
132. Van Dyken SJ, Locksley RM. Interleukin-4- and interleukin-13-mediated alternatively activated macrophages: roles in homeostasis and disease. *Annu Rev Immunol* (2013) **31**:317–43. doi:10.1146/annurev-immunol-032712-095906
133. Chapoval S, Dasgupta P, Dorsey NJ, Keegan AD. Regulation of the T helper cell type 2 (Th2)/T regulatory cell (Treg) balance by IL-4 and STAT6. *J Leukoc Biol* (2010) **87**:1011–8. doi:10.1189/jlb.1209772
134. Quatromoni JG, Eruslanov E. Tumor-associated macrophages: function, phenotype, and link to prognosis in human lung cancer. *Am J Transl Res* (2012) **4**:376–89.
135. LaPorte SL, Juo ZS, Vaclavikova J, Colf LA, Qi X, Heller NM, et al. Molecular and structural basis of cytokine receptor pleiotropy in the interleukin-4/13 system. *Cell* (2008) **132**:259–72. doi:10.1016/j.cell.2007.12.030
136. Oh CK, Geba GP, Molfino N. Investigational therapeutics targeting the IL-4/IL-13/STAT-6 pathway for the treatment of asthma. *Eur Respir Rev* (2010) **19**:46–54. doi:10.1183/09059180.00007609
137. Li Z, Jiang J, Wang Z, Zhang J, Xiao M, Wang C, et al. Endogenous interleukin-4 promotes tumor development by increasing tumor cell resistance to apoptosis. *Cancer Res* (2008) **68**:8687–94. doi:10.1158/0008-5472.CAN-08-0449
138. Humphries A, Cereser B, Gay LJ, Miller DS, Das B, Gutteridge A, et al. Lineage tracing reveals multipotent stem cells maintain human adenomas and the pattern of clonal expansion in tumor evolution. *Proc Natl Acad Sci U S A* (2013) **110**:E2490–9. doi:10.1073/pnas.1220353110
139. Schepers AG, Snippert HJ, Stange DE, van den Born M, van Es JH, van de Wetering M, et al. Lineage tracing reveals Lgr5+ stem cell activity in mouse intestinal adenomas. *Science* (2012) **337**:730–5. doi:10.1126/science.1224676
140. Todaro M, Perez Alea M, Scopelliti A, Medema JP, Stassi G. IL-4-mediated drug resistance in colon cancer stem cells. *Cell Cycle* (2008) **7**:309–13. doi:10.4161/cc.7.3.5389
141. Hershey GK. IL-13 receptors and signaling pathways: an evolving web. *J Allergy Clin Immunol* (2003) **111**:677–90. doi:10.1067/mai.2003.1333 quiz 691,
142. Shimamura T, Fujisawa T, Husain SR, Joshi B, Puri RK. Interleukin 13 mediates signal transduction through interleukin 13 receptor alpha2 in pancreatic ductal adenocarcinoma: role of IL-13 pseudomonas exotoxin in pancreatic cancer therapy. *Clin Cancer Res* (2010) **16**:577–86. doi:10.1158/1078-0432.CCR-09-2015
143. Hall B, Nakashima H, Sun ZJ, Sato Y, Bian Y, Husain SR, et al. Targeting of interleukin-13 receptor alpha2 for treatment of head and neck squamous cell carcinoma induced by conditional deletion of TGF-beta and PTEN signaling. *J Transl Med* (2013) **11**:45. doi:10.1186/1479-5876-11-45
144. Shimamura T, Husain SR, Puri RK. The IL-4 and IL-13 pseudomonas exotoxins: new hope for brain tumor therapy. *Neurosurg Focus* (2006) **20**:E11. doi:10.3171/foc.2006.20.4.6
145. Mut M, Sherman JH, Shaffrey ME, Schiff D. Cintredekin besudotox in treatment of malignant glioma. *Expert Opin Biol Ther* (2008) **8**:805–12. doi:10.1517/14712598.8.6.805
146. Ohka F, Natsume A, Wakabayashi T. Current trends in targeted therapies for glioblastoma multiforme. *Neurol Res Int* (2012) **2012**:878425. doi:10.1155/2012/878425
147. Han D, Cai X, Wen J, Kenyon NS, Chen Z. From biomarkers to a clue of biology: a computation-aided perspective of immune gene expression profiles in human type 1 diabetes. *Front Immunol* (2012) **3**:320. doi:10.3389/fimmu.2012.00320
148. Liseth K, Ersvaer E, Hervig T, Bruserud O. Combination of intensive chemotherapy and anticancer vaccines in the treatment of human malignancies: the hematological experience. *J Biomed Biotechnol* (2010) **2010**:692097. doi:10.1155/2010/692097
149. Finn OJ. Cancer immunology. *N Engl J Med* (2008) **358**:2704–15. doi:10.1056/NEJMra072739
150. Braumüller H, Wieder T, Brenner E, Assmann S, Hahn M, Alkhaled M, et al. T-helper-1-cell cytokines drive cancer into senescence. *Nature* (2013) **494**:361–5. doi:10.1038/nature11824

Conflict of Interest Statement: The authors declare that the research was conducted in the absence of any commercial or financial relationships that could be construed as a potential conflict of interest.

15

A mechanistic model for naive CD4 T cell homeostasis in healthy adults and children

Tharindi Hapuarachchi, Joanna Lewis and Robin E. Callard*

Institute of Child Health and CoMPLEX, University College London, London, UK

Edited by:
Miles Davenport, University of New South Wales, Australia

Reviewed by:
Grant Lythe, University of Leeds, UK
Mark Dowling, Walter and Eliza Hall Institute, Australia

***Correspondence:**
Robin E. Callard, Institute of Child Health and CoMPLEX, University College London, 30 Guilford Street, London WC1N 1EH, UK
e-mail: r.callard@ucl.ac.uk

The size and composition of the T lymphocyte compartment is subject to strict homeostatic regulation and is remarkably stable throughout life in spite of variable dynamics in cell production and death during T cell development and immune responses. Homeostasis is achieved by careful orchestration of lymphocyte survival and cell division. New T cells are generated from the thymus and the number of peripheral T cells is regulated by controlling survival and proliferation. How these processes combine is however very complex. Thymic output increases in the first year of life and then decreases but is crucial for establishing repertoire diversity. Proliferation of new naive T cells plays a crucial role for maintaining numbers but at a potential cost to TCR repertoire diversity. A mechanistic two-compartment model of T cell homeostasis is described here that includes specific terms for thymic output, cell proliferation, and cell death of both resting and dividing cells. The model successfully predicts the homeostatic set point for T cells in adults and identifies variables that determine the total number of T cells. It also accurately predicts T cell numbers in children in early life despite rapid changes in thymic output and growth over this period.

Keywords: naive T cells, homeostasis, CD4 T cells, mathematical modeling, mechanistic modeling, children

INTRODUCTION

The naive T cell compartment in humans is generated early in development by the thymus and then maintained throughout life by continued export from the thymus and cell division in the periphery. In adult humans, the naive T cell compartment is comprised of roughly 10^{11} cells circulating between the blood and the peripheral lymphoid organs. It is estimated to comprise at least 10^8 different T cell receptor specificities (1) providing a broad spectrum of protection in a diverse pathogen environment. The size and composition (T cell receptor diversity) of the naive T cell compartment are subject to strict homeostatic regulation and are remarkably stable throughout adult life despite changing rates of cell production and death during T cell development and immune responses (2, 3). Homeostasis is achieved by control of lymphocyte survival and cell division. Naive T cell survival and peripheral cell division depends on access to the cytokine IL7 (4–7) and TCR signals (8, 9) through contact with self-peptide MHC (spMHC) on dendritic cells (10). In lymphoreplete mice, naive T cells are largely non-cycling (11) whereas homeostatic cell division plays an important role in maintaining naive T cell homeostasis in humans, where cell division is evident in the naive pool (12, 13).

In children, homeostatic control of the T cell compartment may be affected by both the growth of the child with the accompanying increased blood volume (14) and changes in thymic output, which increases to a maximum over the first year of life and then declines to reach an approximately steady level by the age of about 20 years (15). As a result, the CD4 naive T cell count (cells/μl) in children declines over the first 10–20 years of life whereas the total number of naive CD4 cells increases as the child grows (**Figure 1**). This raises important questions about whether the homeostatic mechanisms themselves change during early life or whether the numbers of naive CD4 T cells observed are determined only by the changes in thymic output and growth.

To date, our understanding of the processes controlling survival and proliferation of T cells has been largely qualitative and detailed quantitative knowledge of how homeostatic responses result in the observed equilibrium of the T cell pool with a given size and composition is lacking. Here, a two-compartment mathematical model of homeostasis is presented incorporating specific terms for thymic export into the naive CD4 compartment, rates of entry into cell division and death (survival) rates for both the resting and dividing cell compartments. In this sense, the model can be considered as mechanistic in comparison to empirical or descriptive models where the parameters have no direct biological meaning. The results illustrate the importance of T cell dynamics for the maintenance of constant naive CD4 T cell numbers in adults and the growth of the T cell compartment in children.

MATERIALS AND METHODS

A MODEL OF NAIVE T CELL HOMEOSTASIS

T cell homeostasis can be described using a two-compartment model of resting and dividing cells with input from the thymus into the resting compartment as shown in **Figure 2** (16, 17). In this model we will consider only naive CD4 T cells assuming no antigenic stimulation and maturation of naive to memory cells. The same model could in principle also be applied to memory cells and CD8 T cells.

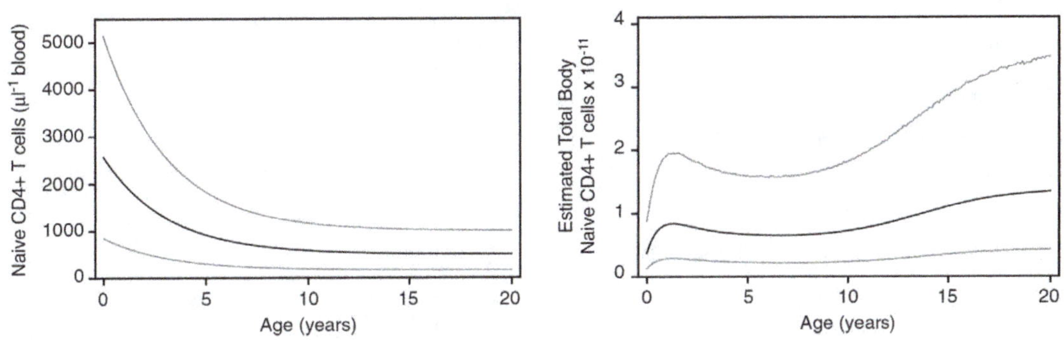

FIGURE 1 | Changes in naive CD4T cell concentration and total whole body numbers with age. Taken from Bains et al. (14).

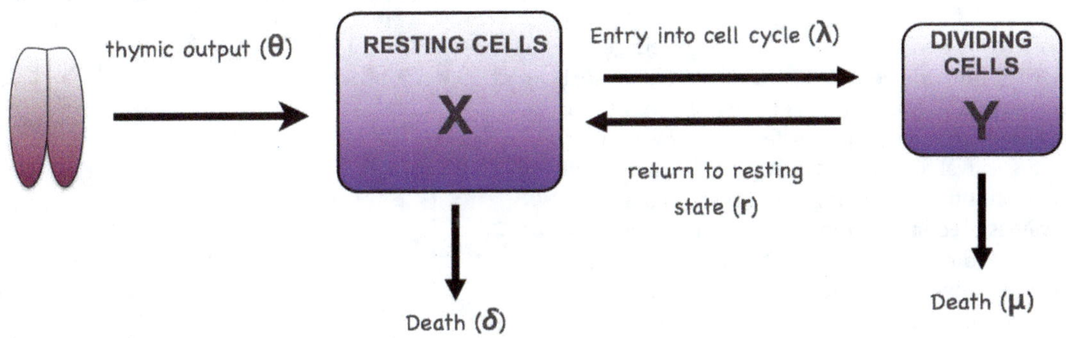

FIGURE 2 | Scheme for two-compartment model of homeostasis

This model can be expressed mathematically using two coupled ordinary non-linear differential equations:

$$\frac{dX}{dt} = \theta + 2rY - \lambda_{(X+Y)}X - \delta_{(X+Y)}X$$
$$\frac{dY}{dt} = \lambda_{(X+Y)}X - rY - \mu_{(Y)}$$

where X is the number of non-dividing (resting) T cells and Y the number of cells undergoing cell division (**Figure 2**). The parameter θ represents T cell export from the thymus, λ the rate at which resting cells enter cell division, r the rate at which dividing cells return to the resting state, δ the death rate of resting cells, and μ the death rate of dividing cells. λ, r, δ, and μ are all first order rate constants, in units of day^{-1}, whereas θ is a zero-order constant, in units of cells day^{-1}.

To develop this model, it is important to have biologically appropriate forms for each of these parameters. Thymic output is known to vary with age with a maximum at about 1 year, which then declines rapidly until about 20 years of age and more slowly thereafter (15, 18). The value of θ for a 20 year old has been estimated to be 3×10^8 CD4 T cells day^{-1} (15). This value was used for modeling CD4 T cell homeostasis in a young adult. In children, the value of θ changes rapidly with age. An expression for θ from 0 to 20 years was determined as described previously (15).

An appropriate form for the rate of entry into cell cycle λ is (19)

$$\lambda = \lambda_0 \exp\left[-N(t)/\varepsilon\right]$$

where $N(t) = X(t) + Y(t)$, i.e., the total number of T cells at time t.

This expression is based on competition between resting naive T cells for signals to enter cell division: TCR signaling by self-peptide MHC and resources such as IL7 (4, 5, 8, 9, 20, 21). The term λ_0 represents the intrinsic ability of a T cell to respond under conditions of no competition (very few cells or an unlimited supply of homeostatic proliferative signals such as IL7), ε is proportional to the amount of resource (IL7) available and N is the total number of T cells competing for the resource. The rate of entry into cell cycle therefore deceases exponentially with decreasing resource or increasing cell number. The rate at which dividing cells return to the resting state r is determined by the length of time taken for one division [known to be about 6 h (19)] and experimental evidence that in homeostatic cell division cells return to the resting state after one division (19, 22). The death rate μ of activated T cells takes the form $\mu = \mu' Y$, which represents density-dependent AICD (activated induced cell death) by Fas–Fas ligand interactions (23, 24). Finally, the death rate of resting cells δ takes the form

$$\delta = \delta_0 \exp\left[N(t)/\rho\right].$$

Table 1 | Parameter values used for the model.

Parameter	Description	Value
Θ	Thymic output for adult 20 years old	3×10^8 cells day^{-1} (15)
λ_0	Rate of entry into cell cycle with infinite resource	0.055 $cell^{-1}day^{-1}$
ε	Resource for entry into cell cycle	1
δ_0	Death rate of resting cells with infinite resource	0.02 $cell^{-1}day^{-1}$
ρ	Resource for resting cell survival	100
r	Rate of return from dividing to resting state	4 day^{-1} (every 6 h)
μ	Death rate of dividing cells	15 day^{-1}

Similar to λ, this term is also derived from the reported dependence of cell survival on competition for a survival signal such as IL7 (resource) where δ_0 is the intrinsic ability of a cell to die under conditions of no competition (very few cells or an unlimited supply of the survival signal) and ρ is proportional to the amount of available resource providing the survival signal (IL7) (21). Parameter values used in the model are shown in **Table 1**.

The model was solved numerically using NDSolve, the proprietary numerical ODE solver in Mathematica that automatically selects the most appropriate method and adapts the step size so that the estimated errors are within the specified tolerance.

RESULTS

HOMEOSTATIC SET POINT IN ADULTS

The homeostatic set point for adults was examined by testing the behavior of the model starting with cell numbers well below and above the equilibrium and with an adult thymic output of 3×10^8 cells day^{-1} (15). Initial conditions were 0 dividing cells and either 0.01 or 2 ($\times 10^{11}$) resting cells. As shown in **Figure 3**, a stable equilibrium of total naïve CD4 T cell numbers (resting plus dividing) was obtained at just over 10^{11} cells, after 200–300 days (see also **Figure 1**). A Jacobian analysis showed that the solutions were stable over a wide range of parameter values for r (>0.281), μ' (<106.79), ε (<1.01), and λ_0 ($>1.05 \times 10^{-14}$) and stability did not depend on thymic output (θ), δ_0, or ρ.

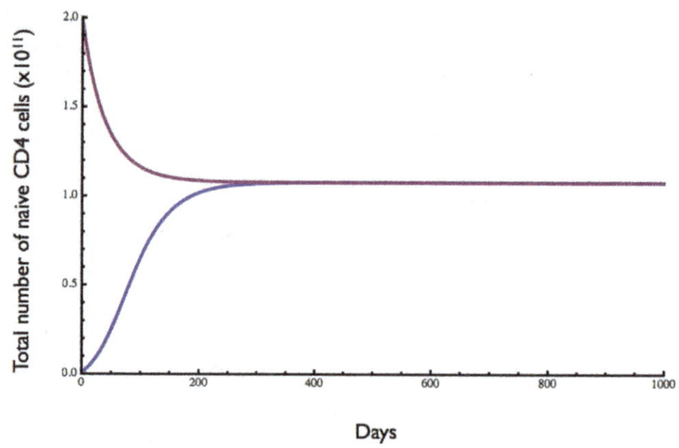

FIGURE 3 | Dynamics of naive CD4T cell homeostasis in adults predicted by the model. Starting with 0.01- or 2-fold the approximate number of naive CD4T cells in a replete young adult, an equilibrium of about 10^{11} cells is reached within 200–300 days. Parameter values are given in **Table 1**.

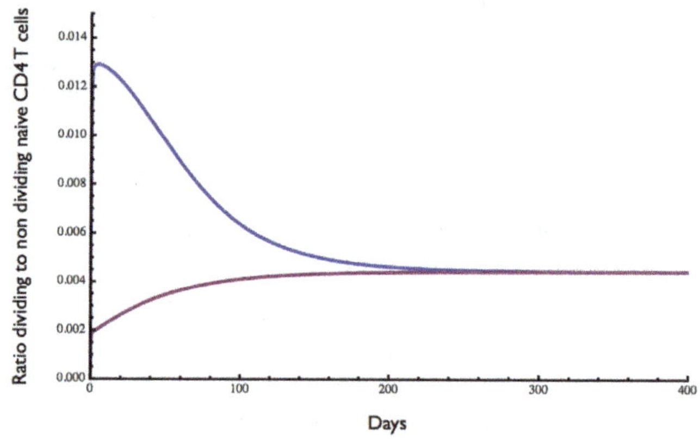

FIGURE 4 | Ratio of dividing to resting cells predicted by the model. Starting with 0.01×10^{11} (blue curve) or 2×10^{11} (red curve) the approximate ratio of dividing to resting cells changes over time to reach an equilibrium of about 0.4%. As expected, the proportion of proliferating cells is greater when the initial cell number is low. Parameter values used in the model are the same as in **Figure 3**.

The ratio of dividing to resting cells is shown in **Figure 4**. With lymphopenic starting conditions of 0.01 ($\times 10^{11}$) resting cells, the proportion of proliferating cells (blue curve) increased very rapidly from 0 to 0.013 and then slowly declined over about 200 days to reach an equilibrium at about 0.5%. In contrast, under starting conditions of excessive T cells, the ratio of dividing to non-dividing cells increased rapidly at first from 0 to about 0.2% and then slowly to reach the same equilibrium of about 0.5%. This equilibrium point is consistent with a low level of cell division in the naive compartment of adult humans as reported previously (25, 26).

EFFECTS OF COMPETITION FOR SURVIVAL AND DIVISION SIGNALS

Next, we investigated the effect of the amount of resource available for cell division (ε) and cell survival (ρ) (**Figure 5**). Consistent with competition between naive CD4 T cells for a resource such as spMHC and/or IL7 in order to survive and undergo cell division, the number of cells at homeostatic equilibrium decreased as the resource terms ε for proliferation and ρ for survival decreased. Interestingly, the rate of entry into cell cycle was significantly more sensitive than survival to changes in resource concentration, consistent with different thresholds for proliferation and survival as previously described (27).

T CELL HOMEOSTASIS IN CHILDREN

Having established the behavior of the two-compartment model for naive CD4 T cell homeostasis in adults, we sought to determine whether it could also be used to explain the changes in T cell numbers that occur during childhood. During the first few years of life as thymic output changes and children grow, the naive CD4 T cell concentration decreases while the total number increases (**Figure 1**). The question is whether the homeostatic mechanism described by the model is in itself enough to explain these variations, or whether different and changing mechanisms apply in children. To examine this question, the model was used to predict the concentration of naive CD4 T cells in cells/μl of blood by converting total numbers to concentration using the estimated blood volume of children at different ages (14). In addition, the changes in thymic output that occur over the first few years of life with a peak at 1 year and then a decline (15) were incorporated into the model. The prediction from the model was then simply compared without parameter fitting to data collected from a cohort of healthy children (born to HIV infected mothers) from the European Collaborative Study on HIV infected pregnant women and their children (28) (**Figure 6**). As can be seen, the model predicted the concentration of T cells over the first 3 years of life extremely well suggesting that the homeostatic mechanisms in children and adults are essentially the same with the only difference being thymic output and growth with a concomitant increase in blood volume.

DISCUSSION

The two-compartment mathematical model presented here is based on the known biology of naive T cell homeostasis. It is derived from an earlier simple model that ignored thymic output and competition for resources (17, 24). Although only naive CD4 T cells are considered here, the same model would essentially be applicable to CD8 T cells. Naive single positive CD4 T cells enter the peripheral pool from the thymus at rates ranging from 4×10^8 to 2×10^9 day^{-1} depending on age from 0 to 20 years, with a peak of 2×10^9 day^{-1} at about 1 year of age (15). In addition to thymic output, maintenance of the naive T cell pool in humans also depends on peripheral T cell division (13). Naive T

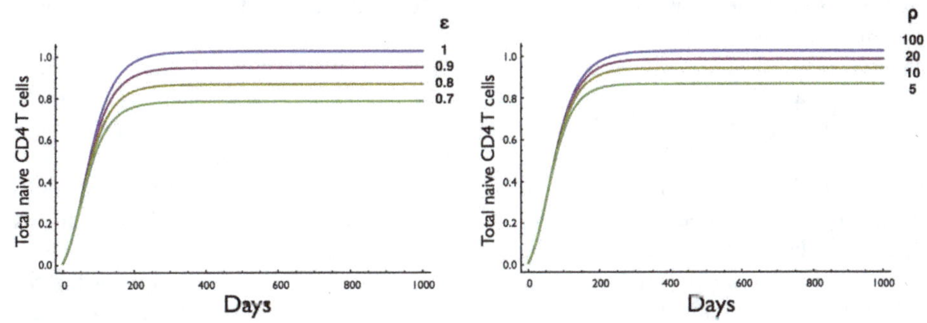

FIGURE 5 | Effect on T cell dynamics of changes in resource concentration for entry into cell division (ε) and survival (ρ). Other parameters are as in **Table 1**. It is noteworthy that the homeostatic equilibrium is more sensitive to changes in the resource parameter (ε) for entry into cell division than the parameter (ρ) for survival.

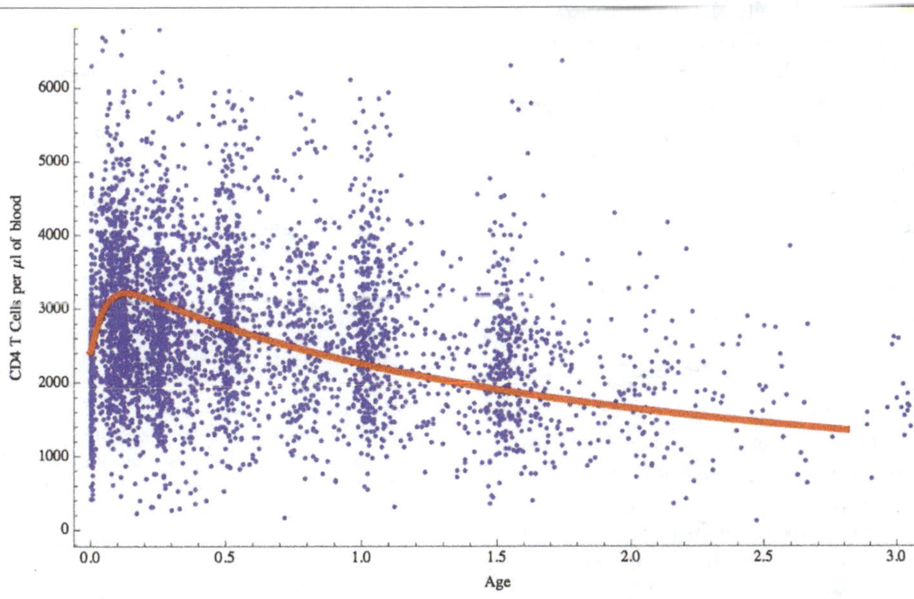

FIGURE 6 | Naive CD4 T cell concentrations (cells/μl of blood) predicted by the model for children aged 0–3 years (red curve) compared with clinical data for normal children.

cell entry into cell division occurs in response to TCR signaling by self-peptide MHC and signals provided by IL7 (4–9, 29). Competition for these resources determines the rate of entry (19, 29). Similarly, survival depends on signaling by IL7 albeit at a different concentration threshold than for proliferation (27). The rate of exit from the cell cycle was taken from the approximate time taken to complete cell division [6 h (19)] and the death rate of the cells in cycle was modeled by the described Fas/Fas ligand mechanism of activated cells (24).

The mathematical model described here consists of two coupled non-linear differential equations representing resting and dividing cell compartments with parameters for thymic export, entry into cell division, return to the resting state and death (at different rates) of resting and dividing cells. Exponential forms were used for entry into cell division and death of cells in the resting compartment to represent the known competition for resources for cell proliferation and survival. Alternative functional forms for density dependence may be worth exploring in the future. The model is a mechanistic model based on the known biology of naïve T cell homeostasis so that the different parameters all have a biological interpretation as indicated in the methods. An alternative but non-mechanistic mathematical model of T cell homeostasis has been described (30), which depends on assumptions about the inheritability of life spans and it cannot therefore be easily compared to the model we describe here. Rather, in our model proliferation and death rates depend on competition for resources as supported by experimental evidence. Our model does however assume the naïve T cell population is homogeneous without taking into account clonal diversity and it would be of interest in the future to develop stochastic ODEs or agent based models.

When T cell export from the thymus was kept constant to represent a young adult, simulated T cell numbers converged from either low or high initial levels to a stable homeostatic equilibrium consistent with cell numbers in a normal, healthy adult. This is concurrent with the increase in T cells observed in response to lymphopenia and the decrease following T cell expansion after infection (16, 17). Consistent with previous studies, the death rate of proliferating cells is higher than that of resting cells in our model (31). The death rate of resting cells found here also agrees approximately with experimental results (32–34). The average time between cell divisions was about 50 days compared to 60 days in the model described by Yates (31). Another interesting aspect of these results was the interdivision time of cells, calculated to be around 30 days. This is comparable to the results of deuterium labeling experiments, which suggest an average of 26 days (16, 17, 34, 35).

The results obtained by altering parameter values gave a clear indication of the effect of the different rates of cell death and proliferation. The corresponding expected rise and fall in the set point of the T cell pool was reassuring. This set point appeared to be more sensitive to increments in the death rate of resting cells than to increases of the same order in the activation rate. Importantly, the T cell numbers at equilibrium decreased as the resource term for entry into cell division (ε) or the resource term for rescue from cell death (ρ) decreased although the equilibrium was less sensitive to changes in the resource required for survival (**Figure 5**). The sensitivity of the homeostatic T cell equilibrium to a resource, such as IL7, is potentially important for understanding conditions resulting in reduced CD4 T cell numbers, such as HIV, and the degree of recovery after treatment with antiretroviral therapy (ART). In a recent study, the degree of CD4 T cell recovery in children on ART was correlated with the initial (pre-ART) CD4 T cell count and the length of time between infection (at birth) and the commencement of treatment (36). One explanation for this finding is that HIV infection compromises lymph node structure and hence the ability to provide resources required for homeostatic T cell division (37, 38). The two-compartment model could then be a valuable tool for exploring T cell homeostasis in HIV and other conditions such as T cell reconstitution following stem cell transplantation.

The other question addressed by the model was whether the incorporated biological mechanisms were in themselves sufficient to explain the known decrease in naive CD4 T cell concentration over the first few years of life when T cell export from the thymus increases to a maximum at 1 year of age and then declines, and the child is growing in size with an accompanying increase in blood volume (**Figure 1**). Total naive CD4 T cell numbers obtained from the model were converted into T cell concentration in the blood using blood volume/age data (14). The model's predictions were found to agree very well with real data from a cohort of children aged 0–3 years (**Figure 6**): the two-compartment model was able to reproduce the initial rise and subsequent slow decline in T cell count observed in healthy individuals over 0–3 years. These findings suggest that the changes in CD4 T cell counts in young children can be explained simply by the change in thymic output and body size as they grow and does not require any additional developmental changes to homeostatic mechanisms. It is important to point out that the thymic export model does not take memory cells into account. However, the proportion of memory cells in the CD4+ T cell pool in children is relatively small and therefore should not have a significant effect on these results (39).

In conclusion, we have presented a mechanistic two-compartment model of naive T cell homeostasis based on the known biology, which reproduces results obtained by other methods with good accuracy. It is likely to be an appropriate model for investigations of T cell reconstitution and homeostasis in diseases such as HIV, in patients given bone marrow transplantation and even for understanding reconstitution after thymic transplants for athymic patients with DiGeorge syndrome.

REFERENCES

1. Arstila TP, Casrouge A, Baron V, Even J, Kanellopoulos J, Kourilsky P. A direct estimate of the human alphabeta T cell receptor diversity. *Science* (1999) **286**:958–61. doi:10.1126/science.286.5441.958
2. Freitas AA, Rocha B. Population biology of lymphocytes: the flight for survival. *Annu Rev Immunol* (2000) **18**:83–111. doi:10.1146/annurev.immunol.18.1.83
3. Jameson SC. T cell homeostasis: keeping useful T cells alive and live T cells useful. *Semin Immunol* (2005) **17**:231–7. doi:10.1016/j.smim.2005.02.003
4. Schluns KS, Kieper WC, Jameson SC, Lefrancois L. Interleukin-7 mediates the homeostasis of naive and memory CD8 T cells in vivo. *Nat Immunol* (2000) **1**:426–32. doi:10.1038/80868
5. Tan JT, Dudl E, Leroy E, Murray R, Sprent J, Weinberg KI, et al. IL-7 is critical for homeostatic proliferation and survival of naive T cells. *Proc Natl Acad Sci USA* (2001) **98**:8732–7. doi:10.1073/pnas.161126098
6. Vivien L, Benoist C, Mathis D. T lymphocytes need IL-7 but not IL-4 or IL-6 to survive in vivo. *Int Immunol* (2001) **13**:763–8. doi:10.1093/intimm/13.6.763

7. Seddon B, Zamoyska R. TCR and IL-7 receptor signals can operate independently or synergize to promote lymphopenia-induced expansion of naive T cells. *J Immunol* (2002) **169**:3752–9.
8. Labrecque N, Whitfield LS, Obst R, Waltzinger C, Benoist C, Mathis D. How much TCR does a T cell need? *Immunity* (2001) **15**:71–82. doi:10.1016/S1074-7613(01)00170-4
9. Seddon B, Zamoyska R. TCR signals mediated by Src family kinases are essential for the survival of naive T cells. *J Immunol* (2002) **169**:2997–3005.
10. Saini M, Pearson C, Seddon B. Regulation of T cell-dendritic cell interactions by IL-7 governs T-cell activation and homeostasis. *Blood* (2009) **113**:5793–800. doi:10.1182/blood-2008-12-192252
11. Tough DF, Sprent J. Turnover of naive- and memory-phenotype T cells. *J Exp Med* (1994) **179**:1127–35. doi:10.1084/jem.179.4.1127
12. Asquith B, Borghans JA, Ganusov VV, Macallan DC. Lymphocyte kinetics in health and disease. *Trends Immunol* (2009) **30**:182–9. doi:10.1016/j.it.2009.07.013
13. den Braber I, Mugwagwa T, Vrisekoop N, Westera L, Mogling R, Bregje De Boer A, et al. Maintenance of peripheral naive T cells is sustained by thymus output in mice but not humans. *Immunity* (2012) **36**:288–97. doi:10.1016/j.immuni.2012.02.006
14. Bains I, Antia R, Callard R, Yates AJ. Quantifying the development of the peripheral naive CD4+ T cell pool in humans. *Blood* (2009) **113**:5480–7. doi:10.1182/blood-2008-10-184184
15. Bains I, Thiebaut R, Yates AJ, Callard RE. Quantifying thymic export: combining models of naive T cell proliferation and TREC dynamics gives an explicit measure of thymic output. *J Immunol* (2009) **183**:4329–36. doi:10.4049/jimmunol.0900743
16. Yates AJ, Callard RE. Cell death and the maintenance of immunological memory. *Discrete Continuous Dyn Syst Ser B* (2001) **1**:43–60. doi:10.3934/dcdsb.2001.1.43
17. Yates AJ, Stark J, Klein N, Antia R, Callard RE. Understanding the slow depletion of memory CD4+ T cells in HIV infection. *PLoS Med* (2007) **4**:e177. doi:10.1371/journal.pmed.0040177
18. Steinmann GG, Klaus B, Muller-Hermelink HK. The involution of the ageing human thymic epithelium is independent of puberty. A morphometric study. *Scand J Immunol* (1985) **22**:563–75. doi:10.1111/j.1365-3083.1985.tb01916.x
19. Hogan T, Shuvaev A, Commenges D, Yates A, Callard R, Thiebaut R, et al. Clonally diverse T cell homeostasis is maintained by a common program of cell-cycle control. *J Immunol* (2013) **190**:3985–93. doi:10.4049/jimmunol.1203213
20. Seddon B, Tomlinson P, Zamoyska R. Interleukin 7 and T cell receptor signals regulate homeostasis of CD4 memory cells. *Nat Immunol* (2003) **4**:680–6. doi:10.1038/ni946
21. Takada K, Jameson SC. Naive T cell homeostasis: from awareness of space to a sense of place. *Nat Rev Immunol* (2009) **9**:823–32. doi:10.1038/nri2657
22. Yates AJ, Saini M, Mathiot A, Seddon B. Mathematical modelling reveals the biological programme regulating lymphopenia-induced proliferation. *J Immunol* (2008) **180**:1414–22.
23. Lynch DH, Ramsdell F, Alderson MR. Fas and FasL in the homeostatic regulation of immune responses. *Immunol Today* (1995) **16**:569–74. doi:10.1016/0167-5699(95)80079-4
24. Callard RE, Stark J, Yates AJ. Fratricide: a mechanism for T memory cell homeostasis. *Trends Immunol* (2003) **24**:370–5. doi:10.1016/S1471-4906(03)00164-9
25. Hellerstein M, Hanley MB, Cesar D, Siler S, Papageorgopoulos C, Wieder E, et al. Directly measured kinetics of circulating T lymphocytes in normal and HIV-1-infected humans. *Nat Med* (1999) **5**:83–9. doi:10.1038/4772
26. Vrisekoop N, Den Braber I, De Boer AB, Ruiter AF, Ackermans MT, Van Der Crabben SN, et al. Sparse production but preferential incorporation of recently produced naive T cells in the human peripheral pool. *Proc Natl Acad Sci U S A* (2008) **105**:6115–20. doi:10.1073/pnas.0709713105
27. Palmer MJ, Mahajan VS, Chen J, Irvine DJ, Lauffenburger DA. Signaling thresholds govern heterogeneity in IL-7-receptor-mediated responses of naive CD8(+) T cells. *Immunol Cell Biol* (2011) **89**:581–94. doi:10.1038/icb.2011.5
28. Bunders M, Thorne C, Newell ML. Maternal and infant factors and lymphocyte, CD4 and CD8 cell counts in uninfected children of HIV-1-infected mothers. *AIDS* (2005) **19**:1071–9. doi:10.1097/01.aids.0000174454.63250.22
29. Kieper WC, Burghardt JT, Surh CD. A role for TCR affinity in regulating naive T cell homeostasis. *J Immunol* (2004) **172**:40–4.
30. Dowling MR, Hodgkin PD. Modelling naive T-cell homeostasis: consequences of heritable cellular lifespan during ageing. *Immunol Cell Biol* (2009) **87**:445–56. doi:10.1038/icb.2009.11
31. Yates AJ, Chan CCT, Callard RE. Modelling T cell activation, proliferation and homeostasis. In: Paton R, Mcnamara L, editors. *Multidisciplinary Approaches to Theory in Medicine*. Elsevier (2006). p. 281–308.
32. Ribeiro RM, Mohri H, Ho DD, Perelson AS. Modeling deuterated glucose labeling of T-lymphocytes. *Bull Math Biol* (2002) **64**:385–405. doi:10.1006/bulm.2001.0282
33. Macallan DC, Wallace D, Zhang Y, De Lara C, Worth AT, Ghattas H, et al. Rapid turnover of effector-memory CD4(+) T cells in healthy humans. *J Exp Med* (2004) **200**:255–60. doi:10.1084/jem.20040341
34. Asquith B, Zhang Y, Mosley AJ, De Lara CM, Wallace DL, Worth A, et al. In vivo T lymphocyte dynamics in humans and the impact of human T-lymphotropic virus 1 infection. *Proc Natl Acad Sci U S A* (2007) **104**:8035–40. doi:10.1073/pnas.0608832104
35. Ganusov VV, Borghans JA, De Boer RJ. Explicit kinetic heterogeneity: mathematical models for interpretation of deuterium labeling of heterogeneous cell populations. *PLoS Comput Biol* (2010) **6**:e1000666. doi:10.1371/journal.pcbi.1000666
36. Lewis J, Walker AS, Castro H, De Rossi A, Gibb DM, Giaquinto C, et al. Age and CD4 count at initiation of antiretroviral therapy in HIV-infected children: effects on long-term T-cell reconstitution. *J Infect Dis* (2012) **205**:548–56. doi:10.1093/infdis/jir787
37. Zeng M, Paiardini M, Engram JC, Beilman GJ, Chipman JG, Schacker TW, et al. Critical role of CD4 T cells in maintaining lymphoid tissue structure for immune cell homeostasis and reconstitution. *Blood* (2012) **120**:1856–67. doi:10.1182/blood-2012-03-418624
38. Zeng M, Southern PJ, Reilly CS, Beilman GJ, Chipman JG, Schacker TW, et al. Lymphoid tissue damage in HIV-1 infection depletes naive T cells and limits T cell reconstitution after antiretroviral therapy. *PLoS Pathog* (2012) **8**:e1002437. doi:10.1371/journal.ppat.1002437
39. Huenecke S, Behl M, Fadler C, Zimmermann SY, Bochennek K, Tramsen L, et al. Age-matched lymphocyte subpopulation reference values in childhood and adolescence: application of exponential regression analysis. *Eur J Haematol* (2008) **80**:532–9. doi:10.1111/j.1600-0609.2008.01052.x

16

Mother and child T cell receptor repertoires: deep profiling study

Ekaterina V. Putintseva[1], Olga V. Britanova[1], Dmitriy B. Staroverov[1], Ekaterina M. Merzlyak[1], Maria A. Turchaninova[1], Mikhail Shugay[1], Dmitriy A. Bolotin[1], Mikhail V. Pogorelyy[1], Ilgar Z. Mamedov[1], Vlasta Bobrynina[2], Mikhail Maschan[2], Yuri B. Lebedev[1] and Dmitriy M. Chudakov[1,3]*

[1] *Shemyakin-Ovchinnikov Institute of Bioorganic Chemistry, Russian Academy of Science, Moscow, Russia*
[2] *Federal Scientific Clinical Center of Pediatric Hematology, Oncology and Immunology, Moscow, Russia*
[3] *Central European Institute of Technology (CEITEC), Masaryk University, Brno, Czech Republic*

Edited by:
Michal Or-Guil, Humboldt University Berlin, Germany

Reviewed by:
Aridaman Pandit, Utrecht University, Netherlands
Nicole Wittenbrink, Humboldt University Berlin, Germany

***Correspondence:**
Dmitriy M. Chudakov, Shemyakin-Ovchinnikov Institute of Bioorganic Chemistry, Russian Academy of Science, Miklukho-Maklaya 16/10, Moscow 117997, Russia
e-mail: chudakovdm@mail.ru

The relationship between maternal and child immunity has been actively studied in the context of complications during pregnancy, autoimmune diseases, and haploidentical transplantation of hematopoietic stem cells and solid organs. Here, we have for the first time used high-throughput Illumina HiSeq sequencing to perform deep quantitative profiling of T cell receptor (TCR) repertoires for peripheral blood samples of three mothers and their six children. Advanced technology allowed accurate identification of 5×10^5 to 2×10^6 TCR beta clonotypes per individual. We performed comparative analysis of these TCR repertoires with the aim of revealing characteristic features that distinguish related mother-child pairs, such as relative TCR beta variable segment usage frequency and relative overlap of TCR beta complementarity-determining region 3 (CDR3) repertoires. We show that thymic selection essentially and similarly shapes the initial output of the TCR recombination machinery in both related and unrelated pairs, with minor effect from inherited differences. The achieved depth of TCR profiling also allowed us to test the hypothesis that mature T cells transferred across the placenta during pregnancy can expand and persist as functional microchimeric clones in their new host, using characteristic TCR beta CDR3 variants as clonal identifiers.

Keywords: TCR repertoires, NGS, maternal-fetal exchange, public clonotypes, T cell receptor, haploidentical transplantation, autoimmune diseases, microchimerism

INTRODUCTION

Closeness and relationship between mother and child immunity have been the focus of studies of pregnancy (1), autoimmunity (2–4) and haploidentical transplantations of hematopoietic stem cells (HSCs) (5), and solid organs (6, 7).

In recent years, the potential of next-generation sequencing (NGS) to reveal the full complexity of human and mouse immune receptor repertoires has inspired numerous efforts to develop optimal techniques for achieving large-scale T cell receptor (TCR) and antibody profiling (8–12) and to decipher various aspects of adaptive immunity (8, 9, 11, 13–17). With appropriate library preparation methods (18), NGS techniques now make it possible to perform quantitative analysis of hundreds of thousands or millions of distinct TCR beta complementarity-determining region 3 (CDR3) variants. This individual diversity of TCR beta CDR3 variants, which is generated in the course of V-D-J recombination and the random addition and deletion of nucleotides in the thymus, largely determines the whole diversity of naïve T cells and specificity of T cell immune responses (19, 20).

In the present study, we have used deep NGS profiling to compare TCR beta repertoires of mothers and their children. We achieved a profiling depth of 500,000–2,000,000 unique TCR beta CDR3 clonotypes per donor, and performed comparative analysis with the aim of revealing specific features of TCR repertoires that distinguish related mother-child pairs from unrelated individuals, and how these familial repertoires manifest the influence of inherited factors, such as the elements of TCR recombination machinery and human leukocyte antigens (HLA). By comparing out-of-frame (i.e., non-functional and thus not subjected to selection) and in-frame TCR beta repertoires, we also show the extent of the impact of thymic selection and the common trends in how this process shapes individual repertoires.

Additionally, the profiling depth that we achieved allowed us to look for the potential presence of maternal or fetal microchimeric T cell clones that may have transmigrated through the placenta as mature α/β T cells and which subsequently persist in both related donors, by using characteristic TCR beta CDR3 variants as clonal identifiers.

MATERIALS AND METHODS

SAMPLE COLLECTION

This study was approved by the ethical committee of the Federal Scientific Clinical Center of Pediatric Hematology, Oncology, and Immunology. Blood donors provided informed consent prior to participating in the study. Ten milliliters of peripheral blood samples were obtained from nine systemically healthy Caucasian donors: three mothers (average age 40 ± 4 years) and their six children (average age 11 ± 4 years). Peripheral blood mononuclear cells (PBMCs) were isolated by Ficoll-Paque (Paneco, Russia) density gradient centrifugation. Total RNA was isolated with Trizol (Invitrogen, USA) in accordance with the manufacturer's protocol.

CONTAMINATION PRECAUTIONS

T cell receptor beta libraries were generated in clean PCR hoods with laminar flow, using reagents of high purity and pipette tips with hydrophobic filters. As an additional precaution, we generated the TCR beta libraries for the two groups being compared – mothers and their children – a month apart, and sequenced the two libraries in two separate Illumina runs to guarantee the absence of inter-library contamination during amplification or on the solid phase of the sequencer.

PREPARING cDNA LIBRARIES FOR QUANTITATIVE TCR BETA PROFILING

cDNA-based library preparation was performed essentially as described previously (9, 12, 16, 18, 21, 22). Briefly, we used the Mint kit (Evrogen, Russia) for first-strand cDNA synthesis. For each donor sample, the whole amount of extracted RNA was used for cDNA synthesis, with 1.5 μg of RNA per 15 μl reaction volume. We incubated the mixture of RNA and priming oligonucleotide BC_R4_short (GTATCTGGAGTCATTGA), which is specific to both variants of the human TCR beta constant (TRBC) segment, at 70°C for 2 min and 42°C for 2 min for annealing. We then added the 5′-adapter for the template switch. The reaction was carried out at 42°C for 2 h, with 5 μl of IP solution added after the first 40 min.

Further cDNA library amplification was performed in two sequential PCRs using Encyclo PCR mix (Evrogen). To capture the maximum number of input cDNA molecules, we used the whole amount of synthesized cDNA for the first PCR amplification. The first PCR totaled 18 cycles with universal primers M1SS (AAGCAGTGGTATCAACGCA) and BC2R (TGCTTCTGATGGCTCAAACAC), which are respectively specific to the 5′-adapter and a nested region of the TRBC segments. The primer annealing temperature was set at 62°C. The products of the first PCR were combined, and a 100-μl aliquot was purified by QIAquick PCR purification Kit (Qiagen) and eluted by 20 μl of EB buffer.

The second PCR amplification was performed for 8–10 cycles with a mix of TCR beta joining (TRBJ)-specific primers and the universal primer M1S ($(N)_{2-4}$(XXXXX)CAGTGGTATCAACGCA GAG), which is specific to the 5′-adapter and is nested relative to the M1SS primer used in the first PCR amplification. XXXXX represents a sample barcode introduced in the second PCR, and $(N)_{2-4}$ are random nucleotides that were added in order to generate diversity for better cluster identification during Illumina sequencing. Primer annealing temperature was set at 62°C.

ILLUMINA HiSeq SEQUENCING

PCR products carrying pre-introduced sample barcodes were mixed together in equal ratio for each of the two groups (mothers and children). Illumina adapters were ligated according to the manufacturer's protocol using NEBNext DNA Library Prep Master Mix Set for Illumina (New England Biolabs, USA). Generated libraries were analyzed using two separate Illumina HiSeq 2000 lanes in separate runs with 100 + 100 nt paired end sequencing using Illumina sequencing primers. Raw sequences deposited in NCBI SRA database (PRJNA229070).

NGS DATA ANALYSIS

TCR beta variable (TRBV) segment identification [using IMGT nomenclature (23)], CDR3 identification (based on the sequence between conserved Cys-104 and Phe-118, inclusive), clonotype clusterization and correction of reverse transcription, PCR, and sequencing errors were performed using our MiTCR software (24)[1]. The sequencing quality threshold of each nucleotide within the CDR3 region was set as Phred >25, with low-quality sequence rescue by mapping to high-quality clonotypes. The strictest "eliminate these errors" correction algorithm was employed to eliminate the maximal number of accumulated PCR and sequencing errors.

STATISTICAL ANALYSIS

We used Jensen–Shannon divergence (JS), which is a symmetrized version of the Kullback–Leibler divergence (KL), to quantify the similarity between the clonotype TRBV gene usage distribution in related and unrelated mother-child pairs. JS and KL are defined as follows (25):

$$\mathrm{JS}\,(P, Q) = \frac{1}{2}\left(\mathrm{KL}\left(P, \frac{P+Q}{2}\right) + \mathrm{KL}\left(Q, \frac{P+Q}{2}\right)\right),$$

$$\mathrm{KL}\,(P, Q) = \sum_i p_i \log_2 \frac{pi}{qi}.$$

Where P and Q correspond to the TRBV gene segment frequency distributions of the two individuals being analyzed, and p_i and q_i stand for the frequency of a particular TRBV gene segment in the first and second individual, correspondingly. For statistical comparison of the JS among related and unrelated mother-child pairs, we used two-tailed, unpaired Student's t-test with P-values <0.05 considered significant. To account for multiple testing, Bonferroni-corrected P-values were used.

We used linear regression to analyze dependency between TRBV CDR3/CDR3 overlap ratio and the number of shared major histocompatibility complex I (MHC-I) alleles, and calculated the Pearson correlation coefficient. The linear model:

$$\mathrm{TRBV-CDR3/CDR3\ overlap\ ratio} = b0 + b1 \times [\mathrm{Number\ of\ shared\ MHC\ alleles}]$$

was fit using the least-squares method. Linear regression and correlation analysis were performed using R programing language[2].

FACS ANALYSIS

We used the following anti-human antibodies: CD3-PC7 (clone UCHT1, eBioscience), CD27-PC5 (clone 1A4CD27, Invitrogen), CD4-PE (clone 13B8.2, Beckman Coulter), CD45RA FITC (eBioscience, clone JS-B3). An aliquot of PBMC was incubated with antibodies for 20 min at room temperature, washed twice with PBS and analyzed via Cytomics FC 500 (Beckman Coulter).

HLA TYPING

The samples were HLA-typed using SSP AllSet Gold HLA-ABC Low Res Kit and SSP AllSet Gold HLA-DRDQ Low Res Kit (Invitrogen) and results were processed using UniMatch software.

---

[1] http://mitcr.milaboratory.com/

[2] http://www.R-project.org/

RESULTS

We obtained at least 1×10^7 TCR beta CDR3-containing sequencing reads for each mother and about 3×10^6 reads for each child. MiTCR software analysis yielded 500,000–2,000,000 distinct TCR beta CDR3 clonotypes per donor (**Table 1**) – representing a significant portion of the total TCR beta diversity for an individual, which lower bound estimate constitutes ~4 million (8). We then subjected these individual TCR beta datasets to comparative analysis in an effort to identify features that distinguish TCR beta repertoires of related mother-child pairs.

TRBV GENE USAGE

We analyzed the relative usage of TRBV gene segments in mother-child pairs at three levels (see **Figure 1**):

Out-of-frame TCR beta variants

The influence of genetic effects on the recombination machinery, which determines the relative frequencies of TRBV gene segment usage in TCRs generated before selection in the thymus, should be reflected by out-of-frame TCR variants that are not subjected to the pressure of further selective processes. Due to nonsense-mediated decay mechanisms, RNA-based libraries generally contain a low percentage of out-of-frame TCR beta variants (9, 12, 26, 27). Nevertheless, out-of-frame CDR3 sequences constituted ~2.5% of all clonotypes (**Table 1**) – 16,048–45,300 clonotypes per donor – which is sufficiently abundant to perform statistical analysis. These subsets were used to compare TRBV gene segment usage in related and unrelated mother-child pairs before thymic selection.

At this level of out-of-frame non-functional TCR beta variants, Jensen–Shannon divergence in TRBV gene usage was comparable for related and unrelated mother-child pairs, albeit with a non-significant increase in divergence for the latter (**Figure 2A**; **Figures 3A,B**, first 2 bars).

Low-frequency in-frame clonotypes

The pressure of thymic selection can be tracked by comparing TRBV gene segment usage in out-of-frame TCR beta variants relative to those variants represented in naïve T cells. In this work, we did not perform separate TCR profiling of FACS-sorted naïve T cells. We aimed to achieve maximal depth of analysis, and sought to avoid the loss of cells and RNA and general quantitative biases that inevitably arise from the cell sorting process. We estimated the pool of TCR beta clonotypes that predominantly belong to the naïve subset as follows. We used FACS analysis to identify the percentage of naïve CD27^{high}CD45RA^{high} CD3+ T cells for each donor (28). This analysis demonstrated that naïve T cells constitute 40–73% of the T cell population in children and 27–55% of the T cell population in mothers (**Table 1**; **Figure 1**). Since each naïve T cell clone is usually represented by minor numbers of TCR-identical cells in an individual (29), for the purposes of bulk analysis, we hypothesized that the subset of the low-frequency clonotypes that occupies the same share of homeostatic space as the FACS-determined share of naïve T cells for that particular donor (433,293–1,797,650 clonotypes per donor) predominantly includes naïve T cells.

At this level of low-frequency, in-frame TCR beta clonotypes, TRBV gene segment usage was significantly less divergent compared to out-of-frame TCR beta variants, both in related and unrelated pairs (**Figures 2B** and **3**). Additionally, TRBV gene segment usage was significantly more similar for related versus unrelated pairs (**Figures 3A,B**, bars 3, 4). In accordance with JS analysis, comparison within related triplets revealed equalization of the usage of particular TRBV gene segments in low-frequency, in-frame TCR clonotypes compared to out-of-frame TCR variants (**Figure 4**). For example, in each triplet, we saw the usage of TRBV gene segments 12-3, 12-4, 20-1, 21-1, and 23-1 equalize in the low-frequency TCR beta clonotypes pool. We also observed an equalizing decrease in TRBV 7-3 usage in triplets A and C, and an equalizing increase in TRBV 28 usage in triplet B.

Notably, the observed changes in TRBV gene segments usage were generally similar in different unrelated donors (compare **Figures 4A–C**), and the convergence of TRBV usage after thymic selection (difference of out-of-frame versus in-frame TRBV usage divergence) was not significantly dependent on the number of shared HLA alleles ($R = 0.12$, $P = 0.63$).

High-frequency in-frame clonotypes

The influence of antigen-specific reactions on selection of TRBV gene segments could be tracked by comparing TRBV gene usage in naïve and antigen-experienced T cells. Following the same logic

Table 1 | Sequencing results: TCR beta reads and clonotypes.

Donor	Sex	Age	Paired end sequencing reads	TCR beta CDR3-containing reads (%)	TCR beta clonotypes before error correction	Final TCR beta clonotypes	% Of out-of-frame clonotypes of all clonotypes	% Of naïve T cells of all T cells (FACS analysis)	% Occupied by >0.001% clonotypes, of all reads
Mother A	F	36	13,656,054	12,513,543 (91.6)	2,044,290	1,708,037	2.7	55.0	19.4
Mother B	F	43	13,872,805	12,901,795 (93.0)	1,213,738	918,557	2.6	27.3	46.2
Mother C	F	43	11,167,059	10,038,463 (89.9)	2,180,886	1,978,745	3.0	39.4	38.2
Child A1	M	11	4,687,578	2,889,352 (61.6)	756,772	729,800	2.6	57.2	16.4
Child A2	M	9	4,202,419	2,467,388 (58.7)	558,173	535,283	2.4	43.0	28.2
Child B1	M	16	4,830,536	3,173,376 (65.7)	821,908	790,592	3.2	60.9	17.2
Child B2	M	10	4,615,093	3,009,961 (65.2)	545,730	517,410	2.3	40.1	34.3
Child C1	F	6	6,081,365	3,940,367 (64.8)	1,104,982	1,060,854	2.3	73.7	13.9
Child C2	M	16	4,564,646	3,008,748 (65.9)	785,164	760,572	2.6	63.7	19.7

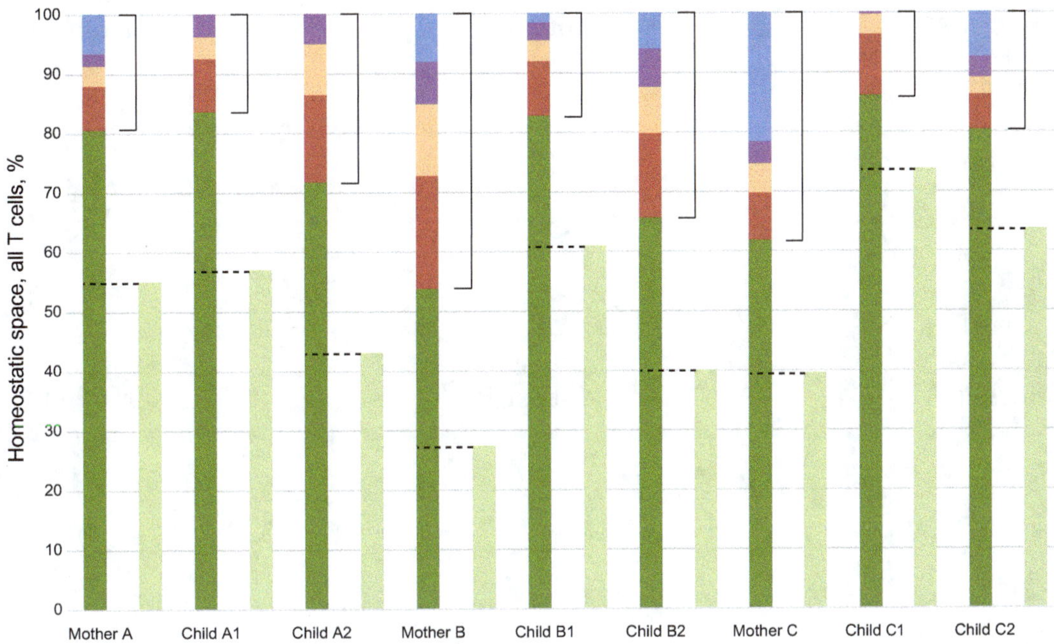

Clone type	Clone Size
Rare	Less than 0.001%
Small	From 0.001% to 0.01%
Medium	From 0.01% to 0.1%
Large	From 0.1% to 1%
Hyperexpanded	More than 1%

FIGURE 1 | Representation of T cell clones of different size in individual TCR beta repertoires. Colored bars represent the share of clonal space occupied by clones of given type (classified by size) for each of the nine donors. Light green bars represent the share of naïve CD27^{high}CD45RA^{high} T cells as determined by FACS analysis. Dashed lines indicate the share of low-frequency TCR beta clonotypes equivalent to this population in each individual, which were included in "low-frequency in-frame clonotypes" analysis. Square brackets indicate the share occupied by high-frequency T cell clones each representing >0.001% of all T cells.

that we used above for the approximate identification of the subset of naïve TCR beta clonotypes, we hypothesized that the most abundant clonotypes predominantly represent antigen-experienced T cell clones. We defined this population as clones representing >0.001% of all CDR3 sequences. Thus, the lower bound for this group was approximately an order of magnitude greater than the upper border set for the low-frequency clones in a given donor's T cell pool (**Figure 1**). Such delineation with a gap between the two subsets minimized "contamination" by naïve TCR beta clonotypes. Still, the pool of high-frequency in-frame clonotypes could contain a portion of naïve clonotypes with TCR beta CDR3 sequence variants of low complexity, that are repetitively produced in thymus due to the convergent recombination events and thus may be highly represented (15).

This set of the 2,803–8,285 most abundant clonotypes per individual cumulatively occupied 13.9–46.2% of the homeostatic T cell space in each donor. These high-frequency TCR beta clonotypes were generally characterized by increased variability in TRBV gene segment usage, and related and unrelated mother-child pairs were nearly indistinguishable (**Figure 2C**; **Figures 3A,B**, bars 5, 6).

OVERLAP OF TCR BETA REPERTOIRES FOR RELATED AND UNRELATED MOTHER-CHILD PAIRS

Several studies in recent years have revealed that unrelated individuals widely share TCR beta repertoires (13–15, 30–32). However, it is presently unclear whether the repertoires of haploidentical individuals are characterized by a higher level of overlap compared to unrelated donors. Additionally, for related mother-child pairs, shared TCR beta variants could conceal microchimeric T cell clones that have been physically shared across the placenta (see below).

To address these questions, we performed comparative analysis of TCR beta repertoire overlap for related and unrelated mother-child pairs by quantifying CDR3 variant identity at the amino acid level, at the nucleotide level, and at the nucleotide level in conjunction with identical TRBV and TRBJ gene segment usage (i.e., fully identical TCR beta chains). We measured overlaps separately for low-frequency and high-frequency in-frame clonotypes (as delineated in **Figure 1**), and all in-frame clonotypes. **Table 2** shows raw, non-normalized numbers of CDR3 variants shared on average by related and unrelated mother-child pairs.

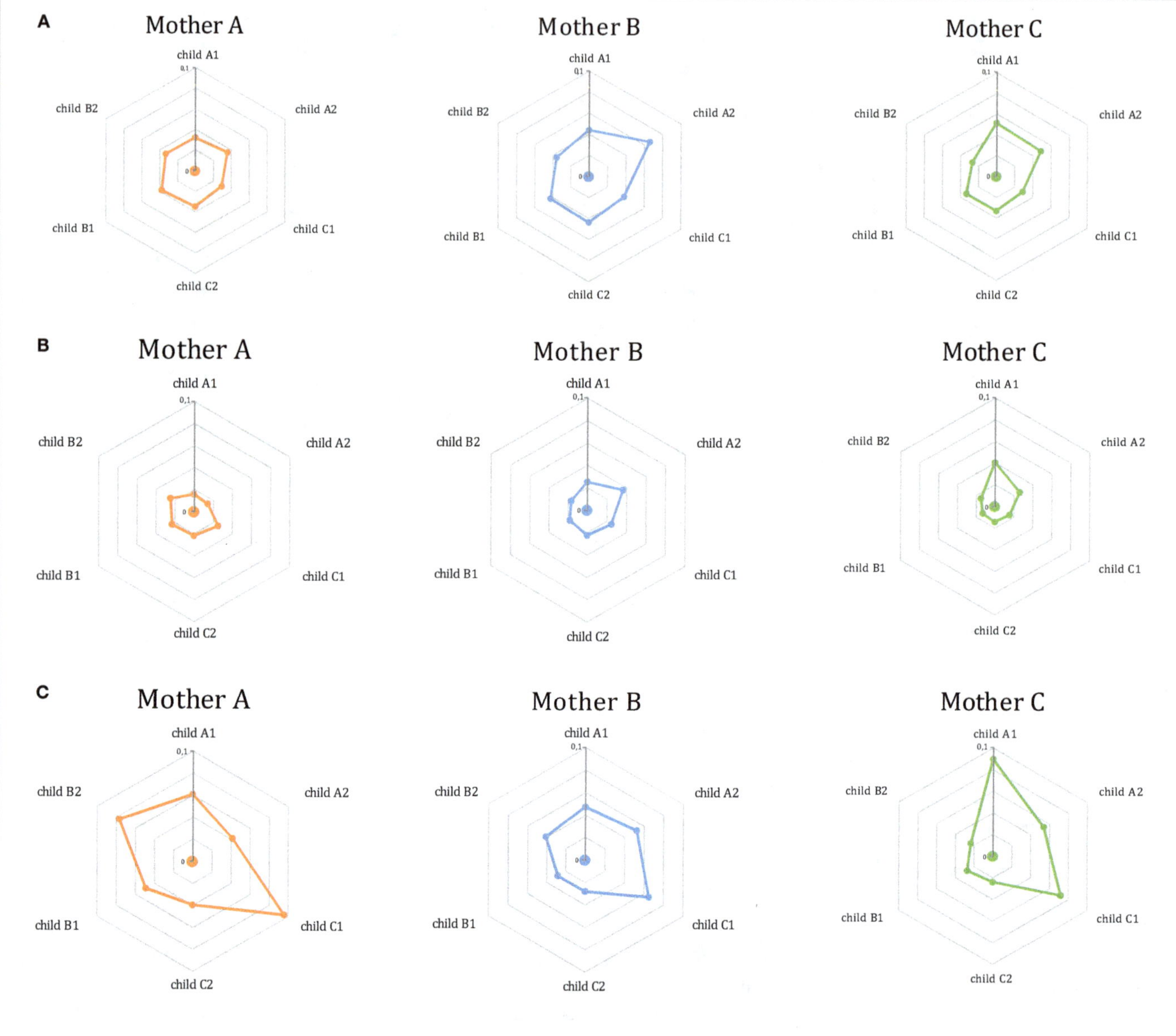

FIGURE 2 | Relative similarity of TRBV gene segments usage analyzed using the Jensen–Shannon divergence method for (A) out-of-frame TCR beta variants; (B) Low-frequency in-frame TCR beta clonotypes; and (C) high-frequency in-frame TCR beta clonotypes. The central dot in each diagram represents Mother **(A)** (orange), **(B)** (blue), or **(C)** (green). Surrounding dots represent the six children. Related children are shown in the same color as their mothers. The closer the "child" dot is to the central "mother" dot, the lower the Jensen–Shannon divergence (i.e., more similar TRBV gene segment usage).

For comparative analysis of relative overlap between subsets of different size, we normalized the number of identical CDR3 variants based on the sizes of the cross-compared samples as follows:

Formula 1: [normalized overlap between TCR sets *A* and *B*] = [overlap between TCR sets *A* and *B*]/([number of clonotypes in set *A*] × [number of clonotypes in set *B*]).

Normalized results are plotted in **Figure 5**. For all CDR3 categories, the degree of overlap was always slightly higher for related pairs, but this difference never approached a significant level compared to unrelated pairs. The highest level of overlap was observed for high-frequency clonotypes, in agreement with the previous work (15).

WITHIN AMINO ACID CDR3 OVERLAPS OF EXPANDED CLONOTYPES, PERCENTAGE OF CLONOTYPES WITH IDENTICAL TRBV GENES IS INCREASED FOR RELATED MOTHER-CHILD PAIRS

The CDR3 region is considered to form interactions mainly with antigenic peptide, while CDR1 and CDR2 encoded in the TRBV segment are mostly responsible for MHC recognition (33–35).

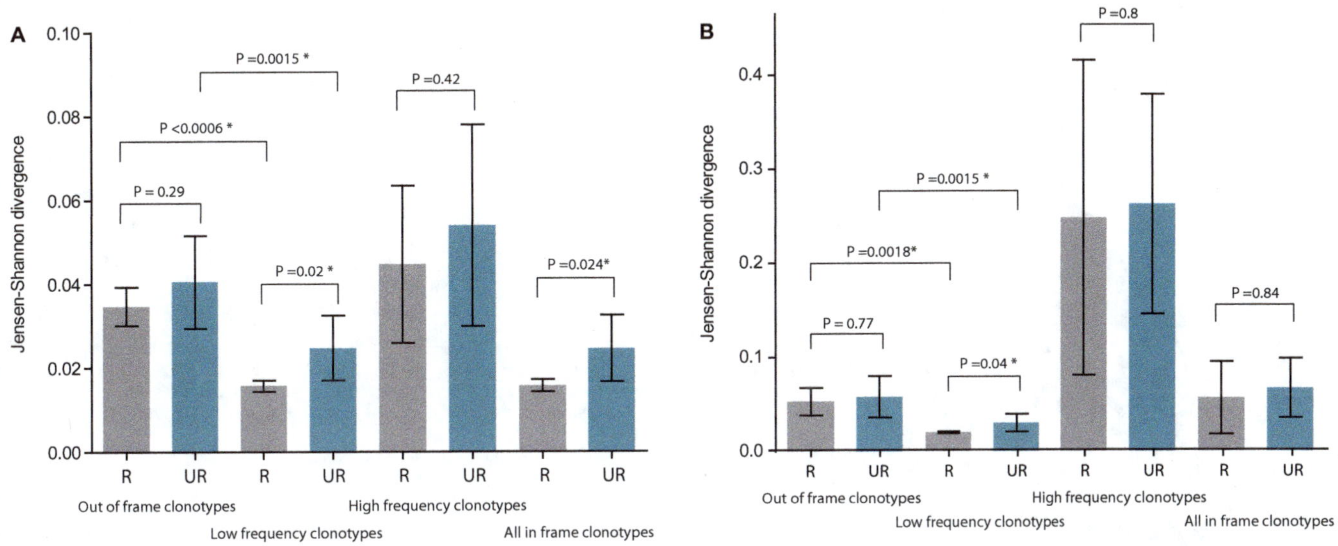

FIGURE 3 | Mean Jensen–Shannon divergence for TRBV gene segment usage for related (R, gray) versus unrelated (UR, blue) mother-child pairs, with SD. Bonferroni-corrected *P*-values are provided to account for multiple testing. **(A)** Comparison of TRBV gene segment usage frequencies at the level of distinct TCR beta clonotypes (but not sequencing reads, so that the influence of relative TCR beta clonotype size within a given repertoire is excluded). **(B)** Comparison of TRBV gene segment usage frequencies at the level of sequencing reads, i.e., considering relative abundance of clonotypes in peripheral blood. The lower the Jensen–Shannon divergence, the more similar the TRBV gene segment usage. *Denotes statistical significance. See **Figure 1** for delineation of low- and high-frequency clonotypes. Please note that "All in-frame clonotypes" include not only low-frequency and high-frequency clonotypes, but also the medium-frequency ones.

Some TRBV segments have nearly identical sequences taking part in CDR3 formation, so two different TRBV segments can often give rise to the same CDR3 amino acid sequence. However, in two individuals with similar or identical HLA alleles, proliferating antigen-specific clones with the same TRBV segment and CDR3 amino acid sequence that recognize the same peptide-MHC complex can be preferentially activated (36). Therefore, since related mother and child pairs share at least 50% of their HLA alleles, we could expect that antigen-experienced clones with identical amino acid CDR3 variants that recognize the same antigenic peptide should more often carry the same TRBV segment encoding CDR1 and CDR2 responsible for MHC recognition.

To verify this hypothesis, we analyzed various repertoire pairs comprising the 10,000 most abundant amino acid CDR3 clonotypes from each individual and computed overlap in terms of shared amino acid CDR3 sequences and shared amino acid CDR3 sequences carrying the same TRBV segment (i.e., identical CDR1, 2, and 3). We then determined the ratio of TRBV-CDR3 overlap to CDR3 overlap for each mother-child pair. In all cases, the ratio was greater for related mother-child pairs (1.3-fold, ±0.16, **Figure 6A**). Moreover, we observed significant positive correlation of this ratio with the number of shared MHC-I alleles between individuals ($R = 0.62$, $P < 0.006$, **Figure 6B**; **Table 3**).

SELECTION IN THE THYMUS DECREASES AVERAGE CDR3 LENGTH COMPARED TO THE INITIALLY GENERATED REPERTOIRE

Comparison of the out-of-frame and in-frame CDR3 repertoires revealed that the former are characterized by higher average length (45.6 ± 0.4 versus 43.3 ± 0.2) and an increased number of added nucleotides (8.6 ± 0.2 versus 7.4 ± 0.1, see **Figure 7A**), in both mothers and children.

This finding indicates that, upon recombination, the initially generated TCR beta CDR3 repertoire (the parameters of which are preserved in the non-functional out-of-frame repertoire) is characterized by higher average length, while further selection in thymus essentially shapes the repertoire toward lower CDR3 length and fewer added nucleotides.

SEARCHING FOR MICROCHIMERIC CLONES TRANSFERRED ACROSS THE PLACENTA AS MATURE T CELLS

It is well established that mother and child exchange cells across the placenta during pregnancy (37–42), and that the progeny of these migrating cells persist in the new host for decades after gestation (43–45).

Most authors agree that lymphoid progenitor cells commonly cross the placenta to populate the new host (45–48). Some observations also indicate that mature T cells can transmigrate through the placenta (see Discussion). However, it remains to be determined whether the transferred mature T cells (hereinafter referred to as mature-microchimeric T cells) can further persist and serve as functional T cell clones in their new host.

We hypothesized that the present deep sequence analysis of such a substantial portion of the maternal and fetal TCR repertoire (including the absolute majority of proliferated antigen-experienced T cell clones) could reveal the presence of transferred and multiplied functional T cell populations, albeit without the immediate ability to distinguish the direction of transfer (i.e., maternal versus fetal microchimerism). Indeed,

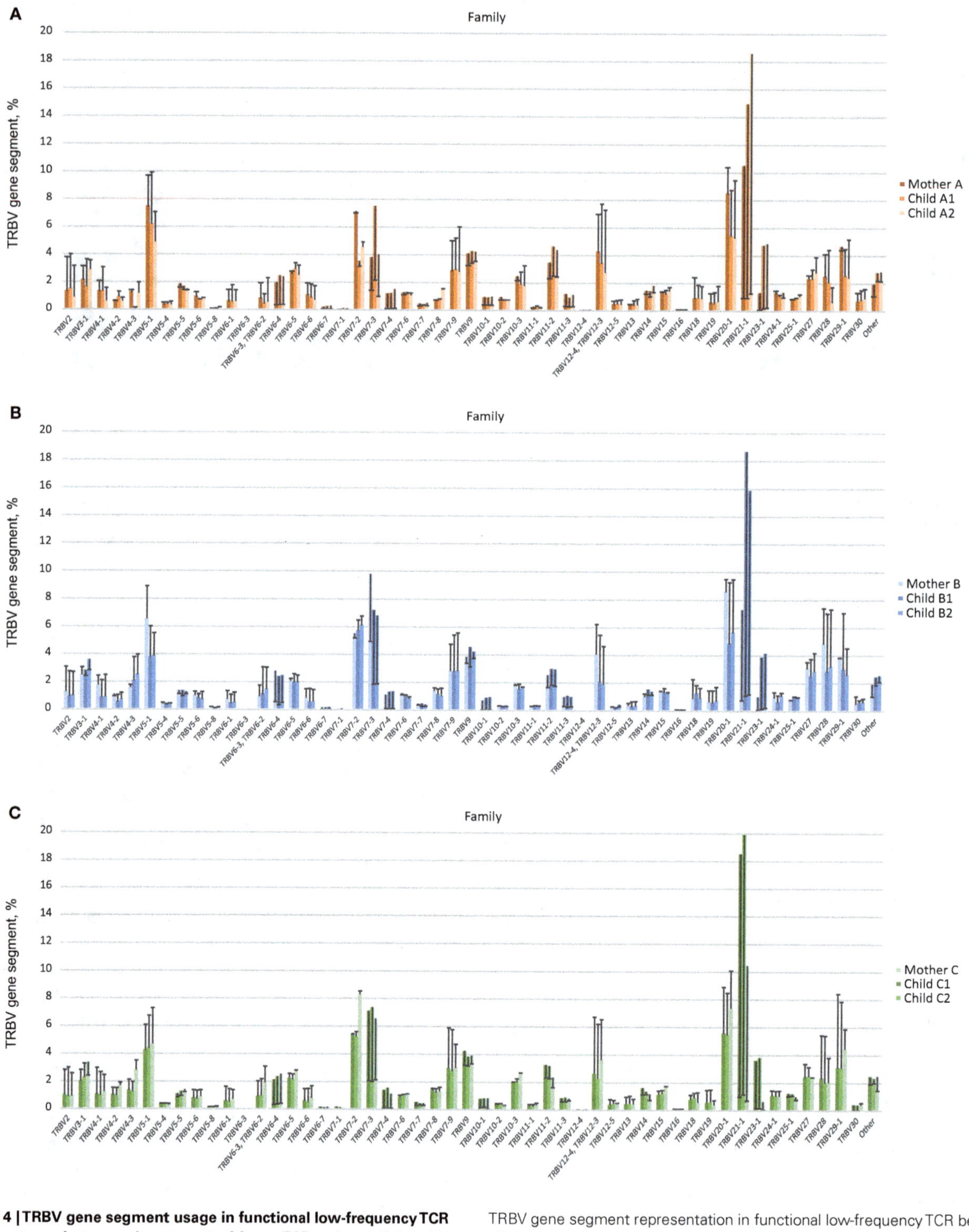

FIGURE 4 | TRBV gene segment usage in functional low-frequency TCR beta clonotypes in comparison to out-of-frame TCR variants. Colored bars indicate the representation of a particular TRBV gene segment family in out-of-frame TCR variants from each individual. Lines represent alterations in TRBV gene segment representation in functional low-frequency TCR beta clonotypes relative to out-of-frame TCR variants. **(A)**, **(B)**, and **(C)** depict TRBV gene segment usage for related donors from family **(A)**, **(B)**, and **(C)**, respectively.

microchimeric T cell clones that were initially transferred across the placenta as mature T cells (mature-microchimeric T cell clones) within a given mother-child pair should be characterized by the same TCR beta CDR3 nucleotide sequence and the same TRBV and TRBJ gene segments, which therefore could serve as a clone-specific identifier.

Table 2 | Average number of shared TCR beta CDR3 clonotypes in related and unrelated pairs.

Pairs	Amino acid			Nucleotide			Nucleotide TRBV, TRBJ identical		
	Low-frequency	High-frequency	All clonotypes	Low-frequency	High-frequency	All clonotypes	Low-frequency	High-frequency	All clonotypes
Related	71,714 ± 25,890	117 ± 34	83,257 ± 26,056	4,938 ± 2,237	69 ± 7	8,407 ± 3,396	2,015 ± 893	40 ± 10	3,456 ± 1,359
Unrelated	68,979 ± 18,822	99 ± 15	80,304 ± 18,626	4,640 ± 1,587	59 ± 12	7,955 ± 2,227	1,823 ± 624	31 ± 11	3,135 ± 897

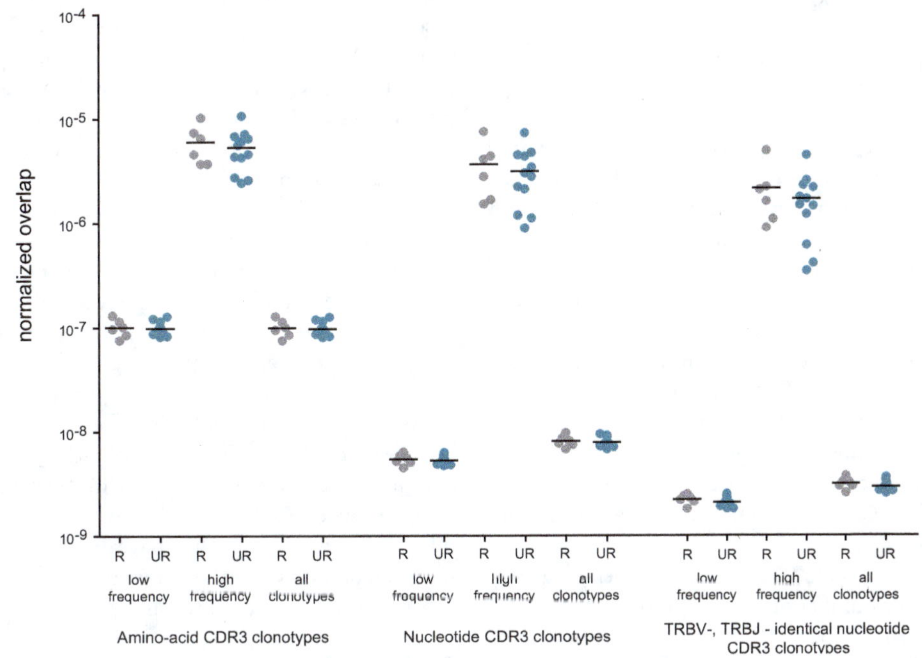

FIGURE 5 | Normalized overlap of individual TCR beta repertoires. Overlaps are shown at the level of CDR3 amino acid sequences, nucleotide sequences, and nucleotide sequences with identical TRBV and TRBJ segments; for related (gray) versus unrelated (blue) mother-child pairs; and for low-frequency, high-frequency, and all in-frame clonotypes. The number of intersections was normalized as described in Formula 1. R, related pairs; UR, unrelated pairs.

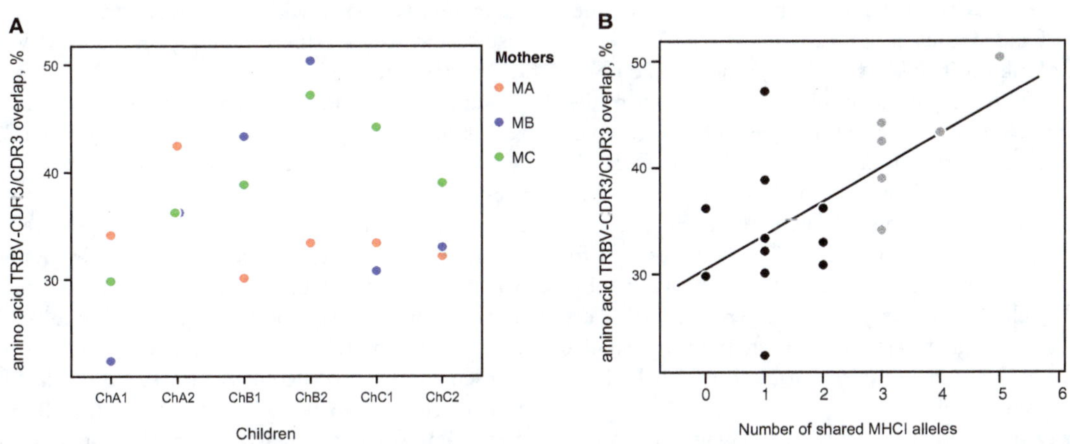

FIGURE 6 | Amino acid TRBV-CDR3/CDR3 overlap ratio. (A) The ratio of TRBV-CDR3 overlap to CDR3 overlap for all possible mother-child pairs, based on the 10,000 most highly represented clonotypes from each donor. Related mother-child pairs had a higher ratio relative to children with either of the unrelated mothers. **(B)** The number of shared MHC-I alleles in mother-child pairs correlates with the TRBV-CDR3/CDR3 overlap ratio for the 10,000 most abundant CDR3 clonotypes. Solid line displays linear regression fit; the Pearson correlation coefficient was 0.62 ($P < 0.006$). Related and unrelated pairs are shown in gray and black, respectively.

Table 3 | HLA typing.

	HLA-A	HLA-B	HLA-C	DRB1	DRB3	DRB4	DQB1
Mother A	02, 24	15, 57	03, 06	07, 14	01–03	01	03, 05
Mother B	02, 23	44, 51	02, 04	07, 11	01–03	01-02	02, 03
Mother C	01, 11	08, 35	04/08, 07	01, 03	01–03	–	02, 05
Child A1	02, 25	15, 18	03, 12	04, 14	01–03	01–02	03, 05
Child A2	02, 02	15, 44	03, 05	11, 14	01–03	–	03, 05
Child B1	02, 23	38, 44	04, 12	07, 13	01–03	01–02	02, 06
Child B2	02, 23	27, 44	02, 04	07, 11	01–03	01–02	02, 03
Child C1	02, 11	35, 38	04, 12	01, 13	01–03	–	05, 06
Child C2	02, 11	35, 38	04, 12	01, 13	01–03	-	05, 06

However, ~40% of the CDR3 nucleotide variants shared between any two individuals were characterized with the same TRBV and TRBJ gene segments, in similar numbers for both related and unrelated mother-child pairs. This means 1,766–5,410 shared clonotype variants across different donor pairs (**Table 2**; **Figure 5**). This widespread sharing of identical TCR beta nucleotide variants makes the TRBV-CDR3-TRBJ identifier insufficient to distinguish clones that were physically transferred across the placenta as mature T cells with recombined TCRs from public TCRs resulting from independent convergent recombination events (15, 32). Thus, if mature-microchimeric T cell clones are present, they are concealed amongst the overwhelming majority of natural public TCRs, and additional characteristics are needed to delineate them.

It has been reported that public TCR beta clonotypes are generally characterized by a low number of added nucleotides in CDR3 (i.e., low complexity) (14, 15, 32). We therefore used the number of added nucleotides as an additional selective characteristic that essentially determines the probability of convergent recombination events leading to CDR3 variants that are identical at the nucleotide level (32, 49). Comparison of this characteristic for all TCR beta CDR3 nucleotide variants and those TRBV-CDR3-TRBJ nucleotide variants that were shared between unrelated mother-child pairs revealed that the latter were characterized by much lower numbers of added nucleotides (**Figure 7A**).

The transfer of mature T cells across the placenta should not be dependent on CDR3 length or the number of added nucleotides. In humans, it has been demonstrated that there is no significant difference between adult blood and cord blood samples in the mean number of added nucleotides (50). Therefore, this characteristic should be essentially identical for both feto-maternal and materno-fetal mature-microchimeric T cell clones and for the general TCR beta repertoire. If the TCR beta repertoires of related mother-child pairs carry mature-microchimeric T cell clones of interest, we would expect to observe shaping of the added nucleotide curve proportional to the contribution of such clones to the repertoire overlap (**Figure 7B**).

The sensitivity of this method to the percentage of mature-microchimeric T cell clones in the shared TCR beta population is therefore limited by the natural dispersion of the added nucleotide curves for unrelated pairs. For example, if mature-microchimeric T cell clones contribute ~0.3% of the TRBV-CDR3-TRBJ overlap for a mother-child pair (i.e., ~10 out of 3,000 overlapping clonotypes, out of the ~1×10^6 total clonotypes sequenced from each donor), the shape of the added nucleotide curve would be indistinguishable from that of an unrelated donor pair – and therefore below the sensitivity threshold of this method. In contrast, the presence of 100 mature-microchimeric T cell clones out of 3,000 clonotypes (i.e., 3.3% of shared variants) per pair of related donors could be clearly distinguished (**Figure 7B**), and this can therefore be considered as the approximate sensitivity limit of the method. We subsequently determined that the presence of mature-microchimeric T cell clones is undetectable in all cases, based on the added nucleotide curves for overlapping TRBV-CDR3-TRBJ nucleotide sequences for our six related mother-child pairs (**Figure 7C**). Correspondingly, the average numbers of added nucleotides in the shared TRBV-CDR3-TRBJ nucleotide variants were indistinguishable for related versus unrelated mother-child pairs (data not shown).

The above-described comparison of added nucleotide curves was performed at the level of distinct TCR beta clonotypes, but not sequencing reads, so that the influence of each T cell clone's relative representation within the repertoire was excluded. Similar albeit noisier results we have obtained when performing the same analysis at the level of sequencing reads (i.e., taking into account relative clonal size).

As such, we have not identified any meaningful difference between the subsets of shared TRBV-CDR3-TRBJ nucleotide variants for related versus unrelated mother-child pairs that would allow us to establish detection of a subpopulation of mature-microchimeric T cells that have been systemically shared during pregnancy as mature naïve or memory T cells, and which subsequently have engrafted and survived for years.

DISCUSSION

TRBV GENE USAGE

For out-of-frame TCR beta variants, which are not expressed and thus avoid any selection, TRBV gene usage was slightly more similar but generally comparable for related versus unrelated mother-child pairs (**Figures 2A** and **3**). This indicates that inherited maternal factors associated with the TCR recombination machinery are insufficient to yield the essentially similar TRBV gene segment selection in the child.

Remarkably, both within related and unrelated pairs, TRBV gene segment usage in low-frequency in-frame TCR beta clonotypes was more similar compared to that in the out-of-frame TCR beta variants (**Figure 3**). The equalization of the usage of TRBV gene segments in functional TCR variants (**Figure 4**) is probably a manifestation of selective pressure during thymic T cell selection, which should distinguish TRBV gene usage in functional TCRs from that preserved in unselected, out-of-frame TCR beta variants. This pressure on relative TRBV usage frequencies was prominent and led to significant convergence in both related ($P = 0.0006$) and unrelated ($P = 0.0015$) pairs, indicating that thymic selection essentially and similarly shapes the initial output of the TCR recombination machinery at the population level.

Interestingly, thymic selection also essentially filters out the longest CDR3 variants with large numbers of added nucleotides, as can be concluded from our comparison of non-functional out-of-frame and in-frame TCR beta CDR3 repertoires (**Figure 7A**).

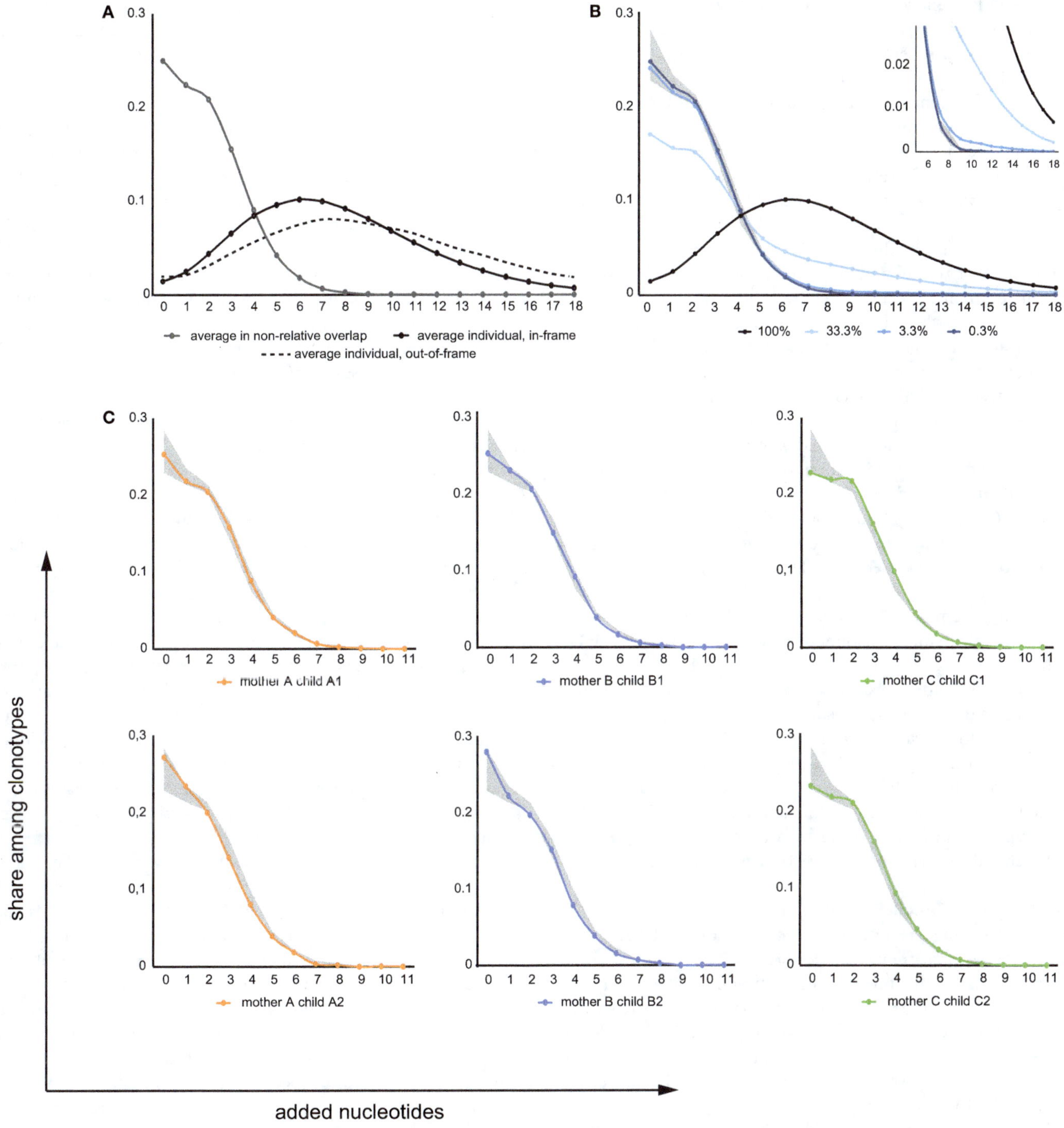

FIGURE 7 | Added nucleotide curves. **(A)** Average distribution of added nucleotides within CDR3 for individual TCR beta repertoires (in-frame: black solid line; out-of-frame: black dashed line) and for TCR beta clonotypes shared between unrelated individuals (gray). **(B)** Modeling of added nucleotide curves for shared TRBV-CDR3-TRBJ variants between mother-child pairs based on input of mature-microchimeric TCR beta CDR3 variants in different proportions. This was derived from the curves in **(A)**, which depict added nucleotide distributions for shared clonotypes between unrelated individuals (gray; equivalent to near-zero contribution to shared clonotypes) and for any individual repertoire (black; equivalent to 100% contribution to shared clonotypes), mixed in different proportions. Lines represent model input where mature-microchimeric TCR beta is equal to 100, 33, 3.3, or 0.3% of shared clonotypes. Shaded region shows the range for unrelated pairs. Inset shows a magnified view. **(C)** Added nucleotide curves for TRBV-CDR3-TRBJ variants shared in each related mother-child pair. Shaded region shows the range for unrelated pairs.

Since TRBV gene segments encode the fragments of TCR chains that interact with MHC (33–35), we would expect that related mother-child pairs, being haploidentical (i.e., sharing at least 50% of HLA alleles), are characterized by more similar TRBV gene segment usage frequencies at the level of functional T cells compared to unrelated donor pairs due to the impact of identical HLA genes in thymic selection. Indeed, we observed that differences in TRBV gene segment usage in related versus unrelated pairs became more pronounced and statistically significant ($P = 0.02$) at the level of low-frequency, in-frame TCR beta CDR3 clonotypes (**Figure 3**). However, the general direction of TCR beta repertoire shaping was similar for related and unrelated donors, suggesting that the pressure of thymic selection is relatively homogenous in the population. The strength of this general pressure was far greater relative to the specific changes that were characteristic of related donors, which only added a minor codirectional trend (**Figures 3** and **4**).

The subset of high-frequency TCR beta clonotypes was characterized by increased variability in TRBV segment usage, and related and unrelated mother-child pairs were indistinguishable at this level (**Figures 2C** and **3**). This is presumably due to the fact that different antigen specificities (but not TRBV segment interaction with MHC) play a dominant role in the priming and expansion of T cell clones, and this semi-random process negates the initial correlations that we observed in TRBV gene usage at the level of naïve T cells.

It should be noted, however, that the above analysis refers to low- and high-frequency clonotypes, which do not fully coincide with the naïve and antigen-experienced T cell subsets, respectively. It was previously demonstrated in other studies that recombinatorial biases might result in relatively high frequencies for certain naïve T cell clones, whereas some memory T cell clones may occur at relatively low frequencies (11, 14, 15). Moreover, these studies have shown a substantial overlap between the naïve and memory T cell repertoires, which suggests that a number of TCR beta CDR3 clonotypes could be associated with both subsets, being paired with either the same or alternative TCR alpha chains.

OVERLAP OF TCR BETA REPERTOIRES

We observed the greatest relative overlap of TCR beta repertoires among high-frequency clonotypes. This observation can be explained by the presence of common expanded antigen-experienced clonotypes recognizing the same antigens, as well as of high-frequency naïve clonotypes carrying the TCR beta CDR3 sequence variants of low complexity that are repetitively produced in thymus and may be highly represented both within and between individuals (15).

In all comparisons, only slightly higher numbers of shared clonotypes were observed in related versus unrelated mother-child pairs (**Figure 5**). This observation is in agreement with the previous report by Robins et al. where the overlap in the naïve CD8+ CDR3 sequence repertoires was suggested to be independent of the degree of HLA matching based on results obtained from three related donors (14). Here, we have achieved a more accurate comparison by studying a larger cohort of related donors, using unbiased library preparation techniques, sequencing the samples being compared on separate Illumina lanes to protect from potential cross-sample contamination on the solid phase and performing deeper individual profiling. Even with these various methodological improvements, we still observed only a subtle trend toward increased TCR beta repertoire overlap in related individuals.

However, among the shared high-frequency amino acid CDR3 variants, the percentage of TRBV-CDR3 identical clonotypes was always higher for related pairs compared to unrelated ones, and correlated with the number of identical MHC-I alleles (**Figure 6**). This finding indicates that optimal recognition of the particular peptide-MHC complex often requires full functional convergence of the TCR beta chain, leading to an increased share of TRBV-identical common CDR3 variants in individuals carrying the same HLA alleles. Notably, this phenomenon was observed for bulk T cell populations, where the input of CD8+ T cells was sufficient to provide correlation. This correlation would probably be much higher if we were to specifically analyze sorted CD8+ T cells.

SEARCHING FOR PERSISTENT MATURE-MICROCHIMERIC CLONES

In humans, maternal T cells are present in different fetal tissues (46, 48, 51), and may be present in the cord blood at a frequency of 0.1–0.5% of total T cells (48, 52). This can represent hundreds of thousands or millions of cells, of which many are likely to be memory T cells (52) capable of further clonal proliferation. Transmigration of maternal differentiated effector/memory Th1 and Th17 cells through the placenta was recently demonstrated in mouse models (53). Transfer of mature T cells is also possible in the opposite direction, and the presence of fetal microchimeric CD4+ and CD8+ T cells was registered in maternal blood during normal pregnancy in humans, predominantly in the third trimester (41) when mature α/β T cells are circulating in the fetus at significant numbers (54). Such mature-microchimeric T cell clones could further affect immunity to solid tumors (55, 56), influence transplantation tolerance (7), cause autoimmune diseases (3, 4, 43, 56–59), or protect the child against infections he/she has never encountered before.

Recent work has demonstrated that, in general, experienced clonal T cells commonly persist in the body for many years (17, 60). We have observed more than 20,000 TCR beta clonotypes that persisted in a patient for at least 7 years – from 2005 until 2012 – even after the patient underwent autologous HSC transplantation in 2009 [Ref. (16) and our unpublished data]. Similarly, naïve T cell clones persist in the body for many years after loss of thymus functionality (61). Therefore, if the engraftment of mature T cell clones transferred from mother to child and/or *vice versa* is a systemic process, we could expect to be able to verify the presence of such clones by using characteristic TCR beta CDR3 variants as clonal identifiers.

In our repertoire analysis, we did not observe mature-microchimeric T cell clones at a level of methodological sensitivity of ~100 mature-microchimeric clones per 10^6 analyzed TCR beta clonotypes. Still, this does not preclude the existence of mature T cell-based maternal or fetal microchimerism at levels below the sensitivity achieved in the current study, in minor number of individuals, or in pathological conditions such as autoimmune disease.

It should be noted that deep TCR beta profiling methodology presently appears to be insufficiently sensitive for identifying particular expanded mature-microchimeric T cell clones, due to the general abundance of common identical TCR beta clonotypes. The following combination of methods could offer a potential way forward: (1) deep TCR beta profiling suggesting the presence of a particular expanded mature-microchimeric T cell clone, preferably with many added nucleotides within CDR3; (2) cell sorting using a TRBV family specific antibody in order to enrich for the hypothetical microchimeric clone of interest; and (3) real-time PCR confirmation of increased microchimerism in the sorted sample.

We also believe that further development of NGS profiling methods – especially in combination with the use of live cell-based emulsion PCR to identify paired TCR alpha-beta chains (62), and to potentially identify TCR beta chains paired with specific HLA molecules serving as an internal marker of microchimeric clones – should greatly facilitate future studies of mature T cell microchimerism in health and disease.

ACKNOWLEDGMENTS

We are grateful to M. Eisenstein for the English editing. This work was supported by the Molecular and Cell Biology program RAS, Russian Foundation for Basic Research (12-04-33139, 13-04-01124, 12-04-00229, 13-04-00998), and European Regional Development Fund (CZ.1.05/1.1.00/02.0068).

REFERENCES

1. Zenclussen AC. Adaptive immune responses during pregnancy. *Am J Reprod Immunol* (2013) **69**:291–303. doi:10.1111/aji.12097
2. Nelson JL, Furst DE, Maloney S, Gooley T, Evans PC, Smith A, et al. Microchimerism and HLA-compatible relationships of pregnancy in scleroderma. *Lancet* (1998) **351**:559–62. doi:10.1016/S0140-6736(97)08357-8
3. Sarkar K, Miller FW. Possible roles and determinants of microchimerism in autoimmune and other disorders. *Autoimmun Rev* (2004) **3**:454–63. doi:10.1016/j.autrev.2004.06.004
4. Lepez T, Vandewoestyne M, Hussain S, Van Nieuwerburgh F, Poppe K, Velkeniers B, et al. Fetal microchimeric cells in blood of women with an autoimmune thyroid disease. *PLoS One* (2011) **6**:e29646. doi:10.1371/journal.pone.0029646
5. Stern M, Ruggeri L, Mancusi A, Bernardo ME, De Angelis C, Bucher C, et al. Survival after T cell-depleted haploidentical stem cell transplantation is improved using the mother as donor. *Blood* (2008) **112**:2990–5. doi:10.1182/blood-2008-01-135285
6. Burlingham WJ, Benichou G. Bidirectional alloreactivity: a proposed microchimerism-based solution to the NIMA paradox. *Chimerism* (2012) **3**:29–36. doi:10.4161/chim.21668
7. Jankowska-Gan E, Sheka A, Sollinger HW, Pirsch JD, Hofmann RM, Haynes LD, et al. Pretransplant immune regulation predicts allograft outcome: bidirectional regulation correlates with excellent renal transplant function in living-related donor-recipient pairs. *Transplantation* (2012) **93**:283–90. doi:10.1097/TP.0b013e31823e46a0
8. Robins HS, Campregher PV, Srivastava SK, Wacher A, Turtle CJ, Kahsai O, et al. Comprehensive assessment of T-cell receptor beta-chain diversity in alphabeta T cells. *Blood* (2009) **114**:4099–107. doi:10.1182/blood-2009-04-217604
9. Mamedov IZ, Britanova OV, Bolotin DA, Chkalina AV, Staroverov DB, Zvyagin IV, et al. Quantitative tracking of T cell clones after haematopoietic stem cell transplantation. *EMBO Mol Med* (2011) **3**:201–7. doi:10.1002/emmm.201100129
10. Nguyen P, Ma J, Pei D, Obert C, Cheng C, Geiger TL. Identification of errors introduced during high throughput sequencing of the T cell receptor repertoire. *BMC Genomics* (2011) **12**:106. doi:10.1186/1471-2164-12-106
11. Warren RL, Freeman JD, Zeng T, Choe G, Munro S, Moore R, et al. Exhaustive T-cell repertoire sequencing of human peripheral blood samples reveals signatures of antigen selection and a directly measured repertoire size of at least 1 million clonotypes. *Genome Res* (2011) **21**:790–7. doi:10.1101/gr.115428.110
12. Bolotin DA, Mamedov IZ, Britanova OV, Zvyagin IV, Shagin D, Ustyugova SV, et al. Next generation sequencing for TCR repertoire profiling: platform-specific features and correction algorithms. *Eur J Immunol* (2012) **42**:3073–83. doi:10.1002/eji.201242517
13. Venturi V, Price DA, Douek DC, Davenport MP. The molecular basis for public T-cell responses? *Nat Rev Immunol* (2008) **8**:231–8. doi:10.1038/nri2260
14. Robins HS, Srivastava SK, Campregher PV, Turtle CJ, Andriesen J, Riddell SR, et al. Overlap and effective size of the human CD8+ T cell receptor repertoire. *Sci Transl Med* (2010) **2**:47ra64. doi:10.1126/scitranslmed.3001442
15. Venturi V, Quigley MF, Greenaway HY, Ng PC, Ende ZS, McIntosh T, et al. A mechanism for TCR sharing between T cell subsets and individuals revealed by pyrosequencing. *J Immunol* (2011) **186**:4285–94. doi:10.4049/jimmunol.1003898
16. Britanova OV, Bochkova AG, Staroverov DB, Fedorenko DA, Bolotin DA, Mamedov IZ, et al. First autologous hematopoietic SCT for ankylosing spondylitis: a case report and clues to understanding the therapy. *Bone Marrow Transplant* (2012) **47**:1479–81. doi:10.1038/bmt.2012.44
17. Klarenbeek PL, Remmerswaal EB, ten Berge IJ, Doorenspleet ME, Van Schaik BD, Esveldt RE, et al. Deep sequencing of antiviral T-cell responses to HCMV and EBV in humans reveals a stable repertoire that is maintained for many years. *PLoS Pathog* (2012) **8**:e1002889. doi:10.1371/journal.ppat.1002889
18. Mamedov IZ, Britanova OV, Zvyagin IV, Turchaninova MA, Bolotin DA, Putintseva EV, et al. Preparing unbiased T cell receptor and antibody cDNA libraries for the deep next generation sequencing profiling. *Front Immunol* (2013) **4**:456. doi:10.3389/fimmu.2013.00456
19. Nemazee D. Receptor editing in lymphocyte development and central tolerance. *Nat Rev Immunol* (2006) **6**:728–40. doi:10.1038/nri1939
20. Venturi V, Rudd BD, Davenport MP. Specificity, promiscuity, and precursor frequency in immunoreceptors. *Curr Opin Immunol* (2013) **25**(5):639–45. doi:10.1016/j.coi.2013.07.001
21. Douek DC, Betts MR, Brenchley JM, Hill BJ, Ambrozak DR, Ngai KL, et al. A novel approach to the analysis of specificity, clonality, and frequency of HIV-specific T cell responses reveals a potential mechanism for control of viral escape. *J Immunol* (2002) **168**:3099–104.
22. Britanova OV, Staroverov DB, Chkalina AV, Kotlobay AA, Zvezdova ES, Bochkova AG, et al. Single high-dose treatment with glucosaminyl-muramyl dipeptide is ineffective in treating ankylosing spondylitis. *Rheumatol Int* (2011) **31**:1101–3. doi:10.1007/s00296-010-1663-3
23. Lefranc MP, Giudicelli V, Busin C, Malik A, Mougenot I, Dehais P, et al. LIGM-DB/IMGT: an integrated database of Ig and TcR, part of the immunogenetics database. *Ann N Y Acad Sci* (1995) **764**:47–9. doi:10.1111/j.1749-6632.1995.tb55805.x
24. Bolotin DA, Shugay M, Mamedov IZ, Putintseva EV, Turchaninova MA, Zvyagin IV, et al. MiTCR: software for T-cell receptor sequencing data analysis. *Nat Methods* (2013) **10**(9):813–4. doi:10.1038/nmeth.2555
25. Lin JT. Divergence measures based on the Shannon entropy. *IEEE Trans Inf Theory* (1991) **37**:145–51. doi:10.1109/18.61115
26. Wang J, Vock VM, Li S, Olivas OR, Wilkinson MF. A quality control pathway that down-regulates aberrant T-cell receptor (TCR) transcripts by a mechanism requiring UPF2 and translation. *J Biol Chem* (2002) **277**:18489–93. doi:10.1074/jbc.M111781200
27. Bhalla AD, Gudikote JP, Wang J, Chan WK, Chang YF, Olivas OR, et al. Nonsense codons trigger an RNA partitioning shift. *J Biol Chem* (2009) **284**:4062–72. doi:10.1074/jbc.M805193200
28. Favre D, Stoddart CA, Emu B, Hoh R, Martin JN, Hecht FM, et al. HIV disease progression correlates with the generation of dysfunctional naive CD8(low) T cells. *Blood* (2011) **117**:2189–99. doi:10.1182/blood-2010-06-288035
29. Arstila TP, Casrouge A, Baron V, Even J, Kanellopoulos J, Kourilsky P. A direct estimate of the human alphabeta T cell receptor diversity. *Science* (1999) **286**:958–61. doi:10.1126/science.286.5441.958
30. Venturi V, Chin HY, Asher TE, Ladell K, Scheinberg P, Bornstein E, et al. TCR beta-chain sharing in human CD8+ T cell responses to cytomegalovirus and EBV. *J Immunol* (2008) **181**:7853–62.
31. Li H, Ye C, Ji G, Han J. Determinants of public T cell responses. *Cell Res* (2012) **22**:33–42. doi:10.1038/cr.2012.1
32. Li H, Ye C, Ji G, Wu X, Xiang Z, Li Y, et al. Recombinatorial biases and convergent recombination determine interindividual TCRbeta sharing in murine thymocytes. *J Immunol* (2012) **189**:2404–13. doi:10.4049/jimmunol.1102087

33. Hogquist KA, Baldwin TA, Jameson SC. Central tolerance: learning self-control in the thymus. *Nat Rev Immunol* (2005) **5**:772–82. doi:10.1038/nri1707
34. Rudolph MG, Stanfield RL, Wilson IA. How TCRs bind MHCs, peptides, and coreceptors. *Annu Rev Immunol* (2006) **24**:419–66. doi:10.1146/annurev.immunol.23.021704.115658
35. Garcia KC, Adams JJ, Feng D, Ely LK. The molecular basis of TCR germline bias for MHC is surprisingly simple. *Nat Immunol* (2009) **10**:143–7. doi:10.1038/ni.f.219
36. Miles JJ, Douek DC, Price DA. Bias in the alphabeta T-cell repertoire: implications for disease pathogenesis and vaccination. *Immunol Cell Biol* (2011) **89**:375–87. doi:10.1038/icb.2010.139
37. Desai RG, Creger WP. Maternofetal passage of leukocytes and platelets in man. *Blood* (1963) **21**:665–73.
38. Herzenberg LA, Bianchi DW, Schroder J, Cann HM, Iverson GM. Fetal cells in the blood of pregnant women: detection and enrichment by fluorescence-activated cell sorting. *Proc Natl Acad Sci U S A* (1979) **76**:1453–5. doi:10.1073/pnas.76.3.1453
39. Iverson GM, Bianchi DW, Cann HM, Herzenberg LA. Detection and isolation of fetal cells from maternal blood using the flourescence-activated cell sorter (FACS). *Prenat Diagn* (1981) **1**:61–73. doi:10.1002/pd.1970010111
40. Nelson JL. Your cells are my cells. *Sci Am* (2008) **298**:64–71.
41. Adams Waldorf KM, Gammill HS, Lucas J, Aydelotte TM, Leisenring WM, Lambert NC, et al. Dynamic changes in fetal microchimerism in maternal peripheral blood mononuclear cells, CD4+ and CD8+ cells in normal pregnancy. *Placenta* (2010) **31**:589–94. doi:10.1016/j.placenta.2010.04.013
42. Nelson JL. The otherness of self: microchimerism in health and disease. *Trends Immunol* (2012) **33**:421–7. doi:10.1016/j.it.2012.03.002
43. Evans PC, Lambert N, Maloney S, Furst DE, Moore JM, Nelson JL. Long-term fetal microchimerism in peripheral blood mononuclear cell subsets in healthy women and women with scleroderma. *Blood* (1999) **93**:2033–7.
44. Maloney S, Smith A, Furst DE, Myerson D, Rupert K, Evans PC, et al. Microchimerism of maternal origin persists into adult life. *J Clin Invest* (1999) **104**:41–7. doi:10.1172/JCI6611
45. Loubiere LS, Lambert NC, Flinn LJ, Erickson TD, Yan Z, Guthrie KA, et al. Maternal microchimerism in healthy adults in lymphocytes, monocyte/macrophages and NK cells. *Lab Invest* (2006) **86**:1185–92.
46. Gotherstrom C, Johnsson AM, Mattsson J, Papadogiannakis N, Westgren M. Identification of maternal hematopoietic cells in a 2nd-trimester fetus. *Fetal Diagn Ther* (2005) **20**:355–8. doi:10.1159/000086812
47. Khosrotehrani K, Leduc M, Bachy V, Nguyen Huu S, Oster M, Abbas A, et al. Pregnancy allows the transfer and differentiation of fetal lymphoid progenitors into functional T and B cells in mothers. *J Immunol* (2008) **180**:889–97.
48. Mold JE, Michaelsson J, Burt TD, Muench MO, Beckerman KP, Busch MP, et al. Maternal alloantigens promote the development of tolerogenic fetal regulatory T cells in utero. *Science* (2008) **322**:1562–5. doi:10.1126/science.1164511
49. Murugan A, Mora T, Walczak AM, Callan CG Jr. Statistical inference of the generation probability of T-cell receptors from sequence repertoires. *Proc Natl Acad Sci U S A* (2012) **109**:16161–6. doi:10.1073/pnas.1212755109
50. Hall MA, Reid JL, Lanchbury JS. The distribution of human TCR junctional region lengths shifts with age in both CD4 and CD8 T cells. *Int Immunol* (1998) **10**:1407–19. doi:10.1093/intimm/10.10.1407
51. Jonsson AM, Uzunel M, Gotherstrom C, Papadogiannakis N, Westgren M. Maternal microchimerism in human fetal tissues. *Am J Obstet Gynecol* (2008) **198**(325):e321–6.
52. Burlingham WJ, Nelson JL. Microchimerism in cord blood: mother as anticancer drug. *Proc Natl Acad Sci U S A* (2012) **109**:2190–1. doi:10.1073/pnas.1120857109
53. Wienecke J, Hebel K, Hegel KJ, Pierau M, Brune T, Reinhold D, et al. Proinflammatory effector Th cells transmigrate through anti-inflammatory environments into the murine fetus. *Placenta* (2012) **33**:39–46. doi:10.1016/j.placenta.2011.10.014
54. Haynes BF, Martin ME, Kay HH, Kurtzberg J. Early events in human T cell ontogeny. Phenotypic characterization and immunohistologic localization of T cell precursors in early human fetal tissues. *J Exp Med* (1988) **168**:1061–80. doi:10.1084/jem.168.3.1061
55. Gadi VK. Fetal microchimerism in breast from women with and without breast cancer. *Breast Cancer Res Treat* (2010) **121**:241–4. doi:10.1007/s10549-009-0548-1
56. Fugazzola L, Cirello V, Beck-Peccoz P. Fetal microchimerism as an explanation of disease. *Nat Rev Endocrinol* (2011) **7**:89–97. doi:10.1038/nrendo.2010.216
57. Willer CJ, Sadovnick AD, Ebers GC. Microchimerism in autoimmunity and transplantation: potential relevance to multiple sclerosis. *J Neuroimmunol* (2002) **126**:126–33. doi:10.1016/S0165-5728(02)00048-6
58. Adams KM, Nelson JL. Microchimerism: an investigative frontier in autoimmunity and transplantation. *JAMA* (2004) **291**:1127–31. doi:10.1001/jama.291.9.1127
59. Lambert NC, Erickson TD, Yan Z, Pang JM, Guthrie KA, Furst DE, et al. Quantification of maternal microchimerism by HLA-specific real-time polymerase chain reaction: studies of healthy women and women with scleroderma. *Arthritis Rheum* (2004) **50**:906–14. doi:10.1002/art.20200
60. Naumova EN, Gorski J, Naumov YN. Two compensatory pathways maintain long-term stability and diversity in CD8 T cell memory repertoires. *J Immunol* (2009) **183**:2851–8. doi:10.4049/jimmunol.0900162
61. den Braber I, Mugwagwa T, Vrisekoop N, Westera L, Mogling R, De Boer AB, et al. Maintenance of peripheral naive T cells is sustained by thymus output in mice but not humans. *Immunity* (2012) **36**:288–97. doi:10.1016/j.immuni.2012.02.006
62. Turchaninova MA, Britanova OV, Bolotin DA, Shugay M, Putintseva EV, Staroverov DB, et al. Pairing of T-cell receptor chains via emulsion PCR. *Eur J Immunol* (2013) **43**(9):2507–15. doi:10.1002/eji.201343453

17

Fallen angels or risen apes? A tale of the intricate complexities of imbalanced immune responses in the pathogenesis and progression of immune-mediated and viral cancers

Beatrice Omusiro Ondondo*

The Jenner Institute, Nuffield Department of Medicine, University of Oxford, Oxford, UK

Edited by:
Fang-Ping Huang, Imperial College London, UK

Reviewed by:
Hua-Chen Chang, Indiana University-Purdue University Indianapolis, USA
Dennis O. Adeegbe, Immunology Frontier Research Center, Japan

Correspondence:
Beatrice Omusiro Ondondo, The Jenner Institute, Nuffield Department of Medicine, University of Oxford, ORCRB, Roosevelt Drive, Oxford OX3 7DQ, UK
e-mail: beatrice.ondondo@ndm.ox.ac.uk

Excessive immune responses directed against foreign pathogens, self-antigens, or commensal microflora can cause cancer establishment and progression if the execution of tight immuno-regulatory mechanisms fails. On the other hand, induction of potent tumor antigen-specific immune responses together with stimulation of the innate immune system is a pre-requisite for effective anti-tumor immunity, and if suppressed by the strong immuno-regulatory mechanisms can lead to cancer progression. Therefore, it is crucial that the inevitable co-existence of these fundamental, yet conflicting roles of immune-regulatory cells is carefully streamlined as imbalances can be detrimental to the host. Infection with chronic persistent viruses is characterized by severe immune dysfunction resulting in T cell exhaustion and sometimes deletion of antigen-specific T cells. More often, this is due to increased immuno-regulatory processes, which are triggered to down-regulate immune responses and limit immunopathology. However, such heightened levels of immune disruption cause a concomitant loss of tumor immune-surveillance and create a permissive microenvironment for cancer establishment and progression, as demonstrated by increased incidences of cancer in immunosuppressed hosts. Paradoxically, while some cancers arise as a consequence of increased immuno-regulatory mechanisms that inhibit protective immune responses and impinge on tumor surveillance, other cancers arise due to impaired immuno-regulatory mechanisms and failure to limit pathogenic inflammatory responses. This intricate complexity, where immuno-regulatory cells can be beneficial in certain immune settings but detrimental in other settings underscores the need for carefully formulated interventions to equilibrate the balance between immuno-stimulatory and immuno-regulatory processes.

Keywords: regulatory T cells, immune dysfunction, immune-regulation, inflammation, cancer, HIV-1

INTRODUCTION

The observation that a sustained and potent immune response to a foreign pathogen, self-antigen, or normal microflora can be the root cause of uncontrolled cancer outgrowth and progression underscores the need for tight immuno-regulatory interventions that could be harnessed for the development of cancer vaccines and cell-based immunotherapies. On the other hand, inflammatory responses characterized by infiltration of tumor-associated antigen (TAA)-specific T cells and other components of the innate immune system are a pre-requisite for effective anti-tumor immunity. Therefore, it is crucial that the inevitable co-existence of these opposing forces is carefully streamlined as imbalances can be detrimental to the host.

Oncogenic viruses such as Epstein–Barr virus (EBV), human papilloma virus (HPV), and Kaposi sarcoma herpes virus (KSHV) express viral oncogenes, which can directly induce tumorigenic cell transformations and initiate the carcinogenesis process. In the case of non-oncogenic viruses such as hepatitis B (HBV) and hepatitis C (HCV), chronic infection and inflammation can lead to carcinogenic mutations in host cells (1), which are manifested by the increased incidences of liver cancer in chronic HBV and HCV patients. In both of these scenarios, the arising transformed tumor cells are genetically altered in a manner that distinguishes them from ordinary healthy self-cells thus conferring the ability to trigger effector immune responses, which in some cases are capable of controlling tumor growth (2, 3). In other instances, however, such modifications may lead to altered antigenicity and escape from immune-surveillance whereby the newly transformed cells are no longer recognized by their original cognate antigen-specific immune cells, thus leading to uncontrolled cancer progression. On a different platform, continuous antigenic stimulation that occurs during chronic virus infections causes severe immune dysfunction characterized by T cell exhaustion, anergy and in some cases deletion of antigen-specific B and T cells (4–6), and a concomitant induction of immuno-regulatory processes, which all result in the loss of tumor immune-surveillance and lead to cancer establishment. This is indeed supported by epidemiological data showing increased incidences of malignancies such as Kaposi sarcoma (KS) and cervical cancer, as well as EBV-associated malignancies such as non-Hodgkin lymphoma (NHL) and Burkitt lymphoma in immunosuppressed HIV/AIDS (7) and transplant patients.

Cancer can also arise due to dysfunctional immuno-regulatory mechanisms that result in uncontrolled excessive inflammatory immune responses. For example, pathogenic immune responses directed at commensal intestinal microflora during inflammatory bowel disease (IBD) are known to increase the risk of colon cancer (8, 9). Indeed prolonged periods of ulcerative colitis (UC) and Crohn's disease (CD) are associated with impaired immuno-regulatory mechanisms, which are in turn linked to colitis-associated colon carcinogenesis (10–12). Under normal circumstances both intrinsic and extrinsic regulatory pathways come into force to limit excessive immune activation and inflammation thus preventing tissue pathology and subsequent risk of cancer. However, as in many cases, failures of these control measures, including reduced frequencies or altered phenotype and function of regulatory T cells (Treg) means that this inflammation progresses in leaps and bounds. These paradoxical scenarios highlight a disruption in the natural homeostatic immuno-regulatory mechanisms that can be switched on to prevent excessive immune activation or turned off to allow execution of effector immune responses and tumor immune-surveillance. However, the exact timing of when a "good" immune response aimed at pathogen or tumor clearance can become a very "bad" response that creates an environment conducive for cancer growth and dissemination remains elusive. Understanding the intricate complexities and the timings of these events will be crucial in designing interventions for immune-mediated and viral cancers.

EXTRINSIC AND INTRINSIC IMMUNO-REGULATORY PATHWAYS

A complex network of finely tuned immune-regulation pathways exists to actively inhibit excessive immune responses during chronic viral infections and inflammation. This is essential for preventing the hyper-proliferation of antigen-specific T cells that could cause immunopathology due to increased release of inflammatory cytokines and targeted killing of infected or antigen-expressing tumor cells by CD8+ T cells. Immuno-regulatory pathways can broadly be divided into extrinsic or intrinsic pathways as depicted in **Figure 1**. Intrinsic mechanisms derive from within the effector cell and usually involve down-regulation of activating receptors and up-regulation of inhibitory receptors as well as activation of antagonist mechanisms, as discussed in the next section. Extrinsic pathways on the other hand usually involve other cells, which exert regulatory functions by cell-to-cell contact or via release of suppressive cytokines and biochemical compounds that inhibit cellular functions.

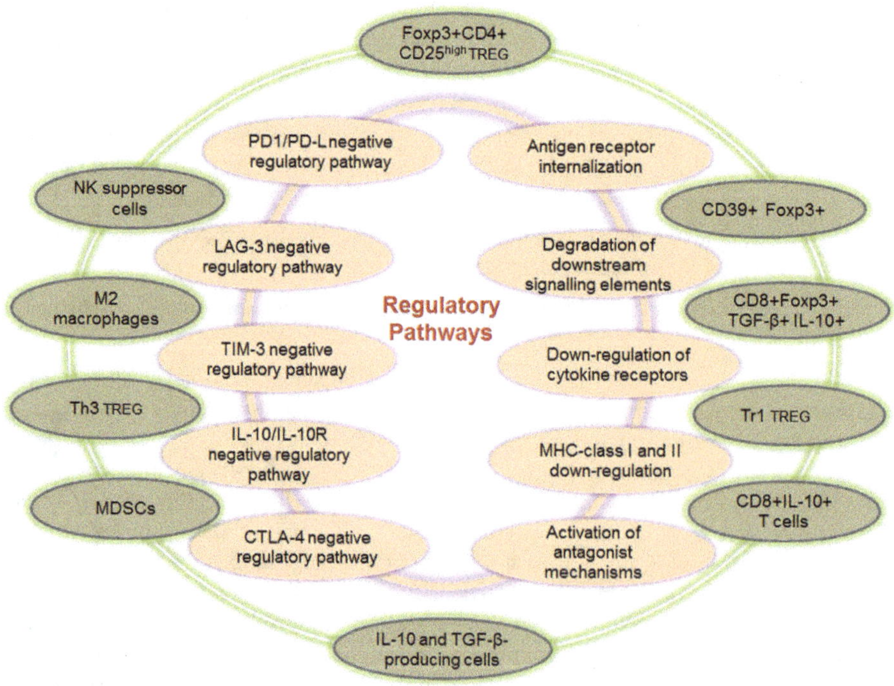

FIGURE 1 | Intrinsic and extrinsic immune-regulatory pathways. Several pathways of immune-regulation exist, and these comprise intrinsic and extrinsic mechanisms. Intrinsic pathways (inner circle) derive from within the effector cell and usually involve up-regulation of inhibitory receptors, down-regulation of cytokine and T cell activation receptors, down-regulation of MHC molecules, as well as the degradation of downstream signaling elements. Although the intrinsic pathways derive mainly from within the effector or antigen presenting cells, interactions with external elements do play a significant role, for instance the down-regulation of MHC class I, which is directly mediated by the HIV-1 Nef protein (13, 14). Extrinsic pathways (outer circle) involve several other cell types that exert immune suppression via cell-to-cell contact or through the release of suppressive cytokines and other biochemical compounds with suppressive activity. These include the various types of regulatory T cells in addition to the Foxp3+ Treg, CD8+ regulatory T cells, MDSCs as well as M2 macrophages and suppressive NK cells.

Of the extrinsic immuno-regulatory pathways, CD4+CD25^{high} Foxp3+ Treg are the most extensively studied and their suppressive mechanisms have been elucidated in greater detail. Existence of other types of immune cells with regulatory functions has been documented, for example CD4+Foxp3− Treg with suppressor functions such as the IL-10 producing Tr1 cells (15) and TGF-β producing Th3 cells (16) have been found in inflammatory environments. Tr1 cells secrete high levels of IL-10 and moderate amounts of TGF-β, and mainly suppress vial IL-10 release, as IL-10 neutralization abrogates their suppressive function (17, 18). On the converse, Th3 cells secrete high levels of TGF-β and low levels of IL-10 and can suppress both Th1 and Th2 responses (16, 17). Other cells with regulatory properties include myeloid-derived suppressor cells (MDSC), which can be induced by cytokines such as IL-6 and growth factors including G-CSF and GM-CSF (19), CD8+Foxp3+ Treg producing both IL-10 and TGF-β, or IL-10-producing CD8+ T cells (20–22), as well as NK cells that possess suppressor functions (23, 24). Activated MDSC can suppress via several mechanisms including IL-10 production as well as via compounds such as arginase 1, reactive oxygen species (ROS), and nitric oxide (NO) among others (19). Moreover, MDSC can indirectly contribute to immuno-regulatory functions by inducing Treg differentiation and expansion.

IMMUNE DYSREGULATION DURING PERSISTENT VIRUS INFECTIONS AND CHRONIC INFLAMMATION

T cells are the key players in many infectious diseases and in eradication of malignant cells. This is well-demonstrated in acute infections where T cells become activated and acquire effector functions, with subsequent clearance of infection and formation of stable memory populations. Moreover, tumors heavily infiltrated with fully functional effector T cells progress less rapidly and in some cases regression can be achieved. However, in the case of persistent antigen stimulation in a chronic setting, memory T cell formation and effector functions are altered, resulting in exhausted, functionally impaired defective T cells incapable of conferring protection. The characteristic properties of these defective cells include diminished cytokine production, decreased cytotoxicity, and reduced proliferative and self-renewal potential. In some cases, mutational escape and/or physical deletion of antigen-specific T cells occurs resulting in inadequate immune control, hence chronic persistence of the viruses. Furthermore, some chronic pathogens directly infect the immune cells, e.g., HIV-1 (CD4+ T cells) and EBV (B cells) leading to loss of immune functions. This state of immunological dysfunction is consistently found in chronic virus infections including HIV, HBV, and HCV (25–27) and is also prevalent in cancer patients. Immune dysregulation can be manifested in several forms, some of which are summarized in **Figure 2** and described below.

T CELL EXHAUSTION

T cell exhaustion refers to a state of progressive loss of immune function, which in some cases, can result in physical deletion of responding cells due to imbalances in the expression of pro-apoptotic and anti-apoptotic factors and the inability to respond to IL-7 and IL-15 (26–28). The dominant mechanism of T cell exhaustion is the up-regulation of several inhibitory receptors, although down-regulation of cytokine receptors such as IL-7Rα and IL-15Rα by exhausted memory T cells is frequently observed. Lower levels of IL-7Rα and IL-15Rα can lead to defective cytokine signaling and consequently impaired homeostatic self-renewal and suboptimal numbers of functional memory T cells (27, 28). Up-regulation of inhibitory receptors such as programed-death 1 (PD-1), T cell immunoglobulin mucin 3 (TIM-3), lymphocyte activation gene 3 (LAG-3), and cytotoxic T-lymphocyte-associated protein-4 (CTLA-4) is a characteristic feature of exhausted T cells. PD-1, an inhibitory receptor of the CD28 superfamily is highly expressed on exhausted CD8+ T cells during progressive chronic viral infections and uncontrolled cancer, making it a major factor in T cell exhaustion. Under normal circumstances, PD-1 is induced following T cell activation to inhibit the TCR signaling cascade and prevent excessive T cell activation, but is then down-regulated following pathogen clearance. In peripheral tolerance, PD-1 is important in inhibiting potentially pathogenic self-reactive T cells as well as promoting Treg development (29, 30) and mice lacking PD-1 succumb to autoimmune diseases (31, 32). However, in chronic infection, the PD-1 pathway mediates pathogen-specific CD8+ T cell dysfunction as demonstrated in HIV (33–35), HCV (36, 37), and HBV (38, 39) infections. For example, the frequency of PD-1+CD8+ T cells is highly elevated in HIV-1 patients where it correlates significantly with viral load and declining CD4+ T cell numbers (33, 40). PD-1 is also up-regulated on HIV-specific CD4+ T cells (40, 41) and inhibits CD4+ T cell responses including proliferation. Interestingly, PD-1 levels are significantly reduced in HIV-1 progressors who initiate highly active antiretroviral therapy (HAART) or in long-term non-progressors (LTNPs), suggesting that antigen persistence drives T cells to exhaustion (33, 34). In chronic HCV infection, increased PD-1 expression on HCV-specific CD8+ T cells is associated with impaired proliferation and cytokine production (37). A part from inhibition of T cell function, PD-1 expression can also lead to spontaneous or FAS-mediated apoptosis of virus-specific T cells (42).

Besides PD-1, other inhibitory receptors such as TIM-3, 2B4 (natural killer cell receptor), and LAG-3 are also up-regulated on virus-specific T cells, and the expression of multiple inhibitory receptors correlates with a severely dysfunctional state (43–45). For example, co-expression of PD-1 and TIM-3 is associated with severely exhausted HIV-specific CD8+ T cells (45) and majority of these also co-express PD-1 and 2B4 (46). CTLA-4 is another inhibitory receptor expressed by activated CD4+ and CD8+ T cells. It has a higher affinity for the B7 ligands (CD80 and CD86) allowing it to out-compete CD28, hence it is a powerful negative regulator of CD28-dependent T cell responses. It is significantly up-regulated on CD4+ T cells during HIV-1 and HCV infections where it correlates positively with disease progression and negatively with antigen-specific IL-2 production (41, 47). CTLA-4 is abundantly expressed on Treg as it is required for optimum suppressive function.

IMPAIRED APC FUNCTION

The fact that fully functional pathogen-specific T cells are rarely found in chronic infections suggests impaired antigen presentation, which could be attributed to either inadequate priming by

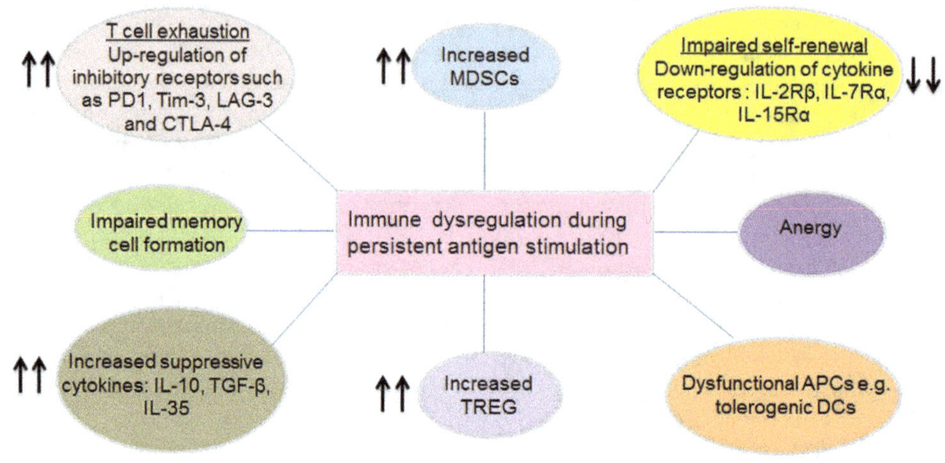

FIGURE 2 | Mechanisms of immune dysregulation during persistent antigen stimulation. Immune dysregulation manifests in several distinct forms, which can occur in isolation or in combination. Persistent antigenic stimulation, especially in settings with high antigen loads can lead to T cell exhaustion (characterized by the up-regulation of several inhibitory receptors and down-regulation of specific T cell activation receptors), anergy (generalized unresponsiveness), impaired memory formation, impaired proliferation, and self-renewal capacity. Besides these, chronic viruses trigger various biochemical pathways that lead to increased frequencies of MDSCs and Treg, which actively suppress effector immune responses via a variety of mechanisms. Immune dysregulation occurring at the T cell priming stage is linked to dysfunctional APCs (for example inadequately activated or tolerogenic DCs), which are likely to skew the immune response toward tolerance. Conceivably, such regulatory mechanisms serve to prevent tissue damage and aberrant immune activation, but they inevitably contribute to the chronic persistence state as a result of inhibiting effector immune responses.

non-professional APCs or possibly altered function of professional APCs during the chronic stages of disease. Indeed, functional impairment of DCs has been associated with T cell exhaustion and progression of disease during HIV, HBV, HCV, and LCMV infection (48–51). Decreased expression of co-stimulatory molecules and lower production of immuno-stimulatory cytokines by APCs can result in functionally tolerant or anergic T cells. Furthermore, chronic infections are associated with loss of DCs, possibly due to direct infection by viruses such as HIV and LCMV. Moreover, DCs can induce T cell exhaustion or tolerance by signaling through inhibitory receptors such as PD-1 and CTLA-4, and also acting via indoleamine 2,3-dioxygenase (IDO)-dependent mechanisms to induce Treg, which further suppress immune responses (52). However, other factors such as virus-induced modulation of the expression of MHC or co-stimulatory molecules have been described and may also significantly affect the generation of fully functional T cells (13, 14).

INCREASED FREQUENCY OF TREG AND MDSC

Increased frequencies of Treg and MDSC are a common feature of persistent chronic viral infections, which is well-documented in infections with HBV (53–55), HCV (56–58), and HIV (52, 59–61). These chronic persistent viruses trigger the production of IL-10 and TGF-β, which in turn increase the frequency and suppressive function of Treg, such as observed in HCV-infected hepatocytes (62). Alternatively, these cytokines may promote the induction of adaptive Treg further reinforcing the immune barrier at sites of infection. HIV and HCV infections also induce plasmacytoid dendritic cells (pDCs) known to induce IL-10-producing Treg via IDO-dependent mechanisms (52, 58). Additionally, the chronic micro-environments created by virus persistence contribute to enhanced Treg proliferation and suppressive function by secreting cytokines and other factors on which Treg thrive. The high frequencies of Treg and MDSC serve an important role of preventing excessive antigen stimulation, persistent inflammatory responses, and viral mediated immunopathology in the chronic stages of viral disease (56, 63). However, the elevated frequencies and enhanced suppressive capacity of Treg and MDSC also contribute to suppression of effector T cells in an antigen-specific or bystander mechanism (64) thus promoting prolonged viral persistence (65, 66) characterized by secondary T cell impairment and exhaustion (67). Thus, counterintuitively, increased expansion and survival of regulatory cells serve to establish, propagate, and maintain the chronic infection state.

INCREASED SUPPRESSIVE CYTOKINES

Apart from Treg and MDSC, increased IL-10 production is another powerful immuno-regulatory mechanism that negatively impacts on the quantity and quality of antigen-specific immune responses. IL-10 is an immuno-regulatory cytokine produced by many cell types and has multiple functions including inhibition of pro-inflammatory cytokine production, dampening T cell responses, blocking APC functions, and also causing B cell dysregulation. Increased IL-10 production is seen in several chronic viruses including HIV, EBV, HCV, HBV, and LCMV (68–75), and IL-10R blockade can induce rapid virus control indicating that excessive levels of IL-10 have a negative influence on the quality of immune responses and disease course (68, 69). TGF-β is yet another immunosuppressive cytokine whose role in limiting immune responses is documented in a number of disease settings (76). Both IL-10 and TGF-β are known to establish highly suppressive micro-environments that are suitable for cancer progression.

DISRUPTION OF IMMUNE-REGULATORY T CELLS IN INFLAMMATORY ENVIRONMENTS

Resolution of inflammation requires swift execution of functional regulatory mechanisms such as the expansion of Treg, a lineage of lymphocytes committed to suppressive functions that maintain self-tolerance and immune homeostasis. Dysregulation of Treg function or induction is linked to a number of chronic inflammatory disorders such as IBD and also fatal autoimmune diseases. Thus, interventions which can restore functional regulation without inducing effector immune responses would be beneficial in such settings. Dysfunctional regulation can manifest as reduced Treg numbers (either due to defective Treg induction or loss of Treg), defective suppressive function (due to loss of Foxp3 expression or reduced production of suppressive cytokines), and impaired migration (due to altered expression of adhesion molecules and chemokine receptors). This section gives a brief description of these mechanisms and the various inflammatory conditions that drive phenotypic and functional modification of Treg.

TREG INSTABILITY: PHENOTYPIC ALTERATION AND FUNCTIONAL IMPAIRMENT

Despite the widely held view of thymic imprinting of Treg cell functions, recent studies indicate developmental plasticity and instability, whereby Treg lose Foxp3 expression and convert to Foxp3− helper T cells (exFoxp3) (77, 78) in certain inflammatory or lymphopenic environments (**Figure 3**). Although exFoxp3 Treg may largely arise from a few promiscuous uncommitted Treg (79), their comparatively higher potential to expand, coupled with the fact that a majority of them are skewed toward self-reactivity suggests potential pathogenicity as a result of altered regulatory functions such as secretion of pro-inflammatory cytokines directed against self-antigens (77). Adoptive transfer studies showed that a large fraction of Treg transferred to lymphopenic recipients lost Foxp3 expression alongside other Treg cell surface markers, and that this was accompanied by acquisition of effector functions including IFN-γ, IL-2, and IL-17-production and a concomitant loss of suppressive function (80–82). Other reports indicated that Foxp3+ Treg effectively lost Foxp3 expression and converted to T helper-type 2 phenotype cells expressing IL-13 and IL-5 (78, 83) or differentiated into follicular helper T cells (Foxp3–T_{FH}-like cells) under the influence of IL-6 and IL-21 (84). Acquisition of T helper features without the simultaneous loss of Foxp3 expression has also been observed. This results in hybrid Treg, which display an activated-memory T cell phenotype and pro-inflammatory properties, such as the IL-17-producing Foxp3+ROR-γt+ IL-17+ (85–90) and IFN-γ-producing Foxp3+T-bet+ IFN-γ+ (91, 92) Treg. Although this hybrid Treg phenotype can exert dual inflammatory and regulatory functions, it has been shown that the phenotypic and transcriptional modifications can reduce their overall suppressive function (81, 93). In other instances however, Treg have been shown to lose their suppressive function without necessarily converting to exFoxp3 or dual function (hybrid) inflammatory Treg (94–100). Such functionally impaired Treg show decreased expression of Foxp3, CTLA-4, and GITR, together with production of very low levels of IL-10 and TGF-β.

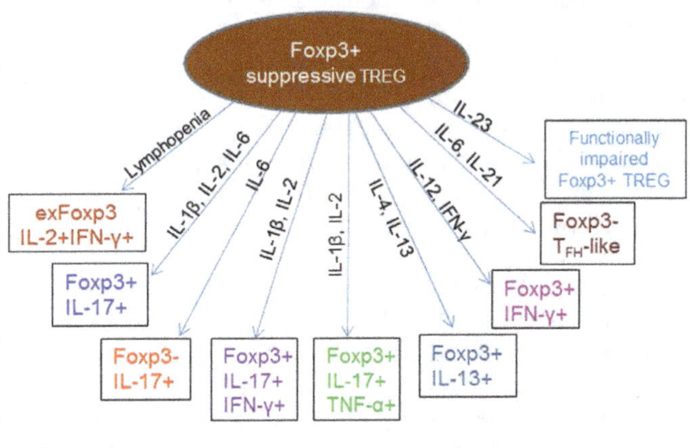

FIGURE 3 | Impaired or altered function of regulatory cells during inflammation. The cytokine and chemokine milieu of inflammatory micro-environments can induce phenotypic and functional modification in Treg, leading to generation of pathogenic exFoxp3 T cells, which express lower levels of Foxp3, CTLA-4, and GITR and produce a combination of Th1, Th2, or Th17 cytokines. Conversion of Foxp3+ Treg into pathogenic IFN-γ-producing Th1 cells or IL-17-producing Th17 exFoxp3 Treg cells is documented in various immunological settings (77, 80, 101). Conversion to a Th2 phenotype expressing IL-13 (Foxp3+IL-13+) and IL-5 (78, 83) as well as differentiation into follicular helper T cells (84) have also been reported. In most cases, the suppressive function of these altered phenotypes is significantly reduced due to decreased Foxp3 expression (81, 82). Certain inflammatory conditions can support the generation of hybrid phenotype Treg, which exhibit dual suppressive and pro-inflammatory functions such as the IL-17-producing Foxp3+IL-17+ (85–90), IFN-γ-producing Foxp3+ IFN-γ+ (91, 92), Foxp3+IL-17+ IFN-γ+, or Foxp3+IL-17+ TNF-α+ (102, 103) Treg. Generally, environments enriched with Th1 cytokines such as IFN-γ, IL-2, and IL-12 favor generation of exFoxp3 Treg producing IFN-γ, those enriched with Th2 cytokines such as IL-4 and IL-13 favor generation of Th2 Treg, while IL-6 favors conversion into the IL-17+Foxp3+ and IL-17+Foxp3− phenotypes.

Several lines of evidence indicate that functional and phenotypic plasticity of Foxp3+ Treg is largely governed by extrinsic signals provided by the inflammatory milieu of their surrounding environments. Increased levels of pro-inflammatory cytokines such as IL-12 or IFN-γ correlate with the frequency of functionally impaired Th1-like Treg (104). In this setting, the Treg suppressive functions were effectively restored by IL-12 withdrawal or IFN-γ blockade suggesting that a pro-inflammatory cytokine milieu not only promotes the Th1-like phenotype, but also inhibits Treg suppressor functions. Overall, inflammatory environments enriched with cytokines such as IL-1β, IL-4, IL-6, IL-21, and IL-23 drive conversion of Foxp3+ Treg into T helper phenotypes (80, 105, 106). As an example, stimulation of peripheral Treg in the presence of IL-6 was shown to result in loss of Foxp3 expression and production of IL-17 (105, 106). Inflammatory environments with IL-1β, IL-2, IL-6, IL-21, IL-23, and TGF-β have been shown to drive conversion of Foxp3+ Treg into IL-17 producing Treg (87, 107), whereas TGF-β, IL-10, and IL-2 help to maintain continued Foxp3 expression, Treg stability, and suppressive function (80, 81, 92, 108–110). Therefore, stable Foxp3 expression and maintenance of optimal Treg suppressive function require the continuous presence of specific signals within the inflammatory environment, without which conversion of Treg into functionally impaired exFoxp3 T cells or hybrid phenotype Treg occurs (102, 103).

Although the various Treg phenomena described above are well-documented in autoimmune settings, it remains possible that the chronic inflammatory environments created by persistent viral infections can also support phenotypic and functional modifications that would render Treg dysfunctional. In favor of this speculation, a recent study has demonstrated that Treg infected with HIV display increased CpG methylation of the Foxp3 locus and a deregulated functional profile, which was characterized by down-regulation of Foxp3 expression, reduced suppressive capacity, and altered cytokine secretion pattern (111). These Treg showed decreased production of TGF-β and increased IL-4 secretion, a characteristic which is thought to orchestrate severe systemic immune hyper-activation that is observed during progressive HIV disease. In chronic infection with HCV, PD-L1 was found to negatively regulate both the function and proliferation of Treg by controlling STAT-5 phosphorylation (112). Although PD-1 was expressed on both Treg and effector T cells, Treg showed significantly higher up-regulation of PD-1, which was correlated with disease progression. These studies highlight the potential of viruses to subvert the induction and function of Treg, but clearly further research is needed to unravel the mechanisms underlying defective regulation during chronic virus infections.

IMPAIRED OR ALTERED MIGRATION OF TREG

Another crucial aspect contributing to Treg dysfunction is their ability to migrate to peripheral sites of chronic inflammation such as the skin, urogenital mucosa, gut-associated lymphoid tissues (GALT), transplanted organs, or tumors for appropriate localization, in close proximity with effector immune cells as suppression is mostly contact-dependent. To do this effectively, activated Treg up-regulate distinct site-specific inflammatory chemokine receptors and adhesion ligands, which facilitate their migration into the inflamed tissues, usually in response to a variety of inflammatory chemokines that serve as migrational cues (113–117). Therefore, altered chemokine receptor and adhesion molecule expression can affect the migrational properties of Treg and impact on their ability to access sites of chronic inflammation. Such attenuated Treg migration can in turn lead to sustained inflammation and increased risk of inflammation-driven cancer in the Treg inaccessible areas, owing to reduced frequency and suppressive activities.

The crucial role of chemokine-receptor-dependent migration in functional regulation is demonstrated in several experiments including a mouse model of colitis and IBD, where CCR4-deficient Treg had impaired migration to the mesenteric lymph nodes and therefore failed to prevent colitis (118). In other settings, a number of chemokine receptors including CCR2, CCR4, CCR5, CCR6, CCR7, and CXCR3 have been implicated in the selective and preferential recruitment of Treg to sites of chronic inflammation and/or tumors (115, 119, 120), thus indicating that alteration in chemokine receptor patterns or blockade of chemokine receptor signaling would have a significant impact on their migration and immuno-regulatory activities. Tumors and their associated stroma are known to express elevated levels of specific inflammatory chemokines, which serve to chemoattract various leukocytes including Treg (121, 122). Although the overall recruitment is also significantly influenced by the type of chemokine receptors expressed by the leukocytes, Treg, especially the "inflammation-seeking" phenotype usually up-regulate multiple chemokine receptors (116), which allow them access to a variety of tumors, where they preferentially accumulate (119). Some studies demonstrate that disruption of key chemokine receptor signaling axes such as CCR4 or CCR5, or the depletion of chemokine receptor-specific Treg can significantly inhibit their migration and prevent accumulation in tumors (123, 124), thus influencing the overall prognosis. Conceivably, while impaired migration and reduced Treg access to tumors would be an awesome advantage in the majority of cancer settings where they impinge on anti-tumor immune responses, it may however be a major setback in certain other settings, which require Treg to limit excessive immune responses, such as in IBD and chronic virus infections.

LOSS OF TREG (IMPAIRED TREG INDUCTION OR TREG DELETION)

In certain disease settings, physical deletion of Treg can result in reduced frequencies. For instance, it is postulated that by virtue of their activated nature, Treg express higher levels of CCR5 and CXCR4, the co-receptors for HIV-1 thus making them preferential targets for HIV-1 infection (125, 126). Since Foxp3+ Treg represent a high proportion of CD4+ T cells (up to 50%) found in mucosal lymphoid organs of HIV-infected individuals (60), it is plausible that HIV infection can subsequently lead to significant depletion of these cells and impaired immuno-regulatory functions (127–129). Furthermore, Treg also express both Fas and Fas ligand and can be targeted and killed by effector T cells without necessarily being infected. Several studies indicate that myeloid dendritic cells (mDCs) can contribute to Treg induction by promoting conversion of conventional CD4+ T cells into Treg (130, 131). However, it has been shown that *in vitro* HIV infection of mDCs not only impairs their capacity to induce Treg but can also trigger preferential targeting and killing of Treg via a caspase-dependent pathway (132), thus contributing to numerical loss of Treg. Changes in the levels of chemokines expressed within certain tissues, together with diminished levels of TGF-β and IL-2 can also result in the loss of Treg in that particular organ. For example, altered expression of ligands for CXCR3, CCR4, and CCR7 was associated with a loss of Treg in lymph nodes during simian immunodeficiency virus (SIV) infection (133). Other mechanisms for reduced Treg frequencies may include increased apoptosis, reduced proliferation and survival, as well as impaired peripheral Treg induction. As discussed earlier, Treg may also be lost by conversion to exFoxp3 T cells under certain inflammatory cytokine milieu.

IMBALANCES IN IMMUNO-REGULATORY AND IMMUNO-STIMULATORY PROCESSES CAN CAUSE CANCER

Increased risk of cancer is often associated with poorly regulated immune responses (**Figure 4**) constituting unresolved inflammation as a result of perturbations in the balance of tumoricidal and tumorigenic activities (134, 135). Treg play a crucial role in maintaining optimum balance between these two arms of the immune response and persistent viruses are known to trigger production of IL-10 and TGF-β (136) to ensure induction and maintenance

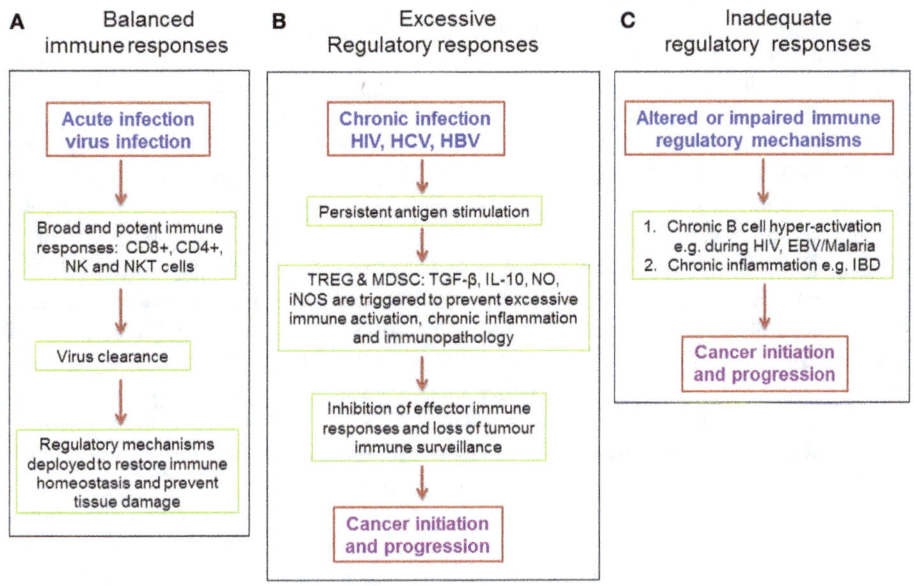

FIGURE 4 | Dysregulated immune responses create a microenvironment suitable for cancer initiation and progression. Perturbations of the balance between effector and regulatory immune responses are often the cause of chronic inflammation and increased risk of cancer (146). Under normal circumstances **(A)**, the immune system mounts a potent and broadly directed immune response following acute virus infection. This immune response, comprising both the innate and adaptive components leads to effective virus clearance and stable memory cell formation, which is effective at rapidly countering subsequent infections. Under this scenario, regulatory mechanisms kick in to prevent tissue damage after virus clearance. However, in the case of persistent antigenic stimulation **(B)** such as caused by HIV, HCV, and HBV, there is continuous generation of effector immune cells that are incapable of clearing the pathogen. This leads to a state of chronic inflammation that in turn triggers regulatory pathways such as increased production of suppressive cytokines and recruitment of Treg and MDSC to dampen excessive immune responses and prevent tissue damage (136). But as fate would have it, such potent regulatory responses also inhibit anti-tumor effector responses leading to loss of tumor immune-surveillance and subsequently cancer initiation and progression. In certain contrasting scenarios such as IBD, impaired regulatory mechanisms **(C)** can result in chronic inflammation, which initiates carcinogenesis. Furthermore, uncontrolled B cell activation during HIV and EBV infections is associated with increased risk of non-Hodgkin's lymphoma (147). NO, nitric oxide; iNOS, nitric oxide synthase.

of adequate numbers of Treg in circulation. In some cases, viruses express homologs of immunosuppressive cytokines or cytokine receptors, such as the well-described human cytomegalovirus (HCMV)-IL-10 and EBV-IL-10 homologs (137, 138), which allow them to directly influence Treg induction or modulate the immune system via other mechanisms including impaired production of pro-inflammatory cytokines and chemokines, as well as MHC class II down-regulation (136). As mentioned earlier, viruses can also promote Treg induction by disrupting the normal activation cascade of dendritic cells and other antigen presenting cells. Furthermore, inflammatory micro-environments are enriched with type 2 macrophages (M2) and MDSC, which also enhance recruitment of Treg, besides directly suppressing antigen-specific effector T cells (19, 139, 140). Additionally, antigen-specific CD8+ Treg are frequently detected in chronic HIV (141, 142), HCV (57, 143), and herpes virus infections (144, 145). The increased numbers of Treg and other immunosuppressive mechanisms serve to actively prevent excessive immune activation and the associated immunopathology, but by so doing, they block antigen-specific effector immune responses that are essential for clearing the pathogen and for tumor immune-surveillance. The resulting immune impairment allows chronic pathogen persistence and an overwhelming state of recurrent inflammation, thus favoring cancer establishment.

Besides the direct disruption of tumor immune-surveillance, establishment of chronic inflammation creates a suppressive tumor-promoting microenvironment, which is enriched with IL-10, TGF-β, and other pro-inflammatory cytokines such as IL-17, known to be angiogenic and to contribute to tumor cell survival and growth (148, 149). In the presence of IL-6, TGF-β can further up-regulate ROR-γt expression leading to enhanced Th17 differentiation (150–152) and increased risk of cancer progression (148, 153–155). Moreover, as discussed earlier, Foxp3+ Treg in certain inflammatory environments can express IL-17, which together with hypoxic conditions could play a role in generation of cancer initiating cells (156). As highlighted in earlier sections, inflammatory environments can also induce phenotypic and functional impairments in immuno-regulatory cells thus leading to dysfunctional immune-regulation and increased risk of cancer. However, whether increased incidence of cancer in individuals with chronic virus infection and inflammation is due to increased suppression of tumor immunity as a result of increased frequency and suppressive activity of immuno-regulatory cells, due to failure of regulatory cells to prevent excessive immune activation and inflammation, or due to enhanced oncogenic potential of the carcinogen remains a subject of intense debate. In this review, I will focus on the contradictory roles of immuno-regulatory cells where they can cause cancer by either exerting potent suppression of effector immune responses that inhibit tumor immune-surveillance (e.g., during chronic virus infections) or through their functional impairment and inability to execute effective suppression of pathogenic effector immune responses (e.g., during IBD).

THE DELICATE BALANCE BETWEEN IMMUNITY AND REGULATION IN HIV INFECTION AND DISEASE

Although HIV can exist in latent reservoirs for many years, it is a chronic persistent virus characterized by the continuous presence of infectious virus and thus chronic immune activation, persistent inflammation, and concurrent CD4+ T cell loss are all observed (157–159). Thus, increased numbers of fully functional regulatory mechanisms become necessary to counteract the ongoing inflammatory processes. However, Treg, which are instrumental in counteracting immune activation and inflammation by actively suppressing effector immune responses can also be detrimental by inhibiting T cell responses that control HIV replication. An appropriate immune response must therefore not disturb this delicate balance, by aiming to maximize the "good" immune responses, which control the virus while minimizing the "bad" immune responses that cause pathology.

Although still a subject of intense debate, a number of studies have demonstrated increased frequencies of Treg during HIV-1 infection and more especially in the chronic stages that mark progression to AIDS (128, 160–163). Studies looking at tissue distribution revealed accumulation of Treg at sites of HIV infection and replication such as the gastrointestinal mucosa and lymph nodes (59, 60, 128, 164). With such increased frequencies and especially given the suppressive role of Treg, it follows that progression of HIV-1 infection to chronic disease could in fact be a consequence of suppressed T cell function. Indeed, robust CD8+ and CD4+ T cell responses (characterized by high proliferation, IFN-γ production, and cytotoxicity), which correlate with HIV control in a minority of infected people usually diminish during chronic infection, coinciding with increased Treg numbers. Depleting Treg was shown to restore the *in vitro* effector immune functions of these cells (59, 165). Lower levels of Treg and a corresponding higher level of HIV-specific T cell responses have been observed in individuals who naturally control HIV-1 in the absence of HAART, i.e., the LTNPs and Elite controllers (160). Furthermore, depletion of Treg in cord blood samples of HIV-exposed uninfected neonates (166) was shown to augment both CD4+ and CD8+ HIV-specific T cell responses. These findings, together with the observation that Treg frequencies are reduced in HIV-infected patients on HAART (160, 164, 167, 168) provide compelling evidence that Treg impinge on immune control of HIV and strongly support immunotherapeutic interventions that reduce their numbers or impair their functions.

Whereas depleting Treg or interfering with their suppressive function might seem plausible in the context of immune function restoration, in fact several studies indicate that reduced Treg frequencies correlate with increased immune activation, which is in turn significantly associated with higher plasma viral loads (169, 170). Treg can therefore prevent collateral damage during chronic HIV infection by limiting immune activation, while at the same time reducing the pool of activated CD4+ T cell targets that would become susceptible to HIV infection. Accordingly, it is thought that the high frequencies of Treg found in highly exposed persistently sero-negative (HESN) individuals (171) and in the *in utero* HIV-exposed uninfected neonates (166) contribute to resistance to HIV infection by significantly reducing the numbers of activated target CD4+ T cells. These studies suggest that Treg may be beneficial at least to some extent, not only in HIV-infected individuals where they could limit immune activation, but also in highly exposed individuals with a greater risk of HIV infection. However, given that LTNPs and elite controllers exhibit both lower levels of immune activation and lower Treg frequencies (172), while at the same time mounting robust HIV-specific immune responses that inhibit virus replication, it is plausible to suggest that Treg are dispensable in HIV immunity, although caution must be exercised as LTNPs and elite controllers represent a very small proportion of HIV-infected individuals, in whom protective HLA alleles are over-represented.

Contrary to these findings, many studies document persistence of immune activation in the presence of elevated Treg frequencies, suggesting that perhaps the suppressive activities of the Treg found in chronic HIV infection are not sufficient to completely reverse the state of chronic immune activation. Indeed, it has been demonstrated that higher frequencies of Treg exist in HIV-infected individuals with progressive disease (173), but their ability to suppress HIV-specific T cells is significantly reduced, which in turn leads to inability to control HIV-associated aberrant immune activation (111, 161, 174). This is in fact discredited by studies demonstrating the existence of functionally suppressive Treg in progressive HIV-1 disease (59, 165, 175), hence suggesting that failure to reduce immune activation may be due to overwhelming levels of persistent stimulation rather than functional impairment of Treg. Thus, it is possible that high Treg frequencies found in chronic HIV infection are a result of failed attempts to reduce the state of chronic persistent antigenic stimulation (176, 177).

Faced with this paradox, timings of when to initiate interventions remain critical to achieving desirable outcomes. Whereas, immune-based therapies aimed at increasing the frequencies of Treg such as IL-2 therapy may only serve to suppress anti-HIV immunity and provide more targets for HIV, and thus not offer clinical benefit earlier in HIV infection (178, 179), they might indeed become useful during the chronic stages in order to limit immune activation (169, 170). Conversely, depleting Treg during the early stages of infection will allow for generation of robust immune responses capable of controlling virus replication and preventing establishment of latent reservoirs (126).

HIV-ASSOCIATED IMMUNE DYSFUNCTION PREDISPOSES TO MALIGNANCIES

The existence of a few HIV-infected individuals with robust HIV-specific immune responses who maintain very low virus loads for many years without treatment and only progress to AIDS following viral immune escape demonstrates constant immune-surveillance that keeps the virus in check. In these individuals, a normal balance between the effector and regulatory immune responses exists, whereby effective immune responses occur without excessive immune hyper-activation that causes T cell exhaustion and functional impairment. However, in a majority of HIV-infected people, the immune system does not control virus replication, leading to continuous immune stimulation with high antigen loads and generates a large pool of immune-effector cells that are by far inadequate in controlling the virus. This can be either due to anergy, functional exhaustion, or immune escape (157), as described earlier. Furthermore, HIV directly infects CD4+ T cells and this leads to the progressive diminution of T helper functions and immune incapacitation that marks progression to AIDS.

Besides these, a number of immuno-regulatory mechanisms triggered to prevent immune activation and inflammation also suppress immune-effector functions and sustain chronic virus persistence. For example, during chronic HIV infection, the expansion of Treg (180) with potent suppressive activity within mucosal tissues not only contributes to persistence of HIV, but also reduces immune vigilance and predisposes to HPV and cervical cancer. Moreover, HIV-1 gp120 has recently been shown to induce IL-6 and a concomitant expansion of MDSC (181), which contribute to immune suppression by modulating cytokine and cellular responses as well as inducing the differentiation and expansion of Treg (182). Large amounts of B cell activation-associated cytokines such as IL-6 and IL-10 are produced during chronic HIV infection and can also increase the numbers and suppressive capacity of MDSC leading to further suppression of effective immune responses. Indeed, higher levels of MDSC are associated with chronic progressive HIV disease (183). The decline of both IL-6 levels and Treg numbers following HAART-mediated immune restoration strongly supports their role in immune modulation during HIV-1 progression. A highly immunosuppressive environment with increased numbers of Treg, MDSC, and suppressive cytokines such as IL-10 and TGF-β is strongly associated with increased risk of cancer (19, 182, 184, 185). Thus, HIV-1 can be classified as indirect carcinogen that perturbs immune balance through immune suppression and a concomitant loss of tumor immune-surveillance to set the stage for oncogenic tumor viruses (186).

Another consequence of HIV-driven impairment of the immune system is the hyper-activation and uncontrolled proliferation of B cells, which not only favors secondary infection by oncogenic viruses (187) such as KSHV and EBV but also increases significantly the potential of chromosomal translocations and oncogenic mutations. A few studies have linked HIV infection with chronic B cell hyper activation (147, 188) and lymphomagenesis, for example, increased incidence of Burkitt lymphoma in HIV-infected individuals or those persistently exposed to *Plasmodium falciparum* in malaria endemic regions where their B cells are in constant stimulation by these antigens (189). HIV-1 can also act directly via gp120 to induce B cell activation and subsequent development of lymphomas (190). Moreover, incorporation of CD40L into HIV virions stimulates B cell activation via interactions with CD40, resulting in production of B cell activating cytokines such as IL-6, IL-8, IL-10, and GM-CSF (191, 192). Indeed, HIV-associated lymphomas are often the aggressive B cell lymphomas, directly supporting a role for HIV in altering the B cell phenotypic and proliferative characteristics.

Therefore, the profound T cell dysfunction, progressive depletion of CD4+ T cells, B cell hyper-activation, together with the increased immuno-regulatory mechanisms all collude to actively impede tumor immune-surveillance and create a permissive environment for cancer initiation and progression. This is a classic example of a "vicious cycle of immune responses" where an effector immune response to a pathogen (in this case HIV) is induced during the initial stages of infection, but somehow fails to eliminate the pathogen, and regulatory mechanisms are triggered in order to restore immune balance and limit excessive inflammation and pathology, yet such regulatory mechanisms actively suppress the anti-tumor immune-surveillance processes and predispose to increased risk of cancer.

HIV-ASSOCIATED MALIGNANCIES

Cancer is a complex multistep process involving many molecular events, which together with the carcinogen or oncogenic virus infection work in concert to generate a transformed cellular phenotype. However, immune response is an important extrinsic factor that determines whether or not cancer occurs following exposure to potential carcinogens. While the immune system of healthy individuals limits proliferation of pre-malignant cells by recognizing and deleting cells that express potentially oncogenic viral proteins, these pre-transformed cells go unchecked and become malignant in immuno-compromised individuals, hence the increased incidence of cancer in transplant patients and those with congenital or secondary immunodeficiency disorders. HIV is not directly oncogenic but it is significantly associated with several lymphoid malignancies known to arise in immuno-compromised individuals who become infected with oncogenic viruses such as HPV, EBV, or KSHV (7). Surveillance data estimates the risk of developing NHL at 60- to 200-fold in people with progressive HIV disease compared to the uninfected population, while that of Hodgkin lymphoma (HL) is 8- to 10-fold, thus supporting the active role of the immune system in controlling cancer. Plausibly, HIV-mediated immune dysregulation contributes to immune escape of these viruses thus allowing for proliferation and emergence of stable populations of virally transformed cells that are not efficiently recognized and eliminated by the host's immune system (187, 193, 194). A wide body of literature documents several AIDS-defining malignancies in the pre-HAART era, but for the purposes of illustrating how immune dysregulation sets a microenvironment conducive for cancer development, this section will draw examples from HIV-associated predisposition to cervical cancer and KS.

HIV-1, KSHV, AND KAPOSI SARCOMA

The non-redundant role of host immunity in the control of viral cancers is well-illustrated by KS, which is more prevalent in untreated HIV/AIDS patients, mainly due to immunosuppression (195). KSHV was discovered as the causative agent of KS in 1994 (196), however, infection with this virus alone is not sufficient to cause KS in healthy immuno-competent individuals. Indeed, the incidence of KS in the general population remains very low (around 1/100,000), but increases dramatically to around 1/20 amongst HIV-infected people (197) and almost 1/3 HIV-infected homosexual men in the pre-HAART era (198). Furthermore, countries in which KS was endemic before the AIDS epidemic have seen a sharp increase in the incidence, with almost half of HIV-infected individuals who acquire KSHV infection going on to develop KS (199). However, within the endemic areas or in the high risk groups, most HIV-negative KSHV-infected individuals do not develop KS, indicating that HIV-associated immune impairment predisposes to KS development.

HIV-1, HPV, AND CERVICAL CANCER

Human papilloma viruses are the main etiological factor for cervical cancer (200). Of these, HPV-16 and HPV-18 are linked with cervical and anogenital cancers hence are classified as high risk genotypes. As with other cancers, the immune system is central in the pathogenesis of HPV and cervical cancer. In immunocompetent individuals, robust HPV-specific immune responses comprising B and T cells are generated and these correlate with spontaneous resolution of HPV (201, 202), demonstrating that host immunity can be sufficient to clear HPV infection. In particular, a Th1 cytokine profile is instrumental in HPV clearance and prevention of viral persistence. Thus, detection of both humoral and cellular responses including T helper cells induces regression of cervical lesions (203, 204), whereas T helper cell impairment leads to cancer development (205). Natural killer cells also play a protective role by directly lysing HPV-infected cells and initiating regression of squamous intraepithelial lesions (SIL) (206, 207).

Despite the existence of strong HPV-specific immune responses in HPV-infected individuals, progression to HPV-associated malignancies does occur in some individuals due to escape from immune-surveillance caused by immune dysfunction as discussed earlier. Central to this is the systemic enrichment of Treg, which correlates with HPV persistence and is frequently detected in patients who develop high grade cervical intraepithelial neoplasia (208, 209). Furthermore, mucosal enrichment of Treg, which is often associated with diminished cellular immunity in the cervical mucosa has been observed and is linked with the severe forms of cervical carcinoma (210, 211). Higher frequencies of HPV-specific Treg are found in the stroma, intraepithelial tissues and tumor draining lymph nodes of cervical cancer patients where they suppress alloreactive CD4+ responder T cells (212, 213). Depletion of Treg in the *in vitro* experiments resulted in increased production of IFN-γ. Besides enhanced Treg-mediated immunosuppression, the profound immune dysfunction resulting from HIV-1 infection and the concomitant loss of CD4+ T cells collude to create an environment permissive for HPV persistence and cervical cancer. This can be directly deduced from the increased incidence of cervical cancer and prolonged persistence of SIL in immunosuppressed women with progressive HIV disease (214–216). In fact, cervical cancer was designated as an AIDS-defining illness in 1993 (217), strongly implicating HIV-driven immune impairment as a major factor favoring the progression from HPV infection to cancer development.

IMMUNE RESTORATION OR HIV SUPPRESSION REDUCES HIV-ASSOCIATED MALIGNANCIES

There is consensus that HIV-associated malignancies arise mainly due to loss of immune-surveillance caused by a dysfunctional immune system. Indeed, the severity of these malignancies correlates positively with the degree of immune impairment as measured by the extent of CD4+ T cell depletion and HIV viral burden. Moreover, the incidence of AIDS-defining malignancies has significantly reduced since the wide-scale implementation of HAART, strongly suggesting better immune control following reconstitution by HAART or perhaps a direct impact of HAART on the replication of EBV, HPV, and KSHV. Therefore, it seems that interventions which limit virus production and prevent chronic antigenic stimulation can effectively reduce immune activation and inflammation, restore effector immune functions through homeostatic equilibration of immuno-stimulatory and regulatory mechanisms, and lead to reduced incidences of HIV-associated malignancies. Recent studies indicate that the increased frequency and suppressive function of Treg observed during chronic HIV infection decreases significantly following HAART initiation (167). This is accompanied by reduced levels of immune activation and enhanced immune-effector functions, which are in turn associated with decreased prevalence and increased regression of cervical lesions in HAART-treated HPV-infected patients (218–220), thus supporting a role for immune reconstitution in the control of HPV and associated cancers. These observations provide evidence for a strong causative link between HIV-mediated immune dysregulation and the onset of HIV-associated cancers (NHL, KS, and cervical cancer) whose incidence has reduced significantly since the introduction of HAART.

HCV/HBV-DRIVEN IMMUNE DYSREGULATION PREDISPOSES TO HEPATOCELLULAR CARCINOMA

Unlike HIV, which directly targets the immune cells (CD4+ T cells) causing their deletion and loss of T helper functions, HBV and HCV target the liver and replicate in hepatocytes. These viruses have also evolved multiple mechanisms to escape immune elimination and can establish chronic persistence and replicate in infected hosts for many years. Epidemiological studies indicate a strong link between chronic HBV/HCV persistence with the development of liver disease, initially manifesting as chronic hepatitis, and leading on to nodular fibrosis that can progress to cirrhosis and eventually hepatocellular carcinoma (HCC). These processes are characterized by inflammation and oxidative stress owing to the influx of several cell types including NK, NKT, and PMN leukocytes, which accumulate in inflammatory lesions in the liver and contribute to inflammation and liver damage. In a majority of infected individuals, robust and poly functional T cell responses are generated causing clearance of acute infection, while in a minority of those infected, both low frequencies and narrowly focused virus-specific CD8+ T cell responses in the liver correlate with persistent chronic infection and increased risk of HCC (221). Furthermore, defects in HBV-specific CD8+ T cells characterized by exhaustion and increased expression of pro-apoptotic mediators have been reported (222). Thus, although virus-specific lymphocytes can be readily detected in inflammatory lesions in the liver, they are often defective and not sufficient to clear virus infection (223). Moreover, weaker CD4+ T cell proliferative responses have been reported (224).

Infection with HBV and HCV is known to induce IL-10 and TGF-β (72, 73), which in turn induce the expansion of Treg to maintain a tolerogenic environment in the liver. HCV-specific impairment of dendritic cell function can also lead to increased numbers of Treg, and these have been found in both the blood and liver of patients with chronic HBV and HCV infection and HCC

(185), where they correlate with *in vitro* suppression of antigen-specific effector responses (225). These effector responses were enhanced by depleting Treg (54, 226). Overall, immune function restoration and inhibition of viral replication following treatment with anti-HBV drugs is associated with diminished Treg expression (227). Thus, persistence of weak, defective, and narrowly directed T cell responses coupled with high numbers of immune-regulatory cells and increased levels of suppressive cytokines act to promote chronic liver disease and progression to HCC. Indeed, patients with HCC often have increased Treg numbers in blood and within tumors, and the tumor-infiltrating CD8+ and CD4+ T cells have been found to be dysfunctional (228), suggesting a possible link between immune disruption and the pathogenesis of HCC. Other factors such as chronic unresolved inflammation can further support tumor growth via induction of angiogenic and tumor survival signals (229).

IMMUNE DYSREGULATION IN INFLAMMATORY BOWEL DISEASE AND COLORECTAL CANCER

Inflammatory bowel disease is characterized by an uncontrolled, microbe-induced chronic inflammatory state that increases the risk of colorectal cancer (CRC) by twofold (8, 9). These chronic inflammatory responses also drive carcinogenesis of colitis-associated cancer (230). Various cell types infiltrate the inflamed mucosa including MDSC, M2 macrophages, and Th17 cells, which promote tumor growth, and NK and CD8+ T cells, which either target and destroy or inhibit proliferation of CRC cells. These effects are mediated by cytokines such as IL-17A, IL-21, IL-6, and TNF-α that create a tumor-permissive environment versus IFN-γ, which exerts tumor-suppressive functions (231). IFN-γ protects from carcinogenesis by activating cytotoxic T cells as well as increasing the susceptibility of pre-malignant cells to cell-mediated cytotoxicity, thus IFN-γ-producing Th1 cells correlate with increased immune-surveillance and better prognosis in CRC patients (232).

Although IL-4- and IL-13-producing Th2 cells have been associated with increased tumor growth in humans (233) and in animal models using IFN-γ−/− and IL-4−/− deficient mice (234, 235), Th17 cells seem to be the most aggressive orchestrators of chronic inflammation during IBD and have a significant role in the initiation of CRC. This has been linked to IL-23, a cytokine known to induce high numbers of Th17 cells and a concomitant accumulation of pathogenic IL-17A+ IFN-γ+ effector T cells, which cause intestinal pathology and correlate with poor prognosis in CRC (153, 236–238). Indeed, high frequencies of activated Th17 cells together with their signature cytokines are found in the intestinal and serum samples of patients with IBD, and also within the colon and blood samples from patients with CD. Furthermore, IL-23-mediated accumulation of IL-17+IL-22+ innate lymphoid cells (ILCs) in inflamed colons is associated with development of invasive colon cancer (239–241), while increased frequencies of IL-17+ILCs are often found in the intestines of patients with CD (242). The tumor-promoting feature of Th17 cells largely arises from secretion of large amounts of IL-17, which in turn induces expression of pro-inflammatory factors such as TNF-α, IL-6, IL-1, and iNOS, known to play a role in CRC pathogenesis (243). Mice that are deficient in ROR-γt, the transcription factor of Th17 cells were shown to be resistant to chronic inflammation in models of colitis (244). Thus, immuno-regulatory pathways capable of limiting the induction and function of pathogenic Th17 effectors cells are required.

TREG PLAY A CRITICAL ROLE IN THE PATHOGENESIS OF IBD AND CRC

The pro-tumoral role of Treg in cancer establishment and progression is well-documented, and in fact a number of interventions that deplete Treg lead to improved prognosis of cancer patients. Furthermore, Treg depletion increases vaccine-mediated anti-tumor immunity (245) and can lead to eradication of established experimental tumors (210, 246). However, Treg play such a critical role in the maintenance of normal gut mucosal immunity by preventing chronic inflammatory responses to food antigens and commensal microflora (247), that inhibition of their function is associated with development of IBD (11, 12). Most astoundingly, increased infiltration of Treg in CRC correlates with a favorable prognosis (10), with several studies in experimental animal models providing evidence that Treg can prevent establishment of CRC (248, 249). This is thought to be through initiation of potent immuno-regulatory functions that prevent chronic inflammation, which would otherwise predispose to cancer establishment and growth. Under normal homeostatic conditions, high frequencies of Treg are found in the gut as it is a preferential site for peripheral Treg induction due to the abundant commensal micro-biota and CD103-producing DCs, which are specialized in inducing the differentiation of Treg from naïve CD4+ T cells (250, 251). However, inadequate regulatory functions are a major characteristic defect during IBD, suggesting alterations in the induction, maintenance, or even suppressive function of Treg. This section highlights some of the mechanisms of immune dysregulation that exacerbate the inflammatory state of IBD to set a stage for CRC.

TREG INDUCTION AND FUNCTION ARE IMPAIRED IN IBD AND CRC

Impaired frequency and function of Treg is one of the mechanisms of immune dysregulation that plays a central role in the pathogenesis of IBD. This is strongly associated with IL-23, a cytokine whose expression is increased in several human cancers including CRC (252). IL-23R signaling suppresses both the differentiation of Treg and IL-10 production by T cells, hence leading to intestinal pathology (236). Such pathology could be prevented by transfer of Treg or administration of Treg-related cytokines such as IL-10 and TGF-β1 (253). TGF-β signaling in tumor-infiltrating lymphocytes is associated with reduced tumor growth in animal models of CRC (254). Crucially, the frequency of Foxp3+ Treg in the colon increases in the absence of IL-23R signaling, indicating a role for IL-23 in controlling the induction and expansion of Treg (255). Since Treg are a source of both IL-10 and TGF-β, the key cytokines in immuno-regulation, it is plausible that IL-23-driven loss of Treg contributes significantly to immune dysregulation by overriding the immunosuppressive pathways in the intestine and favoring IBD and CRC development via generation of pathogenic Th17 effectors cells. Besides reduced numbers, Treg in IBD show altered phenotype and function, attributed to the local cytokine milieu arising from chronic inflammation of the intestinal mucosa. Perhaps, normal Treg in circulation migrate to the lamina propria during active inflammation in order to maintain homeostasis, but on encountering various cytokines within the inflamed mucosa, they undergo phenotypic and functional modifications turning into dual inflammatory and regulatory Foxp3+IL-17+ Treg, which produce large amounts of IFN-γ and IL-17, and moderate amounts of TNF-α and IL-2 (102, 103).

IL-10 PROTECTS AGAINST IBD AND CRC

IL-10 deficiency increases susceptibility to IBD-associated CRC, where it is associated with poor prognosis (256). Mice lacking IL-10 were shown to be highly susceptible to colitis-associated CRC following *Helicobacter hepaticus* infection, and this could be prevented by exogenous administration of IL-10 (257–259), further demonstrating a critical role for IL-10 in the pathogenesis of CRC. It is thought that IL-10 deficiency leads to elevated levels of TNF-α, IL-6, and IL-17, which in turn allow persistence of chronic inflammation (260) thus promoting tumor growth.

BI-FUNCTIONAL IMMUNE-EFFECTOR CELLS CAN PROMOTE IBD AND CRC

Intriguingly, a single cell type can exhibit bi-functional immune characteristics by co-producing effector and suppressor cytokines, thus may have the potential to exert both tumor-promoting and tumor-suppressive functions, depending on the microenvironment. For example, as mentioned above, CD8+ T cells express cytotoxic molecules, which kill CRC cells in addition to secreting IFN-γ, which augments the anti-tumor response (261, 262). However, in some cases of IBD, infiltration of CD8+ T cells does not correlate with improved prognosis (263) and this is linked to elevated perforin and granzyme levels, which sustain the tumor-promoting chronic inflammation (264). Accordingly, perforin deficient mice develop less severe colitis and much fewer tumors in experimental models of colitis-associated CRC (265). Similar bi-functional characteristics have been observed in NKT cells, which exert protective cytotoxic functions, but also secrete Th1, Th2, and Th17 cytokines that could act as enhancers or suppressors of tumor immunity. Increased infiltration of IFN-γ-secreting NKT cells correlates with tumor immunity, which is reflected in increased disease-free survival of CRC patients (266, 267). Conversely, Th2 NKT cells that secrete the immunosuppressive cytokine IL-13, may contribute to colitis-associated CRC (268, 269). These studies demonstrate that CD8+ T cells and NKT cells can simultaneously exert pro-tumoral and anti-tumoral responses, and that perhaps pro-tumoral responses predominate during progressive IBD and CRC. Arguably, intervention strategies targeted at these bi-functional effector cells may result in undesirable outcomes.

INTERVENTIONS

As discussed earlier, some settings such as inflammatory autoimmune diseases will require interventions that boost the immunoregulatory arm of the immune response. Such may include immunotherapeutic agents that expand Treg numbers and enhance suppressive function to effectively curtail chronic inflammation. Therapeutic vaccines to restore immune tolerance could benefit from adjuvants that induce adaptive Treg without generating functional effector cells (270). Other measures such as restoration of TGF-β and IL-10, together with IL-2 administration can help to maintain Treg numbers and Foxp3 expression, thus sustaining functional regulation. In other inflammatory settings such as IBD and colon cancer, measures that enhance Treg differentiation and expansion and restore suppressive function, for example, blockade of IL-23 signaling with the concurrent depletion of IFN-γ and IL-2 to impede generation of pathogenic exFoxp3 Treg might be desirable. Additionally, induction of stable expression of site-specific homing and chemokine receptors in Treg can confer the ability to migrate to preferential sites of chronic inflammation, for example, CCR4 for migration to the lung airways during allergic inflammation, CXCR4 for migration to the bone marrow, and CCR4/CCR9/CD62L/$\alpha_4\beta_7/\alpha_E$(CD103)β_7 for migration to the intestinal mucosa of IBD patients. However, in cases where immuno-regulatory responses are detrimental then immune deregulation interventions are required. Such can include administration of cytokines and/or antibodies that inhibit Treg induction and expansion, suppressive function, and recruitment via blockade of chemokine receptors (124). Interventions such as concurrent CTLA-4 blockade and vaccination (271–273), combined CTLA-4 and PD-1/PD-L1 blockade (274), and Treg depletion (275–277) have been successfully used to ameliorate Treg-mediated immune pathologies and cancer. Measures to reverse exhaustion and restore immune function in chronic infections include blockade of the PD-1:PD-L1/PD-L2 pathway and MDSC development. PD-1/PD-L1 blockade restores HIV-specific T cell function *in vitro* (33, 34, 278), and clinical benefit is also documented in cancer patients (279, 280). In some instances, combined blockade of PD-1 and LAG-3 or PD-1 and TIM-3 synergistically improves T cell responses leading to better virus control (43, 45). Very recently, a study utilizing a mouse model of retrovirus infection showed that combining the blockade of inhibitory receptors PD-1 and Tim-3, together with Treg ablation was more efficient in reducing chronic virus load compared with either strategy on its own (281). Functional blockade, developmental inhibition, or physical deletion of MDSC was shown to enhance the efficacy of cancer vaccines in animal models (282–284).

CONCLUSION

The role of the immune system in inflammation and carcinogenesis is highly influenced by the microenvironment, thus some disease settings can display unique characteristics where immunoregulatory processes are highly beneficial to the host but in other cases quite detrimental and predispose to pathogen persistence and increased risk of cancer. This calls for tailor-matched interventions, which are quite promising, however caution must be exercised since blocking an inhibitory pathway might re-invigorate the immune system to achieve disease control on one hand, but exacerbate immune activation and inflammation on the other. Overall, the timings of these interventions will be crucial in order to achieve favorable outcomes.

ACKNOWLEDGMENTS

Beatrice Omusiro Ondondo is an immunologist employed on a research grant supported by MRC UK.

REFERENCES

1. zur Hausen H. Oncogenic DNA viruses. *Oncogene* (2001) **20**(54):7820–3. doi:10.1038/sj.onc.1204958

2. Pardoll D. Does the immune system see tumors as foreign or self? *Annu Rev Immunol* (2003) **21**:807–39. doi:10.1146/annurev.immunol.21.120601.141135
3. Shankaran V, Ikeda H, Bruce AT, White JM, Swanson PE, Old LJ, et al. IFNgamma and lymphocytes prevent primary tumour development and shape tumour immunogenicity. *Nature* (2001) **410**(6832):1107–11. doi:10.1038/35074122
4. Ramsdell F, Fowlkes BJ. Maintenance of in vivo tolerance by persistence of antigen. *Science* (1992) **257**(5073):1130–4. doi:10.1126/science.257.5073.1130
5. Utzschneider DT, Legat A, Fuertes Marraco SA, Carrie L, Luescher I, Speiser DE, et al. T cells maintain an exhausted phenotype after antigen withdrawal and population reexpansion. *Nat Immunol* (2013) **14**(6):603–10. doi:10.1038/ni.2606
6. Virgin HW, Wherry EJ, Ahmed R. Redefining chronic viral infection. *Cell* (2009) **138**(1):30–50. doi:10.1016/j.cell.2009.06.036
7. Wood C, Harrington W Jr. AIDS and associated malignancies. *Cell Res* (2005) **15**(11–12):947–52. doi:10.1038/sj.cr.7290372
8. Eaden JA, Abrams KR, Mayberry JF. The risk of colorectal cancer in ulcerative colitis: a meta-analysis. *Gut* (2001) **48**(4):526–35. doi:10.1136/gut.48.4.526
9. Bernstein CN, Blanchard JF, Kliewer E, Wajda A. Cancer risk in patients with inflammatory bowel disease: a population-based study. *Cancer* (2001) **91**(4):854–62. doi:10.1002/1097-0142(20010215)91:4<854::AID-CNCR1073>3.0.CO;2-Z
10. Ladoire S, Martin F, Ghiringhelli F. Prognostic role of FOXP3+ regulatory T cells infiltrating human carcinomas: the paradox of colorectal cancer. *Cancer Immunol Immunother* (2011) **60**(7):909–18. doi:10.1007/s00262-011-1046-y
11. Wang Y, Liu XP, Zhao ZB, Chen JH, Yu CG. Expression of CD4+ forkhead box P3 (FOXP3)+ regulatory T cells in inflammatory bowel disease. *J Dig Dis* (2011) **12**(4):286–94. doi:10.1111/j.1751-2980.2011.00505.x
12. Chinen T, Volchkov PY, Chervonsky AV, Rudensky AY. A critical role for regulatory T cell-mediated control of inflammation in the absence of commensal microbiota. *J Exp Med* (2010) **207**(11):2323–30. doi:10.1084/jem.20101235
13. Collins KL, Chen BK, Kalams SA, Walker BD, Baltimore D. HIV-1 Nef protein protects infected primary cells against killing by cytotoxic T lymphocytes. *Nature* (1998) **391**(6665):397–401. doi:10.1038/34929
14. Schwartz O, Marechal V, Le Gall S, Lemonnier F, Heard JM. Endocytosis of major histocompatibility complex class I molecules is induced by the HIV-1 Nef protein. *Nat Med* (1996) **2**(3):338–42. doi:10.1038/nm0396-338
15. Groux H, O'Garra A, Bigler M, Rouleau M, Antonenko S, de Vries JE, et al. A CD4+ T-cell subset inhibits antigen-specific T-cell responses and prevents colitis. *Nature* (1997) **389**(6652):737–42. doi:10.1038/39614
16. Weiner HL. Induction and mechanism of action of transforming growth factor-beta-secreting Th3 regulatory cells. *Immunol Rev* (2001) **182**:207–14. doi:10.1034/j.1600-065X.2001.1820117.x
17. Beissert S, Schwarz A, Schwarz T. Regulatory T cells. *J Invest Dermatol* (2006) **126**(1):15–24. doi:10.1038/sj.jid.5700399
18. Vieira PL, Christensen JR, Minaee S, O'Neill EJ, Barrat FJ, Boonstra A, et al. IL-10-secreting regulatory T cells do not express Foxp3 but have comparable regulatory function to naturally occurring CD4+CD25+ regulatory T cells. *J Immunol* (2004) **172**(10):5986–93.
19. Gabrilovich DI, Nagaraj S. Myeloid-derived suppressor cells as regulators of the immune system. *Nat Rev Immunol* (2009) **9**(3):162–74. doi:10.1038/nri2506
20. Tang XL, Smith TR, Kumar V. Specific control of immunity by regulatory CD8 T cells. *Cell Mol Immunol* (2005) **2**(1):11–9.
21. Cosmi L, Liotta F, Lazzeri E, Francalanci M, Angeli R, Mazzinghi B, et al. Human CD8+CD25+ thymocytes share phenotypic and functional features with CD4+CD25+ regulatory thymocytes. *Blood* (2003) **102**(12):4107–14. doi:10.1182/blood-2003-04-1320
22. Endharti AT, Rifa IM, Shi Z, Fukuoka Y, Nakahara Y, Kawamoto Y, et al. Cutting edge: CD8+CD122+ regulatory T cells produce IL-10 to suppress IFN-gamma production and proliferation of CD8+ T cells. *J Immunol* (2005) **175**(11):7093–7.
23. Ehlers M, Papewalis C, Stenzel W, Jacobs B, Meyer KL, Deenen R, et al. Immunoregulatory natural killer cells suppress autoimmunity by down-regulating antigen-specific CD8+ T cells in mice. *Endocrinology* (2012) **153**(9):4367–79. doi:10.1210/en.2012-1247
24. Ebata K, Shimizu Y, Nakayama Y, Minemura M, Murakami J, Kato T, et al. Immature NK cells suppress dendritic cell functions during the development of leukemia in a mouse model. *J Immunol* (2006) **176**(7):4113–24.
25. Klenerman P, Hill A. T cells and viral persistence: lessons from diverse infections. *Nat Immunol* (2005) **6**(9):873–9. doi:10.1038/ni1241
26. Wherry EJ, Blattman JN, Murali-Krishna K, van der Most R, Ahmed R. Viral persistence alters CD8 T-cell immunodominance and tissue distribution and results in distinct stages of functional impairment. *J Virol* (2003) **77**(8):4911–27. doi:10.1128/JVI.77.8.4911-4927.2003
27. Shin H, Wherry EJ. CD8 T cell dysfunction during chronic viral infection. *Curr Opin Immunol* (2007) **19**(4):408–15. doi:10.1016/j.coi.2007.06.004
28. Shin H, Blackburn SD, Blattman JN, Wherry EJ. Viral antigen and extensive division maintain virus-specific CD8 T cells during chronic infection. *J Exp Med* (2007) **204**(4):941–9. doi:10.1084/jem.20061937
29. Francisco LM, Sage PT, Sharpe AH. The PD-1 pathway in tolerance and autoimmunity. *Immunol Rev* (2010) **236**:219–42. doi:10.1111/j.1600-065X.2010.00923.x
30. Nishimura H, Honjo T. PD-1: an inhibitory immunoreceptor involved in peripheral tolerance. *Trends Immunol* (2001) **22**(5):265–8. doi:10.1016/S1471-4906(01)01888-9
31. Nishimura H, Nose M, Hiai H, Minato N, Honjo T. Development of lupus-like autoimmune diseases by disruption of the PD-1 gene encoding an ITIM motif-carrying immunoreceptor. *Immunity* (1999) **11**(2):141–51. doi:10.1016/S1074-7613(00)80089-8
32. Nishimura H, Okazaki T, Tanaka Y, Nakatani K, Hara M, Matsumori A, et al. Autoimmune dilated cardiomyopathy in PD-1 receptor-deficient mice. *Science* (2001) **291**(5502):319–22. doi:10.1126/science.291.5502.319
33. Day CL, Kaufmann DE, Kiepiela P, Brown JA, Moodley ES, Reddy S, et al. PD-1 expression on HIV-specific T cells is associated with T-cell exhaustion and disease progression. *Nature* (2006) **443**(7109):350–4. doi:10.1038/nature05115
34. Trautmann L, Janbazian L, Chomont N, Said EA, Gimmig S, Bessette B, et al. Upregulation of PD-1 expression on HIV-specific CD8+ T cells leads to reversible immune dysfunction. *Nat Med* (2006) **12**(10):1198–202. doi:10.1038/nm1106-1329b
35. Zhang JY, Zhang Z, Wang X, Fu JL, Yao J, Jiao Y, et al. PD-1 up-regulation is correlated with HIV-specific memory CD8+ T-cell exhaustion in typical progressors but not in long-term nonprogressors. *Blood* (2007) **109**(11):4671–8. doi:10.1182/blood-2006-09-044826
36. Maier H, Isogawa M, Freeman GJ, Chisari FV. PD-1:PD-L1 interactions contribute to the functional suppression of virus-specific CD8+ T lymphocytes in the liver. *J Immunol* (2007) **178**(5):2714–20.
37. Golden-Mason L, Palmer B, Klarquist J, Mengshol JA, Castelblanco N, Rosen HR. Upregulation of PD-1 expression on circulating and intrahepatic hepatitis C virus-specific CD8+ T cells associated with reversible immune dysfunction. *J Virol* (2007) **81**(17):9249–58. doi:10.1128/JVI.00409-07
38. Zhang Z, Zhang JY, Wherry EJ, Jin B, Xu B, Zou ZS, et al. Dynamic programmed death 1 expression by virus-specific CD8 T cells correlates with the outcome of acute hepatitis B. *Gastroenterology* (2008) **134**(7):1938–49. doi:10.1053/j.gastro.2008.03.037
39. Fisicaro P, Valdatta C, Massari M, Loggi E, Biasini E, Sacchelli L, et al. Antiviral intrahepatic T-cell responses can be restored by blocking programmed death-1 pathway in chronic hepatitis B. *Gastroenterology* (2010) **138**(2):e1–4. doi:10.1053/j.gastro.2009.09.052
40. D'Souza M, Fontenot AP, Mack DG, Lozupone C, Dillon S, Meditz A, et al. Programmed death 1 expression on HIV-specific CD4+ T cells is driven by viral replication and associated with T cell dysfunction. *J Immunol* (2007) **179**(3):1979–87.
41. Kaufmann DE, Kavanagh DG, Pereyra F, Zaunders JJ, Mackey EW, Miura T, et al. Upregulation of CTLA-4 by HIV-specific CD4+ T cells correlates with disease progression and defines a reversible immune dysfunction. *Nat Immunol* (2007) **8**(11):1246–54. doi:10.1038/ni1515
42. Petrovas C, Casazza JP, Brenchley JM, Price DA, Gostick E, Adams WC, et al. PD-1 is a regulator of virus-specific CD8+ T cell survival in HIV infection. *J Exp Med* (2006) **203**(10):2281–92. doi:10.1084/jem.20061496
43. Blackburn SD, Shin H, Haining WN, Zou T, Workman CJ, Polley A, et al. Coregulation of CD8+ T cell exhaustion by multiple inhibitory receptors during chronic viral infection. *Nat Immunol* (2009) **10**(1):29–37. doi:10.1038/ni.1679
44. Jones RB, Ndhlovu LC, Barbour JD, Sheth PM, Jha AR, Long BR, et al. Tim-3 expression defines a novel population of dysfunctional T cells with highly elevated frequencies in progressive HIV-1 infection. *J Exp Med* (2008) **205**(12):2763–79. doi:10.1084/jem.20081398

45. Jin HT, Anderson AC, Tan WG, West EE, Ha SJ, Araki K, et al. Cooperation of Tim-3 and PD-1 in CD8 T-cell exhaustion during chronic viral infection. *Proc Natl Acad Sci U S A* (2010) **107**(33):14733–8. doi:10.1073/pnas.1009731107
46. Yamamoto T, Price DA, Casazza JP, Ferrari G, Nason M, Chattopadhyay PK, et al. Surface expression patterns of negative regulatory molecules identify determinants of virus-specific CD8+ T-cell exhaustion in HIV infection. *Blood* (2011) **117**(18):4805–15. doi:10.1182/blood-2010-11-317297
47. Nakamoto N, Cho H, Shaked A, Olthoff K, Valiga ME, Kaminski M, et al. Synergistic reversal of intrahepatic HCV-specific CD8 T cell exhaustion by combined PD-1/CTLA-4 blockade. *PLoS Pathog* (2009) **5**(2):e1000313. doi:10.1371/journal.ppat.1000313
48. Homann D, McGavern DB, Oldstone MB. Visualizing the viral burden: phenotypic and functional alterations of T cells and APCs during persistent infection. *J Immunol* (2004) **172**(10):6239–50.
49. Sevilla N, McGavern DB, Teng C, Kunz S, Oldstone MB. Viral targeting of hematopoietic progenitors and inhibition of DC maturation as a dual strategy for immune subversion. *J Clin Invest* (2004) **113**(5):737–45. doi:10.1172/JCI20243
50. Rodrigue-Gervais IG, Rigsby H, Jouan L, Sauve D, Sekaly RP, Willems B, et al. Dendritic cell inhibition is connected to exhaustion of CD8+ T cell polyfunctionality during chronic hepatitis C virus infection. *J Immunol* (2010) **184**(6):3134–44. doi:10.4049/jimmunol.0902522
51. Chen L, Zhang Z, Chen W, Zhang Z, Li Y, Shi M, et al. B7-H1 up-regulation on myeloid dendritic cells significantly suppresses T cell immune function in patients with chronic hepatitis B. *J Immunol* (2007) **178**(10):6634–41.
52. Manches O, Munn D, Fallahi A, Lifson J, Chaperot L, Plumas J, et al. HIV-activated human plasmacytoid DCs induce Tregs through an indoleamine 2,3-dioxygenase-dependent mechanism. *J Clin Invest* (2008) **118**(10):3431–9. doi:10.1172/JCI34823
53. Franzese O, Kennedy PT, Gehring AJ, Gotto J, Williams R, Maini MK, et al. Modulation of the CD8+-T-cell response by CD4+ CD25+ regulatory T cells in patients with hepatitis B virus infection. *J Virol* (2005) **79**(6):3322–8. doi:10.1128/JVI.79.6.3322-3328.2005
54. Xu D, Fu J, Jin L, Zhang H, Zhou C, Zou Z, et al. Circulating and liver resident CD4+CD25+ regulatory T cells actively influence the antiviral immune response and disease progression in patients with hepatitis B. *J Immunol* (2006) **177**(1):739–47.
55. Barboza L, Salmen S, Goncalves L, Colmenares M, Peterson D, Montes H, et al. Antigen-induced regulatory T cells in HBV chronically infected patients. *Virology* (2007) **368**(1):41–9. doi:10.1016/j.virol.2007.06.030
56. Ebinuma H, Nakamoto N, Li Y, Price DA, Gostick E, Levine BL, et al. Identification and in vitro expansion of functional antigen-specific CD25+ FoxP3+ regulatory T cells in hepatitis C virus infection. *J Virol* (2008) **82**(10):5043–53. doi:10.1128/JVI.01548-07
57. Accapezzato D, Francavilla V, Paroli M, Casciaro M, Chircu LV, Cividini A, et al. Hepatic expansion of a virus-specific regulatory CD8(+) T cell population in chronic hepatitis C virus infection. *J Clin Invest* (2004) **113**(7):963–72. doi:10.1172/JCI20515
58. Dolganiuc A, Paek E, Kodys K, Thomas J, Szabo G. Myeloid dendritic cells of patients with chronic HCV infection induce proliferation of regulatory T lymphocytes. *Gastroenterology* (2008) **135**(6):2119–27. doi:10.1053/j.gastro.2008.07.082
59. Kinter A, McNally J, Riggin L, Jackson R, Roby G, Fauci AS. Suppression of HIV-specific T cell activity by lymph node CD25+ regulatory T cells from HIV-infected individuals. *Proc Natl Acad Sci U S A* (2007) **104**(9):3390–5. doi:10.1073/pnas.0611423104
60. Nilsson J, Boasso A, Velilla PA, Zhang R, Vaccari M, Franchini G, et al. HIV-1-driven regulatory T-cell accumulation in lymphoid tissues is associated with disease progression in HIV/AIDS. *Blood* (2006) **108**(12):3808–17. doi:10.1182/blood-2006-05-021576
61. Bi X, Suzuki Y, Gatanaga H, Oka S. High frequency and proliferation of CD4+ FOXP3+ Treg in HIV-1-infected patients with low CD4 counts. *Eur J Immunol* (2009) **39**(1):301–9. doi:10.1002/eji.200838667
62. Hall CH, Kassel R, Tacke RS, Hahn YS. HCV+ hepatocytes induce human regulatory CD4+ T cells through the production of TGF-beta. *PLoS One* (2010) **5**(8):e12154. doi:10.1371/journal.pone.0012154
63. Ward SM, Fox BC, Brown PJ, Worthington J, Fox SB, Chapman RW, et al. Quantification and localisation of FOXP3+ T lymphocytes and relation to hepatic inflammation during chronic HCV infection. *J Hepatol* (2007) **47**(3):316–24. doi:10.1016/j.jhep.2007.03.023
64. Thornton AM, Shevach EM. Suppressor effector function of CD4+CD25+ immunoregulatory T cells is antigen nonspecific. *J Immunol* (2000) **164**(1):183–90.
65. Cao S, Li Y, Ye J, Yang X, Chen L, Liu X, et al. Japanese encephalitis virus wild strain infection suppresses dendritic cells maturation and function, and causes the expansion of regulatory T cells. *Virol J* (2011) **8**:39. doi:10.1186/1743-422X-8-39
66. Robertson SJ, Hasenkrug KJ. The role of virus-induced regulatory T cells in immunopathology. *Springer Semin Immunopathol* (2006) **28**(1):51–62. doi:10.1007/s00281-006-0019-2
67. Dittmer U, He H, Messer RJ, Schimmer S, Olbrich AR, Ohlen C, et al. Functional impairment of CD8(+) T cells by regulatory T cells during persistent retroviral infection. *Immunity* (2004) **20**(3):293–303. doi:10.1016/S1074-7613(04)00054-8
68. Brooks DG, Trifilo MJ, Edelmann KH, Teyton L, McGavern DB, Oldstone MB. Interleukin-10 determines viral clearance or persistence in vivo. *Nat Med* (2006) **12**(11):1301–9. doi:10.1038/nm1492
69. Ejrnaes M, Filippi CM, Martinic MM, Ling EM, Togher LM, Crotty S, et al. Resolution of a chronic viral infection after interleukin-10 receptor blockade. *J Exp Med* (2006) **203**(11):2461–72. doi:10.1084/jem.20061462
70. Brockman MA, Kwon DS, Tighe DP, Pavlik DF, Rosato PC, Sela J, et al. IL-10 is up-regulated in multiple cell types during viremic HIV infection and reversibly inhibits virus-specific T cells. *Blood* (2009) **114**(2):346–56. doi:10.1182/blood-2008-12-191296
71. Clerici M, Wynn TA, Berzofsky JA, Blatt SP, Hendrix CW, Sher A, et al. Role of interleukin-10 in T helper cell dysfunction in asymptomatic individuals infected with the human immunodeficiency virus. *J Clin Invest* (1994) **93**(2):768–75. doi:10.1172/JCI117031
72. Hyodo N, Nakamura I, Imawari M. Hepatitis B core antigen stimulates interleukin-10 secretion by both T cells and monocytes from peripheral blood of patients with chronic hepatitis B virus infection. *Clin Exp Immunol* (2004) **135**(3):462–6.
73. Kaplan DE, Ikeda F, Li Y, Nakamoto N, Ganesan S, Valiga ME, et al. Peripheral virus-specific T-cell interleukin-10 responses develop early in acute hepatitis C infection and become dominant in chronic hepatitis. *J Hepatol* (2008) **48**(6):903–13. doi:10.1016/j.jhep.2008.01.030
74. Maris CH, Chappell CP, Jacob J. Interleukin-10 plays an early role in generating virus-specific T cell anergy. *BMC Immunol* (2007) **8**:8. doi:10.1186/1471-2172-8-8
75. Ohga S, Nomura A, Takada H, Tanaka T, Furuno K, Takahata Y, et al. Dominant expression of interleukin-10 and transforming growth factor-beta genes in activated T-cells of chronic active Epstein-Barr virus infection. *J Med Virol* (2004) **74**(3):449–58. doi:10.1002/jmv.20197
76. Letterio JJ, Roberts AB. Regulation of immune responses by TGF-beta. *Annu Rev Immunol* (1998) **16**:137–61. doi:10.1146/annurev.immunol.16.1.137
77. Zhou X, Bailey-Bucktrout SL, Jeker LT, Penaranda C, Martinez-Llordella M, Ashby M, et al. Instability of the transcription factor Foxp3 leads to the generation of pathogenic memory T cells in vivo. *Nat Immunol* (2009) **10**(9):1000–7. doi:10.1038/ni.1774
78. Wan YY, Flavell RA. Regulatory T-cell functions are subverted and converted owing to attenuated Foxp3 expression. *Nature* (2007) **445**(7129):766–70. doi:10.1038/nature05479
79. Miyao T, Floess S, Setoguchi R, Luche H, Fehling HJ, Waldmann H, et al. Plasticity of Foxp3(+) T cells reflects promiscuous Foxp3 expression in conventional T cells but not reprogramming of regulatory T cells. *Immunity* (2012) **36**(2):262–75. doi:10.1016/j.immuni.2011.12.012
80. Komatsu N, Mariotti-Ferrandiz ME, Wang Y, Malissen B, Waldmann H, Hori S. Heterogeneity of natural Foxp3+ T cells: a committed regulatory T-cell lineage and an uncommitted minor population retaining plasticity. *Proc Natl Acad Sci U S A* (2009) **106**(6):1903–8. doi:10.1073/pnas.0811556106
81. Duarte JH, Zelenay S, Bergman ML, Martins AC, Demengeot J. Natural Treg cells spontaneously differentiate into pathogenic helper cells in lymphopenic conditions. *Eur J Immunol* (2009) **39**(4):948–55. doi:10.1002/eji.200839196
82. Gavin MA, Rasmussen JP, Fontenot JD, Vasta V, Manganiello VC, Beavo JA, et al. Foxp3-dependent programme of regulatory T-cell differentiation. *Nature* (2007) **445**(7129):771–5. doi:10.1038/nature05543

83. Krishnamoorthy N, Khare A, Oriss TB, Raundhal M, Morse C, Yarlagadda M, et al. Early infection with respiratory syncytial virus impairs regulatory T cell function and increases susceptibility to allergic asthma. *Nat Med* (2012) **18**(10):1525–30. doi:10.1038/nm.2896
84. Tsuji M, Komatsu N, Kawamoto S, Suzuki K, Kanagawa O, Honjo T, et al. Preferential generation of follicular B helper T cells from Foxp3+ T cells in gut Peyer's patches. *Science* (2009) **323**(5920):1488–92. doi:10.1126/science.1169152
85. Zhou L, Lopes JE, Chong MM, Ivanov II, Min R, Victora GD, et al. TGF-beta-induced Foxp3 inhibits T(H)17 cell differentiation by antagonizing RORgammat function. *Nature* (2008) **453**(7192):236–40. doi:10.1038/nature06878
86. Osorio F, LeibundGut-Landmann S, Lochner M, Lahl K, Sparwasser T, Eberl G, et al. DC activated via dectin-1 convert Treg into IL-17 producers. *Eur J Immunol* (2008) **38**(12):3274–81. doi:10.1002/eji.200838950
87. Voo KS, Wang YH, Santori FR, Boggiano C, Wang YH, Arima K, et al. Identification of IL-17-producing FOXP3+ regulatory T cells in humans. *Proc Natl Acad Sci U S A* (2009) **106**(12):4793–8. doi:10.1073/pnas.0900408106
88. Beriou G, Costantino CM, Ashley CW, Yang L, Kuchroo VK, Baecher-Allan C, et al. IL-17-producing human peripheral regulatory T cells retain suppressive function. *Blood* (2009) **113**(18):4240–9. doi:10.1182/blood-2008-10-183251
89. Ayyoub M, Deknuydt F, Raimbaud I, Dousset C, Leveque L, Bioley G, et al. Human memory FOXP3+ Tregs secrete IL-17 ex vivo and constitutively express the T(H)17 lineage-specific transcription factor RORgamma t. *Proc Natl Acad Sci U S A* (2009) **106**(21):8635–40. doi:10.1073/pnas.0900621106
90. Lochner M, Peduto L, Cherrier M, Sawa S, Langa F, Varona R, et al. In vivo equilibrium of proinflammatory IL-17+ and regulatory IL-10+ Foxp3+ RORgamma t+ T cells. *J Exp Med* (2008) **205**(6):1381–93. doi:10.1084/jem.20080034
91. Wei G, Wei L, Zhu J, Zang C, Hu-Li J, Yao Z, et al. Global mapping of H3K4me3 and H3K27me3 reveals specificity and plasticity in lineage fate determination of differentiating CD4+ T cells. *Immunity* (2009) **30**(1):155–67. doi:10.1016/j.immuni.2008.12.009
92. Oldenhove G, Bouladoux N, Wohlfert EA, Hall JA, Chou D, Dos Santos L, et al. Decrease of Foxp3+ Treg cell number and acquisition of effector cell phenotype during lethal infection. *Immunity* (2009) **31**(5):772–86. doi:10.1016/j.immuni.2009.10.001
93. Lindley S, Dayan CM, Bishop A, Roep BO, Peakman M, Tree TI. Defective suppressor function in CD4(+)CD25(+) T-cells from patients with type 1 diabetes. *Diabetes* (2005) **54**(1):92–9. doi:10.2337/diabetes.54.1.92
94. Haas J, Hug A, Viehover A, Fritzsching B, Falk CS, Filser A, et al. Reduced suppressive effect of CD4+CD25high regulatory T cells on the T cell immune response against myelin oligodendrocyte glycoprotein in patients with multiple sclerosis. *Eur J Immunol* (2005) **35**(11):3343–52. doi:10.1002/eji.200526065
95. Huan J, Culbertson N, Spencer L, Bartholomew R, Burrows GG, Chou YK, et al. Decreased FOXP3 levels in multiple sclerosis patients. *J Neurosci Res* (2005) **81**(1):45–52. doi:10.1002/jnr.20522
96. Viglietta V, Baecher-Allan C, Weiner HL, Hafler DA. Loss of functional suppression by CD4+CD25+ regulatory T cells in patients with multiple sclerosis. *J Exp Med* (2004) **199**(7):971–9. doi:10.1084/jem.20031579
97. Fletcher JM, Lonergan R, Costelloe L, Kinsella K, Moran B, O'Farrelly C, et al. CD39+Foxp3+ regulatory T Cells suppress pathogenic Th17 cells and are impaired in multiple sclerosis. *J Immunol* (2009) **183**(11):7602–10. doi:10.4049/jimmunol.0901881
98. Astier AL, Meiffren G, Freeman S, Hafler DA. Alterations in CD46-mediated Tr1 regulatory T cells in patients with multiple sclerosis. *J Clin Invest* (2006) **116**(12):3252–7. doi:10.1172/JCI29251
99. Glick AB, Wodzinski A, Fu P, Levine AD, Wald DN. Impairment of regulatory T-cell function in autoimmune thyroid disease. *Thyroid* (2013) **23**(7):871–8. doi:10.1089/thy.2012.0514
100. Arandi N, Mirshafiey A, Jeddi-Tehrani M, Shaghaghi M, Sadeghi B, Abolhassani H, et al. Alteration in frequency and function of CD4+CD25+FOXP3+ regulatory T cells in patients with immune thrombocytopenic purpura. *Iran J Allergy Asthma Immunol* (2014) **13**(2):85–92.
101. Komatsu N, Okamoto K, Sawa S, Nakashima T, Oh-Hora M, Kodama T, et al. Pathogenic conversion of Foxp3(+) T cells into TH17 cells in autoimmune arthritis. *Nat Med* (2014) **20**(1):62–8. doi:10.1038/nm.3432
102. Hovhannisyan Z, Treatman J, Littman DR, Mayer L. Characterization of interleukin-17-producing regulatory T cells in inflamed intestinal mucosa from patients with inflammatory bowel diseases. *Gastroenterology* (2011) **140**(3):957–65. doi:10.1053/j.gastro.2010.12.002
103. Kryczek I, Wu K, Zhao E, Wei S, Vatan L, Szeliga W, et al. IL-17+ regulatory T cells in the microenvironments of chronic inflammation and cancer. *J Immunol* (2011) **186**(7):4388–95. doi:10.4049/jimmunol.1003251
104. Dominguez-Villar M, Baecher-Allan CM, Hafler DA. Identification of T helper type 1-like, Foxp3+ regulatory T cells in human autoimmune disease. *Nat Med* (2011) **17**(6):673–5. doi:10.1038/nm.2389
105. Xu L, Kitani A, Fuss I, Strober W. Cutting edge: regulatory T cells induce CD4+CD25-Foxp3- T cells or self-induced to become Th17 cells in the absence of exogenous TGF-beta. *J Immunol* (2007) **178**(11):6725–9.
106. Yang XO, Nurieva R, Martinez GJ, Kang HS, Chung Y, Pappu BP, et al. Molecular antagonism and plasticity of regulatory and inflammatory T cell programs. *Immunity* (2008) **29**(1):44–56. doi:10.1016/j.immuni.2008.05.007
107. Nyirenda MH, Sanvito L, Darlington PJ, O'Brien K, Zhang GX, Constantinescu CS, et al. TLR2 stimulation drives human naive and effector regulatory T cells into a Th17-like phenotype with reduced suppressive function. *J Immunol* (2011) **187**(5):2278–90. doi:10.4049/jimmunol.1003715
108. Marie JC, Letterio JJ, Gavin M, Rudensky AY. TGF-beta1 maintains suppressor function and Foxp3 expression in CD4+CD25+ regulatory T cells. *J Exp Med* (2005) **201**(7):1061–7. doi:10.1084/jem.20042276
109. Murai M, Turovskaya O, Kim G, Madan R, Karp CL, Cheroutre H, et al. Interleukin 10 acts on regulatory T cells to maintain expression of the transcription factor Foxp3 and suppressive function in mice with colitis. *Nat Immunol* (2009) **10**(11):1178–84. doi:10.1038/ni.1791
110. Li MO, Sanjabi S, Flavell RA. Transforming growth factor-beta controls development, homeostasis, and tolerance of T cells by regulatory T cell-dependent and -independent mechanisms. *Immunity* (2006) **25**(3):455–71. doi:10.1016/j.immuni.2006.07.011
111. Pion M, Jaramillo-Ruiz D, Martinez A, Munoz-Fernandez MA, Correa-Rocha R. HIV infection of human regulatory T cells downregulates Foxp3 expression by increasing DNMT3b levels and DNA methylation in the FOXP3 gene. *AIDS* (2013) **27**(13):2019–29. doi:10.1097/QAD.0b013e32836253fd
112. Franceschini D, Paroli M, Francavilla V, Videtta M, Morrone S, Labbadia G, et al. PD-L1 negatively regulates CD4+CD25+Foxp3+ Tregs by limiting STAT-5 phosphorylation in patients chronically infected with HCV. *J Clin Invest* (2009) **119**(3):551–64. doi:10.1172/JCI36604
113. Iellem A, Colantonio L, D'Ambrosio D. Skin-versus gut-skewed homing receptor expression and intrinsic CCR4 expression on human peripheral blood CD4+CD25+ suppressor T cells. *Eur J Immunol* (2003) **33**(6):1488–96. doi:10.1002/eji.200323658
114. Wysocki CA, Jiang Q, Panoskaltsis-Mortari A, Taylor PA, McKinnon KP, Su L, et al. Critical role for CCR5 in the function of donor CD4+CD25+ regulatory T cells during acute graft-versus-host disease. *Blood* (2005) **106**(9):3300–7. doi:10.1182/blood-2005-04-1632
115. Yurchenko E, Tritt M, Hay V, Shevach EM, Belkaid Y, Piccirillo CA. CCR5-dependent homing of naturally occurring CD4+ regulatory T cells to sites of *Leishmania major* infection favors pathogen persistence. *J Exp Med* (2006) **203**(11):2451–60. doi:10.1084/jem.20060956
116. Huehn J, Siegmund K, Lehmann JC, Siewert C, Haubold U, Feuerer M, et al. Developmental stage, phenotype, and migration distinguish naive- and effector/memory-like CD4+ regulatory T cells. *J Exp Med* (2004) **199**(3):303–13. doi:10.1084/jem.20031562
117. Luster AD. The role of chemokines in linking innate and adaptive immunity. *Curr Opin Immunol* (2002) **14**(1):129–35. doi:10.1016/S0952-7915(01)00308-9
118. Yuan Q, Bromley SK, Means TK, Jones KJ, Hayashi F, Bhan AK, et al. CCR4-dependent regulatory T cell function in inflammatory bowel disease. *J Exp Med* (2007) **204**(6):1327–34. doi:10.1084/jem.20062076
119. Ondondo B, Jones E, Godkin A, Gallimore A. Home sweet home: the tumor microenvironment as a haven for regulatory T cells. *Front Immunol* (2013) **4**:197. doi:10.3389/fimmu.2013.00197
120. Curiel TJ, Coukos G, Zou L, Alvarez X, Cheng P, Mottram P, et al. Specific recruitment of regulatory T cells in ovarian carcinoma fosters immune privilege and predicts reduced survival. *Nat Med* (2004) **10**(9):942–9. doi:10.1038/nm1093

121. Shields JD, Kourtis IC, Tomei AA, Roberts JM, Swartz MA. Induction of lymphoid like stroma and immune escape by tumors that express the chemokine CCL21. *Science* (2010) **328**(5979):749–52. doi:10.1126/science.1185837
122. Mizukami Y, Kono K, Kawaguchi Y, Akaike H, Kamimura K, Sugai H, et al. CCL17 and CCL22 chemokines within tumor microenvironment are related to accumulation of Foxp3+ regulatory T cells in gastric cancer. *Int J Cancer* (2008) **122**(10):2286–93. doi:10.1002/ijc.23392
123. Tan MC, Goedegebuure PS, Belt BA, Flaherty B, Sankpal N, Gillanders WE, et al. Disruption of CCR5-dependent homing of regulatory T cells inhibits tumor growth in a murine model of pancreatic cancer. *J Immunol* (2009) **182**(3):1746–55.
124. Sugiyama D, Nishikawa H, Maeda Y, Nishioka M, Tanemura A, Katayama I, et al. Anti-CCR4 mAb selectively depletes effector-type FoxP3+CD4+ regulatory T cells, evoking antitumor immune responses in humans. *Proc Natl Acad Sci U S A* (2013) **110**(44):17945–50. doi:10.1073/pnas.1316796110
125. Moreno-Fernandez ME, Zapata W, Blackard JT, Franchini G, Chougnet CA. Human regulatory T cells are targets for human immunodeficiency virus (HIV) infection, and their susceptibility differs depending on the HIV type 1 strain. *J Virol* (2009) **83**(24):12925–33. doi:10.1128/JVI.01352-09
126. Jiang Q, Zhang L, Wang R, Jeffrey J, Washburn ML, Brouwer D, et al. FoxP3+CD4+ regulatory T cells play an important role in acute HIV-1 infection in humanized Rag2-/-gammaC-/- mice in vivo. *Blood* (2008) **112**(7):2858–68. doi:10.1182/blood-2008-03-145946
127. Kinter AL, Hennessey M, Bell A, Kern S, Lin Y, Daucher M, et al. CD25(+)CD4(+) regulatory T cells from the peripheral blood of asymptomatic HIV-infected individuals regulate CD4(+) and CD8(+) HIV-specific T cell immune responses in vitro and are associated with favorable clinical markers of disease status. *J Exp Med* (2004) **200**(3):331–43. doi:10.1084/jem.20032069
128. Andersson J, Boasso A, Nilsson J, Zhang R, Shire NJ, Lindback S, et al. The prevalence of regulatory T cells in lymphoid tissue is correlated with viral load in HIV-infected patients. *J Immunol* (2005) **174**(6):3143–7.
129. Chase AJ, Sedaghat AR, German JR, Gama L, Zink MC, Clements JE, et al. Severe depletion of CD4+ CD25+ regulatory T cells from the intestinal lamina propria but not peripheral blood or lymph nodes during acute simian immunodeficiency virus infection. *J Virol* (2007) **81**(23):12748–57. doi:10.1128/JVI.00841-07
130. Presicce P, Shaw JM, Miller CJ, Shacklett BL, Chougnet CA. Myeloid dendritic cells isolated from tissues of SIV-infected Rhesus macaques promote the induction of regulatory T cells. *AIDS* (2012) **26**(3):263–73. doi:10.1097/QAD.0b013e32834ed8df
131. Banerjee DK, Dhodapkar MV, Matayeva E, Steinman RM, Dhodapkar KM. Expansion of FOXP3high regulatory T cells by human dendritic cells (DCs) in vitro and after injection of cytokine-matured DCs in myeloma patients. *Blood* (2006) **108**(8):2655–61. doi:10.1182/blood-2006-03-011353
132. Presicce P, Moreno-Fernandez ME, Rusie LK, Fichtenbaum C, Chougnet CA. In vitro HIV infection impairs the capacity of myeloid dendritic cells to induce regulatory T cells. *PLoS One* (2012) **7**(8):e42802. doi:10.1371/journal.pone.0042802
133. Qin S, Sui Y, Soloff AC, Junecko BA, Kirschner DE, Murphey-Corb MA, et al. Chemokine and cytokine mediated loss of regulatory T cells in lymph nodes during pathogenic simian immunodeficiency virus infection. *J Immunol* (2008) **180**(8):5530–6.
134. Khatami M. Inflammation, aging, and cancer: tumoricidal versus tumorigenesis of immunity: a common denominator mapping chronic diseases. *Cell Biochem Biophys* (2009) **55**(2):55–79. doi:10.1007/s12013-009-9059-2
135. Khatami M. 'Yin and Yang' in inflammation: duality in innate immune cell function and tumorigenesis. *Expert Opin Biol Ther* (2008) **8**(10):1461–72. doi:10.1517/14712598.8.10.1461
136. Rouse BT, Sehrawat S. Immunity and immunopathology to viruses: what decides the outcome? *Nat Rev Immunol* (2010) **10**(7):514–26. doi:10.1038/nri2802
137. Moore KW, Vieira P, Fiorentino DF, Trounstine ML, Khan TA, Mosmann TR. Homology of cytokine synthesis inhibitory factor (IL-10) to the Epstein-Barr virus gene BCRFI. *Science* (1990) **248**(4960):1230–4. doi:10.1126/science.2161559
138. Slobedman B, Barry PA, Spencer JV, Avdic S, Abendroth A. Virus-encoded homologs of cellular interleukin-10 and their control of host immune function. *J Virol* (2009) **83**(19):9618–29. doi:10.1128/JVI.01098-09
139. Liu J, Zhang N, Li Q, Zhang W, Ke F, Leng Q, et al. Tumor-associated macrophages recruit CCR6+ regulatory T cells and promote the development of colorectal cancer via enhancing CCL20 production in mice. *PLoS One* (2011) **6**(4):e19495. doi:10.1371/journal.pone.0019495
140. Doedens AL, Stockmann C, Rubinstein MP, Liao D, Zhang N, DeNardo DG, et al. Macrophage expression of hypoxia-inducible factor-1 alpha suppresses T-cell function and promotes tumor progression. *Cancer Res* (2010) **70**(19):7465–75. doi:10.1158/0008-5472.CAN-10-1439
141. Elrefaei M, Barugahare B, Ssali F, Mugyenyi P, Cao H. HIV-specific IL-10-positive CD8+ T cells are increased in advanced disease and are associated with decreased HIV-specific cytolysis. *J Immunol* (2006) **176**(2):1274–80.
142. Elrefaei M, Ventura FL, Baker CA, Clark R, Bangsberg DR, Cao H. HIV-specific IL-10-positive CD8+ T cells suppress cytolysis and IL-2 production by CD8+ T cells. *J Immunol* (2007) **178**(5):3265–71.
143. Dolganiuc A, Szabo G. T cells with regulatory activity in hepatitis C virus infection: what we know and what we don't. *J Leukoc Biol* (2008) **84**(3):614–22. doi:10.1189/jlb.1107770
144. Nordstrom I, Nurkkala M, Collins LV, Eriksson K. CD8+ T-cells suppress antigen-specific and allogeneic CD4+ T-cell responses to herpes simplex virus type 2-infected human dendritic cells. *Viral Immunol* (2005) **18**(4):616–26. doi:10.1089/vim.2005.18.616
145. Popescu I, Macedo C, Abu-Elmagd K, Shapiro R, Hua Y, Thomson AW, et al. EBV-specific CD8+ T cell reactivation in transplant patients results in expansion of CD8+ type-1 regulatory T cells. *Am J Transplant* (2007) **7**(5):1215–23. doi:10.1111/j.1600-6143.2007.01740.x
146. Kundu JK, Surh YJ. Inflammation: gearing the journey to cancer. *Mutat Res* (2008) **659**(1–2):15–30. doi:10.1016/j.mrrev.2008.03.002
147. Grulich AE, Wan X, Law MG, Milliken ST, Lewis CR, Garsia RJ, et al. B-cell stimulation and prolonged immune deficiency are risk factors for non-Hodgkin's lymphoma in people with AIDS. *AIDS* (2000) **14**(2):133–40. doi:10.1097/00002030-200001280-00008
148. Wang L, Yi T, Kortylewski M, Pardoll DM, Zeng D, Yu H. IL-17 can promote tumor growth through an IL-6-Stat3 signaling pathway. *J Exp Med* (2009) **206**(7):1457–64. doi:10.1084/jem.20090207
149. Numasaki M, Watanabe M, Suzuki T, Takahashi H, Nakamura A, McAllister F, et al. IL-17 enhances the net angiogenic activity and in vivo growth of human non-small cell lung cancer in SCID mice through promoting CXCR-2-dependent angiogenesis. *J Immunol* (2005) **175**(9):6177–89.
150. Veldhoen M, Hocking RJ, Atkins CJ, Locksley RM, Stockinger B. TGF-beta in the context of an inflammatory cytokine milieu supports de novo differentiation of IL-17-producing T cells. *Immunity* (2006) **24**(2):179–89. doi:10.1016/j.immuni.2006.01.001
151. Bettelli E, Carrier Y, Gao W, Korn T, Strom TB, Oukka M, et al. Reciprocal developmental pathways for the generation of pathogenic effector TH17 and regulatory T cells. *Nature* (2006) **441**(7090):235–8. doi:10.1038/nature04753
152. Mangan PR, Harrington LE, O'Quinn DB, Helms WS, Bullard DC, Elson CO, et al. Transforming growth factor-beta induces development of the T(H)17 lineage. *Nature* (2006) **441**(7090):231–4. doi:10.1038/nature04754
153. Liu J, Duan Y, Cheng X, Chen X, Xie W, Long H, et al. IL-17 is associated with poor prognosis and promotes angiogenesis via stimulating VEGF production of cancer cells in colorectal carcinoma. *Biochem Biophys Res Commun* (2011) **407**(2):348–54. doi:10.1016/j.bbrc.2011.03.021
154. Iida T, Iwahashi M, Katsuda M, Ishida K, Nakamori M, Nakamura M, et al. Tumor-infiltrating CD4+ Th17 cells produce IL-17 in tumor microenvironment and promote tumor progression in human gastric cancer. *Oncol Rep* (2011) **25**(5):1271–7. doi:10.3892/or.2011.1201
155. Su Z, Sun Y, Zhu H, Liu Y, Lin X, Shen H, et al. Th17 cell expansion in gastric cancer may contribute to cancer development and metastasis. *Immunol Res* (2014) **58**(1):118–24. doi:10.1007/s12026-013-8483-y
156. Yang S, Wang B, Guan C, Wu B, Cai C, Wang M, et al. Foxp3+IL-17+ T cells promote development of cancer-initiating cells in colorectal cancer. *J Leukoc Biol* (2011) **89**(1):85–91. doi:10.1189/jlb.0910506
157. Bentwich Z, Kalinkovich A, Weisman Z, Grossman Z. Immune activation in the context of HIV infection. *Clin Exp Immunol* (1998) **111**(1):1–2. doi:10.1046/j.1365-2249.1998.00483.x
158. Hazenberg MD, Hamann D, Schuitemaker H, Miedema F. T cell depletion in HIV-1 infection: how CD4+ T cells go out of stock. *Nat Immunol* (2000) **1**(4):285–9. doi:10.1038/79724

cachectic patients with colorectal and gastric cancer. *J Clin Gastroenterol* (2002) **34**(4):416–20. doi:10.1097/00004836-200204000-00006

234. Osawa E, Nakajima A, Fujisawa T, Kawamura YI, Toyama-Sorimachi N, Nakagama H, et al. Predominant T helper type 2-inflammatory responses promote murine colon cancers. *Int J Cancer* (2006) **118**(9):2232–6. doi:10.1002/ijc.21639
235. Kettunen HL, Kettunen AS, Rautonen NE. Intestinal immune responses in wild-type and Apcmin/+ mouse, a model for colon cancer. *Cancer Res* (2003) **63**(16):5136–42.
236. Ahern PP, Schiering C, Buonocore S, McGeachy MJ, Cua DJ, Maloy KJ, et al. Interleukin-23 drives intestinal inflammation through direct activity on T cells. *Immunity* (2010) **33**(2):279–88. doi:10.1016/j.immuni.2010.08.010
237. McGeachy MJ, Chen Y, Tato CM, Laurence A, Joyce-Shaikh B, Blumenschein WM, et al. The interleukin 23 receptor is essential for the terminal differentiation of interleukin 17-producing effector T helper cells in vivo. *Nat Immunol* (2009) **10**(3):314–24. doi:10.1038/ni.1698
238. Duerr RH, Taylor KD, Brant SR, Rioux JD, Silverberg MS, Daly MJ, et al. A genome-wide association study identifies IL23R as an inflammatory bowel disease gene. *Science* (2006) **314**(5804):1461–3. doi:10.1126/science.1135245
239. Liang SC, Tan XY, Luxenberg DP, Karim R, Dunussi-Joannopoulos K, Collins M, et al. Interleukin (IL)-22 and IL-17 are coexpressed by Th17 cells and cooperatively enhance expression of antimicrobial peptides. *J Exp Med* (2006) **203**(10):2271–9. doi:10.1084/jem.20061308
240. Kirchberger S, Royston DJ, Boulard O, Thornton E, Franchini F, Szabady RL, et al. Innate lymphoid cells sustain colon cancer through production of interleukin-22 in a mouse model. *J Exp Med* (2013) **210**(5):917–31. doi:10.1084/jem.20122308
241. Buonocore S, Ahern PP, Uhlig HH, Ivanov II, Littman DR, Maloy KJ, et al. Innate lymphoid cells drive interleukin-23-dependent innate intestinal pathology. *Nature* (2010) **464**(7293):1371–5. doi:10.1038/nature08949
242. Geremia A, Arancibia-Carcamo CV, Fleming MP, Rust N, Singh B, Mortensen NJ, et al. IL-23-responsive innate lymphoid cells are increased in inflammatory bowel disease. *J Exp Med* (2011) **208**(6):1127–33. doi:10.1084/jem.20101712
243. Fouser LA, Wright JF, Dunussi-Joannopoulos K, Collins M. Th17 cytokines and their emerging roles in inflammation and autoimmunity. *Immunol Rev* (2008) **226**:87–102. doi:10.1111/j.1600-065X.2008.00712.x
244. Leppkes M, Becker C, Ivanov II, Hirth S, Wirtz S, Neufert C, et al. RORgamma-expressing Th17 cells induce murine chronic intestinal inflammation via redundant effects of IL-17A and IL-17F. *Gastroenterology* (2009) **136**(1):257–67. doi:10.1053/j.gastro.2008.10.018
245. Dannull J, Su Z, Rizzieri D, Yang BK, Coleman D, Yancey D, et al. Enhancement of vaccine-mediated antitumor immunity in cancer patients after depletion of regulatory T cells. *J Clin Invest* (2005) **115**(12):3623–33. doi:10.1172/JCI25947
246. Litzinger MT, Fernando R, Curiel TJ, Grosenbach DW, Schlom J, Palena C. IL-2 immunotoxin denileukin diftitox reduces regulatory T cells and enhances vaccine-mediated T-cell immunity. *Blood* (2007) **110**(9):3192–201. doi:10.1182/blood-2007-06-094615
247. Littman DR, Rudensky AY. Th17 and regulatory T cells in mediating and restraining inflammation. *Cell* (2010) **140**(6):845–58. doi:10.1016/j.cell.2010.02.021
248. Erdman SE, Sohn JJ, Rao VP, Nambiar PR, Ge Z, Fox JG, et al. CD4+CD25+ regulatory lymphocytes induce regression of intestinal tumors in ApcMin/+ mice. *Cancer Res* (2005) **65**(10):3998–4004. doi:10.1158/0008-5472.CAN-04-3104
249. Sugai M, Aoki K, Osato M, Nambu Y, Ito K, Taketo MM, et al. Runx3 is required for full activation of regulatory T cells to prevent colitis-associated tumor formation. *J Immunol* (2011) **186**(11):6515–20. doi:10.4049/jimmunol.1001671
250. Coombes JL, Siddiqui KR, Arancibia-Carcamo CV, Hall J, Sun CM, Belkaid Y, et al. A functionally specialized population of mucosal CD103+ DCs induces Foxp3+ regulatory T cells via a TGF-beta and retinoic acid-dependent mechanism. *J Exp Med* (2007) **204**(8):1757–64. doi:10.1084/jem.20070590
251. Sun CM, Hall JA, Blank RB, Bouladoux N, Oukka M, Mora JR, et al. Small intestine lamina propria dendritic cells promote de novo generation of Foxp3 T reg cells via retinoic acid. *J Exp Med* (2007) **204**(8):1775–85. doi:10.1084/jem.20070602
252. Langowski JL, Zhang X, Wu L, Mattson JD, Chen T, Smith K, et al. IL-23 promotes tumour incidence and growth. *Nature* (2006) **442**(7101):461–5. doi:10.1038/nature04808
253. Li MO, Flavell RA. Contextual regulation of inflammation: a duet by transforming growth factor-beta and interleukin-10. *Immunity* (2008) **28**(4):468–76. doi:10.1016/j.immuni.2008.03.003
254. Becker C, Fantini MC, Schramm C, Lehr HA, Wirtz S, Nikolaev A, et al. TGF-beta suppresses tumor progression in colon cancer by inhibition of IL-6 trans-signaling. *Immunity* (2004) **21**(4):491–501. doi:10.1016/j.immuni.2004.07.020
255. Izcue A, Hue S, Buonocore S, Arancibia-Carcamo CV, Ahern PP, Iwakura Y, et al. Interleukin-23 restrains regulatory T cell activity to drive T cell-dependent colitis. *Immunity* (2008) **28**(4):559–70. doi:10.1016/j.immuni.2008.02.019
256. Boivin GP, Washington K, Yang K, Ward JM, Pretlow TP, Russell R, et al. Pathology of mouse models of intestinal cancer: consensus report and recommendations. *Gastroenterology* (2003) **124**(3):762–77. doi:10.1053/gast.2003.50094
257. Erdman SE, Rao VP, Poutahidis T, Ihrig MM, Ge Z, Feng Y, et al. CD4(+)CD25(+) regulatory lymphocytes require interleukin 10 to interrupt colon carcinogenesis in mice. *Cancer Res* (2003) **63**(18):6042–50.
258. Berg DJ, Davidson N, Kuhn R, Muller W, Menon S, Holland G, et al. Enterocolitis and colon cancer in interleukin-10-deficient mice are associated with aberrant cytokine production and CD4(+) TH1-like responses. *J Clin Invest* (1996) **98**(4):1010–20. doi:10.1172/JCI118861
259. Kuhn R, Lohler J, Rennick D, Rajewsky K, Muller W. Interleukin-10-deficient mice develop chronic enterocolitis. *Cell* (1993) **75**(2):263–74.
260. Kullberg MC, Jankovic D, Feng CG, Hue S, Gorelick PL, McKenzie BS, et al. IL-23 plays a key role in *Helicobacter hepaticus*-induced T cell-dependent colitis. *J Exp Med* (2006) **203**(11):2485–94. doi:10.1084/jem.20061082
261. Dunn GP, Old LJ, Schreiber RD. The immunobiology of cancer immunosurveillance and immunoediting. *Immunity* (2004) **21**(2):137–48. doi:10.1016/j.immuni.2004.07.017
262. Tannenbaum CS, Hamilton TA. Immune-inflammatory mechanisms in IFNgamma-mediated anti-tumor activity. *Semin Cancer Biol* (2000) **10**(2):113–23. doi:10.1006/scbi.2000.0314
263. Michael-Robinson JM, Pandeya N, Walsh MD, Biemer-Huttmann AE, Eri RD, Buttenshaw RL, et al. Characterization of tumour-infiltrating lymphocytes and apoptosis in colitis-associated neoplasia: comparison with sporadic colorectal cancer. *J Pathol* (2006) **208**(3):381–7. doi:10.1002/path.1895
264. Muller S, Lory J, Corazza N, Griffiths GM, Z'Graggen K, Mazzucchelli L, et al. Activated CD4+ and CD8+ cytotoxic cells are present in increased numbers in the intestinal mucosa from patients with active inflammatory bowel disease. *Am J Pathol* (1998) **152**(1):261–8.
265. Waldner MJ, Wirtz S, Becker C, Seidel D, Tubbe I, Cappel K, et al. Perforin deficiency attenuates inflammation and tumor growth in colitis-associated cancer. *Inflamm Bowel Dis* (2010) **16**(4):559–67. doi:10.1002/ibd.21107
266. Berzofsky JA, Terabe M. The contrasting roles of NKT cells in tumor immunity. *Curr Mol Med* (2009) **9**(6):667–72. doi:10.2174/156652409788970706
267. Kitamura H, Iwakabe K, Yahata T, Nishimura S, Ohta A, Ohmi Y, et al. The natural killer T (NKT) cell ligand alpha-galactosylceramide demonstrates its immunopotentiating effect by inducing interleukin (IL)-12 production by dendritic cells and IL-12 receptor expression on NKT cells. *J Exp Med* (1999) **189**(7):1121–8. doi:10.1084/jem.189.7.1121
268. Fuss IJ, Heller F, Boirivant M, Leon F, Yoshida M, Fichtner-Feigl S, et al. Nonclassical CD1d-restricted NK T cells that produce IL-13 characterize an atypical Th2 response in ulcerative colitis. *J Clin Invest* (2004) **113**(10):1490–7. doi:10.1172/JCI19836
269. Mandal D, Levine AD. Elevated IL-13Ralpha2 in intestinal epithelial cells from ulcerative colitis or colorectal cancer initiates MAPK pathway. *Inflamm Bowel Dis* (2010) **16**(5):753–64. doi:10.1002/ibd.21133
270. Keijzer C, van der Zee R, van Eden W, Broere F. Treg inducing adjuvants for therapeutic vaccination against chronic inflammatory diseases. *Front Immunol* (2013) **4**:245. doi:10.3389/fimmu.2013.00245
271. Hurwitz AA, Foster BA, Kwon ED, Truong T, Choi EM, Greenberg NM, et al. Combination immunotherapy of primary prostate cancer in a transgenic mouse model using CTLA-4 blockade. *Cancer Res* (2000) **60**(9):2444–8.
272. Hurwitz AA, Yu TF, Leach DR, Allison JP. CTLA-4 blockade synergizes with tumor-derived granulocyte-macrophage colony-stimulating factor for treatment of an experimental mammary carcinoma. *Proc Natl Acad Sci U S A* (1998) **95**(17):10067–71. doi:10.1073/pnas.95.17.10067
273. Bajor DL, Vonderheide RH. Cracking the stone: combination vaccination and CTLA-4 blockade in pancreatic cancer. *J Immunother* (2013) **36**(7):362–4. doi:10.1097/CJI.0b013e31829fb7c8

274. Ott PA, Hodi FS, Robert C. CTLA-4 and PD-1/PD-L1 blockade: new immunotherapeutic modalities with durable clinical benefit in melanoma patients. *Clin Cancer Res* (2013) **19**(19):5300–9. doi:10.1158/1078-0432.CCR-13-0143
275. Kadin ME, Vonderheid EC. Targeted therapies: denileukin diftitox – a step towards a 'magic bullet' for CTCL. *Nat Rev Clin Oncol* (2010) **7**(8):430–2. doi:10.1038/nrclinonc.2010.105
276. Dao H Jr, Barr PM, Honda K. Regression of CD30+ cutaneous anaplastic large-cell lymphoma with denileukin diftitox. *J Am Acad Dermatol* (2011) **64**(6):e123–5. doi:10.1016/j.jaad.2010.11.001
277. Gritzapis AD, Voutsas IF, Baxevanis CN. Ontak reduces the immunosuppressive tumor environment and enhances successful therapeutic vaccination in HER-2/neu-tolerant mice. *Cancer Immunol Immunother* (2012) **61**(3):397–407. doi:10.1007/s00262-011-1113-4
278. Porichis F, Kwon DS, Zupkosky J, Tighe DP, McMullen A, Brockman MA, et al. Responsiveness of HIV-specific CD4 T cells to PD-1 blockade. *Blood* (2011) **118**(4):965–74. doi:10.1182/blood-2010-12-328070
279. Brahmer JR, Drake CG, Wollner I, Powderly JD, Picus J, Sharfman WH, et al. Phase I study of single-agent anti-programmed death-1 (MDX-1106) in refractory solid tumors: safety, clinical activity, pharmacodynamics, and immunologic correlates. *J Clin Oncol* (2010) **28**(19):3167–75. doi:10.1200/JCO.2009.26.7609
280. Berger R, Rotem-Yehudar R, Slama G, Landes S, Kneller A, Leiba M, et al. Phase I safety and pharmacokinetic study of CT-011, a humanized antibody interacting with PD-1, in patients with advanced hematologic malignancies. *Clin Cancer Res* (2008) **14**(10):3044–51. doi:10.1158/1078-0432.CCR-07-4079
281. Dietze KK, Zelinskyy G, Liu J, Kretzmer F, Schimmer S, Dittmer U. Combining regulatory T cell depletion and inhibitory receptor blockade improves reactivation of exhausted virus-specific CD8+ T cells and efficiently reduces chronic retroviral loads. *PLoS Pathog* (2013) **9**(12):e1003798. doi:10.1371/journal.ppat.1003798
282. Bose A, Taylor JL, Alber S, Watkins SC, Garcia JA, Rini BI, et al. Sunitinib facilitates the activation and recruitment of therapeutic anti-tumor immunity in concert with specific vaccination. *Int J Cancer* (2011) **129**(9):2158–70. doi:10.1002/ijc.25863
283. Nakashima H, Terabe M, Berzofsky JA, Husain SR, Puri RK. A novel combination immunotherapy for cancer by IL-13Ralpha2-targeted DNA vaccine and immunotoxin in murine tumor models. *J Immunol* (2011) **187**(10):4935–46. doi:10.4049/jimmunol.1102095
284. Ishizaki H, Manuel ER, Song GY, Srivastava T, Sun S, Diamond DJ, et al. Modified vaccinia Ankara expressing survivin combined with gemcitabine generates specific antitumor effects in a murine pancreatic carcinoma model. *Cancer Immunol Immunother* (2011) **60**(1):99–109. doi:10.1007/s00262-010-0923-0

Conflict of Interest Statement: The author declares that the research was conducted in the absence of any commercial or financial relationships that could be construed as a potential conflict of interest.

18

Self-tolerance in a minimal model of the idiotypic network

Robert Schulz, Benjamin Werner*[†] and Ulrich Behn*

Institute for Theoretical Physics, University of Leipzig, Leipzig, Germany

Edited by:
Rob J. De Boer, Utrecht University, Netherlands

Reviewed by:
Gennady Bocharov, Russian Academy of Sciences, Russia
Véronique Thomas-Vaslin, Centre National de la Recherche Scientifique, France

***Correspondence:**
Benjamin Werner, Max Planck Institute for Evolutionary Biology, August-Thienemann-Street, 2, D-24306 Plön, Germany
e-mail: werner@evolbio.mpg.de;
Ulrich Behn, Institute for Theoretical Physics, University of Leipzig, POB 100 900, D-04009 Leipzig, Germany
e-mail: behn@itp.uni-leipzig.de

We consider the problem of self-tolerance in the frame of a minimalistic model of the idiotypic network. A node of this network represents a population of B-lymphocytes of the same idiotype, which is encoded by a bit string. The links of the network connect nodes with (nearly) complementary strings. The population of a node survives if the number of occupied neighbors is not too small and not too large. There is an influx of lymphocytes with random idiotype from the bone marrow. Previous investigations have shown that this system evolves toward highly organized architectures, where the nodes can be classified into groups according to their statistical properties. The building principles of these architectures can be analytically described and the statistical results of simulations agree very well with results of a modular mean-field theory. In this paper, we present simulation results for the case that one or several nodes, playing the role of self, are permanently occupied. These self nodes influence their linked neighbors, the autoreactive clones, but are themselves not affected by idiotypic interactions. We observe that the group structure of the architecture is very similar to the case without self antigen, but organized such that the neighbors of the self are only weakly occupied, thus providing self-tolerance. We also treat this situation in mean-field theory, which give results in good agreement with data from simulation. The model supports the view that autoreactive clones, which naturally occur also in healthy organisms are controlled by anti-idiotypic interactions, and could be helpful to understand network aspects of autoimmune disorders.

Keywords: idiotypic network, self-tolerance, control of autoreactive idiotypes, autoimmunity, bitstring model, mean-field theory

1. INTRODUCTION

B-lymphocytes express Y-shaped receptor molecules, antibodies, on their surface. These antibodies have specific binding sites which determine their idiotype. All receptors of a given B-cell have the same idiotype. B-cells with random idiotypes of remarkable diversity are produced in the bone marrow.

A B-cell is stimulated to proliferate if its receptors are cross-linked by complementary structures, unstimulated B-cells die. Proliferation occurs if the concentration of complementary structures is not too low or not too high, see e.g., Ref. (1). The latter condition refers to a steric hindrance for cross-linking if too many complementary molecules are around. Stimulating complementary structures can be found on foreign antigens and on other, so-called anti-idiotypic antibodies of complementary specificity. Thus B-lymphocytes can stimulate each other and form a functional network, the idiotypic network, as first proposed in Ref. (2), see also Ref. (3, 4).

The potential repertoire includes idiotypes that can recognize other complementary structures, e.g., on the active sites of enzymes, hormones, and neurotransmitters. Further, there are idiotypic interactions of B-lymphocytes with T-lymphocytes and between T-cells (5). Thus, the idiotypic network is not an autonomous entity of the adaptive immune system, but is coupled to many other networks.

Even for a hypothetical autonomous B-lymphocyte system, we have the requisites of evolution, random innovation, and selection. So the architecture of the idiotypic network can be conceived as the result of an evolution during the life time of an individual. In a revised version of the idiotypic network paradigm, the second generation idiotypic network (6–8), it was suggested that this architecture comprises a densely connected central part with autonomous dynamics and a hereto disconnected (or only sparsely connected) periphery. The periphery is able to clonal expansion in (an adaptive) response to external antigen, and since it is disconnected to the central part, the stimulation does not percolate through the network.

Already Jerne thought the idiotypic network to play an essential role in the control of autoreactive idiotypes (3). Today, the concept of idiotypic networks is still popular in the research on autoimmune diseases, both in theoretical studies and clinical context. Indeed, autoreactive antibodies are regularly found in healthy individuals though in low concentrations. Antibodies which escape other regulatory mechanisms can be controlled by the idiotypic network (9). Anti-idiotypic antibodies specific to potentially autoreactive clones are found in healthy individuals or in patients during remission, they are absent during periods of active autoimmune disease (10). Autoimmune diseases can be related to perturbations of the control of autoreactive clones (10–17), as for example in Myasthenia gravis, a well known B-cell associated autoimmune disease (18).

There are many alternative or complementary concepts to explain self-tolerance and a multitude of possible mechanisms to cause autoimmune diseases. It is of course beyond the scope of this paper to give an exhaustive review over this rapidly expanding field. We can list only a necessarily subjective selection of a few major concepts and mechanisms. Several theoretical concepts of self-nonself discrimination are presented in a topical issue of Seminars in Immunology (19), including the Two-signal theory (20), the Danger model (21), the context dependent tuning of T-cell antigen recognition (22), cf. also (23, 24), and the Immunological homunculus (25), cf. also (26, 27). Zinkernagel (28) emphasizes the importance of localization, dose, and time of antigens: antigen that does not reach secondary lymphoid organs in minimum doses or for sufficiently long times is immunologically ignored.

Regulatory T-cells have been identified to suppress a variety of immune responses and playing a crucial role in self-tolerance and in controlling the balance of T-helper cells such as Th1, Th2, and Th17 (29, 30). Various mechanisms how infections can trigger autoimmunity are reviewed in Ref. (31). Superantigens may cause a polyclonal T-cell response with an excessive cytokine release, which in turn can induce autoimmune disorders. Chronic tissue damage can, regardless of the initial stimulus, lead to a spreading of the specificity of the T-cell response (epitope spreading) including self-epitopes (32). More recently, epigenetic mechanisms which may cause a breakdown of immune tolerance have been identified in the context of several autoimmune diseases, for a review see Ref. (33), cf. also Ref. (34).

Recent progress in the understanding of autoimmune diseases is reviewed in a topical section of Current Opinion in Immunology edited by Wucherpfennig and Noel (35). The T-cell system and the B-cell system interact in various ways at different stages of an immune response and the distinction between B-cell mediated and T-cell mediated autoimmune disorders appears to erode (36). For T-independent features of B-cell response confer however (37). Also idiotype driven interactions exist between B-cells and T-cells, as reviewed in Ref. (38). Very recently, regulatory B-cells are brought into discussion (36, 39).

There are early attempts to model self-tolerance and autoimmunity mathematically within the network paradigm. We can distinguish papers which consider networks with predefined architecture from work, which studies the (ontogenic) evolution of the networks architecture.

In Ref. (40), based on experimental results (41), an idealized architecture of 26 clones was proposed, which comprises four groups of B-cell clones, a multi-affine group A, two mirror groups B and C with mutual coupling but no intra-group affinity, and a group D which couples with low affinity only to A. Based on this *ad hoc* architecture, a set of non-linear ordinary differential equations (ODEs) is proposed (42) that describes the continuous dynamics of B-cells and antibodies in the presence of self. The proliferation and maturation of by idiotypic interactions activated B-cells is modeled by the non-linear terms of the ODEs. Computer simulations of these ODEs reveal that the response of clones, which couple to self antigen depends on their connectivity to other clones of the network: the higher the connectivity the greater the degree of tolerance; poorly connected clones show unlimited growth.

In Ref. (43), an analytical theory for the dynamics of clones in the mirror groups B and C, which feel the mean-field exerted by the clones of group A that couple to self antigen is considered. The model describes a switching between tolerant and autoimmune states and reverse, induced by infection with external antigen.

Also a paper by Calenbuhr et al. (44) studies the behavior of idiotypic networks with predefined architecture in the presence of self. There, using a similar continuous dynamics as (42) the interaction between N clones of different idiotypes is determined by an $N \times N$ connectivity matrix ($N = 2, \ldots, 25$) with entries zero and one. The maximum number of interactions C of a single clone with other clones is varied between 1 and $N - 1$ and open (chain like) and closed architectures are distinguished. The autonomous system shows oscillatory or chaotic behavior with parameter depending amplitudes. The response to a self-antigen depends on its concentration, and on the parameters of the autonomous system. The state of the system is called tolerant (safe) if the clones which couple to the self have low concentration, otherwise, for a large or even unbounded response, it is called dangerous. The study confirms that more densely connected networks tend to provide tolerant states.

Our work describing the *evolution* of the idiotypic network in the presence of self antigens is similar in spirit to previous work by De Boer and Perelson (45), Stewart and Varela (46), and Takumi and De Boer (47).

De Boer and Perelson (45) investigated a model which describes the population dynamics of antibodies and B-cells by a set of non-linear ODEs. The idiotype is modeled in a discrete shape space by bitstrings of length L ($L = 32$), two idiotypes match if the two aligned bitstrings are complementary in at least T adjacent positions (T is varied from 6 to 11, mainly $T = 8$) which mimics the presence of several idiotopes on an antibody with certain idiotype. For exactly T complementary positions an affinity of 0.1 is assigned, for more than T an affinity of 1. The stimulation of B-cells is described by a bell-shaped activation function, and the production of antibodies by stimulated B-cells by a gearing-up mechanism. There is an input of 10 new clones per day. They are incorporated in the network if at least one other clone is complementary. Clones with too high connectivity are suppressed. Simulations show that the network reaches a stationary regime where the idiotypes that are incorporated in the network are more similar than to be expected for a completely random choice. This gives an advantage because the incorporated B-cells feel a similar stimulating field and their (similar) antibodies do not form complexes. Among the clones which do not expand there are about 25% which have no sufficient stimulation. They are not incorporated in the network and can be considered as the clonal (peripheral) component of the immune system (similar to the singletons in our work, see below). Self antigen is also modeled by bitstrings. In high concentration it suppresses all clones which recognize the antigen, in stimulative concentrations (i.e., if their field is in the stimulating region of the bell-shaped activation function) it gives rise to unlimited self aggression. The authors mention that some of the self-reactive clones, especially those with a high connectivity, are controlled by overstimulation, clones with few connections escape the control.

Stewart and Varela (46) considered a model, which describes the presence or absence of clones of a given idiotype, not distinguishing B-cells and antibodies, using a discrete dynamics. A clone of idiotype i survives if it receives a stimulus σ_i within an allowed window, $\sigma_L \leq \sigma_i \leq \sigma_U$. If σ_i is outside the window, the clone does not survive the next step of a parallel update. The stimulus an idiotype i receives from clones of complementary idiotype is calculated in a double-sheeted two-dimensional continuous shape space as $\sigma_i = \sum_j m_{ij}$ where $m_{ij} = \exp\{-a_{ij}/c\}^2$. An idiotype is represented by a point on one of the sheets (say, the white one) while the perfectly complementary idiotype has the same coordinates on the other (black) sheet. a_{ij} is the Euklidian distance of two points at different sheets and c is a characteristic distance below which idiotypic interactions are relevant. Simulations for periodic boundary conditions show that stationary patterns on the shape space emerge which consist of nested (concentric) black and white ellipses. They can be conceived as mirror groups where members of one group have only idiotypic interactions with the other group but not within their own group. Idiotypes disconnected from these groups (clonal components) only occur before saturation. The system needs a longer time to reach saturation as smaller c is. Self antigen is represented as points on the two-dimensional shape space. If located on the black (white) sheet it is incorporated in the black (white) elliptic lines. So if the bone marrow is able to produce idiotypes similar to the self, they buffer the self against aggressive autoimmunity.

Takumi and De Boer (47) investigated the evolution of a model network on a double-sheeted two-dimensional discrete shape space in the presence of self-epitopes. Self-reactive clones are deleted by hand assuming some not closer characterized self-tolerance process. Each idiotype has several determinants (idiotopes). New B-cell clones are generated randomly. The dynamics of B-cells is described by a system of ODEs with a log-bell-shaped activation function. A buffering term prohibits the explosion of the clone size, clones are removed if their size falls below an extinction threshold. Their main finding is that the network organizes such that most self-epitopes are embedded in an antibody repertoire of intermediate concentration. Without the explicit deletion of self-reactive clones the authors were unable to obtain robust self-tolerance.

The B-cell models mentioned above, describing the evolution of the network, have in common that they do not show an appropriate partitioning into network and disconnected fraction, and are not reliably stable when coupled to permanently present self antigen. Motivated by these drawbacks (48, 49) proposed to extend their previous models to include the cooperation with T-lymphocytes. Indeed, simulations of the ontogenic evolution of the network in the presence of self antigens ("founder" antigens) show that the system differentiates in several stages into two coexisting compartments, the central immune system that couples to and tolerates self antigens, and the peripheral immune system that could respond to "late" antigen. In the first stage, T-cells which become activated by the initial founding set of antigens, activate in turn B-cells. This continues until the B-cell repertoire is complete and the B-cells start to exert a regulatory feedback on the T-cells. In the second stage, the B-cells compete for T-cell help and their repertoire shrinks to B-cells of an idiotype, which directly recognize a T-cell receptor. After this, a single new antigen would elicit a response only of clones, which are not mounted to the network. However it turned out, that the peripheral system is too tolerant to a later antigen. This motivated (50) to further modify this model making the idiotypic connectivity an explicit function of time, and introducing a log-bell-shaped activation function also for the T-cells. Stewart and Coutinho (51) reviewed the state of modeling and the development of the paradigm, and critically mentioned the lack of experimental evidence supporting the physiological significance of idiotypic interactions between B-cell and T-cell receptors.

For more detailed reviews on the history of the paradigm, mathematical modeling, and new immunological and clinical developments the reader is referred to Ref. (52, 53). For very interesting personal accounts on the development of the network paradigm and the concept of immunological self, see Ref. (8, 54–57).

In the present paper, we consider a model of the idiotypic B-cell network proposed in Ref. (58) which describes the evolution toward complex, functional architectures. The model uses a discrete shape space spanned by bitstrings which represent idiotypes. The discrete dynamics describes presence or absence of idiotypic clones, which survive if their stimulus is within an allowed window. In a sense, the model combines the simplest features of the models previously proposed by De Boer and Perelson (45) and Stewart and Varela (46) and therefore can be considered as a minimal model.

The most interesting architecture emerging in this model comprises (i) densely linked core groups, (ii) peripheral groups without intra-group linking, (iii) groups of suppressed clones, and (iv) groups of singletons which potentially interact only with the suppressed clones. The expressed clones of the core and periphery groups build the actual network, the central part. The expressed clones of the singleton groups are not mounted to the network and can be considered as the peripheral or clonal component. This is clearly very close to the architecture envisaged in the concept of second generation idiotypic networks (6–8) and similar to the idealized *ad hoc* architecture of (40) but in our model these properties evolve from simple principles.

In the steady state, the size of these groups and their linking does not change with time. The groups are built from clones of different idiotypes, which have an individual dynamics but share certain statistical properties. The building principles of these architectures can be described analytically (59, 60), and the statistical properties can be calculated within a mean-field theory in good agreement with simulations (61).

Whereas the preceding work by Brede and Behn (58), Schmidtchen and Behn (59), Schmidtchen et al. (60), and Schmidtchen and Behn (61) considered the autonomous idiotypic network, i.e., the network of B-lymphocytes and their antibodies without foreign or self antigen, we investigate here the evolution of the idiotypic network, in the presence of self, toward an architecture where the expansion of autoreactive clones is controlled by idiotypic interactions. Self is modeled by permanently present idiotypes which influence the evolution of the network but are themselves not affected by idiotypic interactions. Our model avoids the above reviewed drawbacks of previous attempts, and the results clearly support the view that the idiotypic network is instrumental in the control of autoreactive clones.

The paper is organized as follows. In Section 2, we describe essential features of the model, its update rules, the general building principles which allow to understand the structural properties of the expressed networks architecture, and a tool which allows a real time identification of patterns in simulations. In Section 3, we sketch the derivation of the mean-field theory which allows to compute statistical properties if the structural properties of the pattern are known. In Section 4, we describe how the model should be modified in the presence of self. We report on simulations where the network in the presence of self evolves to an architecture such that the self is linked only to groups with very low population. Results of a modified mean-field theory are in good agreement with simulations. Finally, we give some conclusions and discuss problems for further research. There is a glossary where major key terms are briefly explained in a logical order.

2. THE MODEL

In this paper, we consider a minimal model of the idiotypic network (58), which is a coarse simplification of the real biological system but retains most important features and reveals a surprising complexity. The model has only few parameters and allows an analytical understanding of many of its properties.

2.1. POTENTIAL REPERTOIRE AND IDIOTYPIC INTERACTIONS

We model the repertoire of all possible idiotypes and their interactions by an undirected network, where each node v of the network represents a distinct clone of B-lymphocytes of a given idiotype together with its antibodies. The idiotype is encoded by a bitstring of length d with entries 0 or 1. The number of different bitstrings 2^d is the size of the potential repertoire. Note that the bitstrings are not thought to represent the genetic code or the sequence of amino acids but are meant as a caricature of the phenotype allowing an easy notion of complementarity. Interpreting the entries of the bitstrings as coordinates in a d-dimensional space each node can be conceived as a corner of a d-dimensional unit hypercube.

B-lymphocytes receive a stimulus to proliferate if their receptors are cross-linked by complementary structures, which can be situated on antigen but also on antibodies of complementary idiotype. We represent possible idiotypic interactions by links between nodes of nearly complementary idiotype. Assuming only perfect complementary receptor structures seems unrealistic and it appears reasonable to allow small variations. Therefore, two nodes v and u of our model are linked if their bitstrings are complementary allowing for up to m mismatches. We denote the undirected graph with 2^d nodes labeled by bitstrings of length d and links between complementary nodes with up to m mismatches as base graph $G_d^{(m)}$. Each node of the graph is linked to $\kappa = \sum_{k=0}^{m} \binom{d}{k}$ nodes, which we will call the neighborhood of a node in the following. For example, consider in $d = 12$ the bitstring **1 1 1 1 1 1 1 1 1 1 1 1**, which is perfect complementary to the bitstring **0 0 0 0 0 0 0 0 0 0 0 0**. Replacing anyone of the zero's in the latter by **1**, we obtain the 12 bitstrings which are complementary to the former except for one mismatch.

We only account whether an idiotypic clone is present or not and the corresponding node v is either occupied $n(v) = 1$ or empty $n(v) = 0$. The subgraph of occupied nodes, the expressed repertoire, with its links represents the expressed idiotypic network at a certain time. In the following subsection, we describe how the expressed idiotypic repertoire is generated.

2.2. METADYNAMICS AND LOCAL DYNAMICS

There is a continuous influx of new B-lymphocytes from the bone marrow. There, by somatic random reshuffling of the VDJ genes, which are responsible for the binding sites of the variable regions of an antibody, different idiotypes of an enormous diversity are generated. The potential repertoire is estimated to exceed the order of 10^{10} (62). We model this metadynamics by occupying, in each step of an iteration procedure, empty nodes of the expressed network with probability p.

The stimulation of a B lymphocyte to proliferate is a non-monotonous, log-bell-shaped, function of the concentration of complementary structures (63). The number of cross-linked receptors increases with the concentration of complementary structures. However, if their concentration is too high, cross-linking becomes less likely due to a steric hindrance and the stimulation decreases. An unstimulated B-lymphocyte dies. In our model an occupied node, i.e., a clone of a certain idiotype only survives if the number of its occupied neighbors is in an allowed window between two thresholds, t_L and t_U. The survival of a clone depends in a deterministic way on its local neighborhood in the shape space.

The dynamics is described in discrete time, the time step should be chosen such that an unstimulated cell will die within this time span and a stimulated cell can proliferate. The temporal evolution of the network is induced by the following update rules:

(i) Influx: occupy empty nodes with probability p.
(ii) Window rule: count the number of occupied neighbors $n(\partial v)$ of node v. If $n(\partial v)$ is outside the window $[t_L, t_U]$, set the node v empty. This step is performed in parallel.
(iii) Iterate.

All three steps, the random global metadynamics, the deterministic local selection, and the iteration are of equal importance to describe an evolution of the network toward a complex architecture. Technically, our model can be categorized as a probabilistic cellular automaton, and also as a Boolean network, see Ref. (60) for a more detailed discussion.

Figure 1 illustrates the construction of the base graph and the application of the update rules for the case $d = 3$, $m = 1$, $[t_L, t_U] = [1,3]$.

Here, we report mainly on results for the following parameter setting, which is best investigated. The length of the bitstring is $d = 12$, then the network has $2^{12} = 4096$ nodes. We allow $m = 2$ mismatches, which make the linking neither too sparse nor too dense, each node has $\kappa = 79$ neighbors. The lower threshold t_L of the window rule has its minimal non-trivial value $t_L = 1$: for survival of a clone the stimulation by at least one anti-idiotypic clone is required. The upper threshold of the window rule is chosen as $t_U = 10$ that excludes very regular static patterns, which are in our context not interesting, for more details, see Ref. (60). Given these values, the influx probability p remains as main control parameter. In previous work (60, 61), we have studied a range for p from 0 to 0.1 and found that the architecture, which is of interest here evolves for p from 0.026 to 0.078. The results presented here explicitly are for p close to 0.078, where it is easier to initiate a reorganization of the pattern, but we have also studied a broader range of p. Simulations for longer bitstrings up to $d = 22$ have shown that many features are also found in larger networks and the major concepts of structural analysis are still applicable

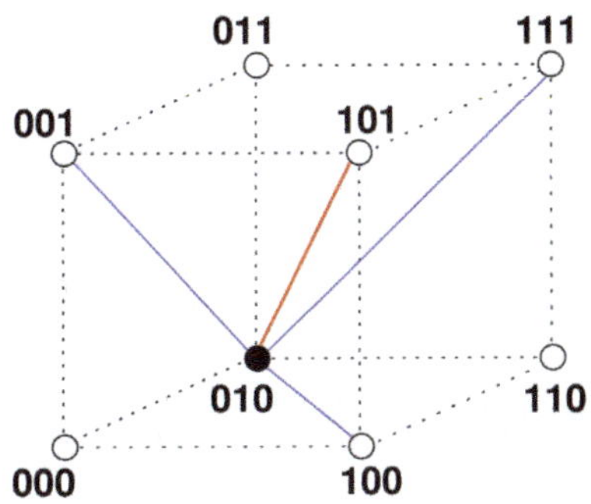

FIGURE 1 | Potential and expressed idiotypic repertoire. The figure shows all nodes whose idiotypes are encoded by bitstrings of length $d=3$. The nodes can be thought as the corners of a 3-dimensional cube. Also shown are the links of node 010 (filled circle) to the node with perfect complementary idiotype 101 (red line), and to the nodes with idiotypes 100, 001, and 111, which are complementary allowing for one mismatch (blue lines). The dotted lines are only to visualize the edges of the cube. The base graph $G_d^{(m)}$ for $d=3$ and $m=1$ consists of these $2^d=8$ nodes and all links connecting complementary nodes allowing for up to one mismatch. It represents the potential idiotypic repertoire and the possible idiotypic interactions. The influx of B cells from the bone marrow is modeled occupying empty nodes with probability p. Assume that node 010 is occupied. If the neighboring nodes representing clones of complementary idiotypes are empty, it receives no stimulation and will die. It will also die if there are too many, say all 4, nodes of complementary idiotype occupied. So the node 010 survives the update only if the number of occupied neighbor nodes is within a window $[t_L, t_U]=[1,3]$. These steps, random influx and parallel application of the window rule for all nodes, are repeated and lead for larger dimensions d and appropriate parameters to a steady state with a complex architecture of the expressed idiotypic network, see text.

(64). The program code is implemented in C++. For small base graphs ($d\approx 12$) optimization is not necessary. Larger base graphs ($d\approx 20$) require optimization and parallel computing.

2.3. BUILDING PRINCIPLES OF THE NETWORK ARCHITECTURE

Extensive simulations have shown that the network evolves, depending on the parameter choice, toward quasistationary states of possibly complex architecture (58). This architecture is characterized by groups of nodes that share statistical properties such as the mean occupation $\langle n(v)\rangle$ and the mean occupation of neighbors $\langle n(\partial v)\rangle$. The mean occupation of the nodes, the groups, and of the whole base graph, i.e., the size of the expressed idiotypic repertoire, all are stationary – which implies homeostasis. Although, the mean occupation of a single node is stationary, its actual occupation switches in time between 0 and 1. These switches are induced by both the random influx from the bone marrow and the deterministic window rule. A statistical characteristics of this behavior is the mean life time, which is also stationary and the same for all nodes of a group.

There are general building principles of the network's architecture which have been found by observing regularities in the bitstrings of nodes, which belong to the same group (59, 60). These principles make it possible to calculate the number of groups, their size, and the linkage between groups. Here, we only introduce the key terms and describe the essential results which are used in the following. For a deeper understanding of the derivation the reader should consult the original papers.

For a given architecture, the nodes can be classified according to their entries in the so-called determinant positions of the bitstrings. Different architectures have a different number $d_M \le d$ of determinant positions. The group S_1 is defined as the set of all nodes with the same entries in all determinant positions, the entries in the non-determinant positions run through all 2^{d-d_M} possible combinations. Nodes in group S_2 differ in one determinant position compared to nodes in S_1, nodes in group S_3 in two determinant positions, and so on. Consequently we have d_M+1 groups of size

$$|S_g| = 2^{d-d_M}\binom{d_M}{g-1} \tag{1}$$

for $g=1,\ldots,d_M+1$ and we can immediately observe that groups S_g and S_{d_M+2-g} have the same size.

The whole architecture can be build from smaller units, so-called pattern modules. These modules are the corners of a d_M-dimensional hypercube labeled by the determinant bits, together with the allowed links. Since the number of non-determinant bits is $d-d_M$, the whole architecture is obtained by arranging 2^{d-d_M} identical pattern modules and adding the allowed links between the nodes of these modules.

Next, we discuss the linkage of our idiotypic network in a pattern with d_M determinant bits on a base graph $G_d^{(m)}$. Each node in group S_i has a fixed number L_{ij} of links to nodes in group S_j. The L_{ij} are the elements of the link matrix $\mathbb{L}$. Since the update rule counts the number of occupied neighbors and all nodes of a group have the same mean occupation these data are of obvious interest to formulate a mean-field theory. A careful analysis of the bitstrings which encode the nodes of groups S_i and S_j allows to derive an explicit expression (59, 60) which can be written as

$$L_{ij} = \sum_{k=0}^{m}\sum_{r=0}^{k}\binom{i-1}{r}\binom{d_M-i+1}{j-1-r} \times \binom{d-d_M}{k+j-1-2r-(d_M-i+1)}. \tag{2}$$

Given a pattern with d_M determinant bits there are d_M+1 groups, therefore in equation (2) both i and j run from 1 to d_M+1. As every node has κ neighbors, the row sum of $\mathbb{L}$ yields κ. Since $L_{ij} = L_{d_M+2-i,d_M+2-j}$ the link matrix is centrosymmetric, i.e., it fulfills the identity $\mathbb{L}J = J\mathbb{L}$ where the exchange matrix J has entries 1 on the counterdiagonal and 0 elsewhere. $\mathbb{L}$ describes a directed graph.

2.4. REAL TIME PATTERN IDENTIFICATION

In simulations, huge amounts of data are produced describing the occupation of each of the 2^d nodes of the network in every single time step. An enormous, namely logarithmic reduction of information can be reached by introducing a center of mass vector $\mathbf{R}$ in dimension d which allows a real time identification of patterns and detection of pattern changes (60). Instead of monitoring 2^d

data per time step it is enough to observe the d components of R. The center of mass vector is defined as

$$\mathbf{R} = \frac{1}{n(G)} \sum_{v} n(v)\mathbf{r}(v), \tag{3}$$

where the position vector $\mathbf{r}(v)$ of a node v, which is encoded by the bitstring $\mathbf{b}_d\mathbf{b}_{d-1}\cdots\mathbf{b}_1$ with $\mathbf{b}_i \in \{0, 1\}$ has components $r_i(v) = 2\mathbf{b_i} - 1$. $n(\mathrm{G})$ is the total occupation of the basegraph G. By definition, for a symmetrically occupied base graph, we have $\mathbf{R} = \mathbf{0}$, a symmetry breaking pattern is easy to identify.

In **Figure 2**, we see the time series of the components of $\mathbf{R}$ for the evolution toward a stationary 12-group pattern. The trajectory of R_2 fluctuates around zero. Since, the entries of non-determinant bits take for every group all possible values, and supposing that all nodes of a group are occupied with the same probability, the corresponding bit position can be identified as non-determinant. The trajectories of the five components R_7, R_9, R_{10}, R_{11}, R_{12} fluctuate around 0.4 and those of the 6 components R_1, R_3, R_4, R_5, R_6, R_8 around -0.4, The corresponding 11 bit positions are determinant. The dimension of the pattern module is $d_M = 11$, thus we have a 12-group architecture. Furthermore, we can readily identify the determinant bits of the group S_1. As explained below, S_1 is a peripheral group with high occupation. The observation that five components of $\mathbf{R}$ fluctuate around a positive value indicates that the five determinant bits at the corresponding positions should have entry 1, and the other six should have entry 0. Thus, the nodes of group S_1 have a bitstring **1 1 1 1 0 1 0 0 0 0 • 0**, where the • represents the only non-determinant bit. The determinant bits of S_{12} are complementary, and also nodes of the other groups are easily identified knowing their bitstrings. The reader who is interested in further technical details should consult (60).

The procedure is fast, robust against defects of patterns, and allows to identify pattern changes. Needless to say, the method hinges by construction on the encoding of the idiotype by bitstrings, which is only a gross caricature of the phenotype. Here, we use this tool to characterize the behavior of the network if several nodes become permanently occupied to mimic the presence of self.

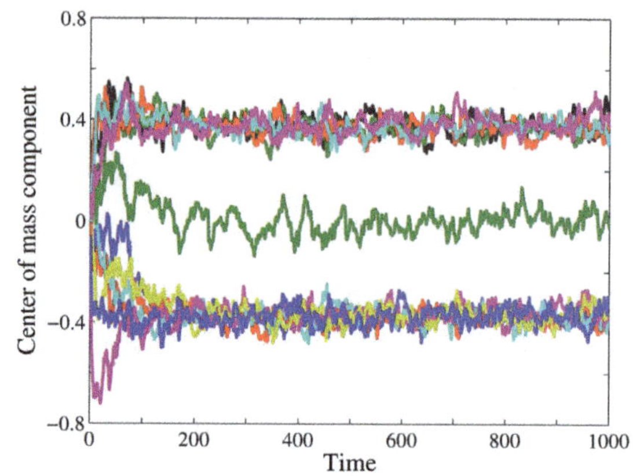

FIGURE 2 | Real time pattern identification. Time series of the components of the center of mass vector **R** given by equation (3), here on the base graph $G_{12}^{(2)}$ for a window $[t_L, t_U] = [1,10]$ and influx probability $p = 0.074$. Every color corresponds to one component of the center of mass vector. We start from an empty base graph, which is gradually occupied. A stationary state has evolved after about 200 time steps. The trajectory of R_2 (green) fluctuates around zero. The corresponding bit position is non-determinant, see text. The trajectories of the five components R_7, R_9, R_{10}, R_{11}, R_{12} fluctuate around 0.4 and those of the 6 components R_1, R_3, R_4, R_5, R_6, R_8 around -0.4, The corresponding bit positions are determinant. Together there are 11 determinant bits, hence the dimension of the pattern module is $d_M = 11$, and we can infer that the system has evolved toward a stationary 12-group architecture.

3. MEAN-FIELD THEORY

Once established, an architecture, characterized by the number of groups, their size, and their linking remains stationary for long periods of time and over some range of the main control parameter p. As shortly sketched above, for most architectures found in simulations their characteristics can be computed knowing the number of determinant bits d_M, which can be inferred from the time series of the center of mass coordinates.

The statistical properties of the nodes, which belong to the same group, such as the mean occupation and the mean life time, depend however on the actual value of p. They can be calculated (61) adopting the concept of mean-field theories, which was developed in statistical physics to describe phase transitions and has been transferred to many other problems in different fields. The main argument goes as follows.

The window rule (ii) for update of the occupation of a node counts only the total of the occupied neighbors. All nodes of a group have the same number of neighbors in the other groups given by the elements of the link matrix. The occupation of these neighbors typically fluctuates in time, and if they are many, it appears natural to replace the actual occupation of the neighbors by the average occupation. This works the better, the more neighbors are involved. In this view, a node feels only the different mean-fields, the modular mean-fields, exerted by the occupied neighboring nodes belonging to the different groups.

We now shortly describe the derivation in a more formal way to make the modifications understandable which are necessary when modeling the presence of self. Consider an architecture, which can be described by pattern modules of dimension d_M. Then, we have $d_M + 1$ groups of nodes S_g which share the mean occupation $\langle n(v_g)\rangle = n_g$ where $v_g \in S_g$, their linking is described by the link matrix $\mathbb{L}$. The set of mean occupations $\mathbf{n} = (n_1, \cdots, n_{d_M+1})^{\mathrm{T}}$ defines the state of the network in the reduced mean-field description at a certain time. Application of the update rules to $\mathbf{n}$ leads to a new state $\mathbf{n}'$ given by

$$\mathbf{n}' = \mathbf{f}(\mathbf{n}), \tag{4}$$

where the non-linear function $\mathbf{f}$ depends on the update rules and on the pattern we want to describe. We know that a node v_g of group S_g has L_{gl} neighbors in S_l. If the mean occupation in S_l is n_l, the new mean occupation after the influx with probability p is $\tilde{n}_l = n_l + p(1 - n_l)$. The probability that k_l nodes of the neighborhood in S_l are occupied after the influx is

$$\binom{L_{gl}}{k_l} \tilde{n}_l^{\,k_l}(1 - \tilde{n}_l)^{L_{gl}-k_l}. \tag{5}$$

Supposing that the groups are independent, the probability that for a micro-configuration with fixed $k_l, l = 1, \ldots, d_M + 1$, a total of $\sum_{l=1}^{d_M+1} k_l$ neighbors is occupied is simply the product of factors (5) for each group. Summing over all micro-configurations and taking into account the window rule leads to

$$\left[\sum_{k_l=0}^{L_{gl}}\right]_{l=1}^{d_M+1} \mathbb{1}\left(t_L \leq \sum_{l=1}^{d_M+1} k_l \leq t_U\right) \prod_{l=1}^{d_M+1} \binom{L_{gl}}{k_l} \tilde{n}_l^{k_l} (1-\tilde{n}_l)^{L_{gl}-k_l}, \tag{6}$$

where the indicator function $\mathbb{1}(\cdot)$ gives one, when the window rule in the parameters is fulfilled, otherwise zero. The last result should be multiplied with the mean occupation of a node of the considered group after the influx $\tilde{n}_g = n_g + p(1 - n_g)$ which gives

$$n'_g = \tilde{n}_g \left[\sum_{k_l=0}^{L_{gl}}\right]_{l=1}^{d_M+1} \mathbb{1}\left(t_L \leq \sum_{l=1}^{d_M+1} k_l \leq t_U\right) \times \prod_{l=1}^{d_M+1} \binom{L_{gl}}{k_l} \tilde{n}_l^{k_l} (1-\tilde{n}_l)^{L_{gl}-k_l}. \tag{7}$$

Iterating equation (7), for $g = 1, \ldots, d_M + 1$, the $\mathbf{n}'$ converge to a fixed point $\mathbf{n}^*$. Since $\mathbf{f}(\mathbf{n})$ is a non-linear function, several fixed points may exist. As a thumb rule, initial values close to the stationary average values seen in simulations are in the basin of attraction of fixed points of equation (7), which reproduce the simulation results. There may exist other fixed points, which were not found in simulations, for details see Ref. (61).

4. IDIOTYPIC NETWORK AND SELF

The 12-group architecture is of particular interest, as it strongly resembles the central and peripheral parts of the second generation idiotypic network. A scheme of these architecture is given in **Figure 3**. The 12-group architecture evolves on the base graph $G_{12}^{(2)}$ for $[t_L, t_U] = [1,10]$ and a range of p from 0.026 to 0.078. The groups comprise two self coupled core groups, two peripheral groups, which couple only to the core and five groups of stable holes. Stable holes are typically unoccupied since their occupied neighbors exceed t_U. Finally, there are three groups of singletons which are neighbored only by stable holes. Nodes of the singleton groups have an average occupation of 0.2–0.8, nodes of the periphery groups have 0.4–0.8 depending on p. The average occupation of the densely linked core groups is kept below 0.07, and the holes are almost empty, for details see Figure 8 in Ref. (61). Note that the singletons have no links to the connected part of the occupied network, which is built of the core and periphery groups. In terms of the second generation idiotypic networks, core, and periphery groups form the central part. The singletons, disconnected from the central part, form the clonal component (the peripheral part) of the second generation network.

The simplest possible way we can imagine to mimic the presence of self is to permanently occupy one or several nodes of the base graph and investigate their influence on the network architecture. The self nodes contribute to the number of occupied neighbors counted in the window rule but are themselves not affected by idiotypic interactions. The window rule does not apply to self nodes. We performed two types of computer experiments, inserting permanently occupied nodes in a fully developed 12-group architecture and monitoring the induced changes, or in an empty base graph and observing from scratch the evolution of the networks architecture.

A

	S_1	S_2	S_3	S_4	S_5	S_6	S_7	S_8	S_9	S_{10}	S_{11}	S_{12}
v_1	0	0	0	0	0	0	0	0	0	55	22	2
v_2	0	0	0	0	0	0	0	0	45	20	12	2
v_3	0	0	0	0	0	0	0	36	18	20	4	1
v_4	0	0	0	0	0	0	28	16	26	6	3	0
v_5	0	0	0	0	0	21	14	30	8	6	0	0
v_6	0	0	0	0	15	12	32	10	10	0	0	0
v_7	0	0	0	10	10	32	12	15	0	0	0	0
v_8	0	0	6	8	30	14	21	0	0	0	0	0
v_9	0	3	6	26	16	28	0	0	0	0	0	0
v_{10}	1	4	20	18	36	0	0	0	0	0	0	0
v_{11}	2	12	20	45	0	0	0	0	0	0	0	0
v_{12}	2	22	55	0	0	0	0	0	0	0	0	0

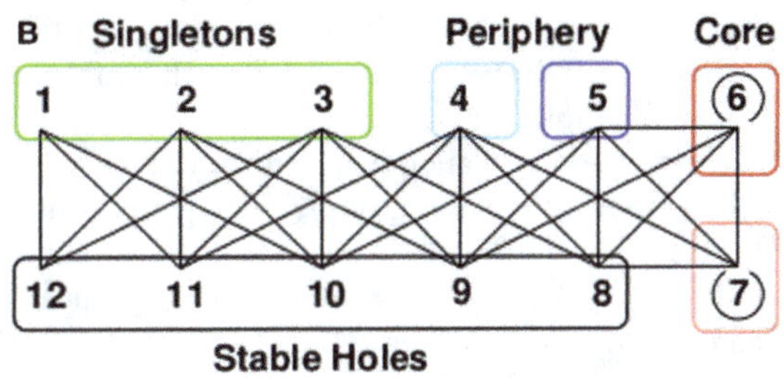

FIGURE 3 | 12-group architecture. **(A)** The entries L_{ij} of the link matrix, given by equation (2), show the number of neighbors a node v_i of group S_i has in group S_j. For example, the first row of the matrix tells that every node of the singleton group S_1 (denoted by v_1) is linked only to nodes of the hole groups S_{10}, S_{11}, and S_{12}, namely to 55, 22, and 2 nodes, respectively. Only nodes of S_6 and S_7 (red box) have links to other nodes of the own group. **(B)** The architecture generated by this link matrix together with a phenomenological classification into singletons (green), periphery (blue), core (red), and stable holes (black). The lines symbolize the existence of links between nodes of the connected groups, i.e., possible idiotypic interactions between the corresponding clones. The number of links which a node in S_i has to nodes in S_j is given by the element L_{ij} of the link matrix shown in **(A)**. The weakly occupied core groups have links within the own groups (open circles). The periphery groups are highly occupied and couple to the core and to the group of stable holes. The group of singletons is highly occupied and couples only to the stable holes. This architecture evolves on the base graph $G_{12}^{(2)}$ for a window $[t_L, t_U] = [1,10]$ and a range of the influx probability p from 0.026 to 0.078. See also Glossary.

Naturally, the influence of the permanently occupied nodes increases with their number. Their impact also depends on the influx rate p since the 12-group architecture becomes unstable for $p \gtrsim 0.08$. Inserting self nodes in the established architecture, close to this threshold the strongest impact is to be expected.

4.1. SIMULATIONS

We performed extensive simulations for different protocols. Here, we describe only few most instructive cases.

We permanently occupy one node of the hole group S_{10} of an established 12-group pattern for $p = 0.076$, i.e., close but below the upper threshold of stability of the pattern. The hole groups have many occupied neighbors and a self node staying there would be subject of a heavy autoimmune response. After few iterations, the former stable pattern destabilizes under the presence of the self and collapses. Thereafter, a new 12-group architecture evolves where the self node is now located in a group with only weakly occupied neighbors, which could be one of the singleton or periphery groups. **Figure 4A** shows the time series of the center of mass components for an example where the permanent occupied node (the self) is after a reorganization of the architecture finally in the periphery group S_5.

If we permanently occupy more than one node the scenario is similar. **Figure 4B** shows an example where we have permanently occupied 10 nodes of the hole group S_{10} of an established 12-group pattern for $p = 0.076$. The reorganization of the architecture is faster and in the new steady state the self nodes are found in singleton and periphery groups.

We also performed simulations where for a stationary 12-group pattern all members of the hole group S_{10} are permanently occupied. After reorganization of the architecture, in the steady state all self nodes belong to singletons and periphery groups and are never seen in a core or a hole group. If we start from an established 12-group pattern and permanently occupy one of the singletons or periphery groups this state will be stable for very long periods of time.

Starting from an empty base graph with several permanently occupied nodes, one observes that the architecture evolves from the very beginning such that the self nodes have only weakly occupied neighbors and thus are tolerated. This evolution from scratch toward a tolerant architecture occurs for a much broader range of p than the reorganization of an established architecture.

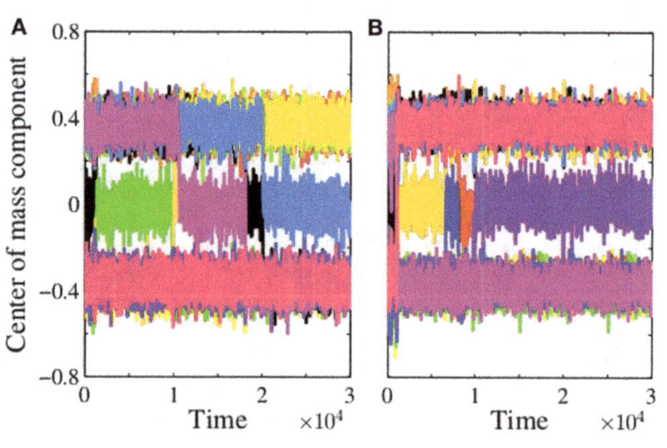

FIGURE 4 | Reorganization of the 12-group architecture with self. The figures displays the time series of the components of the center of mass vector obtained from simulations for an influx probability $p = 0.076$ when at $t = 0$ one node **(A)** or 10 nodes **(B)** of the hole group S_{10} are permanently occupied. Each of the 12 components is drawn with a different color. They are plotted one after another, only the last printed color is visible. The trajectories mainly fluctuate around ± 0.4 and zero. Jumps between these values indicate changes of the determinant bits associated with a reorganization of the architecture. For one self node **(A)** we see five jumps and for $t \gtrsim 2 \times 10^4$ a stationary state is reached. For 10 self nodes **(B)**, after a few jumps, the stationary state is already reached for $t \gtrsim 10^4$, obviously the impact of 10 self nodes is stronger than the impact of one. A closer look at the data (not discussed here) shows that the new stationary pattern has indeed a 12-group architecture where the self node in case **(A)** belongs to periphery group S_5 and in case **(B)** four self nodes belong to the singleton group S_3 and the remaining six self nodes belong to the periphery group S_5.

4.2. MEAN-FIELD THEORY WITH SELF

It is possible to modify the mean-field theory to describe a stationary architecture in the presence of self. We thus can describe situations where in an established pattern nodes are permanently occupied and the impact is so small that no reorganization sets in. If the impact is strong enough that a reorganization occurs and a new steady state emerges, we also can describe statistical properties of this steady state, such as the mean occupation of nodes and its neighbors, provided that we know its architecture.

We first consider one permanently occupied node of group S_s. It is linked to nodes of group S_g if $L_{sg} > 0$. The group S_g contains L_{sg} nodes that see the self. For these nodes we should modify the mean-field mapping, equation (7). The node of S_s which is permanently occupied should be exempted from the combinatorics of possible and allowed micro-configurations. Thus, we need to replace L_{gs} by $L_{gs} - 1$. Observe that $\binom{L_{gs} - 1}{k_s}$ in the modified equation (7) is zero if $L_{gs} - 1$ is smaller than zero or k_s. To account for the permanently occupied self node, we should decrease both thresholds of the window condition by 1. For the $|S_g| - L_{sg}$ nodes of S_g which do not see the self node, the mapping is not modified. For example, for an influx with $p = 0.07$ and one permanently occupied node in a hole group or in a core group, $\langle n(\partial v)\rangle$ increases by about 1 and $\langle n(v)\rangle$ decreases by about 20% if v is linked to the self node. The mean-field theory agrees with the simulation within 3–5%.

The case that all nodes of a group S_s are permanently occupied is even simpler because all nodes in group S_g see the same number L_{sg} of self nodes. We only have to modify the window condition decreasing both thresholds by L_{sg}. Note that if $t_U - L_{sg} < 0$ the modified window condition cannot be fulfilled and the indicator function $\mathbb{1}(\cdot)$ in the modified equation (7) returns 0. **Table 1** gives a detailed comparison of simulation and mean-field theory for the case that all 110 nodes of the singleton group S_{10}, cf. equation (1) for $d = 12$, $d_M = 11$, are occupied for $p = 0.074$.

For N_s self nodes with $1 < N_s < |S_s|$ the modification is also possible but more intricate and will not be reported here.

Encouraged by the good quantitative agreement between the steady states obtained in simulations and mean-field theory, we also looked at the time series of **n** generated by the mean-field mapping for a $d_M = 11$ pattern at $p = 0.074$ to see the effect induced by permanently occupying a group of nodes. We start with the fixed point $\mathbf{n}^*$, which describes a 12-group pattern where the groups are ordered as in **Figure 5A**. In the steady state, at an arbitrary iteration step, we permanently occupy the hole group S_{10}. The time series, cf. **Figure 6**, shows that this state immediately destabilizes and that a reorganization sets in. The pattern converges to a new state where the self belongs to the new singleton group S_{10}. These singletons have only neighbors in the new unoccupied hole groups, see **Figure 5B**. The network controls the expansion of the autoreactive idiotypes in the hole groups – thus providing self-tolerance. Analogous results (not shown here) are obtained if we permanently occupy the hole group S_9, after reorganization

Table 1 | 12-Group architecture with self after reorganization.

Group	$\langle n(v)\rangle$		$\langle n(\partial v)\rangle$	
	Simulation	MFT	Simulation	MFT
S_1	0.0	0.0	71.75 (54.01)	71.40 (53.99)
S_2	0.0	0.0	60.34 (53.86)	60.29 (53.96)
S_3	0.0	0.0	59.62 (53.50)	59.85 (53.52)
S_4	0.0	0.0	36.70 (34.86)	36.62 (34.72)
S_5	0.0	0.0	31.5 (29.62)	31.63 (29.73)
S_6	0.002 (0.001)	0.0	13.52 (13.53)	13.63 (13.63)
S_7	0.01	0.003	10.12 (10.09)	10.10
S_8	0.677 (0.661)	0.6708	0.15 (0.14)	0.07
S_9	0.706 (0.681)	0.6827	0.025 (0.018)	0.01
S_{10}	1.0 (0.685)	1.0 (0.685)	0.02 (0.0)	0.0
S_{11}	0.685 (0.684)	0.6835 (0.685)	0.001 (0.0)	0.0
S_{12}	0.685 (0.682)	0.6835 (0.685)	0.001 (0.0)	0.0

The 110 nodes of the singleton group S_{10} are permanently occupied to mimic the presence of self antigen, see ***Figure 5B****. The table shows the mean occupation $\langle n(v)\rangle$ and the mean occupation of neighbors $\langle n(\partial v)\rangle$ for all groups as obtained for $p = 0.074$ from simulations and from mean-field theory (MFT) with a $d_M = 11$ module. When deviating, the data for the case without self are given in parentheses. The groups $S_1, \ldots, S_6$ have direct neighbors in S_{10}, where S_1 has the most ones. Therefore, the change in $\langle n(\partial v)\rangle$ due to self is largest for S_1. Results from simulation and mean-field theory are in good agreement. The simulation data are obtained as follows. We first computed the temporal average of each node's occupation from 30,000 time steps. Then the mean of these data over all nodes of the same group is calculated. The variance of the mean over the group members is of the order 10^{-3}.*

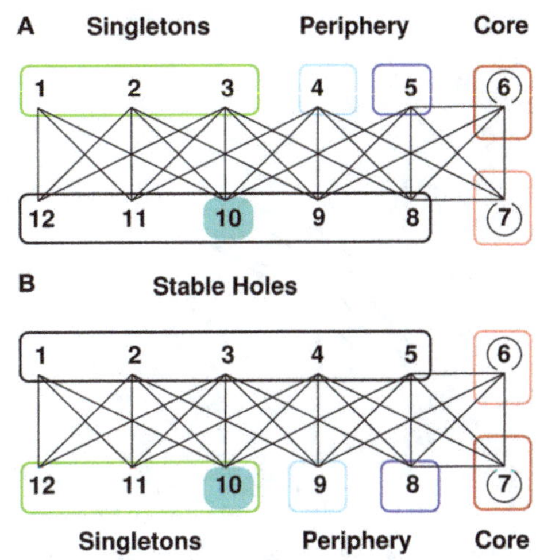

FIGURE 5 | 12-group architecture with self. (A) We permanently occupy one of the hole groups, group 10 (cyan), thus mimicking the permanent presence of self. This state is not favorable since the self couples to singletons and periphery, which have a high occupation. **(B)** Letting the thus prepared system evolve, it soon reaches a new steady state, still a 12-group architecture, but organized such that the self now belongs to the singletons and thus couples only to the almost empty stable holes. The self-recognizing idiotypes are controlled by the network, thus providing self-tolerance.

group S_9 is a periphery group coupling only to the holes and to the weakly occupied core.

We note in this context that due to the centrosymmetry of the link matrix of the autonomous network without self, given a fixed point $\mathbf{n}^* = (n_1^*, n_2^*, \ldots, n_{d_M+1}^*)^T$, there exists always a mirrored fixed point $\mathbf{n}^*_{\text{mirror}} = (n_{d_M+1}^*, \ldots, n_2^*, n_1^*)^T$. Obviously this symmetry is broken if self is present.

5. CONCLUSION AND OUTLOOK

We have extended a minimal model of the idiotypic network (58, 60, 61) to study the evolution of the network in the presence of self. Self is represented by permanently occupied nodes of certain idiotypes. These self nodes can stimulate autoreactive clones and thus influence the evolution of the network but are themselves not affected by the idiotypic interactions. We report on simulation results for the case that the self nodes are permanently occupied already at the initial state. Then, the network evolves toward an architecture where the permanently occupied self nodes are incorporated into groups of nodes which have, in a sense, a similar idiotype. These groups can idiotypically interact only with other groups that are either completely suppressed by the network (stable holes) or only weakly occupied. The network controls the expansion of self-reactive clones thus providing self-tolerance.

We also studied the response of a network with an already established architecture to a sudden appearance of self antigen. Nodes of the hole groups were permanently occupied, which is most unfavorable since these groups are linked to highly occupied clones. Provided that the influx from the bone marrow is sufficiently high the network reorganizes its architecture such that in the end the self nodes belong to groups, which have only empty ore weakly occupied neighbors, as in the previous case.

For the simplest cases that only one node or all nodes of a group are permanently occupied, we have modified the mean-field theory and found good agreement of analytical and simulation results.

As discussed in the introduction to some extent, there are preceding attempts in the literature, which aim in the same direction but were not really satisfying. Our results strongly support the view that idiotypic interactions can be instrumental in the control of autoreactive clones.

The network in the presence of self has been previously studied by one of us in simulations for one self node on the base graph $G_{12}^{(3)}$ with weighted links. The weights were given according to the number of mismatches of the linked nodes and the window condition was modified accordingly. The patterns are slightly easier to destabilize which explains why the phenomenon of self-tolerance was first observed in that version of the model (65).

Further studies should systematically explore the system's behavior for other protocols, e.g., for arbitrary numbers of self nodes possibly distributed over the whole base graph, desirably in both simulations and an accordingly extended mean-field approach.

It is of obvious interest to investigate in the frame of the model possible reasons for failure of self-tolerance. Transitions from a healthy self-tolerant state to an autoimmune state by a perturbation, possibly an ordinary infection, of the clones that

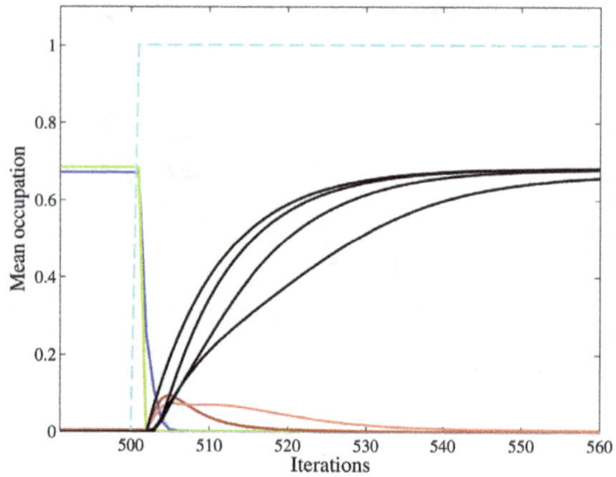

FIGURE 6 | Mean-field theory of a 12-group architecture with self. The figure shows the time series of the mean occupation per node of the 12 groups as obtained from iterating equation (7) for an influx probability $p = 0.074$. We start with the autonomous system in the steady state where singletons (green) and periphery (blue) have a mean occupation per node $\langle n \rangle \approx 0.68$, whereas core (red) and stable holes (black) have $\langle n \rangle \approx 0$. The color code is the same as in **Figure 5A**. At some arbitrary iteration step (here 500), we permanently occupy the 110 nodes of the hole group S_{10} (dashed cyan line). The fixed point of equation (7) looses its stability and a new mirrored architecture emerges where the permanently occupied nodes, the self, now belong to the singletons, which have neighbors only in the empty hole groups, cf. **Figure 5B**. The occupation of the previous singleton (green line) and periphery (blue line) groups drops down to almost zero, whereas the previous hole groups (black lines) become occupied as typical for singletons and periphery. (The light blue line of the periphery group S_4 is not visible here since it is covered by the green line up to iteration step 500, and thereafter by the blue line.) After an temporary increase the core groups (red lines) return to its previous occupation. For a detailed comparison of steady state results of mean-field theory and simulation see **Table 1**.

control the autoreactive idiotypes should be considered, together with the reverse phenomenon of 'spontaneous' remission from an autoimmune to a healthy state. Therapeutic strategies adopting the network paradigm (66), which consist in stimulating the protective clones that control the autoreactive clones, instead of applying immunosuppressive drugs, could be modeled.

To study age induced effects, it would be very interesting to consider an influx rate p from the bone marrow, which decreases over the lifespan of an individual. The architecture which controls autoreactive clones is found for a certain range of p. However, if we suddenly stop the influx at all, the group of singletons, which is only sustained by the influx would be depopulated, and the other, connected part of the network would, in a sense, freeze. Since the singletons play an important part in controlling the autoreactive clones this should have consequences for maintaining self-tolerance. A small influx outside the range mentioned above would lead to less complex architectures which may be not functional.

The renewal rate of the expressed idiotypic repertoire is certainly relevant in the physiological context. Therefore, it would be interesting to determine this characteristics in the frame of our model. It is of course related to the influx from the bone marrow but also depending on the population dynamics of the B-cell clones. It would be collective characteristics of a group and is more difficult to determine than the mean life of a single clone.

Motivation to develop our mathematical model further comes also from experimental and clinical medicine and from the progress of microarray technologies.

Hampe (10) reviewed the role of anti-idiotypic antibodies in autoimmunity, including Type 1 Diabetes. There is experimental evidence of anti-Id mediated neutralization of autoantibodies, e.g., in Myasthenia gravis, or suppression of autoantibody secretion, e.g., in Idiopathic thrombocytopenic purpura. For a number of autoimmune diseases including systemic lupus erythematosus and autoimmune thyroid diseases it has been shown that anti-Id specific to autoantibodies are present in patients during remission and/or in healthy individuals, whereas it is absent during periods of active disease. The formation of anti-Id-autoantibody complexes makes it difficult to detect the single constituents by conventional assays, but several methods have been developed to overcome this problem.

Monoclonal antibodies become rapidly important in clinical therapies of autoimmune and inflammatory diseases, see e.g., Ref. (67). This gives a strong motivation to improve our understanding of systemic consequences of immunomanipulation.

The rapid technological progress makes large scale studies of the expressed idiotypic repertoire feasible. The use of antigen microarrays to profile the autoantibody repertoire in health and disease is reviewed in Ref. (68), for an application of network theory to detect antibody trees associated with antigen see (69). Immunosignaturing, reviewed in Ref. (70) uses random-sequence peptide microarrays. Microarrays using antibodies or proteins are however still expensive and complicated (70). In addition, inferring the network architecture from a sample, which is only a snapshot of a subset of the expressed idiotypic repertoire is a very demanding task.

Our model, which provides an analytical understanding of the network architecture, could be helpful to formulate conditions for a new generation of experiments with the aim to infer the networks architecture and to elucidate its role in healthy conditions and disease. From the viewpoint of statistical physics or systems biology, the question appears natural and most interesting whether there is a general principle which guides the evolution of the idiotypic network.

6. GLOSSARY

- **Nodes:** A node of the network represents a clone of B-lymphocytes of a certain idiotype together with its antibodies. At a given time a node can be either occupied or empty, the corresponding clone is present or absent, respectively.
- **Bitstrings:** An idiotype is encoded by a bitstring of length d with entries 0 or 1. There is a total of 2^d different bitstrings, which is the size of the potential idiotypic repertoire.
- **Links:** A link of the network connects two nodes with complementary idiotype, i.e., with complementary bitstrings. We do not require perfect complementarity but allow for up to m mismatches. The links represent the possible idiotypic interactions between the clones of the potential idiotypic repertoire.
- **Base graph:** The base graph consists of all nodes and their links for a given choice of d and m. It represents the potential idiotypic

repertoire and the possible idiotypic interactions, which take place if the linked nodes are occupied.

- **Influx:** The influx of new B-lymphocytes with random idiotype from the bone marrow is modeled by occupying empty nodes with a certain probability p in each iteration of an update procedure.
- **Window rule:** The window rule decides whether an occupied node will survive the update or not. It will only remain occupied if the number of its occupied neighbors is neither too small nor too high but lies within an allowed window with lower and upper thresholds, t_L and t_U. The window rule is applied in parallel for all nodes of the network in each iteration of an update.
- **Evolution:** Iterating the steps of random innovation (influx) and deterministic selection (window rule) induces an evolution which leads, after a transient period, toward a quasistationary state of the network which may have, depending on the parameter setting, a very complex architecture.
- **Architecture:** In the steady state, groups of nodes can be identified which share statistical properties such as mean occupation and mean occupation of neighbors. The number of groups, their size, and their linking remain constant and characterize the architecture. The most interesting architecture, considered in this paper, comprises a connected part (core and periphery), a hereof disconnected part (singletons), and groups of suppressed clones (stable holes).
- **Pattern modules:** The architecture can be build by arranging identical smaller units, the pattern modules which are constructed like the base graph but have a smaller dimension d_M. A pattern module contains at least one node from every group. Given d_M, the number of groups, their size, and their linking can be calculated.
- **Stable Holes:** Group of nodes that are mainly unoccupied because the number of their occupied neighbors typically exceeds by far the upper threshold of the window rule, therefore we call this group stable holes. The mean occupation is close to zero.
- **Core:** Groups consisting of nodes with links to nodes in the same group build the core. The mean occupation is very low.
- **Periphery:** Groups consisting of nodes linked to the core and to stable holes, but not to nodes in its own group. The core and periphery correspond to the central part of the network. The mean occupation is high.
- **Singletons:** Groups of nodes that are only connected to stable holes. An occupied singleton can survive if it has, after the influx step, an occupied neighbor (in the group of stable holes) which typically does not survive applying the window rule. The mean occupation is high.
- **Mean-field theory:** The mean-field theory allows for a given architecture to calculate statistical properties of the groups, independent of simulations. The main simplification is that the actual occupation of neighboring nodes is replaced by their mean occupation which works the better the more neighbors are involved.
- **Self:** In the extended version of the model, self is represented by permanently occupied nodes of the network that exert influence on the linked neighbor nodes but are themselves not affected by idiotypic interactions. The window rule does not apply to self nodes.

ACKNOWLEDGMENTS

The authors thank Holger Schmidtchen and Rüdiger Kürsten for valuable discussions, and Nicolas Preuß for carefully checking the numerical results in **Table 1**.

REFERENCES

1. Coutinho A. Beyond clonal selection and network. *Immunol Rev* (1989) **110**(1):63–88. doi:10.1111/j.1600-065X.1989.tb00027.x
2. Jerne NK. Towards a network theory of the immune system. *Ann Immunol* (1974) **125C**:373–89.
3. Jerne NK. Idiotypic networks and other preconceived ideas. *Immunol Rev* (1984) **79**(1):5–24. doi:10.1111/j.1600-065X.1984.tb00484.x
4. Jerne NK. The generative grammar of the immune system. *EMBO J* (1985) **4**:847–52.
5. Sim GK, MacNeil IA, Augustin A. T helper cell receptors: idiotypes and repertoire. *Immunol Rev* (1986) **90**:49–72. doi:10.1111/j.1600-065X.1986.tb01477.x
6. Huetz F, Jacquemart F, Peña Rossi C, Varela F, Coutinho A. Autoimmunity: the moving boundaries between physiology and pathology. *J Autoimmun* (1988) **1**(6):507–18. doi:10.1016/0896-8411(88)90044-3
7. Varela FJ, Coutinho A. Second generation immune networks. *Immunol Today* (1991) **12**(5):159–66. doi:10.1016/S0167-5699(05)80046-5
8. Coutinho A. A walk with Francisco Varela from first- to second-generation networks: in search of the structure, dynamics and metadynamics of an organism-centered immune system. *Biol Res* (2003) **36**(1):17–26. doi:10.4067/S0716-97602003000100004
9. Urbain J, Wikler M, Franssen J, Collignon C. Idiotypic regulation of the immune system by the induction of antibodies against anti-idiotypic antibodies. *Proc Natl Acad Sci U S A* (1977) **74**(11):5126–30. doi:10.1073/pnas.74.11.5126
10. Hampe CS. Protective role of anti-idiotypic antibodies in autoimmunity – lessons for type 1 diabetes. *Autoimmunity* (2012) **45**(4):320–31. doi:10.3109/08916934.2012.659299
11. Avrameas S. Natural autoantibodies: from 'horror autotoxicus' to 'gnothi seauton'. *Immunol Today* (1991) **12**(5):154–9. doi:10.1016/0167-5699(91)90080-D
12. Shoenfeld Y, George J. Induction of autoimmunity. A role for the idiotypic network. *Ann N Y Acad Sci* (1997) **815**:342–9. doi:10.1111/j.1749-6632.1997.tb52080.x
13. Shoenfeld Y. The idiotypic network in autoimmunity: antibodies that bind antibodies that bind antibodies. *Nat Med* (2004) **10**(1):17–8. doi:10.1038/nm0104-17
14. Pendergraft WF, Preston GA, Shah RR, Tropsha A, Carter CW, Jennette JC, et al. Autoimmunity is triggered by cPR-3(105-201), a protein complementary to human autoantigen proteinase-3. *Nat Med* (2003) **10**(1):72–9. doi:10.1038/nm968
15. McGuire KL, Holmes DS. Role of complementary proteins in autoimmunity: an old idea re-emerges with new twists. *Trends Immunol* (2005) **26**(7):367–72. doi:10.1016/j.it.2005.05.001
16. Tzioufas AG, Routsias JG. Idiotype, anti-idiotype network of autoantibodies. *Autoimmun Rev* (2010) **9**(9):631–3. doi:10.1016/j.autrev.2010.05.013
17. Routsias JG, Tzioufas AG. B-cell epitopes of the intracellular autoantigens Ro/SSA and La/SSB: tools to study the regulation of the autoimmune response. *J Autoimmun* (2010) **35**(3):256–64. doi:10.1016/j.jaut.2010.06.016
18. Dwyer DS, Vakil M, Kearney J. Idiotypic network connectivity and a possible cause of myasthenia gravis. *J Exp Med* (1986) **164**(4):1310–8. doi:10.1084/jem.164.4.1310
19. Langman R, Cohn M. Editorial introduction. *Semin Immunol* (2000) **12**(3):159–62. doi:10.1006/smim.2000.0227
20. Langman R, Cohn M. A minimal model for the self-nonself discrimination: a return to the basics. *Semin Immunol* (2000) **12**(3):189–95. doi:10.1006/smim.2000.0231
21. Anderson CC, Matzinger P. Danger: the view from the bottom of the cliff. *Semin Immunol* (2000) **12**(3):231–8. doi:10.1006/smim.2000.0236
22. Grossman Z, Paul WE. Self-tolerance: context dependent tuning of T cell antigen recognition. *Semin Immunol* (2000) **12**(3):197–203. doi:10.1006/smim.2000.0232
23. Grossman Z, Paul WE. Autoreactivity, dynamic tuning and selectivity. *Curr Opin Immunol* (2001) **13**(6):687–98. doi:10.1016/S0952-7915(01)00280-1
24. Grossman Z, Min B, Meier-Schellersheim M, Paul WE. Opinion: concomitant regulation of T-cell activation and homeostasis. *Nat Rev Immunol* (2004) **4**(5):387–95. doi:10.1038/nri1355

25. Cohen I. Discrimination and dialogue in the immune system. *Semin Immunol* (2000) **12**(3):215–9. doi:10.1006/smim.2000.0234
26. Cohen IR. Biomarkers, self-antigens and the immunological homunculus. *J Autoimmun* (2007) **29**(4):246–9. doi:10.1016/j.jaut.2007.07.016
27. Poletaev AB, Stepanyuk VL, Gershwin EM. Integrating immunity: the immunculus and self-reactivity. *J Autoimmun* (2008) **30**(1-2):68–73. doi:10.1016/j.jaut.2007.11.012
28. Zinkernagel R. Localization dose and time of antigens determine immune reactivity. *Semin Immunol* (2000) **12**(3):163–71. doi:10.1006/smim.2000.0253
29. Sakaguchi S, Wing K, Miyara M. Regulatory T cells – a brief history and perspective. *Eur J Immunol* (2007) **37**(S1):S116–23. doi:10.1002/eji.200737593
30. Sakaguchi S, Wing K, Onishi Y, Prieto-Martin P, Yamaguchi T. Regulatory T cells: how do they suppress immune responses? *Int Immunol* (2009) **21**(10):1105–11. doi:10.1093/intimm/dxp095
31. Shoenfeld Y, Rose NR editors. *Infection and Autoimmunity.* Amsterdam: Elsevier (2004).
32. Vanderlugt CL, Miller SD. Epitope spreading in immune-mediated diseases: implications for immunotherapy. *Nat Rev Immunol* (2002) **2**(2):85–95. doi:10.1038/nri724
33. Meda F, Folci M, Baccarelli A, Selmi C. The epigenetics of autoimmunity. *Cell Mol Immunol* (2011) **8**(3):226–36. doi:10.1038/cmi.2010.78
34. Zouali M editor. *The Epigenetics of Autoimmune Diseases.* Chichester: Wiley (2009).
35. Wucherpfennig KW, Noel RJ. Editorial overview. *Curr Opin Immunol* (2011) **23**(6):699–701. doi:10.1016/j.coi.2011.10.003
36. Pillai S, Mattoo H, Cariappa A. B cells and autoimmunity. *Curr Opin Immunol* (2011) **23**(6):721–31. doi:10.1016/j.coi.2011.10.007
37. Fagarasan S, Honjo T. T-independent immune response: new aspects of B cell biology. *Science* (2000) **290**(5489):89–92. doi:10.1126/science.290.5489.89
38. Bogen B, Ruffini P. Review: to what extent are T cells tolerant to immunoglobulin variable regions? *Scand J Immunol* (2009) **70**(6):526–30. doi:10.1111/j.1365-3083.2009.02340.x
39. Salinas GF, Braza F, Brouard S, Tak P-P, Baeten D. The role of B lymphocytes in the progression from autoimmunity to autoimmune disease. *Clin Immunol* (2013) **146**(1):34–45. doi:10.1016/j.clim.2012.10.005
40. Stewart J, Varela FJ. Exploring the meaning of connectivity in the immune network. *Immunol Rev* (1989) **110**:37–61. doi:10.1111/j.1600-065X.1989.tb00026.x
41. Kearney J, Vakil M, Nicholson A. Non-random VH gene expression and idiotype anti-idiotype expression in early B cells. In: Kelsoe G, Schulze D editors. *Evolution and Vertebrate Immunity: The Antigen Receptor and MHC Gene Families.* Austin: Texas University Press (1987). p. 175–90.
42. Stewart J, Varela FJ, Coutinho A. The relationship between connectivity and tolerance as revealed by computer simulation of the immune network: some lessons for an understanding of autoimmunity. *J Autoimmun* (1989) **2**:15–23. doi:10.1016/0896-8411(89)90113-3
43. Sulzer B, van Hemmen JL, Behn U. Central immune system, the self and autoimmunity. *Bull Math Biol* (1994) **56**(6):1009–40. doi:10.1016/S0092-8240(05)80331-3
44. Calenbuhr V, Varela F, Bersini H. Natural tolerance as a function of network connectivity. *Int J Bifurcat Chaos* (1996) **06**(09):1691–702. doi:10.1142/S0218127496001041
45. De Boer RJ, Perelson AS. Size and connectivity as emergent properties of a developing immune network. *J Theor Biol* (1991) **149**(3):381–424. doi:10.1016/S0022-5193(05)80313-3
46. Stewart J, Varela FJ. Morphogenesis in shape-space. Elementary meta-dynamics in a model of the immune network. *J Theor Biol* (1991) **153**(4):477–98. doi:10.1016/S0022-5193(05)80152-3
47. Takumi K, De Boer RJ. Self assertion modeled as a network repertoire of multideterminant antibodies. *J Theor Biol* (1996) **183**:55–66. doi:10.1006/jtbi.1996.0201
48. Carneiro J, Coutinho A, Faro J, Stewart J. A model of the immune network with B-T cell co-operation. I – prototypical structures and dynamics. *J Theor Biol* (1996) **182**(4):513–29. doi:10.1006/jtbi.1996.0193
49. Carneiro J, Coutinho A, Stewart J. A model of the immune network with B-T cell co-operation. II – the simulation of ontogenesis. *J Theor Biol* (1996) **182**(4):531–47. doi:10.1006/jtbi.1996.0193
50. Leon K, Carneiro J, Perez R, Montero E, Lage A. Natural and induced tolerance in an immune network model. *J Theor Biol* (1998) **193**(3):519–34. doi:10.1006/jtbi.1998.0720
51. Stewart J, Coutinho A. The affirmation of self: a new perspective on the immune system. *Artif Life* (2004) **10**:261–76. doi:10.1162/1064546041255593
52. Behn U. Idiotypic networks: toward a renaissance? *Immunol Rev* (2007) **216**(1):142–52. doi:10.1111/j.1600-065X.2006.00496.x
53. Behn U. Idiotype network. In: Delves P, editor. *Encyclopedia of Life Sciences (ELS).* Chichester: John Wiley & Sons, Ltd (2011). p. 1–11. doi:10.1002/9780470015902.a0000954.pub2
54. Bersini H. Self-assertion versus self-recognition: a tribute to Francisco Varela. In: Timmis J, Bentley PJ editors. *Proceedings of the 1st International Conference on Artificial Immune Systems (ICARIS).* Canterbury: University of Kent at Canterbury Printing Unit (2002). p. 107–112.
55. Vaz NM. Francisco Varela and the immunological self. *Syst Res Behav Sci* (2011) **28**(6):696–703. doi:10.1002/sres.1126
56. Vaz NM. The specificity of immunologic observations. *Construct Found* (2011) **6**(3):334–42. Available from: http://www.univie.ac.at/constructivism/journal/6/3/334.vaz
57. Vaz NM, Ramos GC, deCastro AB. The enactive paradigm 33 years later. Response to Alfred Tauber. *Construct Found* (2011) **6**(3):345–51. Available from: http://www.univie.ac.at/constructivism/journal/6/3/345.vaz
58. Brede M, Behn U. Patterns in randomly evolving networks: idiotypic networks. *Phys Rev E* (2003) **67**(3):031920. doi:10.1103/PhysRevE.67.031920
59. Schmidtchen H, Behn U. Randomly evolving idiotypic networks: analysis of building principles. In: Bersini H, Carneiro J editors. *Artificial Immune Systems, Volume 4163 of Lecture Notes in Computer Science.* Berlin: Springer (2006). p. 81–94.
60. Schmidtchen H, Thüne M, Behn U. Randomly evolving idiotypic networks: structural properties and architecture. *Phys Rev E* (2012) **86**(1):011930. doi:10.1103/PhysRevE.86.011930
61. Schmidtchen H, Behn U. Randomly evolving idiotypic networks: modular mean field theory. *Phys Rev E* (2012) **86**(1):011931. doi:10.1103/PhysRevE.86.011931
62. Berek C, Milstein C. The dynamic nature of the antibody repertoire. *Immunol Rev* (1988) **105**:5–26. doi:10.1111/j.1600-065X.1988.tb00763.x
63. Perelson A, Weisbuch G. Immunology for physicists. *Rev Mod Phys* (1997) **69**:1219. doi:10.1103/RevModPhys.69.1219
64. Sachsenweger H. *Bitstring Model for the Idiotypic Network: Automatized Pattern Identification and Simulation of Large Systems.* Master's thesis. Leipzig: University Leipzig, Institute for Theoretical Physics (2012).
65. Werner B. *Idiotypische Netzwerke mit Antigenen: Gedächtnis und Selbsttoleranz.* Diplomarbeit. Leipzig: University Leipzig, Institute for Theoretical Physics (2010).
66. Feldmann M, Steinman L. Design of effective immunotherapy for human autoimmunity. *Nature* (2005) **435**(7042):612–9. doi:10.1038/nature03727
67. Chan AC, Carter PJ. Therapeutic antibodies for autoimmunity and inflammation. *Nat Rev Immunol* (2010) **10**:301–16. doi:10.1038/nri2761
68. Cohen IR. Autoantibody repertoires, natural biomarkers, and system controllers. *Trends Immunol* (2013) **34**(12):620–5. doi:10.1016/j.it.2013.05.003
69. Madi A, Kenett DY, Bransburg-Zabary S, Merbl Y, Quintana FJ, Tauber AI, et al. Network theory analysis of antibody-antigen reactivity data: the immune trees at birth and adulthood. *PLoS One* (2011) **6**(3):e17445. doi:10.1371/journal.pone.0017445
70. Stafford P, Halperin R, Legutki JB, Magee DM, Galgiani J, Johnston SA. Physical characterization of the "immunosignaturing effect." *Mol Cell Proteom* (2012) **11**(4):M111.011593. doi:10.1074/mcp.M111.011593

19

Dendritic cells in cancer immunotherapy clinical trials: are we making progress?

Lisa H. Butterfield**

Departments of Medicine, Surgery and Immunology, University of Pittsburgh Cancer Institute, University of Pittsburgh, Pittsburgh, PA, USA

Edited by:
Penelope Anne Morel, University of Pittsburgh, USA

Reviewed by:
Antonella Sistigu, Istituto Superiore di Sanità, Italy
Shikhar Mehrotra, Medical University of South Carolina, USA

****Correspondence:***
Lisa H. Butterfield, Departments of Medicine, Surgery and Immunology, Hillman Cancer Center, University of Pittsburgh Cancer Institute, University of Pittsburgh, 5117 Centre Avenue, Suite 1.27, Pittsburgh, PA 15213, USA
e-mail: butterfieldl@upmc.edu

Dendritic cells (DC) have been tested in cancer immunotherapy clinical trials for two decades. Over this time, the methods of DC culture (or manufacture) have evolved, the approaches for antigen loading have broadened, the maturation signals have varied and different sites of administration have been tested. The post-vaccination immunologic questions asked have also varied between trials and over time. In this review, I will consider multiple aspects of DC-based vaccines tested in cancer patients, including the cell culture, antigen loading, maturation, and delivery, as well as what we have learned from testing immune responses in vaccinated patients who have benefited clinically, and those who have not measurably benefited.

Keywords: cancer vaccines, tumor immunology, antigen presentation, dendritic cells, antigen loading

INTRODUCTION

BEGINNINGS

Dendritic cells (DC) were first identified in the early 1970s (1). However, the extremely low frequency of these cells in peripheral blood and many tissues made experimentation with DC challenging. General agreement on cell surface markers to uniquely identify "DC" from other myeloid lineage cells was another early hurdle in the field that was surmounted (DC are, at a minimum, large, granular lymphocytes that are MHC class I, MHC class II, and CD86 high, **Figure 1**). The more widespread investigation of DC identity and biology, and subsequent clinical testing of DC-based vaccines required methods for small and large-scale culture and expansion of DC progenitors *in vitro* (2). Methods were initially identified for expanding DC from human peripheral blood monocytes with granulocyte-macrophage-colony stimulating factor (GM-CSF) (3, 4) and eventually, similar approaches and surface markers were found that could be utilized for both human and murine systems. After these advances, the field was wide open.

In one of the earliest trials, Mukherji et al. (5) used intradermal injection of MHC class I-restricted MAGE-1 peptide-pulsed and GM-CSF-cultured monocytes to treat three HLA-A1^{+} patients with advanced metastatic melanoma. They observed autologous melanoma-reactive and peptide-specific CD8^{+} T cell responses, but no significant therapeutic responses. Such very early clinical results supported the safety and immunologic activity of these cells in cancer patients.

FIRST GENERATION CLINICAL TRIALS

The early clinical trials of DC-based cancer immunotherapy established the general safety and feasibility of this cancer vaccine strategy, and its lack of toxicity compared with other cancer treatment approaches (e.g., chemotherapy, radiation). Importantly, a small number of positive clinical responses and the clear demonstration that the goal of anti-tumor immune activation was achieved, bolstered the field, and supported additional trials. There have been several recent DC vaccine reviews published that are excellent, and that give additional details (6–8). The few early trials highlighted below are important, but small, and did not utilize standardized manufacture procedures throughout the clinical trial.

One of the first reported clinical trials that described the ability of tumor antigen-pulsed DCs to elicit a tumor-specific T cell response and yield a clinical response was published by Hsu et al. (9). In this study, four patients were treated with low-grade follicular B-cell lymphoma resistant to chemotherapy. The DCs were pulsed with target antigens of clonal immunoglobulin (idiotype) expressed by the non-Hodgkin's lymphoma, a tumor-specific, unique antigen. Patients were immunized with DC followed by booster injections of idiotype protein and keyhole limpet hemocyanin (KLH, as an immunogenic xenoantigen as well as heterologous "help" to activate CD4^{+} T cells) as well as a final DC boost infusion given 5–6 months later. All four patients developed cellular proliferative responses specific to their own idiotype protein. More importantly, one patient had a complete tumor regression, a second patient had a partial regression, and a third patient resolved all evidence of disease. This very small study was an important proof of principal for the clinical potential of DC vaccines.

While the study performed by Mukherji et al. (above) evaluated monocyte-derived antigen presenting cells (APC), it may not have formally tested a more fully differentiated DC because the culture contained GM-CSF, but it lacked IL-4. The first clinical trial using the monocyte-derived DC that have been most commonly used in clinical trials (including both GM-CSF and IL-4 in the monocyte precursor culture) was performed by Nestle et al. (10). Sixteen melanoma patients were treated using autologous monocyte-derived DC pulsed with a cocktail of gp100, MART-1, tyrosinase, MAGE-1, or MAGE-3 peptides chosen to suit the individual patient's class I HLA molecules. In addition, DC pulsed with autologous tumor lysate were used to treat another four patients. To provide antigen non-specific CD4$^+$ T cell-mediated help for the CD8$^+$ T cells, KLH was included during antigen pulsing. DC were injected directly into uninvolved lymph nodes. Patients received 6–10 injections of 1×10^6 cells every 1–4 weeks. Tumor regression was seen in 5 of the 16 patients, including two complete responses lasting over 15 months. Tumor regressions occurred in skin, soft tissue, lung, and pancreas indicating an impact on the clinical course of metastasizing melanoma, regardless of metastatic site.

As with many of the early trials (examples here and others), a variable number of DC vaccine administrations, consisting of different cell numbers and boost injections were delivered, and multiple types of antigen loading strategies were used. These earliest clinical studies were more proof of principle for the *in vivo* activity of DC, and less a formal testing of a specific DC vaccine approach.

In another melanoma clinical trial, Banchereau et al. (11) evaluated immune and clinical responses in 18 patients with metastatic melanoma after injecting DCs pulsed with peptides (MART-1, tyrosinase, MAGE-A3, and gp100) subcutaneously. They utilized CD34$^+$ hematopoietic progenitor cells as an alternative source of DC. DC were administered in a dose-escalation design. Enhanced antigen-specific immune responses to at least one of the peptides were seen in 16 or 18 patients, and 6 of 7 patients with immunity to two or fewer antigens had progressive disease after the study ended, while only 1 of 10 patients who responded to more than two antigens had tumor progression. This larger and more standardized study showed that broad immune responses to multiple tumor antigen-derived peptides correlated with better clinical outcome, one of the first studies showing that statistically significant correlation between immunity induced from DC vaccines and clinical outcome.

It is clear from the clinical trials described above, that most clinical trials are unique, they involve individual patient vaccination approaches and single clinical trial arms, and it is difficult to compare them. Monocytes and CD34$^+$ progenitors; complex tumor lysates containing normal, tumor-associated/shared and tumor-specific/private antigens, or synthetic MHC class I-restricted peptides; injection into blood (i.v.), skin (s.c. or i.d.), or lymph nodes (i.n.); are all parameters playing unclear roles in any clinical responses seen (**Figure 2**). The initial lessons learned were simply that DC-based vaccines were safe, feasible, and had the potential to promote clinically significant tumor regressions.

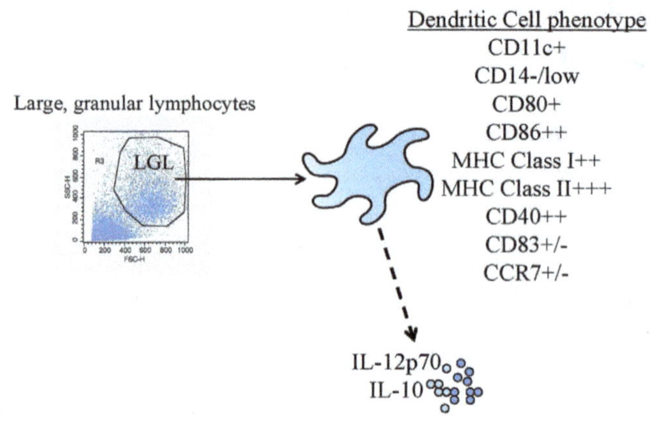

FIGURE 1 | Common DC vaccine phenotypic and functional assessments. The diagram shows the most common identity (flow cytometric phenotyping) and potency (cytokine production) tests performed.

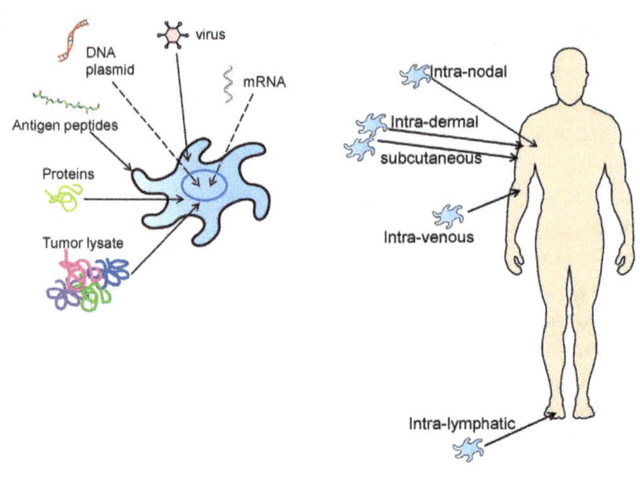

FIGURE 2 | DC vaccine loading and administration approaches that have previously been tested in clinical trials, and which are still being investigated today.

LIMITED CLINICAL RESULTS FOR DC-BASED VACCINES

In 2004, Rosenberg et al. published an article on the state of active specific immunotherapy cancer trials (12). They analyzed 9 years of data (1995–2004), essentially all of the early, or "first generation" trials. Overall, they reviewed 1,306 solid tumor patients using the modified Response Evaluation Criteria in Solid Tumors (RECIST) in which clinical response is defined as at least 50% reduction in the sum of the products of the perpendicular diameters of all lesions without 25% growth of any lesion or the appearance of new lesions. With an overall therapy-induced tumor regression rate of only 3.3% in patients vaccinated with synthetic peptides, "naked" DNA, peptide-pulsed DC, recombinant vaccinia viruses, recombinant fowlpox viruses, or recombinant adenoviruses expressing various tumor-associated antigen (TAA), the results were grim for vaccine approaches in general. Of these immunization methods, peptide-pulsed DCs seemed to be the most effective strategy, with 7.1% of treated patients exhibiting tumor regression. While this frequency of response was higher than those frequencies found for other vaccination strategies, the clinical response was still low.

DC VACCINE COMPLEXITIES

Unlike chemotherapy, immunological vaccines have not followed a linear dose-response effect. Instead, because immunologic vaccines depend on the complex interactions of a large number of variables, many of which are difficult to test: (1) the administration route (s.c., i.d., i.v., i.n., and more recently, intra-lymphatic, i.l.),

(2) minimum immunogenic dose, (3) higher dose effects, (4) vaccination schedule (weekly, monthly, or multiple times in a week or month), (5) immunological adjuvant type, and (6) the existing state of host immunological competence. There have been attempts to make "immune competence" a criterion for trial enrollment. A standardized skin test to recall antigens like tetanus and mumps was investigated, but the results were unrelated to vaccine immune response. Better measures of "immune health" are under investigation (13) but there are no clear definitions to date that might serve to identify patients who are most likely to benefit. Any alterations of these many variables can impact the patient immunologic as well as clinical outcome following therapeutic immunization.

The majority of patients treated in these earlier studies were late-stage metastatic patients that were heavily pretreated with conventional chemotherapeutic drugs prior to immunizations. Not only do late-stage tumors have potent immune-inhibitory functions well established both in the tumor microenvironment and systemically, but many traditional chemotherapies have also been shown to non-specifically decrease the number of leukocytes in recipients, making metastatic patients severely immune-compromised. Such patients would also be expected to have multiple tumor resistance mechanisms in place (e.g., infiltrated regulatory T cells, myeloid-derived suppressor cells, and other immature and skewed macrophages, immuno-inhibitory cytokines, and genetic heterogeneity in tumor subclones). Assessment of tumor infiltration and inflammation is being investigated as a biomarker for responsiveness to not only vaccines, but also other immunotherapy approaches and traditional cancer treatments (14, 15), but these areas of investigation are relatively recent and still being validated.

There are several other possibilities to explain the poor clinical response to these vaccines. The immune system, while potentially effective, is limited by the frequency of responders that can be stimulated by vaccinations. Even if TAA-specific responses were stimulated by immunization, it is possible that the bulk tumor mass was too large at the time of treatment for the available effector T cell population to infiltrate it and eliminate it efficiently. It is also possible that while the vaccine-targeted antigens are expressed by the tumors, their derivative peptides are not presenting on the cell surface in the context of MHC class I molecules, making the tumor cells effectively invisible to $CD8^+$ T cell recognition. Tumors can down-regulate antigen processing machinery molecules, including β-2-microglobulin (16, 17). Another possibility is that TAA used for vaccinations were not expressed by targeted tumors because metastatic deposits do not necessarily express the same repertoire of antigens as the primary tumor or that TAA-derived peptides used were not effective at eliciting high-avidity T cell responders. This heterogeneity has been observed in melanoma (18). The highest avidity T cells specific for self antigens may have been deleted during the development of the immune system by normal negative selection. Therefore, for some patients treated in early DC vaccine trials, instead of receiving a vaccine tailored to the individual patient's TAA repertoire, these individuals may have been treated with arguably irrelevant non-presented or weakly immunogenic antigens that led to a clinically meaningless immune response. Vaccines targeting only $CD8^+$ T cells, with short MHC class I-restricted peptides, may have only been able to activate "helpless" $CD8^+$ T cells with functional defects (19). Lastly, some tumors have evolved cell-autonomous resistance to immune-mediated killing.

SOURCES OF TUMOR ANTIGEN: IMMUNE TARGET COMPLEXITIES

Tumors are not homogenous tissues that can be effectively treated with a single antigen epitope vaccination tactic. Tumors vary in physiological location (primary tumor sites and metastatic sites), TAA repertoire, vascularization, surrounding stroma, and other properties. Some tumor types are considered more "immunogenic" due to spontaneous immune infiltration and have, therefore, been an early focus for many DC-based immunotherapy trials (melanoma, renal cell cancer). These variations in tumor biology, immune infiltration, and microenvironment biology are observed between patients, the tissues affected, and at different time points in the malignant process. For example, when considering inclusion criteria, "stage IV cancer patients" are not a homogeneous group. Whether patients with brain metastases can be included, or those with LDH levels above normal limits must be considered, as immunotherapy vaccine clinical responses can need time to evolve, and not all clinical settings are expected to allow for immune response evolution.

When considering autologous tumor-based immunization strategies, there are types of cancer that are not generally surgically removed (pancreatic cancer, hepatocellular cancer treated with ablative techniques), so the ability to load DC with autologous tumor as a source of all potential public and private TAA may not be feasible. Established cell lines are an immortal source of antigen, but may have limited antigenic overlap with a specific patient's tumor. Cell lines may express a few known, shared TAAs, however they may not express any tumor-specific and/or mutated/private antigens that the patient's tumor expresses and which may be critical to clinical outcomes. Similarly, some tumor types may have only a few characterized shared TAA with even fewer well-defined HLA-matched peptide epitopes. Importantly, since the expression of TAA is not uniform among tumor cells and metastases, it may be critical to co-administer several antigens, rather than a single one, to avoid the possibility that the sole TAA will prove non-immunogenic or that its epitopes may not be adequately presented on the tumor cell. A long term goal in the field has been to identify the "best" TAA for targeting with vaccines. The optimal TAA would be critical to survival of the tumor cells, expressed at distant metastatic sites (not downregulatable), specific to the tumor (not expressed on normal tissues), and immunogenic. Characterized TAA were ranked by a group of experts (20), but the ideal, defined, shared targets have not been identified for many tumor types, and there remains some disagreement in the field exactly what type of antigen should be targeted.

TECHNICAL ISSUES AND REMAINING QUESTIONS REGARDING DC VACCINES

MATURATION

An early lesson learned in DC vaccine development was that the DC obtained after 5–7 days of culture with GM-CSF+IL-4 were not in an optimal state for T cell activation. These DC were subsequently referred to as "immature" and potentially tolerogenic until triggered by a pathogen and/or inflammatory signal. Such signals serve to upregulate antigen presentation and co-stimulation molecules and function, and reduce antigen uptake. Early cocktails were sometimes donor-specific and undefined (monocyte-conditioned medium), weakly stimulatory (TNF), or contained molecules which were subsequently shown to have some negative effects (PGE_2). Currently employed cocktails can incorporate specific pathogen-derived molecules, toll-like-receptor ligands (TLRs) and other "type 1" skewing agents including interferons (21). Conversely for clinical settings other than cancer, immune suppressive cocktails can be used to push DC toward their tolerizing capabilities, for autoimmune or transplantation settings. For example, anti-sense oligo co-culture of DC with anti-sense CD80, CD86, and CD40 for treatment of autoimmune diabetes has been tested, or DC culture with vitamin A for inhibition of transplant-specific immunity is being developed (22, 23). Overall, as environmental sensors, DC can be significantly modulated by instructions delivered by maturation signals and optimal signals for DC vaccines are still being developed.

DOSE AND ROUTE

Many new therapeutic drugs are tested for the effective, maximum tolerated, and toxic doses in early clinical trials. Their routes of administration are often intravenous for quick dissemination to many anatomic sites. DC vaccine development has not yet shown significant toxicity at any dose delivered (24, 25), and there have been few suggestions of minimum required dose. Doses are largely defined as the "maximally feasible dose" from a blood draw or leukapheresis procedure of a specific duration (90 min to 4 h). Regarding route of delivery, many options have been tested and questions remain, each has positive and negative aspects to consider. For intradermal delivery, too many DC in a small volume might die *in situ*. Intra-nodal delivery may deliver the DC to an optimal site, unless they are not injected into a cellular region and are injected in fat or stroma instead (26). Intravenous delivery may send cells to lungs and liver and not secondary lymphoid tissues. Not all tumors are accessible for intra-tumoral injection (which has been tested with unloaded DC to allow DC to directly sample TAA), and that environment might be harsh and result in quick loss of DC function or viability *in vivo*. Intra-lymphatic delivery may also be immunologically ideal (like intra-nodal), but is clinically challenging to administer. The optimal DC vaccine dose and route also remains to be established for human clinical trials.

SECOND GENERATION TRIALS AND LESSONS LEARNED

A new generation of clinical trials was conducted from 2004 to 2012, testing new hypotheses based on the lessons learned from the first generation, proof-of-principle studies. One key area of change has been the use of defined, optimized cytokine cocktails and pathogen-derived agonists to mature DC. The individual constituents of these cocktails have an important impact on DC biology, including the relative level of cell surface molecules (e.g., co-stimulatory molecules CD80, CD86, or maturation markers CD83 or CCR7), the amount, timing, and duration of cytokine production by DC (e.g., IL-12p70, IL-12p40, IL-10), DC lifespan, and the trafficking potential and response to chemokine gradients (21). Early, high level production of IL-12p70 may not be as optimal for T cell activation *in vivo* as delayed IL-12 production until after DC have arrived from the site of injection to the lymph node. Newer DC vaccines are not simply "mature" by a few phenotypic markers, but are treated to elicit specific types of "maturity" or immunologic skewing, based on culture conditions, and planned antigen loading and injection route strategies. Some trials testing more optimal cocktails have been performed and published results should be available soon. Other cytokine culture conditions have been tested *in vitro* [with IL-15 or IL-13 (7, 8)] but access to clinical grade reagents has been a limitation until more relaxed guidelines from the US FDA, at least for the earliest stage trials ("Guidance for Industry: CGMP for Phase I Investigational Drugs" http://www.fda.gov/downloads/Drugs/GuidanceComplianceRegulatoryInformation/Guidances/ucm070273.pdf).

Shorter duration of DC cell culture (2–3 days instead of 5–7 days with different DC maturation triggers has also been tested (27). It is difficult to identify superior DC *in vitro* given that DC differentiation may not be fixed once the DC are administered, and very few randomized trials have been performed which compare different DC *in vivo*. This also leads to one of the major limitations in DC trials. The size of most trials is quite small and hence, there are not multiple trial arms to compare experimental groups and learn the answers to important questions (with any statistical confidence). Even when trials are "negative," showing minimal positive clinical effects, there are still many variables which might explain weak results, including unavoidable patient–patient variation in generation of an autologous cellular product, and insufficient funding available to run larger, randomized trials testing specific variables, like maturation cocktails, antigen choice, antigen loading, dose, and route (28).

A blow to the field was the result of the randomized Phase III trial comparing DTIC chemotherapy for melanoma (which has a very poor efficacy record) with a matured, peptide-pulsed DC vaccine (29). The trial was stopped early due to lack of differences between the trial arms, which had similar overall clinical response rates of <6%. Many of the variables discussed above have been hypothesized to have played a part in the disappointing DC vaccine results, including DC vaccine quality and consistency in manufacture between different manufacturing sites, site of delivery (s.c. instead of i.d.), and lack of tumor-specific helper epitopes or heterologous help to promote $CD4^+$ T cell activation. With so many open questions on how best to prepare DC vaccines, there are still many possible causes for minimal clinical responses.

However, there have been a number of more successful trials published in this period. Objective clinical responses and significant immunologic responses were observed in a trial in renal cell carcinoma patients testing Muc-1 peptide+heterologous PADRE pulsed DC (s.c.) (30). These DC vaccines were combined with low dose IL-2. In another study, acute myeloid leukemia patients in remission from previous standard therapy receiving WT-1 mRNA-loaded DC vaccines showed immune activation and improved clinical outcomes (31). Another trial tested DC-tumor fusions in myeloma patients before or after autologous stem cell transplant, and observed both anti-tumor immune activation and reduction of disease (32). Interestingly, these trials all employed a DC vaccine combination strategy.

NEXT GENERATION TRIALS: WHERE ARE WE GOING?

DC FOR CANCER PREVENTION?

A new clinical setting for tumor antigen vaccination has been proposed, focused on prevention of cancer development in high risk patients without current disease (33). This vaccination setting was recently reported for a Muc-1 peptide-based vaccine in subjects with advanced colonic adenomas (but not yet colorectal cancer). The results showed that the peptide vaccine was immunogenic in 43% of the subjects and response was inversely correlated with circulating MDSC levels (34). A related Muc-1 vaccine improved survival in a murine model of colitis-associated colorectal cancer (35), supporting the further testing of preventative cancer vaccination, including utilizing DC, in a prevention setting.

ANTIGEN LOADING

For antigen loading, peptide-pulsing, transfection/transduction, and protein-pulsing continue to be used, as well as tumor lysate loading. The procedure followed for tumor lysate preparation has recently been examined. The simplest approach has been multiple rounds of freezing (in a dry ice/ethanol bath or at −80°C) and thawing (by 37° water bath). This procedure can break open cells in a manner mimicking necrosis and allow subsequent tumor protein isolation. However, there are other approaches. Tumor cell exposure to UV and gamma irradiation has been shown to mimic apoptosis, which delivers different signals to DC than necrotic cells. Recently, tumor treatment with hypochlorous acid before lysate purification was tested (36), and this method of oxidation and rapid necrosis may be superior for DC vaccine loading. Another important element may be the changes in tumor antigen expression when tumors are cultured in hypoxic conditions (5% instead of 20%) specifically mimicking *in situ* hypoxic tumor oxygen levels (37). Such improved antigen preparation approaches may yield improved clinical outcomes.

ROUTE OF DELIVERY

Based on data demonstrating that DC vaccines delivered intradermally (i.d.) show very low level (<2%) migration to lymph nodes (based most often on ^{111}In-labeling (38, 39), and that ultrasound-guided intra-nodal delivery has a risk of the vaccine being injected into fat instead of a cellular area (26), other routes of delivery have been tested. The results have varied between mice and humans, and in patients, and all tested routes of delivery have proven to be immunogenic in terms of T cell response induction. Without higher rates of objective clinical responses, identification of superior routes of delivery remain unknown. Thus far, there has also been no strict correlation between phenotypic measures, like CCR7 level on the DC surface (40), and subsequent migration. There are suggestions that the maturation cocktail used impacts migration (40) but there are no definitive answers yet. More recently, newer MRI-based DC vaccine labels have been tested (41) (D. Bartlett and P. Kalinski, personal communication, 2013) and prolonged, semi-continuous intra-lymphatic delivery of DC has been tested [(42), and P. Kalinski, personal communication, 2013]. Continued efforts at tracking DC migration *in vivo* and optimizing routes of delivery may yield more potent DC vaccines. A few such DC trials are underway.

SUPPRESSIVE DC

While the cancer and infectious disease communities have investigated optimally immune stimulating DC, the organ transplantation and autoimmunity fields have sought approaches to either maintain an "immature" DC status, or differentiate DC toward a tolerogenic or immune suppressive activity. Such strategies include pulsing DC with anti-sense oligonucleotides for co-stimulatory molecules CD40, CD80, and CD86 to downregulate these molecules (22) for prevention and treatment of diabetes, or culture with vitamin D3 and IL-10 for allograft tolerance (23). A recent Phase I clinical trial testing anti-sense CD40/80/86 oligo pulsed DC in type 1 diabetic patients showed that the cells were safe, well-tolerated, and resulted in a reduction in a subset of B cells (22). In recent preclinical primate modeling of kidney allograft survival, i.v. infusion of vitamin D3/IL-10 regulatory DC was also safe and resulted in significantly improved allograft survival (23). Further clinical development of these strategies are underway.

DC VACCINE COMBINATIONS

The field of cancer immunotherapy is now in the position of having more effective drugs encompassing not only vaccines in development, but small molecule inhibitors of key signal transduction pathways and immunologic checkpoint inhibiting antibodies. While all of these modalities, like the traditional standards of care (surgery, chemotherapy, radiation) have strengths and weaknesses, the current generation of clinical trials focuses on combinations of these approaches. DC vaccines may have limitations as stand-alone therapeutics, but in combinations they could play a role in initiating and boosting anti-tumor immunity, promoting *in vivo* cross-presentation, and promoting long term immunologic memory. Cytotoxic treatments can have multiple positive effects on the immune system, from simple release of tumor antigens as cancer cells die, to cytotoxic agent-specific effects. Release of tumor antigens allows endogenous DC to take up and present them, or for larger numbers of tumor bed injected DC to take up the broad array of released tumor antigens for T cell activation. Cytotoxic agent-specific immune effects can include: upregulation of immune stimulatory molecule expression on tumor cells (e.g., DAMPs), increased tumor antigen expression, reduced suppressor cells frequencies, as well as increased CTL proliferation and activation. The pioneering studies in this area have largely been performed in murine models, but the immune-promoting effects of non-immune-based therapeutics are now being assessed in clinical trials. Future DC vaccine combinations with rationally chosen agents may increase the effectiveness of DC vaccines (43, 44).

DC TRANSCRIPTOME ANALYSIS

An important technological breakthrough has been the ability to test the DC vaccine transcriptome. This detailed molecular characterization allows for a broader understanding of DC vaccines. Manufacturing conditions, different maturation cocktails (45, 46), and their impact on DC biology, over and above even a very thorough examination of DC surface phenotype and cytokine production (47) can be examined on a molecular basis. To date, surface expression of standard DC markers (CD80, CD83, CD86, MHC class I, MHC class II, CCR7) has not correlated significantly with *in vivo* vaccine effects. The type-1-skewing cytokine produced by DC, IL-12p70, is actively being investigated as a potency assessment, based on its significant correlation with clinical outcome was demonstrated (48). This assay was employed after it was standardized for both spontaneous and induced expression of IL-12p70 heterodimers (47). Transcriptome analysis allows for a much broader assessment of DC vaccines, and may prove informative for predictive biomarkers of immune and/or clinical response. Such profiling has identified a type-1-skewing genetic profile expressed by DC matured with IFNγ+LPS (45), and a list of candidate genes that may be helpful for identity, stability, and potency measures of DC vaccines (46). This approach may also identify patient-to-patient variation of immunologic significance.

IMMUNOLOGIC MONITORING

Each DC vaccine clinical trial is based on the hypothesis that optimal tumor antigen presentation will promote clinically effective anti-tumor immunity. Understanding the effects of the vaccines on each patient's immune system is of utmost importance in moving the field forward. Most trials examine effector T cells activated by antigen-pulsed DC, but the cross-talk between DC and innate immune cells may also be mechanistically very important. Vaccine cell interaction with innate immune cells is expected to be variable with different types of DC cultured and loaded in different ways. DC modulation of suppressor cells, like regulatory T cells and myeloid-derived suppressor cells, may occur, and the overall immune effects may vary in magnitude and quality between peripheral blood and the tumor site. Some studies have found similar results in blood and tumor, while others have not, and studies examining DC vaccine effects at the tumor site are limited. Obtaining tumor biopsies can be challenging but well is worth the difficulties in order to understand the direct tumor site impact. Larger sized DC trials may involve multiple clinical sites, as well as vaccine manufacture sites, which necessitates careful standardization of blood processing vaccine culture and immune monitoring assay methodologies (49) as well as data reporting (50). Despite the technical challenges, careful immunologic monitoring, particularly with multiple functional assays, yields critical mechanistic insights.

CONCLUSION

Yes, we are making progress in the DC vaccine field. A more rational, defined, and data-driven approach is being employed in culturing, maturing, and antigen loading of DC (51). Fully characterizing DC vaccine transcription profiles moves far beyond the limited cell surface phenotypes previously employed. Performing more standardized trial designs where patients receive the same type of vaccine reduces variables to patient-to-patient variation instead of adding variables and may identify the most critical vaccine parameters to carry forward. More thorough, robust and standardized immune monitoring assessments are allowing to field to draw more meaningful conclusions from each trial. In the future, the next generation of optimized vaccines identified may selectively be used for individual patients, based on their tumor biology. A new generation of DC vaccine trials are underway (52) which have the potential to move this area of personalized medicine forward.

ACKNOWLEDGMENTS

This work was supported by the University of Pittsburgh Skin SPORE Grant, P50 CA121973 (PI: J. M. Kirkwood; Project 2 PI: Lisa H. Butterfield) and also in part by the UPCI CCSG award, P30 CA047904.

REFERENCES

1. Steinman RM, Cohn ZA. Identification of a novel cell type in peripheral lymphoid organs of mice. I. Morphology, quantitation, tissue distribution. *J Exp Med* (1973) **137**:1142–62. doi:10.1084/jem.137.5.1142
2. Inaba K, Steinman RM, Pack MW, Aya H, Inaba M, Sudo T, et al. Identification of proliferating dendritic cell precursors in mouse blood. *J Exp Med* (1992) **175**:1157–67. doi:10.1084/jem.175.5.1157
3. Markowicz S, Engleman EG. Granulocyte-macrophage colony-stimulating factor promotes differentiation and survival of human peripheral blood dendritic cells in vitro. *J Clin Invest* (1990) **85**:955–61. doi:10.1172/JCI114525
4. Romani N, Gruner S, Brang D, Kampgen E, Lenz A, Trockenbacher B, et al. Proliferating dendritic cell progenitors in human blood. *J Exp Med* (1994) **180**:83–93. doi:10.1084/jem.180.1.83
5. Mukherji B, Chakraborty NG, Yamasaki S, Okino T, Yamase H, Sporn JR, et al. Induction of antigen-specific cytolytic T cells in situ in human melanoma by immunization with synthetic peptide-pulsed autologous antigen presenting cells. *Proc Natl Acad Sci U S A* (1995) **92**:8078–82. doi:10.1073/pnas.92.17.8078
6. Palucka K, Ueno H, Fay J, Banchereau J. Dendritic cells and immunity against cancer. *J Intern Med* (2011) **269**:64–73. doi:10.1111/j.1365-2796.2010.02317.x
7. Palucka K, Banchereau J. Cancer immunotherapy via dendritic cells. *Nat Rev Cancer* (2012) **12**:265–77. doi:10.1038/nrc3258
8. Palucka K, Banchereau J. Dendritic-cell-based therapeutic cancer vaccines. *Immunity* (2013) **39**:38–48. doi:10.1016/j.immuni.2013.07.004
9. Hsu FJ, Benike C, Fagnoni F, Liles TM, Czerwinski D, Taidi B, et al. Vaccination of patients with B-cell lymphoma using autologous antigen-pulsed dendritic cells. *Nat Med* (1996) **2**:52–8. doi:10.1038/nm0196-52
10. Nestle FO, Alijagic S, Gilliet M, Sun Y, Grabbe S, Dummer R, et al. Vaccination of melanoma patients with peptide- or tumor lysate-pulsed dendritic cells. *Nat Med* (1998) **4**:328–32. doi:10.1038/nm0398-328
11. Banchereau J, Palucka AK, Dhodapkar M, Burkeholder S, Taquet N, Rolland A, et al. Immune and clinical responses in patients with metastatic melanoma to CD34(+) progenitor-derived dendritic cell vaccine. *Cancer Res* (2001) **61**:6451–8.
12. Rosenberg SA, Yang JC, Restifo NP. Cancer immunotherapy: moving beyond current vaccines. *Nat Med* (2004) **10**:909–15. doi:10.1038/nm1100
13. Davis MM. A prescription for human immunology. *Immunity* (2008) **29**:835–8. doi:10.1016/j.immuni.2008.12.003
14. Fuertes MB, Woo SR, Burnett B, Fu YX, Gajewski TF. Type I interferon response and innate immune sensing of cancer. *Trends Immunol* (2013) **34**:67–73. doi:10.1016/j.it.2012.10.004
15. Galon J, Pages F, Marincola FM, Angell HK, Thurin M, Lugli A, et al. Cancer classification using the immunoscore: a worldwide task force. *J Transl Med* (2012) **10**:205. doi:10.1186/1479-5876-10-205
16. Chang CC, Ferrone S. Immune selective pressure and HLA class I antigen defects in malignant lesions. *Cancer Immunol Immunother* (2007) **56**:227–36. doi:10.1007/s00262-006-0183-1
17. Lopez-Albaitero A, Nayak JV, Ogino T, Machandia A, Gooding W, Deleo AB, et al. Role of antigen-processing machinery in the in vitro resistance of squamous cell carcinoma of the head and neck cells to recognition by CTL. *J Immunol* (2006) **176**:3402–9.
18. Trefzer U, Hofmann M, Reinke S, Guo YJ, Audring H, Spagnoli G, et al. Concordant loss of melanoma differentiation antigens in synchronous and asynchronous melanoma metastases: implications for immunotherapy. *Melanoma Res* (2006) **16**:137–45. doi:10.1097/01.cmr.0000200489.55099.20
19. Janssen EM, Droin NM, Lemmens EE, Pinkoski MJ, Bensinger SJ, Ehst BD, et al. CD4+ T-cell help controls CD8+ T-cell memory via TRAIL-mediated activation-induced cell death. *Nature* (2005) **434**:88–93. doi:10.1038/nature03337
20. Cheever MA, Allison JP, Ferris AS, Finn OJ, Hastings BM, Hecht TT, et al. The prioritization of cancer antigens: a national cancer institute pilot project for

the acceleration of translational research. *Clin Cancer Res* (2009) **15**:5323–37. doi:10.1158/1078-0432.CCR-09-0737

21. Mailliard RB, Wankowicz-Kalinska A, Cai Q, Wesa A, Hilkens CM, Kapsenberg ML, et al. alpha-type-1 polarized dendritic cells: a novel immunization tool with optimized CTL-inducing activity. *Cancer Res* (2004) **64**:5934–7. doi:10.1158/0008-5472.CAN-04-1261
22. Giannoukakis N, Phillips B, Finegold D, Harnaha J, Trucco M. Phase I (safety) study of autologous tolerogenic dendritic cells in type 1 diabetic patients. *Diabetes Care* (2011) **34**:2026–32. doi:10.2337/dc11-0472
23. Ezzelarab MB, Zahorchak AF, Lu L, Morelli AE, Chalasani G, Demetris AJ, et al. Regulatory dendritic cell infusion prolongs kidney allograft survival in nonhuman primates. *Am J Transplant* (2013) **13**:1989–2005. doi:10.1111/ajt.12310
24. Butterfield LH, Ribas A, Dissette VB, Amarnani SN, Vu HT, Oseguera D, et al. Determinant spreading associated with clinical response in dendritic cell-based immunotherapy for malignant melanoma. *Clin Cancer Res* (2003) **9**:998–1008.
25. Grover A, Kim GJ, Lizee G, Tschoi M, Wang G, Wunderlich JR, et al. Intralymphatic dendritic cell vaccination induces tumor antigen-specific, skin-homing T lymphocytes. *Clin Cancer Res* (2006) **12**:5801–8. doi:10.1158/1078-0432.CCR-05-2421
26. de Vries IJ, Lesterhuis WJ, Barentsz JO, Verdijk P, van Krieken JH, Boerman OC, et al. Magnetic resonance tracking of dendritic cells in melanoma patients for monitoring of cellular therapy. *Nat Biotechnol* (2005) **23**:1407–13. doi:10.1038/nbt1154
27. Kvistborg P, Boegh M, Pedersen AW, Claesson MH, Zocca MB. Fast generation of dendritic cells. *Cell Immunol* (2009) **260**:56–62. doi:10.1016/j.cellimm.2009.09.003
28. Engell-Noerregaard L, Hansen TH, Andersen MH, Thor Straten P, Svane IM. Review of clinical studies on dendritic cell-based vaccination of patients with malignant melanoma: assessment of correlation between clinical response and vaccine parameters. *Cancer Immunol Immunother* (2009) **58**:1–14. doi:10.1007/s00262-008-0568-4
29. Schadendorf D, Hauschild A, Ugurel S, Thoelke A, Egberts F, Kreissig M, et al. Dose-intensified bi-weekly temozolomide in patients with asymptomatic brain metastases from malignant melanoma: a phase II DeCOG/ADO study. *Ann Oncol* (2006) **17**:1592–7. doi:10.1093/annonc/mdl148
30. Wierecky J, Muller MR, Wirths S, Halder-Oehler E, Dorfel D, Schmidt SM, et al. Immunologic and clinical responses after vaccinations with peptide-pulsed dendritic cells in metastatic renal cancer patients. *Cancer Res* (2006) **66**:5910–8. doi:10.1158/0008-5472.CAN-05-3905
31. Van Tendeloo VF, van de Velde A, van Driessche A, Cools N, Anguille S, Ladell K, et al. Induction of complete and molecular remissions in acute myeloid leukemia by Wilms' tumor 1 antigen-targeted dendritic cell vaccination. *Proc Natl Acad Sci U S A* (2010) **107**:13824–9. doi:10.1073/pnas.1008051107
32. Rosenblatt J, Avivi I, Vasir B, Uhl L, Munshi NC, Katz T, et al. Vaccination with dendritic cell/tumor fusions following autologous stem cell transplant induces immunologic and clinical responses in multiple myeloma patients. *Clin Cancer Res* (2013) **19**:3640–8. doi:10.1158/1078-0432.CCR-13-0282
33. Finn OJ. Cancer immunology. *N Engl J Med* (2008) **358**:2704–15. doi:10.1056/NEJMra072739
34. Kimura T, Mckolanis JR, Dzubinski LA, Islam K, Potter DM, Salazar AM, et al. MUC1 vaccine for individuals with advanced adenoma of the colon: a cancer immunoprevention feasibility study. *Cancer Prev Res (Phila)* (2013) **6**:18–26. doi:10.1158/1940-6207.CAPR-12-0275
35. Beatty P, Ranganathan S, Finn OJ. Prevention of colitis-associated colon cancer using a vaccine to target abnormal expression of the MUC1 tumor antigen. *Oncoimmunology* (2012) **1**:263–70. doi:10.4161/onci.18950
36. Chiang CL, Kandalaft LE, Tanyi J, Hagemann AR, Motz GT, Svoronos N, et al. A dendritic cell vaccine pulsed with autologous hypochlorous acid-oxidized ovarian cancer lysate primes effective broad antitumor immunity: from bench to bedside. *Clin Cancer Res* (2013) **19**:4801–15. doi:10.1158/1078-0432.CCR-13-1185
37. Olin MR, Andersen BM, Zellmer DM, Grogan PT, Popescu FE, Xiong Z, et al. Superior efficacy of tumor cell vaccines grown in physiologic oxygen. *Clin Cancer Res* (2010) **16**:4800–8. doi:10.1158/1078-0432.CCR-10-1572
38. Morse MA, Coleman RE, Akabani G, Niehaus N, Coleman D, Lyerly HK. Migration of human dendritic cells after injection in patients with metastatic malignancies. *Cancer Res* (1999) **59**:56–8.
39. De Vries IJ, Krooshoop DJ, Scharenborg NM, Lesterhuis WJ, Diepstra JH, van Muijen GN, et al. Effective migration of antigen-pulsed dendritic cells to lymph nodes in melanoma patients is determined by their maturation state. *Cancer Res* (2003) **63**:12–7.
40. Quillien V, Moisan A, Carsin A, Lesimple T, Lefeuvre C, Adamski H, et al. Biodistribution of radiolabelled human dendritic cells injected by various routes. *Eur J Nucl Med Mol Imaging* (2005) **32**:731–41. doi:10.1007/s00259-005-1825-9
41. Helfer BM, Balducci A, Nelson AD, Janjic JM, Gil RR, Kalinski P, et al. Functional assessment of human dendritic cells labeled for in vivo (19)F magnetic resonance imaging cell tracking. *Cytotherapy* (2010) **12**:238–50. doi:10.3109/14653240903446902
42. Kalinski P, Edington H, Zeh HJ, Okada H, Butterfield LH, Kirkwood JM, et al. Dendritic cells in cancer immunotherapy: vaccines or autologous transplants? *Immunol Res* (2011) **50**:235–47. doi:10.1007/s12026-011-8224-z
43. Zitvogel L, Kepp O, Kroemer G. Immune parameters affecting the efficacy of chemotherapeutic regimens. *Nat Rev Clin Oncol* (2011) **8**:151–60. doi:10.1038/nrclinonc.2010.223
44. Galluzzi L, Senovilla L, Zitvogel L, Kroemer G. The secretally: immunostimulation by anticancer drugs. *Nat Rev Drug Discov* (2012) **11**:215–33. doi:10.1038/nrd3626
45. Jin P, Han TH, Ren J, Saunders S, Wang E, Marincola FM, et al. Molecular signatures of maturing dendritic cells: implications for testing the quality of dendritic cell therapies. *J Transl Med* (2010) **8**:4. doi:10.1186/1479-5876-8-4
46. Castiello L, Sabatino M, Zhao Y, Tumaini B, Ren J, Ping J, et al. Quality controls in cellular immunotherapies: rapid assessment of clinical grade dendritic cells by gene expression profiling. *Mol Ther* (2013) **21**:476–84. doi:10.1038/mt.2012.89
47. Butterfield LH, Gooding W, Whiteside TL. Development of a potency assay for human dendritic cells: IL-12p70 production. *J Immunother* (2008) **31**:89–100. doi:10.1097/CJI.0b013e318158fce0
48. Okada H, Kalinski P, Ueda R, Hoji A, Kohanbash G, Donegan TE, et al. Induction of CD8+ T-cell responses against novel glioma-associated antigen peptides and clinical activity by vaccinations with {alpha}-type 1 polarized dendritic cells and polyinosinic-polycytidylic acid stabilized by lysine and carboxymethylcellulose in patients with recurrent malignant glioma. *J Clin Oncol* (2011) **29**:330–6. doi:10.1200/JCO.2010.30.7744
49. Butterfield LH, Palucka AK, Britten CM, Dhodapkar MV, Hakansson L, Janetzki S, et al. Recommendations from the iSBTc-SITC/FDA/NCI Workshop on Immunotherapy Biomarkers. *Clin Cancer Res* (2011) **17**:3064–76. doi:10.1158/1078-0432.CCR-10-2234
50. Britten CM, Janetzki S, Butterfield LH, Ferrari G, Gouttefangeas C, Huber C, et al. T cell assays and MIATA: the essential minimum for maximum impact. *Immunity* (2012) **37**:1–2. doi:10.1016/j.immuni.2012.07.010
51. Nicolette CA, Healey D, Tcherepanova I, Whelton P, Monesmith T, Coombs L, et al. Dendritic cells for active immunotherapy: optimizing design and manufacture in order to develop commercially and clinically viable products. *Vaccine* (2007) **25**(Suppl 2):B47–60. doi:10.1016/j.vaccine.2007.06.006
52. Galluzzi L, Senovilla L, Vacchelli E, Eggermont A, Fridman WH, Galon J, et al. Trial watch: dendritic cell-based interventions for cancer therapy. *Oncoimmunology* (2012) **1**:1111–34. doi:10.4161/onci.21494

20

Reconstructing a B-cell clonal lineage. II. mutation, selection, and affinity maturation

Thomas B. Kepler[1,2]*, Supriya Munshaw[3], Kevin Wiehe[4], Ruijun Zhang[4], Jae-Sung Yu[4,5], Christopher W. Woods[5,6,7,8], Thomas N. Denny[4,5], Georgia D. Tomaras[4,5,9], S. Munir Alam[4,5], M. Anthony Moody[3,4], Garnett Kelsoe[4,9], Hua-Xin Liao[4,5] and Barton F. Haynes[4,5]

[1] Department of Microbiology, Boston University School of Medicine, Boston, MA, USA
[2] Department of Mathematics and Statistics, Boston University, Boston, MA, USA
[3] Center for Viral Hepatitis Research, Johns Hopkins University, Baltimore, MD, USA
[4] Duke Human Vaccine Institute, Duke University Medical Center, Durham, NC, USA
[5] Department of Medicine, Duke University Medical Center, Durham, NC, USA
[6] Department of Pathology, Duke University Medical Center, Durham, NC, USA
[7] Hubert-Yeargan Center for Global Health, Duke University Medical Center, Durham, NC, USA
[8] Department of Pediatrics, Duke University Medical Center, Durham, NC, USA
[9] Department of Immunology, Duke University Medical Center, Durham, NC, USA

Edited by:
Ramit Mehr, Bar-Ilan University, Israel

Reviewed by:
Ramit Mehr, Bar-Ilan University, Israel
Andrew M. Collins, University of New South Wales, Australia
Uri Hershberg, Drexel University, USA

***Correspondence:**
Thomas B. Kepler, Departments of Microbiology, Mathematics and Statistics, Boston University, 72 East Concord Street, L-504, Boston, MA 02118, USA
e-mail: tbkepler@bu.edu

Affinity maturation of the antibody response is a fundamental process in adaptive immunity during which B-cells activated by infection or vaccination undergo rapid proliferation accompanied by the acquisition of point mutations in their rearranged immunoglobulin (Ig) genes and selection for increased affinity for the eliciting antigen. The rate of somatic hypermutation at any position within an Ig gene is known to depend strongly on the local DNA sequence, and Ig genes have region-specific codon biases that influence the local mutation rate within the gene resulting in increased differential mutability in the regions that encode the antigen-binding domains. We have isolated a set of clonally related natural Ig heavy chain–light chain pairs from an experimentally infected influenza patient, inferred the unmutated ancestral rearrangements and the maturation intermediates, and synthesized all the antibodies using recombinant methods. The lineage exhibits a remarkably uniform rate of improvement of the effective affinity to influenza hemagglutinin (HA) over evolutionary time, increasing 1000-fold overall from the unmutated ancestor to the best of the observed antibodies. Furthermore, analysis of selection reveals that selection and mutation bias were concordant even at the level of maturation to a single antigen. Substantial improvement in affinity to HA occurred along mutationally preferred paths in sequence space and was thus strongly facilitated by the underlying local codon biases.

Keywords: somatic hypermutation, experimental influenza infection, antibody selection, antibody affinity maturation, phylogenetics

INTRODUCTION

B-cells that respond to infection or vaccination are induced by signaling through their B-cell receptors to proliferate and differentiate into plasmacytes and memory cells. Short-lived plasmacytes secrete antibody and provide immediate protection from the eliciting agent; memory cells and long-lived plasmacytes persist clonally for very long times, providing protection against recurring challenges from the same or closely related agents (1). Cells that go on to find persistent clones are subject to affinity maturation in their post-exposure development. During affinity maturation, the affinity of the B-cell receptor for antigens on the eliciting agent is substantially increased, resulting in a more potent response on recall (2).

Affinity maturation proceeds through somatic hypermutation, the introduction of point mutations into the rearranged immunoglobulin (Ig) genes that encode the B-cell receptor. Those B-cells that thereby acquire an increased affinity for the antigen gain a proliferative advantage and come to dominate the activated B-cell population. Affinity maturation is crucial for humoral immune protection, conferring greater neutralization capacity (3) and opsonization efficiency (4), and is generally correlated with higher vaccine efficacy (5). In fact, lack of effective affinity maturation has been directly implicated in adverse outcomes for at least one vaccine (6).

The rate of somatic hypermutation at a given position with an Ig variable region is significantly influenced by the local DNA sequence – both the nucleotide at that position and sequence of nucleotides containing it (7). Codon usage in Ig V-gene segments is strongly biased, with zones of high mutability largely overlapping with the complementarity-determining regions (CDR), which encode the antibody's antigen-binding residues (8, 9). Thus, somatic mutation drives Ig genes along statistically favored paths through the genotype space. Some combinations of substitutions will therefore be visited much more rapidly than others involving the same number of changes. Each Ig gene segment has been involved in the response to a huge number of antigens over the course of its evolutionary history and has experienced selection pressure to enhance its role as a template for affinity maturation.

Technology for the isolation of native heavy-chain/light-chain pairs and their subsequent recombinant synthesis have recently been developed (10, 11) and refined (12), making it feasible to determine the biophysical properties of large numbers of monoclonal antibodies (mAb). We have complemented this technology with the development of computational tools that substantially improve our ability to infer the unmutated common ancestor of a set of clonally related antibodies, and the corresponding maturation intermediates (13).

We have now applied these methods to the detailed study of the maturation pathways of a B-cell clone whose antibody genes were isolated from a human experimental influenza infection study, providing an elucidation of the interplay of mutational constraints and selection on antigen-binding affinity. One of our aims in this study is to examine the influence that this differential mutability has on a specific instance of affinity maturation to a given antigen: the immune response to influenza hemagglutinin (HA) in a human subject. This question clearly goes beyond the issue of codon bias as a statistical regularity to inquire about influence of codon bias in a specific case. The relationship between these two questions is analogous to the phenomenon of HCDR3 length in autoimmune disease. There one has the statistical observation that B-cells with long HCDR3 are counter-selected during development (14), yet the role of long HCDR3 for individual autoantibodies is rarely understood. In our case, we know that the mutation frequency is higher on average in regions that encode amino acids that are more likely, on average, to contact epitopes. In this study, we examine the interplay of differential mutation frequency and selection in the evolution of a single antibody lineage.

Specifically, we demonstrate that intraclonal affinity maturation proceeded by stepwise accumulation of affinity-enhancing mutations and that mutation and selection interacted synergistically. These insights and others gained by application of the tools we have developed promise to facilitate the effective harnessing of affinity maturation for vaccine engineering.

RESULTS

ISOLATION AND IDENTIFICATION OF ANTI-INFLUENZA HEMAGGLUTININ A B-CELL CLONE CL2569

Human subjects were experimentally infected intranasally with influenza virus (15). Eighty-six natural heavy-chain/light-chain gene pairs were isolated from one subject (subject EI13) on day 4 after exposure. Among these, we found three clonally related sets. Two of the clones contained two antibodies each; the other contained five. The members of this five-member clone, designated CL2569, all bind HA in the $K_d = 1$–20 nM range. Four of these antibodies are of the IgM isotype while the other is IgA1. The light chain in each antibody is Ig kappa. The remainder of this study describes our analysis of CL2569.

The antibodies are highly diversified. The heavy chains have a mean (±SD) pairwise difference of 28.0 ± 5.4 nucleotides (nt) and 16.7 ± 3.6 amino acids (aa); the light chains have an average pairwise difference of 18.0 ± 2.5 nt and 8.2 ± 1.5 aa.

We inferred the unmutated ancestor (UA) and intermediates along the affinity maturation pathways by computing the Bayesian posterior probability mass function on nucleotide states at each position of the heavy and light chains conditioned by the data and the maximum-likelihood phylogram as described in the companion study (13). The mutations acquired along each branch were enumerated and classified according to the IMGT classification (16) (**Table 1**). The UA and all intermediates for both heavy and light chains were synthesized using the same recombinant technology used to synthesize the observed antibodies.

The probable error profile for the heavy-chain UA is shown in **Figure 1**. Briefly, the sum of the probable errors over all positions is 3.2. There are five nucleotide positions where the marginal posterior probability of the modal nucleotide is <0.8, all of which occur in CDR3. Importantly, at these somewhat lower-confidence positions, the inferred modal CDR3 is identical to all five observed sequences. The summed probable errors for each of the inferred intermediates is less than that of the inferred UA and decreases as one gets closer to the observed sequences. The kappa chain UA is known with high confidence. The sum of the probable errors is 0.33.

THE DISSOCIATION CONSTANT DECREASES EXPONENTIALLY WITH UNIFORM RATE OVER THE DURATION OF THE PROCESS

The dissociation constant K_d for binding to HA of the Brisbane strain of influenza virus was measured using ELISA on solutions of monoclonal antibody prepared at known concentrations. K_d

Table 1 | Classification of mutations in CL2569 heavy- and light-chain histories.

	Heavy chains		Light chains	
	Non	Synon	Non	Synon
FR	40	20	14	7
CDR	17	11	11	4

FR, framework region; CDR, complementarity-determining region; Non, non-synonymous; Synon, synonymous.

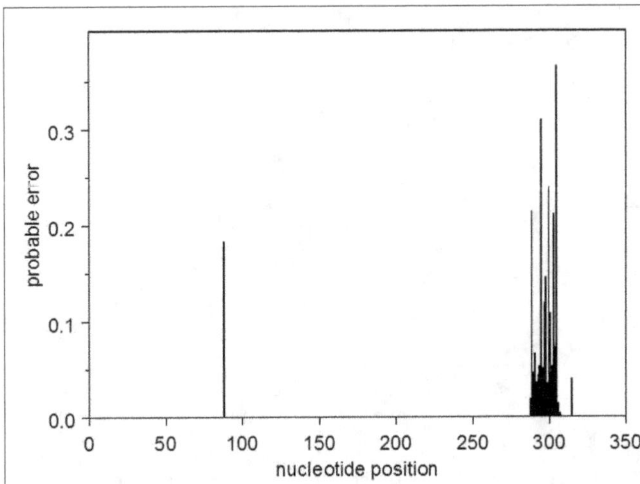

FIGURE 1 | The profile of the probable error in the modal heavy chain UA.

was estimated by non-linear curve fitting simultaneously on all data for each plate. The UA binds to HA very weakly but measurably, $K_d = 2.6\ \mu M$. Throughout the evolutionary process, K_d declines uniformly and exponentially ($R^2 = 0.92$), falling 50–74% (95% confidence interval) for each 1% increase in evolutionary distance (**Figure 2**). The affinities of the observed antibodies are approximately three orders of magnitude higher than that of the ancestor, an improvement that occurs over a total evolutionary distance of 6–9% nucleotide differences.

INTERACTION BETWEEN SELECTION AND MUTABILITY

To gage the force of selection in molecular evolution, deviations in the ratio of the number of synonymous mutations to the number of non-synonymous mutations from that expected under the null hypothesis of selection-free evolution are often used for statistical testing (17). For antibody somatic evolution, mutations are further classified by region, occurring in the CDR or framework regions (FR) and various combinations specific deviations from expected values within these classifications used in statistical tests [see, e.g., Ref. (18)]. Crucially, the distribution expected under the no selection null hypothesis for Ig somatic evolution is not trivially

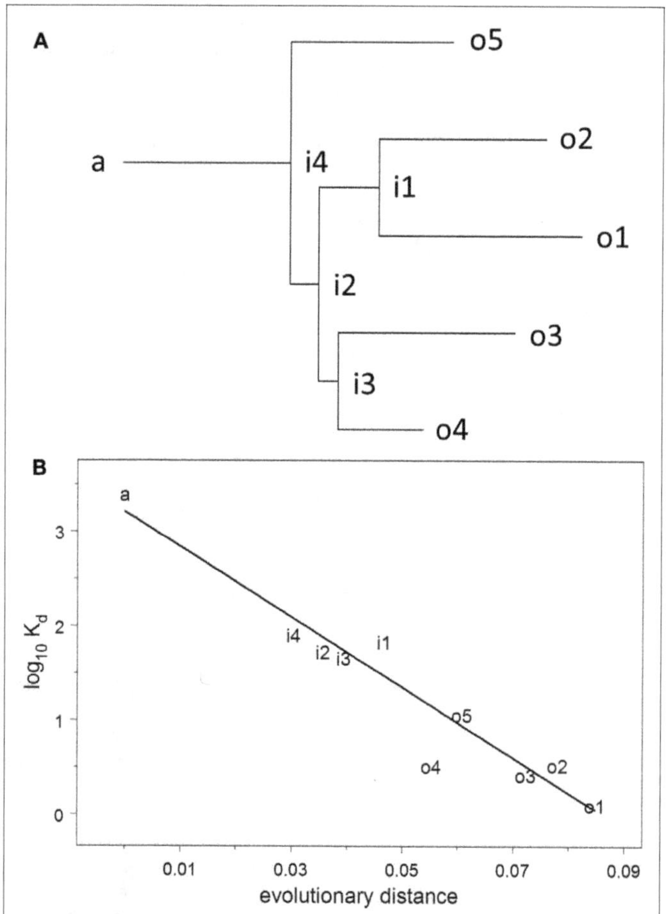

FIGURE 2 | (A) Maximum-likelihood clonal tree showing observed (o), intermediate (i), and ancestral (a) sequences. The tree was inferred using both heavy and light chains. **(B)** Regression analysis of $\log_{10} K_d$ vs. evolutionary distance.

computed. Because the codon bias has been adapted for Ig plasticity, empirical estimation of the distributions under the null cannot be avoided.

The model we use to estimate parameters and perform tests is straightforwardly derived using likelihood-based methods in statistics. We nevertheless describe the model in some detail below so that the argument may be essentially self-contained.

In order to explore the interplay of selection and mutability, we use a non-linear regression model and multiple independent categorical distributions[1] in which every gene position along each branch of the clonal tree can either be unmutated, mutated synonymously, or mutated non-synonymously. That is, there are three possible classifications for each nucleotide, and the "mutation type" variable takes one of the two values: $T \in \{S, N\}$. For the ith nucleotide in gene g, the variable x_{gi}^T is an indicator for the mutation type. For example, if the nucleotide in question has been mutated non-synonymously along the branch leading up to g from its parent sequence $a(g)$, we have $x_{gi}^N = 1$ and $x_{gi}^S = 0$. If the nucleotide is not mutated at all, we have $x_{gi}^N = 0$ and $x_{gi}^S = 0$.

The relevant likelihood function is the product of independent categorical distributions, whose log (we work with the log of the likelihood function for convenience) is

$$\log L = \sum_{gi}\left[\sum_{T} x_{gi}^{T} \log P_{a(g)i}^{T} + \left(1 - x_{gi}^{\bullet}\right)\log\left(1 - P_{a(g)i}^{\bullet}\right)\right] \tag{1}$$

where $P_{a(g)i}^T$ is the probability that the ith nucleotide in the parent of gene g would have mutation type T. The dot in place of an index indicates summation over that index, for example, $1 - P_{a(g)i}^{\bullet}$ is the probability that the nucleotide in question is not mutated. It is the dependency of these probabilities on the covariates that we model.

The covariates are themselves properties of the specific nucleotide expressed in terms of probabilities. There is first the probability that a given nucleotide mutates at all. This probability is the product of the sequence-specific mutation rate μ_{ai} and the effective evolutionary time τ along the relevant branch. Then, we have the probability σ_{ai}^T that a mutation occurring at the position and gene in question will have type T (that is, conditional on there being a mutation at all). This probability depends on the codon in which the nucleotide is found and its position within the codon. But it also depends on the local sequence (19); these influences have to be estimated for the nucleotide at each position of the gene. Finally, there is the impact of selection. Once a mutation has occurred, it must survive to fixation in order to be observed.

The covariates we will consider for predicting the survival of mutations at the ith position of gene a are the type T of the mutation, the region $R(i) \in \{\text{FR,CDR}\}$ that contains position i, and the mutability μ_{ai}. Note that the dependence of the survival probability on mutability is over and above the role of the mutability in inducing the mutation initially. Indeed, it is the dependence of survival on mutability that is of primary concern for this study. The dependence of survival probability on region is given by the

[1]Such a product distribution is similar to a multinomial distribution, but has different probabilities at each site.

terms γ_R^T. The ratios of these terms give the relative survival probabilities. Because they are introduced as multiplicative rather than additive effects, they are subject, without loss of generality, to the multiplicative constraint $\gamma_{FR}^{Syn}\gamma_{CDR}^{Syn}\gamma_{FR}^{Non}\gamma_{CDR}^{Non} = 1$.

Combining all the component probabilities then gives the probability that gene g has acquired an observed mutation of type T at position i and has survived. It is given by

$$P_{gi}^{T} = \tau\mu_{a(g)i}\sigma_{a(g)i}^{T}\left(\gamma_{R(i)}^{T} + \beta_T\mu_{a(g)i}\right). \quad (2)$$

The local sequence specificity of μ_{ai} and σ_{ai}^T are estimated using external data as described in the supplementary information.

For each hypothesis being tested, we impose the specific constraints on the model parameters in Eq. 2 that correspond to the hypothesis, estimate the remaining parameters by maximizing the likelihood. We then test hypotheses using the likelihood ratio test (20) where applicable, and compare models using the Akaike information criterion (AIC). The AIC is a penalized likelihood, appropriate for model selection where the likelihood ratio test is inapplicable because the respective models are not nested (21).

Local mutability is strongly informative. We compare two models: in the first (Model 0), the mutability is constant over positions $\mu_i = \mu_j$ for all positions i and j. In the second (Model 1), the mutability is determined by the local sequence $\mu_i = m_j$ where m_i is the mutability for the local sequence context at position i, estimated from an independent dataset (see Materials and Methods section). For this test, assume that selection is based on the covariate region × type, and allow γ_R^T to vary subject to the multiplicative constraint above, whereas $\beta_T = 0$ for both T. The models are not nested, so we use AIC and relative likelihood for the comparison. The model with empirical mutability is substantially better supported by the data than is the constant-mutability model (relative likelihood $= 3 \times 10^8$).

Region × type is informative in selection. If region and type are used to classify each potential mutation into one of the four classes that are then used to model the selection process, the predictive power of the model is increased. On comparing the selection-free null model with empirical local mutability (Model 1) with the alternative model in which γ_R^T are fit to the data (Model 2: $\beta_T = 0$, $\mu_i = m_i$), we reject the null model (likelihood ratio test, $p = 0.014$).

Mutability × type is informative in selection. In addition to the mutability that is used to predict the generation of mutations, we may use mutability as a covariate for predicting selection. The resulting model has both linear and quadratic terms in the mutability. On comparing the null model that recognizes type, but not region (Model 3: $\gamma_{FR}^T = \gamma_{CDR}^T$, $\beta_T = 0$ and $\mu_i = m_i$), with the alternative model in which β_T are fit to the data (Model 4: $\gamma_{FR}^T = \gamma_{CDR}^T$ $\mu_i = m_i$), we reject the null model (likelihood ratio test, $p = 0.010$).

Mutability × type is slightly more informative than region × type in selection. Both region × type and mutability × type have been shown to be predictive. To determine which covariate is more effective as a predictor, we perform a model comparison by AIC; comparing the region × type model (Model 2) with the mutability × type model (Model 4). Both have four degrees of freedom, so by AIC, the comparison favors the mutability × type model (relative likelihood = 1.35).

This result is illustrated in **Figure 3**, which shows the distribution of relative mutabilities in relation to region and the distribution of observed non-synonymous mutations over both gene position and evolutionary time.

The AIC-optimal model uses both mutability × type and region × type to predict mutations. Given the covariates to which we have access, the largest model has $\mu_i = m_i$, and both γ_R^T and β_T are free to vary. This model (Model 5) has the minimum AIC of all models, and all those models that are nested within it are rejected by likelihood ratio tests ($p < 0.05$). The coefficients of the optimal model are shown in **Table 2**.

The selection observed is predominantly purifying. Having determined that selection is measurably occurring, we investigate the nature of the selection by examining the coefficients of the model fit (**Table 2**). In both CDR and FR, the coefficients for non-synonymous mutations are significantly smaller than those for synonymous mutations, consistent with a scenario in which deleterious mutations were introduced in cells that did not survive selection.

Mutability × type is more informative than mutability alone. We have shown that mutability × type is informative. An informative test, the meaning of which will be elaborated on in the discussion, is whether the contribution of mutability to the survival of a mutation depends on the mutation type. For this comparison, we take the null model (Model 6) to have $\beta_{FR} = \beta_{CDR}$ and $\gamma_{FR}^T = \gamma_{CDR}^T$, and the alternative model (Model 4) with β_T free to vary. The null model is rejected (likelihood ratio test, $p = 8 \times 10^{-3}$).

It is crucial here to understand that this last test is a test of whether type (synonymous vs. non-synonymous) interacts in the statistical sense with mutability (the evolved biases in the targeting of somatic hypermutation) to influence the probability that a mutation survives to fixation. It is taken as given that type alone does influence a mutation's survival probability. It is further taken as given that mutability alone influences whether a mutation occurs in the first place or not. This test is a test of whether mutability is informative regarding the probability that a mutation survives selection. Selection cannot act on synonymous mutations, so evidence that mutability is correlated with selective survival must come from examination of the interaction term between mutability and type. This interaction term is equivalent to $\beta_{FR} - \beta_{CDR}$. The rejected null hypothesis is that this quantity is zero.

DISCUSSION

In this study, by inference and expression of the UA and inferred intermediate antibodies of a single clone, we have directly demonstrated the stepwise maturation of antibodies. Such stepwise maturation has been assumed on theoretical grounds (22), but the technology to observe it has not been utilized before now.

The antibodies of clone CL2569 bind influenza HA and are highly mutated. For these reasons, they almost certainly represent a secondary response. In fact, the most likely scenario for the ontogeny of this lineage is that it was formed via affinity maturation during an earlier infection or vaccination

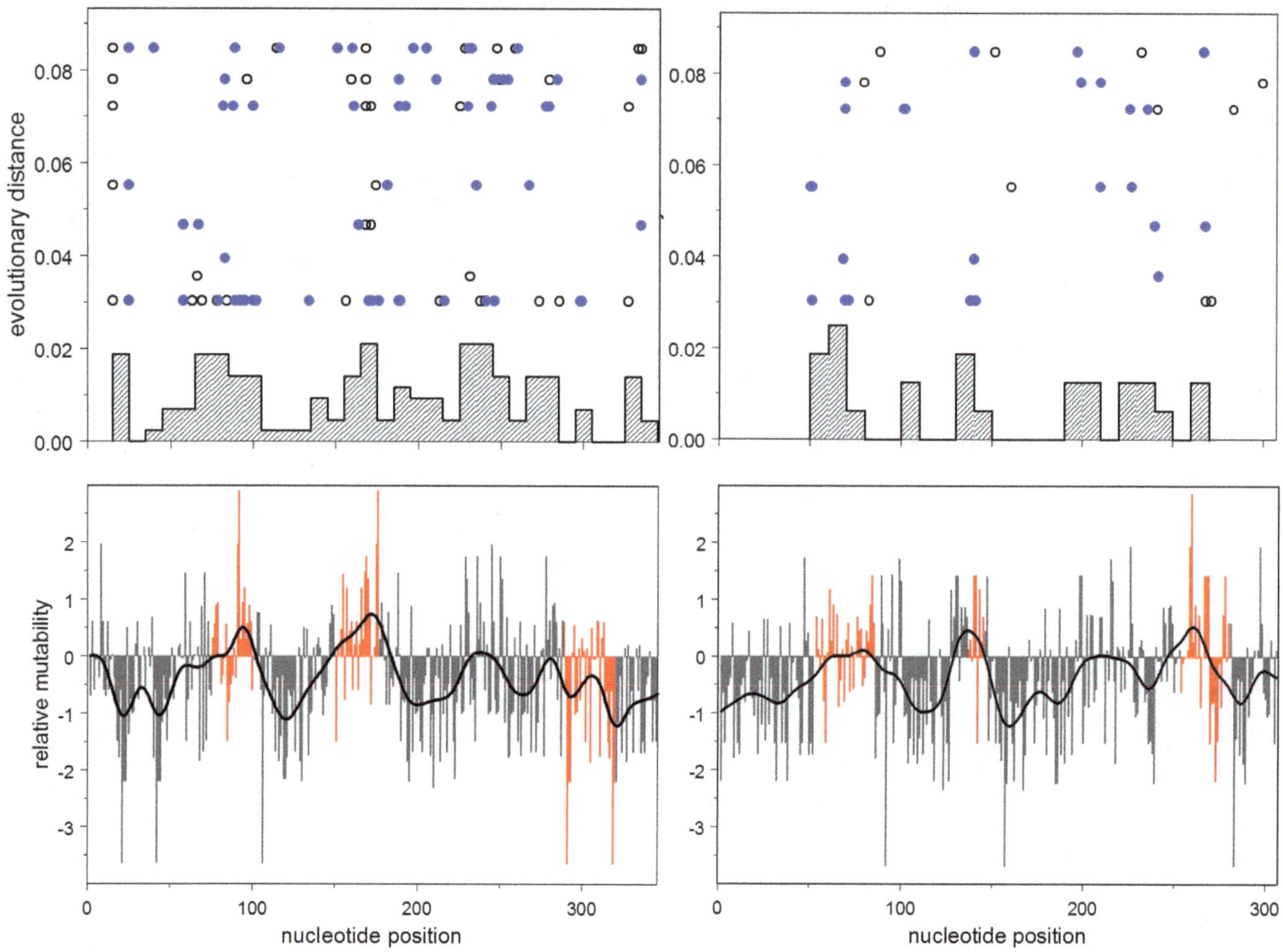

FIGURE 3 | Lower: mutability by position for heavy (left) and light (right) chains. Mutability at CDR nucleotides is shown in red. Upper: histogram by position of accumulated non-synonymous mutations; evolutionary distance vs. position for each synonymous (open disks), and non-synonymous (closed disks) mutation.

Table 2 | Maximum-likelihood estimates for the coefficients in the optimal model.

Model	Mutability	γ_{FR}^{Syn}	γ_{CDR}^{Syn}	γ_{FR}^{Non}	γ_{CDR}^{Non}	β_{Syn}	β_{Non}	AIC
0	Constant	(1)	(1)	(1)	(1)	(0)	(0)	640.0
1	Empirical	(1)	(1)	(1)	(1)	(0)	(0)	589.2
2	Empirical	0.75	2.12	0.67	(0.94)	(0)	(0)	584.6
3	Empirical	1.18	(1.18)	(0.85)	(0.85)	(0)	(0)	589.2
4	Empirical	2.25	(2.25)	(0.44)	(0.44)	−25.8	16.6	584.0
5	Empirical	1.58	3.23	0.34	(0.58)	−21.4	13.8	579.0
6	Empirical	1.29	(1.29)	(0.78)	(0.78)	9.63	(9.63)	589.0

Parentheses indicate that the parameter is invariant at the indicated value in the model considered.

and was subsequently activated into differentiation to plasmacytes by the experimental infection without undergoing further affinity maturation. The subject was infected with the H3N2 A/Wisconsin/67/2005 strain of influenza virus; preliminary binding assays were done on HA from several strains including the infecting strain, H1 A/Brisbane/59/2007, and several others. Although the maturation patterns were similar across several of the strains, the affinities measured against H1 A/Brisbane/59/2007 were generally higher (15). The infection study was performed in 2008, so previous infection in the subject with influenza strains circulating in 2007 is consistent with this observed reactivity to H1 A/Brisbane/59/2007.

The recovered mAb in this clonal lineage were mostly IgM with a single member that was IgA1, and all the members had a degree of somatic hypermutation consistent with one or more prior rounds of antigen-driven germinal center maturation. Recent work by Pape et al. (23) has shown that in mice IgM-memory B-cells and class-switched memory B-cells have different circulation kinetics, such that IgM-memory B-cells persist after class-switched memory B-cells have disappeared from circulation. Furthermore, upon restimulation with antigen, IgM-memory B-cells were less likely to produce a secondary response in the presence of antigen-specific plasma antibody. Thus, it is interesting that the members of this clonal lineage bind to various previously circulating strains including the older H3 A/Johannesburg/33/1994 strain, that the antibodies were predominantly IgM, were hypermutated, and did not significantly contribute to the plasma antibody pool 4 weeks after experimental infection (15). All these findings suggest that this lineage is an example of such an IgM-memory B-cell clone isolated from an influenza-infected human subject.

Like other Darwinian processes, affinity maturation arises in the interplay between the generation of diversity and the subsequent selection of fitter variants. Affinity maturation, however, is a somatic process; properties of the germline gene segments that facilitate efficient maturation are preserved for the next germline generation (8). Thus, mutation and selection in affinity maturation are very strongly intertwined with mutations that are more likely on average to confer advantage, produced more frequently than those that are more likely on average to confer disadvantage. This circumstance has a practical consequence, complicating the analysis of selective pressure. We have overcome that problem by estimating the relevant characteristics of somatic hypermutation from a collection of human heavy chain genes rearranged out of frame and insusceptible to selection.

SELECTION AND MUTABILITY SYNERGIZE DURING AFFINITY MATURATION TO HA

The local codon bias that is present in Ig V-gene segments and increases mutability in the CDR creates a strongly non-uniform probability distribution over the links between Ig genes in the genotype space (**Figure 4**). Each of the Ig genes at the nodes of this space has an effective affinity for the antigen HA associated with it, which presumably determines the relative fitness of B-cells expressing the antibody encoded by that gene. Because of the mutational bias, from any starting node there are preferred nodes, which are visited with greater probability and in less time on average, than others. The question addressed here is whether the sequences more likely to be visited during somatic hypermutation because of this bias are also more likely to encode antibodies that confer a selective advantage.

Figure 4 is a simple cartoon intended to illustrate the idea. The grid represents the genotype space (although the topology is not at all realistic). The dark arrows indicate the directions of preferred mutations. We consider the node 1 to be the starting node. The other nodes 2–4 are each six mutations away from node 1, but they differ in the number of non-preferred mutations that are required to reach them. In the real system, we can estimate the mutation rate for each link, and in particular can estimate the mutation rates over the links connecting the nodes actually occupied during affinity maturation. We also have measured the affinity at each of these nodes, and know that they represent increases over time. So the question is, "are the visited nodes largely close to the preferred paths (as are nodes 2 and 3 in **Figure 4**), or randomly placed with respect to the preferred paths (illustrated by node 4)?"

We expect that such correlation between mutational preference and selective advantage holds on average over the history of antigens encountered by the gene segment in question. It is hypothesized that this is the reason why such local codon bias exists in the first place. The question addressed here is whether such a correlation exists, not on average, but in this particular instance, for this one specific antigen.

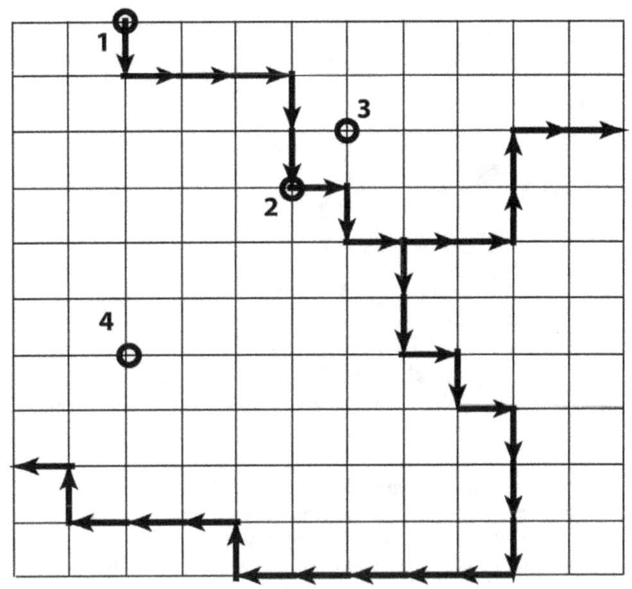

FIGURE 4 | Simplified illustration of genotype space with preferred directions. Each node is a DNA sequence, and neighbors differ by one nucleotide. The dark arrows show preferred directions, meaning the mutation along the direction of the arrow occurs at a higher rate than mutations along the regular paths. The nodes labeled 2, 3, and 4 are all six steps from node 1, but differ in the number of non-preferred steps that must be taken to arrive there from 1.

The mutability is defined at each nucleotide position as the probability of a mutation at that position conditional on there being exactly one mutation in the gene, and no selection on the gene product. In the presence of selection, the probability that a mutation will be fixed is the product of the probability that the mutation occurs at all and the probability that, once it has occurred, it is preserved through selection. The hypothesis we are testing is that the second of these probabilities, the probability of preservation, is itself functionally depending on the mutability. The order of the causality would be that the mutabilities have been adjusted, largely through codon usage, to make evolution toward the potentially advantageous genes more rapidly and more reliably.

We address the question in **Figure 5**, which shows the empirical cumulative distribution plots of synonymous and non-synonymous mutations as a function of mutability, compared to three theoretical models: zero order (mutability has no influence, even on the probability of having a mutation in the first place), first order (mutability has the influence expected under selection-free conditions), and second-order (probability of selection is directly proportional to mutability). The plots show that the synonymous mutations are consistent, as expected, with the first-order model. Indeed, this plot should be regarded as a test of the accuracy of the estimated mutability, which appears to be adequate, although the mutabilities of the higher-mutability positions may be somewhat over-estimated. In contrast, the observed non-synonymous mutations fall between the first- and second-order curves, consistent with synergy between local codon bias and selection. **Figure 5** is merely suggestive; the direct test of the relevant hypothesis (Model 4 vs. Model 6) provides stronger evidence.

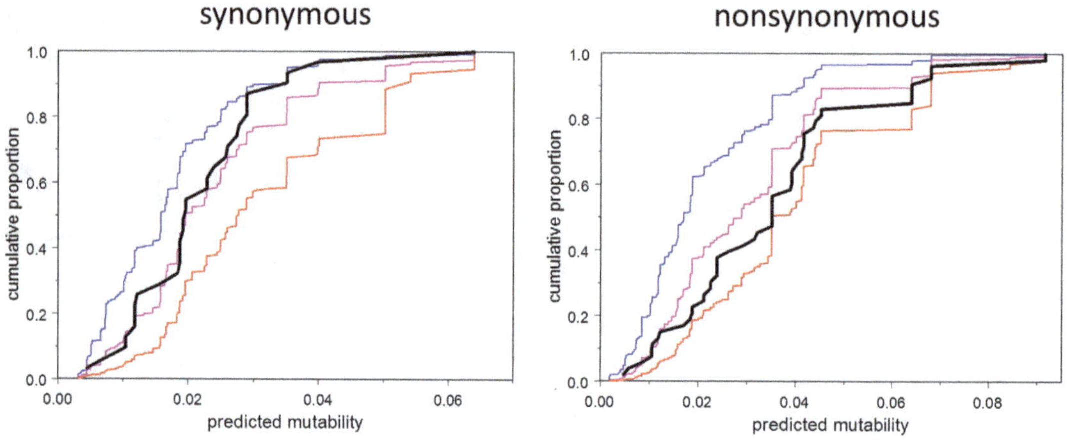

FIGURE 5 | Cumulative distribution function (CDF) of mutability among observed mutations (black), and corresponding to three models: order 0 (no effect of mutability at all, blue), order 1 (consistent with selection random with respect to mutability, magenta), second order (selection proportional to mutability, red). Note that the observed CDF for synonymous mutations is approximately consistent with the order one model, and falls between the order zero and order one curves in any case. The CDF for non-synonymous mutations falls between the order one and order two curves.

This test says that the influence of mutability on the survival of a mutation depends on the type of mutation, whether synonymous or non-synonymous. If the mutation is non-synonymous, the mutability has greater positive predictive power than that of synonymous type.

CONCLUSION

Strikingly, despite the fact that the dissociation constant changed by three orders of magnitude from the common ancestor to the observed mature antibodies, the distribution of mutations is heavily biased toward those with high intrinsic mutability, suggesting that selection worked in synergy with local codon bias in the maturation of CL2569. This analysis suggests that affinity maturation is strongly constrained to occur by mutational diffusion along preferred paths in genotype space, with selection acting negatively on genotypes in this network that fail to confer enhanced antigen-binding affinity. There is no evidence for selection pulling the evolving clone substantially out of the mutationally preferred paths.

There are many highly effective vaccines that work through the induction of a potent humoral response, but there are many devastating infectious diseases for which no effective vaccine is yet available in spite of intense research efforts, including malaria, hepatitis C, and HIV-1. The agents of these diseases do not typically elicit protective natural immunity, so new approaches to vaccine development may be indicated. One such approach is predicated on the observation that the efficiency of immunogen stimulation of germinal center naïve and intermediate B-cell antibodies is determined by immunogen affinity for B-cell precursor B-cell receptor (24–26). Design of immunogens with high-affinity binding for antibody UAs and their intermediates is now possible with the computational methods described in this study (27). It is our hope that the emerging understanding of the intertwined mechanisms of diversification and selection in affinity maturation will open new avenues for vaccine engineering.

MATERIALS AND METHODS

STATISTICAL AND COMPUTATIONAL

All analyses and computational manipulations were performed using software developed in the Kepler laboratory.

ELISA data analysis

The data from the ELISA dilution series were fit to a Hill function with Hill coefficient = 1 and additive background (28). The maximum value of the optical density and the value of the background optical density were taken to be equal over all wells on a given plate.

Inference of unobserved antibodies: ancestral rearrangement and maturation intermediates

We compute the posterior probability mass function on the nucleotides at each position of the unmutated common ancestor given the set of clonally related observed Ig genes of CL2569, as described in detail in Ref. (13).

Inference of somatic hypermutation sequence specificity

We searched NCBI Genbank for rearranged human Ig heavy-chain variable-region genes and retrieved and validated 34,546 genes. We eliminated genes with possible clonal relatives in the set by randomly eliminating all but one of each sequence within groups likely to be clonally related. Two antibodies were considered likely to be related if they shared the same inferred IGHV and IGHJ genes (without regard to allele) and shared at least 75% nucleotide identity in CDR3[2]. From these, we selected those that were likely to have been rearranged out of frame as evidenced by the number of

[2]This is admittedly a crude estimation procedure, but sequence set is small enough that we expect few if any errors from its use. Furthermore, we are unconcerned about falsely excluding unrelated sequences, which is the only likely error to be made by this method. Finally, the proper statistical procedure for testing clonal relatedness is sufficiently complex (Thomas B. Kepler, in preparation) that to put aside the space in a paper that does not require its full power would be distracting.

nucleotides between the intact invariant cysteine in VH FR 3 and the intact invariant tryptophan in JH being other than a multiple of three.

By counting frame-shift mutations in the VH-encoded part of the gene, which have resulted from somatic mutations or sequencing error, we estimate the likely number of genes that would have frame-shift mutations in CDR3 to be about 195 genes. That is about 11% of our candidate non-productively rearranged genes are likely to have been rearranged in-frame and to have acquired their frame-shift mutations subsequently.

To ameliorate the impact this contamination could have on the downstream analysis, we removed all genes inferred to have been rearranged to a VH1 family member. The reason for this filtering step is that the positions of pentanucleotides in the remaining sequences will be significantly de-correlated from the positions of the corresponding pentanucleotides in the target sequences, which are rearranged to a VH1 family member.

After this filtering step, 1707 sequences remained, containing 9961 nucleotide substitutions in 423,654 total bases.

The mutation frequency for the central position at each pentanucleotide motif was computed by scanning each inferred UA. Of the 4^5 (1024) possible pentanucleotides, 938 motifs were present in the total dataset, 922 in the out of frame dataset. Of the motifs with at least 100 observations among the UAs in the non-productive set, 24 of them had no mutations. In contrast, the motif AGCTA, which is consistent with the canonical "hot-spot" RGYW, was mutated at the center position 112 out of 618 times for a frequency of 18%.

For comparison to other such datasets previously assembled, we also computed the trinucleotide mutation frequencies. The spearman correlation between our trinucleotide mutation frequencies and the corresponding mutability indices from unselected sequences in the study by Shapiro et al. (29) is 0.80, indicating a high level of agreement between the two sets.

Rather than use, the raw count ratios for the mutability and mutation spectrum estimates directly (which is likely to result in over- or under-fitting), we chose to fit these data to a variable-motif length model using regression trees. The first statistical treatment of sequence specificity in somatic mutation produced hot-spot motifs of different lengths (7) and it seems natural to fit such a model now that much more data are available.

The end result of this estimation procedure is a set of nucleotide motifs that are mutually exclusive and complete (every nucleotide in any DNA sequence will belong to exactly one motif) to each member of which is assigned a mutation rate. Each motif may be up to 5 nt long. The procedure is as follows.

Each node in the decision tree contains a pentanucleotide motif of the form n_1, n_2, n_3, n_4, n_5 in which each $n_i = \{A, G, T, C, R, Y, S, W, N\}$ where R, Y, S, W, N are the IUPAC symbols respectively for purine (A or G), pyrimidine (T or C), weak (A or T), strong (G or C), and any (A, G, T, or C) nucleotide.

The function to be maximized, the objective function, is the log of the marginal likelihood summed over all nodes in the tree. The overall likelihood is the product of the binomial likelihoods at each node. At each node, the prior distribution on mutations is a beta distribution with parameters $\alpha = 1, \beta = 47$. The beta distribution is chosen because it is conjugate to the binomial distribution, and the specific parameters are chosen because they maximize the information entropy at the observed average mutation frequency in the set, 2.1%. As such, this prior is the most uninformative prior consistent with the average mutation frequency.

The marginal likelihood for a node with m mutations and u unmutated bases is computed by integrating over the mutation probabilities in the product of the likelihood and prior density functions giving:

$$L_{\mathrm{MU}}(m, u|\alpha, \beta) = \frac{\Gamma(\alpha + m)\,\Gamma(\beta + u)\,\Gamma(\alpha + \beta + 1)}{\Gamma(\alpha)\,\Gamma(\beta)\,\Gamma(\alpha + \beta + m + u + 1)} \qquad (3)$$

where Γ is the gamma function.

The tree-building algorithm is greedy, choosing the best available split at each node. Allowed splits at any step in the algorithm at any single position in the motif are as follows:

$$N \to R/Y, N \to S/W, R \to A/G, Y \to T/C,$$
$$S \to G/C, W \to A/T.$$

This scheme ensures that each pentanucleotide is mapped to exactly one terminal node on the tree at all stages of the procedure. A node is declared terminal if the product of the marginal likelihoods for the two daughter nodes in the optimal split is less than the marginal likelihood of the parent node, that is, if the likelihood cannot be increased any further at that node.

The result of applying this process to our count data is a tree with 55 terminal nodes. Among these, the one with the lowest relative mutability is with YT<u>G</u>GS with posterior mean $\widehat{p} = 7.9 \times 10^{-4}$. The AID "hot-spot" motif A<u>G</u>CT is assigned to the NA<u>G</u>CW node, with $\widehat{p} = 8.8 \times 10^{-2}$.

Regression model for the dependence of selection on mutability

The model scheme for analysis of selection is described in the main text. The data used are all nucleotide position in the heavy-chain variable regions up to and including the nucleotides of the FR3 invariant cysteine codon. The fitting of parameters by maximum likelihood was performed by numerical optimization using the Nelder–Mead simplex algorithm using a software implementation based largely on that described in Numerical Recipes (30).

Statistical hypothesis tests are based on the likelihood ratio test when models are nested. Model comparison is done by differential AIC expressed as relative likelihoods (31).

EXPERIMENTAL

Clinical protocol

The clinical EI protocol study was performed at Retroscreen Virology Ltd. (Brentwood, UK) as previously described (32) using a protocol approved by their local ethics board and the Duke IRB. Subjects were prescreened and provided informed consent before being given a nasal challenge with influenza A/Wisconsin/67/2005 (H3N2) challenge stock manufactured under current good manufacturing practices by Baxter BioScience (Vienna, Austria). Intranasal challenge was given using $10^{3.08}$ TCID50 to subject EI13 from whom the antibodies described in this study were derived. In this protocol, blood was drawn before challenge, then daily on days 0–7, and on day 28 after challenge. Symptoms were recorded twice daily using a modified Jackson scoring system (33). Productive infection was confirmed by active viral shedding detected by assays of nasal washes obtained during the 7-day quarantine period.

Single-cell flow cytometry sorting strategy

Human peripheral blood mononuclear cell samples collected 7 days after infection with A/Wisconsin/67/2005 (H3N2) were labeled with panels of fluorochrome-antibody conjugates specific for human CD3 (PE-Cy5), CD16 (PE-Cy5), CD19 (APC-Cy7), CD20 (PE-Cy7), CD27 (Pacific Blue), CD235a (PE-Cy5), IgD (PE), IgM (FITC) (all, BD Biosciences, San Jose, CA, USA), CD14 (PE-Cy5), and CD38 (APC-Cy5.5) (both Invitrogen, Carlsbad, CA, USA). Plasma cells/plasmablasts were sorted into 20 μl/well RT/PCR buffer in 96-well plates as described (10, 12) by gating on $CD3^{-}$ $CD14^{-}$ $CD16^{-}$ $CD235a^{-}$ $CD19^{+}$ $CD20^{-/lo}$ $CD27^{hi}$ $CD38^{hi}$ cells. All antibody reagents were tittered and used at optimal concentrations for flow cytometry.

PCR amplification of plasmablast/plasma cell immunoglobulin VH and VL variable-region genes

The Ig VH and VL variable-region genes of the sorted plasmablast were amplified by RT and nested PCR using the method as reported (11). The PCR products amplified by this method contain enough coding region sequences for the constant regions of either heavy- or light-chain genes for allowing the identification of IgH subclass and light-chain types (12). Isolated VH and VL variable-region genes were used to assemble full-length Ig IgG1 heavy- and light-chain expression cassette by overlapping to express recombinant IgG1 antibodies using the method as described (12).

Expression of VH and VL variable-region genes as IgG1 recombinant mAb

The isolated Ig VH and VL gene pairs were assembled by PCR into the linear full-length Ig heavy- and light-chain gene expression cassettes for production of recombinant mAbs by transfection in the human embryonic kidney cell line, 293T (ATCC, Manassas, VA, USA) using the methods as described (12). The purified PCR products of the paired Ig heavy- and light-chain gene expression cassettes were co-transfected into near confluent 293T cells grown in 6-well (2 μg of DNA for each cassettes per well) tissue culture plates (Becton Dickson, Franklin Lakes, NJ, USA) using PolyFect (Qiagen, Valencia, CA, USA) or Effectene (Qiagen Valencia, CA, USA) using protocols recommended by the manufacturers. Six to eight hours after transfection, the 293T cells were fed with fresh culture medium supplemented with 2% FCS and were incubated at 37°C in a 5% CO_2 incubator. Culture supernatants were harvested 3 days after transfection and quantified for expressed IgG levels and screened for antibody specificity.

Antibodies that bound HA in a screening assay as well as the inferred UA and intermediate clonal antibodies were produced on a larger scale so that screening assays could be replicated and broadened to more fully define the range of binding activity of expressed plasma cell derived-antibodies. Purified recombinant antibodies were produced in bulk cultures by transient transfection using Ig heavy- and light-chain genes cloned in pcDNA plasmids (12). The Ig heavy- and light-chain gene expression cassettes used for production of recombinant antibodies for initial screening were cloned into pcDNA 3.3 (Invitrogen, Carlsbad, CA, USA) for production of purified recombinant mAbs using standard molecular protocol, and co-transfected into 293T cells cultured in T175 flasks using PolyFect (Qiagen, Valencia, CA, USA) or polyethylenimine (34), cultured in DMEM supplemented with 2% FCS. Recombinant mAbs were purified from culture supernatants of the transfected-293T cells using anti-human Ig heavy-chain-specific antibody–agarose beads (Sigma, St. Louis, MO, USA) using the method as previously described (12, 34). Purified antibodies used in the study were confirmed having typical patterns of predominant whole IgG in SDS-PAGE and Western blots under reducing and non-reducing conditions (12).

Binding antibody multiplex assay

Concentration of recombinant mAbs secreted in the transfected-293T cell culture in the supernatants was determined using a method previously described (12). The expressed recombinant mAb were assayed for antibody reactivity by a standardized binding antibody multiplex assay (35) performed in a GCLP compliant manner. Binding specificities to influenza vaccine 2007 (Fluzone® 2007), trivalent influenza vaccine 2008 (Fluzone® 2008), and baculovirus-derived HA proteins (H1N1 A/Brisbane/59/2007, H1N1 A/California/04/2009, H1N1 A/Solomon Islands/03/06, H3N2 A/Brisbane/10/2007, H3N2 A/Johannesburg/33/1994, H3N2 A/Johannesburg/33/1994, H3N2 A/Wisconsin/67/05, B/Florida/04/06; Protein Sciences, Meriden, CT, USA) were determined using purified mAb diluted serially starting at 50 μg/ml.

ELISA data analysis for estimation of K_d

Purified mAb prepared at known concentrations were evaluated by ELISA against baculovirus-expressed purified hemagglutinin (H1 A/Brisbane/59/2007; Protein Sciences, Meriden, CT, USA). Samples were diluted serially for the analysis and data were analyzed using the model

$$y_i = \log\left[\alpha + (\beta - \alpha)\frac{c_i}{K_d + c_i}\right] + \varepsilon_i \tag{4}$$

where y_i is the log of the optical density measured at the ith dilution, α is the background optical density, β is the maximum optical density, K_d is the equilibrium dissociation constant, c_i is the known concentration of analyte at the ith dilution, and the ε are independent, identically distributed Gaussian errors. For each antibody studied, the parameters of this model were fit using software developed for the purpose (28).

ACKNOWLEDGMENTS

We are grateful for fruitful discussions with the members of the Center for Computational Immunology, and the members of the Duke Human Vaccine Institute's Antibodyome research group. Grant Information: this work was supported by NIH/NIAID research contract HHSN272201000053C (to Thomas B. Kepler, PI) and a Vaccine Development Center grant in the Collaboration for AIDS Vaccine Discovery Program from the Bill and Melinda Gates Foundation (Barton F. Haynes, PI).

Datasheet 1 | Sequence alignment for CL2569 heavy chain, including observed and inferred sequences.

Datasheet 2 | Sequence alignment for CL2569 light chain, including observed and inferred sequences.

Datasheet 3 | Tables of results for sequence specificity of mutation frequency.

REFERENCES

1. Yoshida T, Mei H, Dörner T, Hiepe F, Radbruch A, Fillatreau S, et al. Memory B and memory plasma cells. *Immunol Rev* (2010) **237**:117–39. doi:10.1111/j.1600-065X.2010.00938.x
2. Di Noia JM, Neuberger MS. Molecular mechanisms of antibody somatic hypermutation. *Annu Rev Biochem* (2007) **76**:1–22. doi:10.1146/annurev.biochem.76.061705.090740
3. Brown LE, Murray JM, White DO, Jackson DC. An analysis of the properties of monoclonal antibodies directed to epitopes on influenza virus hemagglutinin. *Arch Virol* (1990) **114**:1–26. doi:10.1007/BF01311008
4. Usinger WR, Lucas AH. Avidity as a determinant of the protective efficacy of human antibodies to pneumococcal capsular polysaccharides. *Infect Immun* (1999) **67**:2366–70.
5. Lambert P-H, Liu M, Siegrist C-A. Can successful vaccines teach us how to induce efficient protective immune responses? *Nat Med* (2005) **11**(4 Suppl):S54–62. doi:10.1038/nm1216
6. Delgado MF, Coviello S, Monsalvo AC, Melendi GA, Hernandez JZ, Batalle JP, et al. Lack of antibody affinity maturation due to poor toll-like receptor stimulation leads to enhanced respiratory syncytial virus disease. *Nat Med* (2009) **15**:34–41. doi:10.1038/nm.1894
7. Rogozin IB, Kolchanov NA. Somatic hypermutagenesis in immunoglobulin genes. II. Influence of neighbouring base sequences on mutagenesis. *Biochim Biophys Acta* (1992) **1171**:11–8. doi:10.1016/0167-4781(92)90134-L
8. Kepler TB. Codon bias and plasticity in immunoglobulins. *Mol Biol Evol* (1997) **14**:637–43. doi:10.1093/oxfordjournals.molbev.a025803
9. Wagner SD, Milstein C, Neuberger MS. Codon bias targets mutation. *Nature* (1995) **376**:732–732. doi:10.1038/376732a0
10. Wrammert J, Smith K, Miller J, Langley WA, Kokko K, Larsen C, et al. Rapid cloning of high-affinity human monoclonal antibodies against influenza virus. *Nature* (2008) **453**:667–71. doi:10.1038/nature06890
11. Tiller T, Meffre E, Yurasov S, Tsuiji M, Nussenzweig MC, Wardemann H. Efficient generation of monoclonal antibodies from single human B cells by single cell RT-PCR and expression vector cloning. *J Immunol Methods* (2008) **329**:112–24. doi:10.1016/j.jim.2007.09.017
12. Liao HX, Levesque MC, Nagel A, Dixon A, Zhang R, Walter E, et al. High-throughput isolation of immunoglobulin genes from single human B cells and expression as monoclonal antibodies. *J Virol Methods* (2009) **158**:171–9. doi:10.1016/j.jviromet.2009.02.014
13. Kepler TB. Reconstructing a B-cell clonal lineage. I. Statistical inference of unobserved ancestors. *F1000Res* (2013) **2**:103. doi:10.12688/f1000research.2-103.v1
14. Wardemann H, Yurasov S, Schaefer A, Young JW, Meffre E, Nussenzweig MC. Predominant autoantibody production by early human B cell precursors. *Science* (2003) **301**:1374–7. doi:10.1126/science.1086907
15. Moody MA, Zhang R, Walter EB, Woods CW, Ginsburg GS, McClain MT, et al. H3N2 influenza infection elicits more cross reactive and less clonally expanded anti-hemagglutinin antibodies than influenza vaccination. *PLoS One* (2011) **6**(10):e25797. doi:10.1371/journal.pone.0025797
16. Lefranc M-P, Giudicelli V, Ginestoux C, Jabado-Michaloud J, Folch G, Bellahcene F, et al. IMGT®, the international ImMunoGeneTics information system®. *Nucleic Acids Res* (2009) **37**:D1006–12. doi:10.1093/nar/gkn838
17. Kreitman M, Akashi H. Molecular evidence for natural selection. *Annu Rev Ecol Syst* (1995) **26**:403–22. doi:10.1146/annurev.es.26.110195.002155
18. Hershberg U, Uduman M, Shlomchik MJ, Kleinstein SH. Improved methods for detecting selection by mutation analysis of Ig V region sequences. *Int Immunol* (2008) **20**:683–94. doi:10.1093/intimm/dxn026
19. Cowell LG, Kepler TB. The nucleotide-replacement spectrum under somatic hypermutation exhibits microsequence dependence that is strand-symmetric and distinct from that under germline mutation. *J Immunol* (2000) **164**:1971–6.
20. Neyman J, Pearson ES. On the problem of the most efficient tests of statistical hypotheses. *Philos Trans R Soc Lond A* (1933) **231**:289–337. doi:10.1098/rsta.1933.0009
21. Akaike H. A new look at the statistical model identification. *IEEE Trans Automat Contr* (1974) **19**:716–23. doi:10.1109/TAC.1974.1100705
22. Kepler TB, Perelson AS. Somatic hypermutation in B cells: an optimal control treatment. *J Theor Biol* (1993) **164**:37–64. doi:10.1006/jtbi.1993.1139
23. Pape KA, Taylor JJ, Maul RW, Gearhart PJ, Jenkins MK. Different B cell populations mediate early and late memory during an endogenous immune response. *Science* (2011) **331**:1203–7. doi:10.1126/science.1201730
24. Dal Porto JM, Haberman AM, Kelsoe G, Shlomchik MJ. Very low affinity B cells form germinal centers, become memory B cells, and participate in secondary immune responses when higher affinity competition is reduced. *J Exp Med* (2002) **195**:1215–21. doi:10.1084/jem.20011550
25. Shih TA, Meffre E, Roederer M, Nussenzweig MC. Role of BCR affinity in T cell dependent antibody responses in vivo. *Nat Immunol* (2002) **3**:570–5. doi:10.1038/ni776
26. Schwickert TA, Victora GD, Fooksman DR, Kamphorst AO, Mugnier MR, Gitlin AD, et al. A dynamic T cell-limited checkpoint regulates affinity-dependent B cell entry into the germinal center. *J Exp Med* (2011) **208**(6):1243–52. doi:10.1084/jem.20102477
27. Haynes BF, Kelsoe G, Harrison SC, Kepler TB. B-cell-lineage immunogen design in vaccine development with HIV-1 as a case study. *Nat Biotechnol* (2012) **30**:423–33. doi:10.1038/nbt.2197
28. Feng F, Sales AP, Kepler TB. A Bayesian approach for estimating calibration curves and unknown concentrations in immunoassays. *Bioinformatics* (2011) **27**:707–12. doi:10.1093/bioinformatics/btq686
29. Shapiro GS, Aviszus K, Murphy J, Wysocki LJ. Evolution of Ig DNA sequence to target specific base positions within codons for somatic hypermutation. *J Immunol* (2002) **168**:2302–6.
30. Press WH, Teukolsky SA, Vetterling WT, Flannery BP. *Numerical Recipes: The Art of Scientific Computing.* New York: Cambridge University Press (2007).
31. Burnham KP, Anderson DR. *Model Selection and Multi-Model Inference: A Practical Information-Theoretic Approach.* 2nd ed. New York: Springer (2002). p. 49–97.
32. Zaas AK, Chen M, Varkey J, Veldman T, Hero AO3rd, Lucas J, et al. Gene expression signatures diagnose influenza and other symptomatic respiratory viral infections in humans. *Cell Host Microbe* (2009) **6**:207–17. doi:10.1016/j.chom.2009.07.006
33. Jackson GG, Dowling HF, Spiesman IG, Boand AV. Transmission of the common cold to volunteers under controlled conditions. I. The common cold as a clinical entity. *AMA Arch Intern Med* (1958) **101**:267–78. doi:10.1001/archinte.1958.00260140099015
34. Smith K, Garman L, Wrammert J, Zheng NY, Capra JD, Ahmed R, et al. Rapid generation of fully human monoclonal antibodies specific to a vaccinating antigen. *Nat Protoc* (2009) **4**:372–84. doi:10.1038/nprot.2009.3
35. Tomaras GD, Yates NL, Liu P, Qin L, Fouda GG, Chavez LL, et al. Initial B-cell responses to transmitted human immunodeficiency virus type 1: virion-binding immunoglobulin M (IgM) and IgG antibodies followed by plasma anti-gp41 antibodies with ineffective control of initial viremia. *J Virol* (2008) **82**:12449–63. doi:10.1128/JVI.01708-08

Permissions

All chapters in this book were first published in DCCIR, by Frontiers; hereby published with permission under the Creative Commons Attribution License or equivalent. Every chapter published in this book has been scrutinized by our experts. Their significance has been extensively debated. The topics covered herein carry significant findings which will fuel the growth of the discipline. They may even be implemented as practical applications or may be referred to as a beginning point for another development.

The contributors of this book come from diverse backgrounds, making this book a truly international effort. This book will bring forth new frontiers with its revolutionizing research information and detailed analysis of the nascent developments around the world.

We would like to thank all the contributing authors for lending their expertise to make the book truly unique.

They have played a crucial role in the development of this book. Without their invaluable contributions this book wouldn't have been possible. They have made vital efforts to compile up to date information on the varied aspects of this subject to make this book a valuable addition to the collection of many professionals and students.

This book was conceptualized with the vision of imparting up-to-date information and advanced data in this field. To ensure the same, a matchless editorial board was set up. Every individual on the board went through rigorous rounds of assessment to prove their worth. After which they invested a large part of their time researching and compiling the most relevant data for our readers.

The editorial board has been involved in producing this book since its inception. They have spent rigorous hours researching and exploring the diverse topics which have resulted in the successful publishing of this book. They have passed on their knowledge of decades through this book. To expedite this challenging task, the publisher supported the team at every step. A small team of assistant editors was also appointed to further simplify the editing procedure and attain best results for the readers.

Apart from the editorial board, the designing team has also invested a significant amount of their time in understanding the subject and creating the most relevant covers. They scrutinized every image to scout for the most suitable representation of the subject and create an appropriate cover for the book.

The publishing team has been an ardent support to the editorial, designing and production team. Their endless efforts to recruit the best for this project, has resulted in the accomplishment of this book. They are a veteran in the field of academics and their pool of knowledge is as vast as their experience in printing. Their expertise and guidance has proved useful at every step. Their uncompromising quality standards have made this book an exceptional effort. Their encouragement from time to time has been an inspiration for everyone.

The publisher and the editorial board hope that this book will prove to be a valuable piece of knowledge for researchers, students, practitioners and scholars across the globe.

List of Contributors

Andrew J. Yates
Departments of Systems and Computational Biology, Microbiology and Immunology, Albert Einstein College of Medicine, NewYork, NY, USA

Boris M. Hartmann, Nada Marjanovic, German Nudelman and Stuart C. Sealfon
Department of Neurology, Mount Sinai School of Medicine, Center for Translational Systems Biology, New York, NY, USA

Thomas M. Moran
Department of Microbiology, Mount Sinai School of Medicine, Center for Translational Systems Biology, New York, NY, USA

Tianxiang Chen
W. M. Keck Center for Collaborative Neuroscience, Rutgers, The State University of New Jersey, New Jersey, NJ, USA
Department of Thoracic Surgery, First Affiliated Hospital, School of Medicine, Zhejiang University, Hangzhou, China

Xi Wang
W. M. Keck Center for Collaborative Neuroscience, Rutgers, The State University of New Jersey, New Jersey, NJ, USA
Institute of Neurosciences, The Fourth Military Medical University, Xian, China

Lei Guo
Department of Biomedical Sciences, Florida State University College of Medicine, Tallahassee, FL, USA
Department of Orthopedic Surgery, The Second Hospital of Xian Jiaotong University, Xian, China

Jing Lv, Wenjiao Tai, Ruth Didier and Yi Ren
Department of Biomedical Sciences, Florida State University College of Medicine, Tallahassee, FL, USA

Hemamalini Renganathan, Dongming Sun, Wise Young, Mingmei Wu and Zhaoxia Duan
W. M. Keck Center for Collaborative Neuroscience, Rutgers, The State University of New Jersey, New Jersey, NJ, USA

Xiaoming Chen
Institute of Translational Medicine, First Affiliated Hospital, Wenzhou Medical University, Wenzhou, China

Xijing He
Department of Orthopedic Surgery, The Second Hospital of Xian Jiaotong University, Xian, China

Jianqing Fan
Statistics Laboratory, Princeton University, Princeton, NJ, USA

Maria Sawicka, Joseph Reynolds, Niloufar Abourashchi, Grant Lythe and Carmen Molina-París
Department of Applied Mathematics, School of Mathematics, University of Leeds, Leeds, UK

Gretta L. Stritesky and Kristin A. Hogquist
Department of Laboratory Medicine and Pathology, Center for Immunology, University of Minnesota, Minneapolis, MN, USA

Harm Westdorp and I. Jolanda M. de Vries
Department of Tumor Immunology, Radboud Institute for Molecular Life Sciences, Radboud University Medical Center, Nijmegen, Netherlands
Department of Medical Oncology, Radboud University Medical Center, Nijmegen, Netherlands

Annette E. Sköld, Berit A. Snijer and Sebastian Franik
Department of Tumor Immunology, Radboud Institute for Molecular Life Sciences, Radboud University Medical Center, Nijmegen, Netherlands

Sasja F. Mulder and Winald R. Gerritsen
Department of Medical Oncology, Radboud University Medical Center, Nijmegen, Netherlands

Pierre P. Major and Ronan Foley
Juravinski Hospital and Cancer Centre, Hamilton, ON, Canada

Priyanka Nair-Gupta
Department of Medicine, Immunology Institute, Graduate School of Biological Sciences, Icahn School of Medicine at Mount Sinai, New York, NY, USA

J. Magarian Blander
Department of Medicine, Immunology Institute, Graduate School of Biological Sciences, Icahn School of Medicine at Mount Sinai, New York, NY, USA
Tisch Cancer Institute, Icahn School of Medicine at Mount Sinai, New York, NY, USA

Gur Yaari
Bioengineering Program, Faculty of Engineering, Bar Ilan University, Ramat Gan, Israel
Department of Pathology, Yale School of Medicine, New Haven, CT, USA

Jason A. Vander Heiden, Daniel Gadala-Maria and Namita Gupta
Interdepartmental Program in Computational Biology and Bioinformatics, Yale University, New Haven, CT, USA

Mohamed Uduman
Department of Pathology, Yale School of Medicine, New Haven, CT, USA

Joel N. H. Stern
Department of Neurology, Yale School of Medicine, New Haven, CT, USA
Department of Science Education, Hofstra North Shore-LIJ School of Medicine, Hempstead, NY, USA

Kevin C. O'Connor
Department of Neurology, Yale School of Medicine, New Haven, CT, USA
Human and Translational Immunology Program, Yale School of Medicine, New Haven, CT, USA

David A. Hafler
Department of Neurology, Yale School of Medicine, New Haven, CT, USA
Department of Immunobiology, Yale School of Medicine, New Haven, CT, USA

Uri Laserson
Department of Genetics, Harvard Medical School, Boston, MA, USA

Francois Vigneault
AbVitro, Inc., Boston, MA, USA

Steven H. Kleinstein
Department of Pathology, Yale School of Medicine, New Haven, CT, USA
Interdepartmental Program in Computational Biology and Bioinformatics, Yale University, New Haven, CT, USA

Yi-chi M. Kong
Department of Immunology and Microbiology, Wayne State University School of Medicine, Detroit, MI, USA

Jeffrey C. Flynn
Department of Orthopaedic Surgery, Providence Hospital and Medical Centers, Southfield, MI, USA

Douglas M. Marvel and Olivera J. Finn
Department of Immunology, University of Pittsburgh School of Medicine, Pittsburgh, PA, USA

Eric Shifrut, Hilah Gal, Wilfred Ndifon and Nir Friedman
Department of Immunology, Weizmann Institute of Science, Rehovot, Israel

Kuti Baruch, Aleksandra Deczkowska and Michal Schwartz
Department of Neurobiology, Weizmann Institute of Science, Rehovot, Israel

Penelope A. Morel
Department of Immunology, University of Pittsburgh, Pittsburgh, PA, USA

Lily A. Chylek
Department of Chemistry and Chemical Biology, Cornell University, Ithaca, NY, USA
Los Alamos National Laboratory, Theoretical Division, Center for Non-linear Studies, Los Alamos, NM, USA

David A. Holowka and Barbara A. Baird
Department of Chemistry and Chemical Biology, Cornell University, Ithaca, NY, USA

William S. Hlavacek
Los Alamos National Laboratory, Theoretical Division, Center for Non-linear Studies, Los Alamos, NM, USA

Sebastian Gerdes, Ingmar Glauche and Ingo Roeder
Institute for Medical Informatics and Biometry, Medical Faculty Carl Gustav Carus, Dresden, Germany

Sebastian Newrzela and Martin-Leo Hansmann
Senckenberg Institute of Pathology, Goethe-University Hospital Frankfurt, Frankfurt, Germany

Dorothee von Laer
Department of Hygiene, Medical University Innsbruck, Innsbruck, Austria

Kevin H. Toomer
Department of Microbiology and Immunology, University of Miami Miller School of Medicine, Miami, FL, USA

Zhibin Chen
Department of Microbiology and Immunology, University of Miami Miller School of Medicine, Miami, FL, USA
Sylvester Comprehensive Cancer Center, University of Miami Miller School of Medicine, Miami, FL, USA

Tharindi Hapuarachchi, Joanna Lewis and Robin E. Callard
Institute of Child Health and CoMPLEX, University College London, London, UK

EkaterinaV. Putintseva, OlgaV. Britanova, Dmitriy B. Staroverov, Ekaterina M. Merzlyak, Maria A. Turchaninova, Mikhail Shugay, Dmitriy A. Bolotin, Mikhail V. Pogorelyy, Ilgar Z. Mamedov and Yuri B. Lebedev
Shemyakin-Ovchinnikov Institute of Bioorganic Chemistry, Russian Academy of Science, Moscow, Russia

Vlasta Bobrynina and Mikhail Maschan
Federal Scientific Clinical Center of Pediatric Hematology, Oncology and Immunology, Moscow, Russia

Dmitriy M. Chudakov
Shemyakin-Ovchinnikov Institute of Bioorganic Chemistry, Russian Academy of Science, Moscow, Russia
Central European Institute of Technology (CEITEC), Masaryk University, Brno, Czech Republic

Beatrice Omusiro Ondondo
The Jenner Institute, Nuffield Department of Medicine, University of Oxford, Oxford, UK

Robert Schulz, Benjamin Werner and Ulrich Behn
Institute for Theoretical Physics, University of Leipzig, Leipzig, Germany

Lisa H. Butterfield
Departments of Medicine, Surgery and Immunology, University of Pittsburgh Cancer Institute, University of Pittsburgh, Pittsburgh, PA, USA

Thomas B. Kepler
Department of Microbiology, Boston University School of Medicine, Boston, MA, USA
Department of Mathematics and Statistics, Boston University, Boston, MA, USA

Supriya Munshaw
Center for Viral Hepatitis Research, Johns Hopkins University, Baltimore, MD, USA

Kevin Wiehe and Ruijun Zhang
Duke Human Vaccine Institute, Duke University Medical Center, Durham, NC, USA

Christopher W. Woods
Department of Medicine, Duke University Medical Center, Durham, NC, USA
Department of Pathology, Duke University Medical Center, Durham, NC, USA
Hubert-Yeargan Center for Global Health, Duke University Medical Center, Durham, NC, USA
Department of Pediatrics, Duke University Medical Center, Durham, NC, USA

Georgia D. Tomaras and Garnett Kelsoe
Duke Human Vaccine Institute, Duke University Medical Center, Durham, NC, USA
Department of Medicine, Duke University Medical Center, Durham, NC, USA
Department of Immunology, Duke University Medical Center, Durham, NC, USA

M. Anthony Moody
Center for Viral Hepatitis Research, Johns Hopkins University, Baltimore, MD, USA
Duke Human Vaccine Institute, Duke University Medical Center, Durham, NC, USA

Jae-Sung Yu, Thomas N. Denny, S. Munir Alam, Hua-Xin Liao and Barton F. Haynes
Duke Human Vaccine Institute, Duke University Medical Center, Durham, NC, USA
Department of Medicine, Duke University Medical Center, Durham, NC, USA

Index

www.ingramcontent.com/pod-product-compliance
Lightning Source LLC
LaVergne TN
LVHW080956210926
848485LV00004B/837